MRI
ATLAS
OF NORMAL
ANATOMY

NOTICE

MRI ATLAS OF NORMAL ANATOMY

ANNA K. CHACKO, M.D.

Army Medical Department
Colonel, MC USA

RICHARD W. KATZBERG, M.D.

Professor and Chairman
Department of Radiology
Oregon Health Sciences University
Portland, Oregon

AILEEN MacKAY, M.S.R.

Department of Magnetic Resonance Imaging
University of Rochester School of Medicine
Rochester, New York

McGRAW-HILL, INC. • Health Professions Division

New York St. Louis San Francisco Colorado Springs Auckland Bogotá Caracas Hamburg Lisbon London Madrid Mexico Milan Montreal New Delhi Paris San Juan São Paulo Singapore Sydney Tokyo Toronto

MRI Atlas of Normal Anatomy

1 2 3 4 5 6 7 8 9 0 HALHAL 9 8 7 6 5 4 3 2 1 0

ISBN 0-07-010425-5

This book was set in ITC Korinna by York Graphic Services, Inc. The editors were William Day and Peter McCurdy; the production supervisor was Annette Mayeski; the cover and text were designed by José Fonfrias. Halliday Lithographic Corporation was printer and binder.

LIBRARY OF CONGRESS CATALOGING-IN-PUBLICATION DATA

Chacko, Anna K.

MRI atlas of normal anatomy / Anna K. Chacko, Richard W. Katzberg, Aileen MacKay.

p. cm.

ISBN 0-07-010425-5

1. Human anatomy—Atlases. 2. Magnetic resonance imaging—Atlases. I. Katzberg, Richard W. II. MacKay, Aileen. III. Title.

[DNLM: 1. Anatomy—atlases. 2. Magnetic Resonance Imaging—atlases. QS 17 C431m]

QM25.C43 1990

611′ .0022—dc20

DLC

for Library of Congress 90-13221

CIP

To my mother and my late father, Mary and Isaac Kuruvilla, and to Major General Edward J. Huycke, M.D. Their guidance, support, and example have shaped my life, and I owe them an undying debt of gratitude. AKC

To Harry W. Fischer, M.D., former Chairman of the Department of Radiology, the University of Rochester School of Medicine and Dentistry, Rochester, New York, for his inspiration as a great academician and teacher. RWK

To Catherine Cunningham, my mother. AM

CONTENTS

PREFACE

The initial excitement over magnetic resonance imaging sprang from the dream that an imaging modality had been developed that could provide tissue-specificity. That dream has not come to pass, but an even more exciting capability of MRI is now well appreciated. The clinical power of magnetic resonance that *has* been realized is the exquisite anatomic depiction of the human body. This atlas is dedicated to the effective use of that power in daily clinical practice. It provides a basic overview of the important anatomic landmarks encountered in the daily use of MRI. The material presented here is not meant to be exhaustive: it covers only the essentials to the performance of good clinical interpretation.

Most of these magnetic resonance images were obtained utilizing sequences commonly used at our institution. In some instances we have incorporated images that were not normal so that the reader could detect the location of structures not normally visualized. For example, in some of the axial sections of the head, scans were included that depicted the tip of the petrous temporal bone. In some other instances we have included more than one sequence because we felt that not all of the important structures could be seen if only one sequence were chosen.

Now that the superb resolution of magnetic resonance is widely available, a more in-depth knowledge of anatomy will be expected of the radiologist than has been the case in the past. Most of us are in a situation where our knowledge of normal anatomy has become rusty through long years of disuse. We hope that this book will be useful in rekindling the reader's interest in normal anatomy and opening eyes to the new possibilities of diagnosis through MRI. It will provide a quick and ready reference, obviating the need to refer to many textbooks and articles on gross anatomy, cross sectional imaging, and magnetic resonance.

Choice of Images in the Head, Neck, and Spine Section

The choice of images in this section is based on our intent to provide the fundamental anatomic detail necessary for an understanding of basic neuroanatomy. We have erred toward more rather than fewer images for the sake of completeness.

We have used, wherever possible, sequences and weightings that depict the largest number of anatomic structures. In many instances, we have used more than one type of pulse sequence. This should not, however, be interpreted to mean that the sequences used to demonstrate the anatomy are necessarily those recommended for daily clinical practice.

ACKNOWLEDGMENTS

The authors would like to thank the many people who have made this endeavor possible. We would first like to credit the technologists at the University of Rochester Magnetic Resonance Imaging Center: Anna Wicks, Connie White, and Bill Badger. Special thanks is also given to Mrs. Elizabeth Pender for her excellent assistance.

Many thanks for helpful suggestions are due to Drs. Dave Nelson, Mike Polise, and Bill Weidner of the Oregon Health Sciences University Department of Radiology, Portland, Oregon.

We would also like to thank Dr. Jack Simon, Dr. Jerzy Szumowski, and Mr. Tom Foster.

We hope that this atlas will provide the anatomic fundamentals for clinical magnetic resonance at its best.

MRI ATLAS OF NORMAL ANATOMY

Head, Sagittal

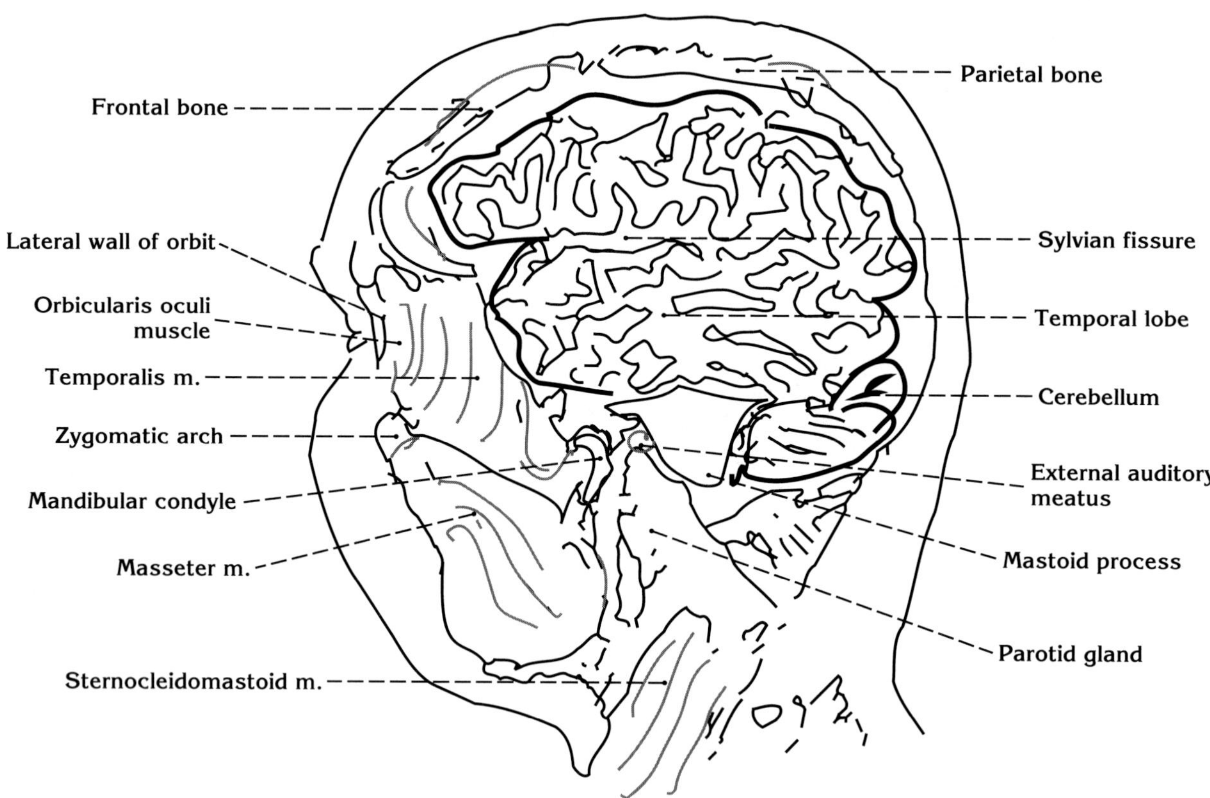

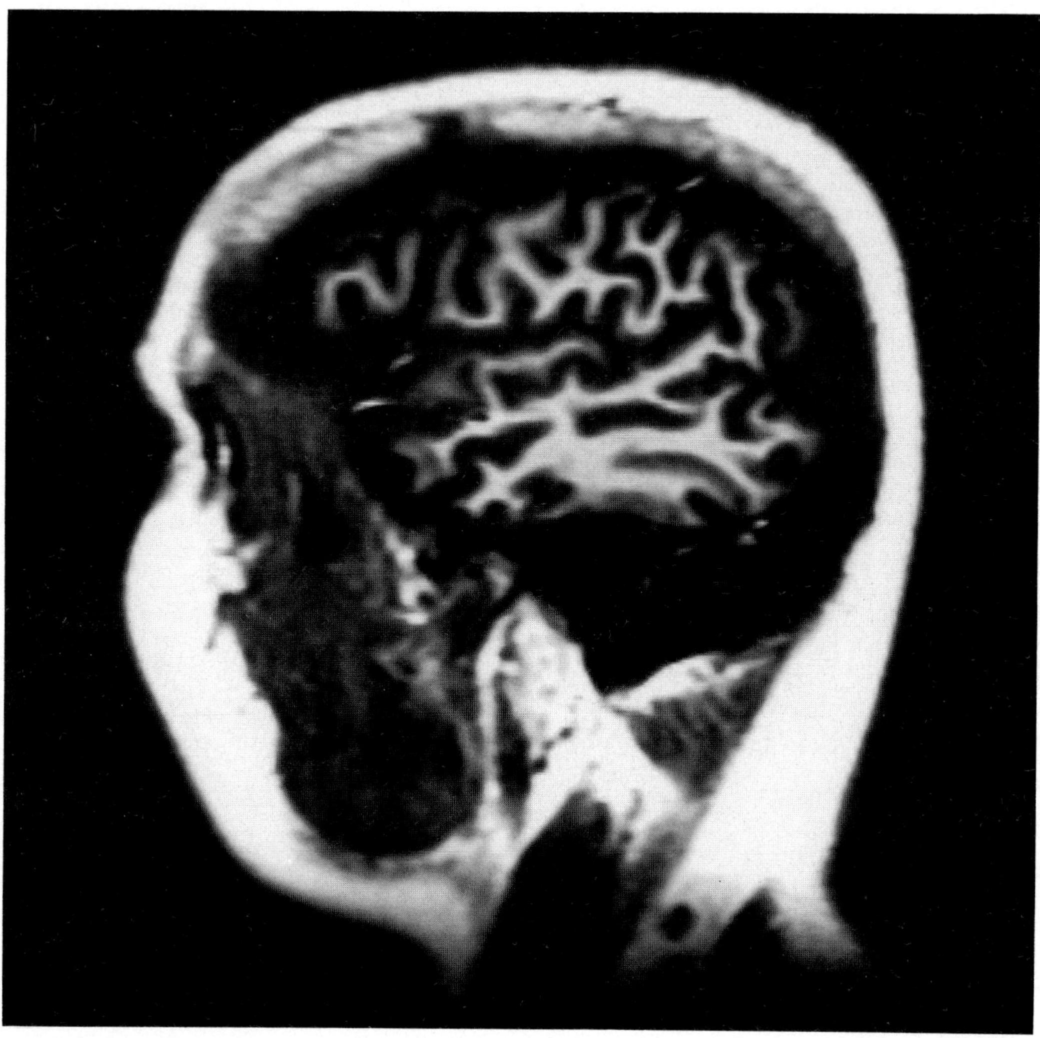

1-1 Head, sagittal view (inversion recovery).

Head, Sagittal

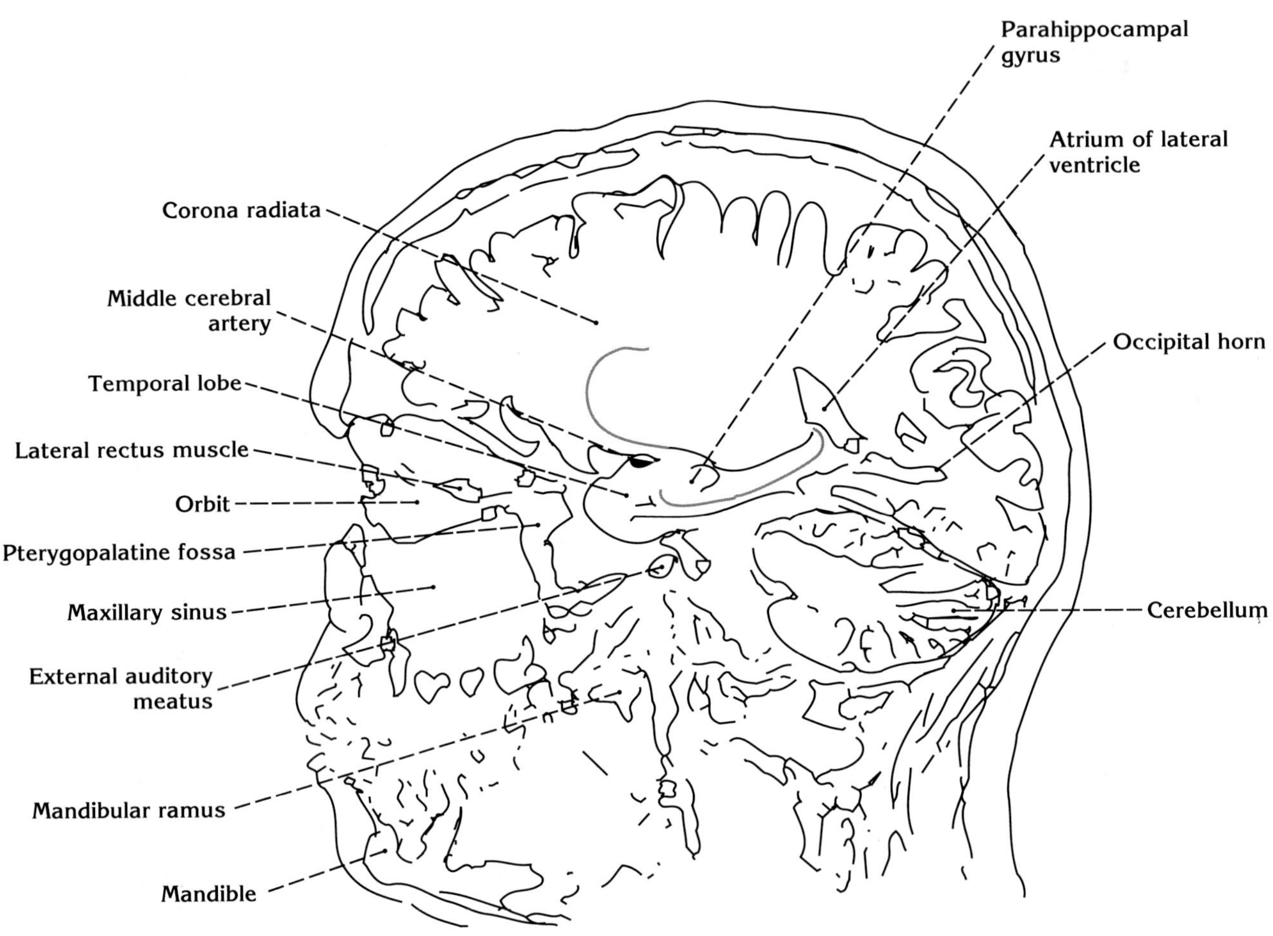

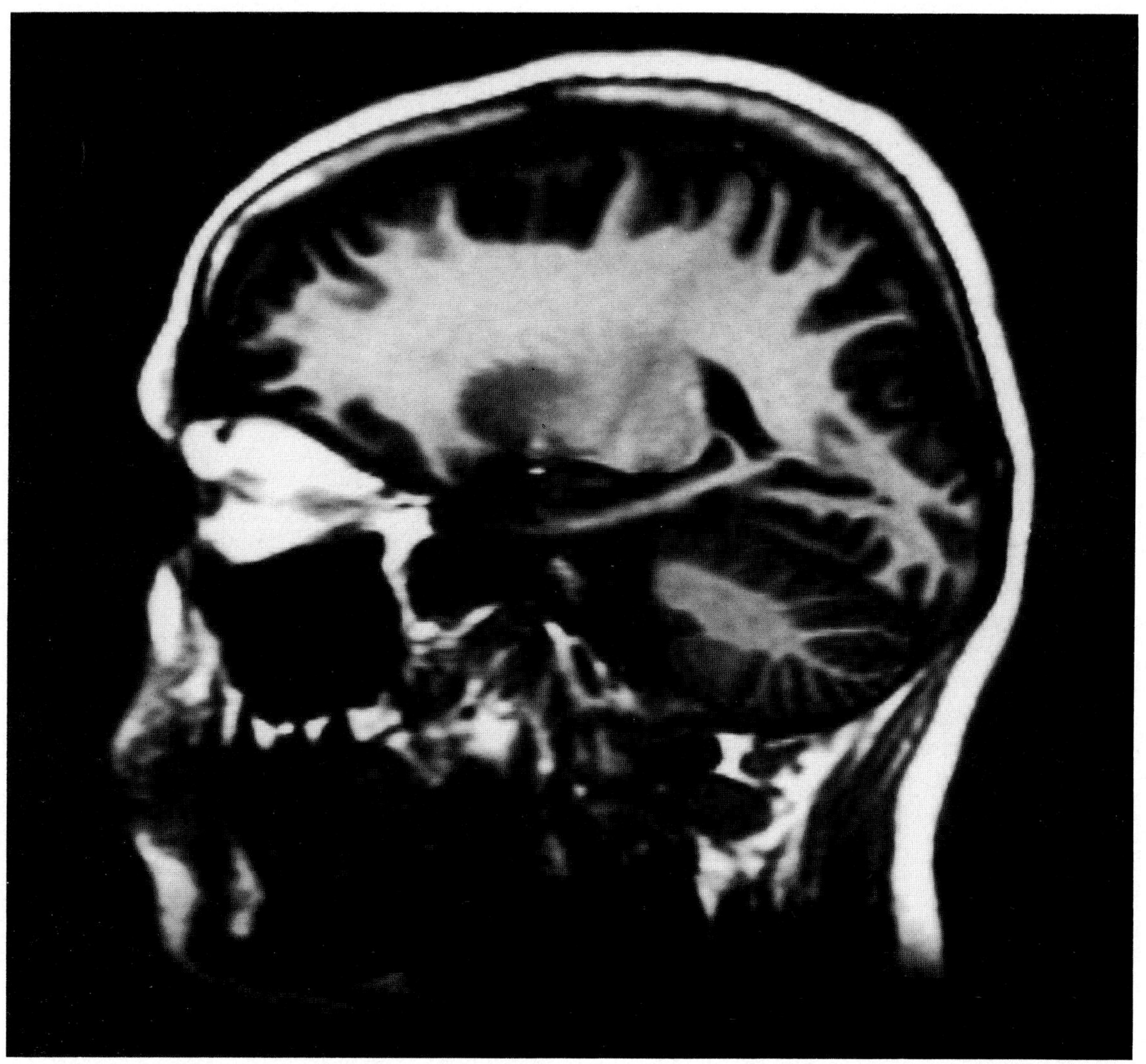

1-2 Head, sagittal view (inversion recovery).

Head, Sagittal

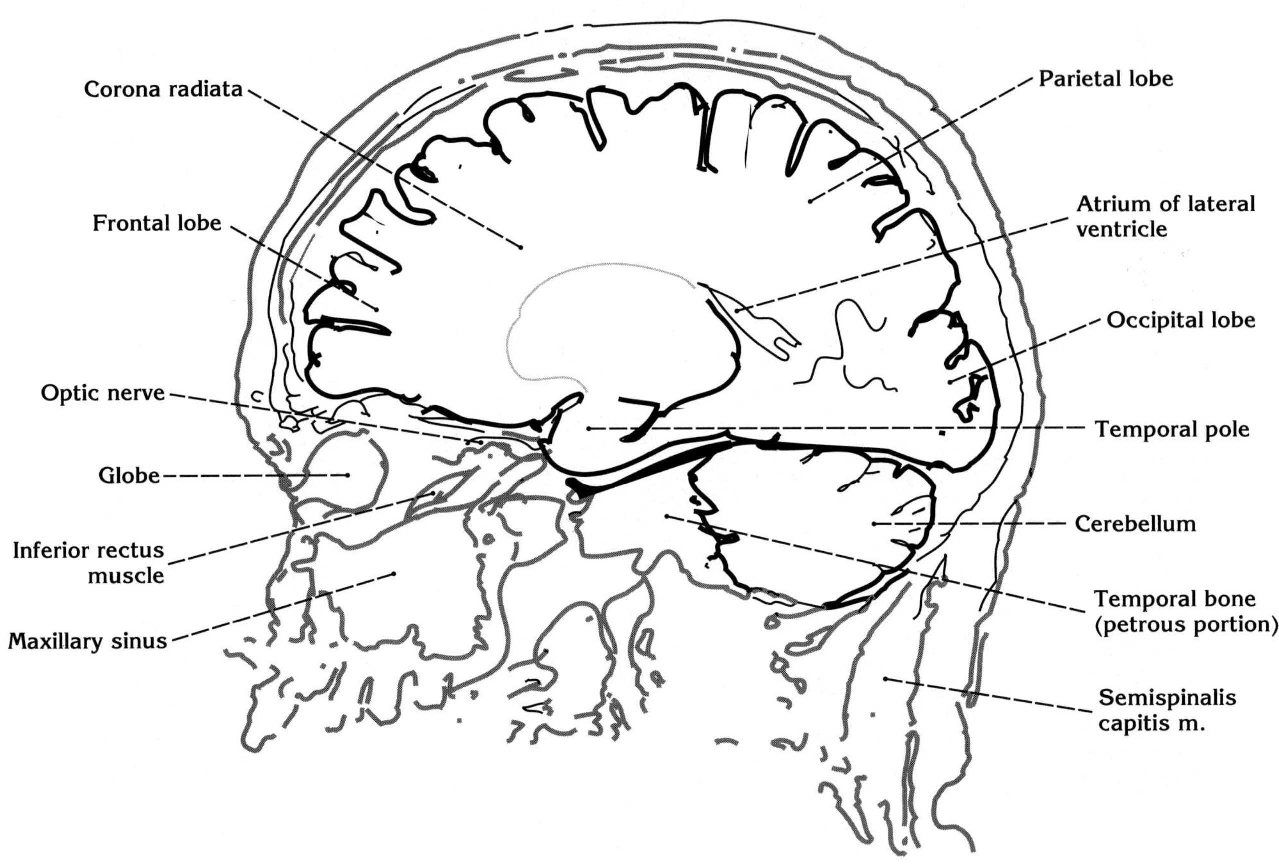

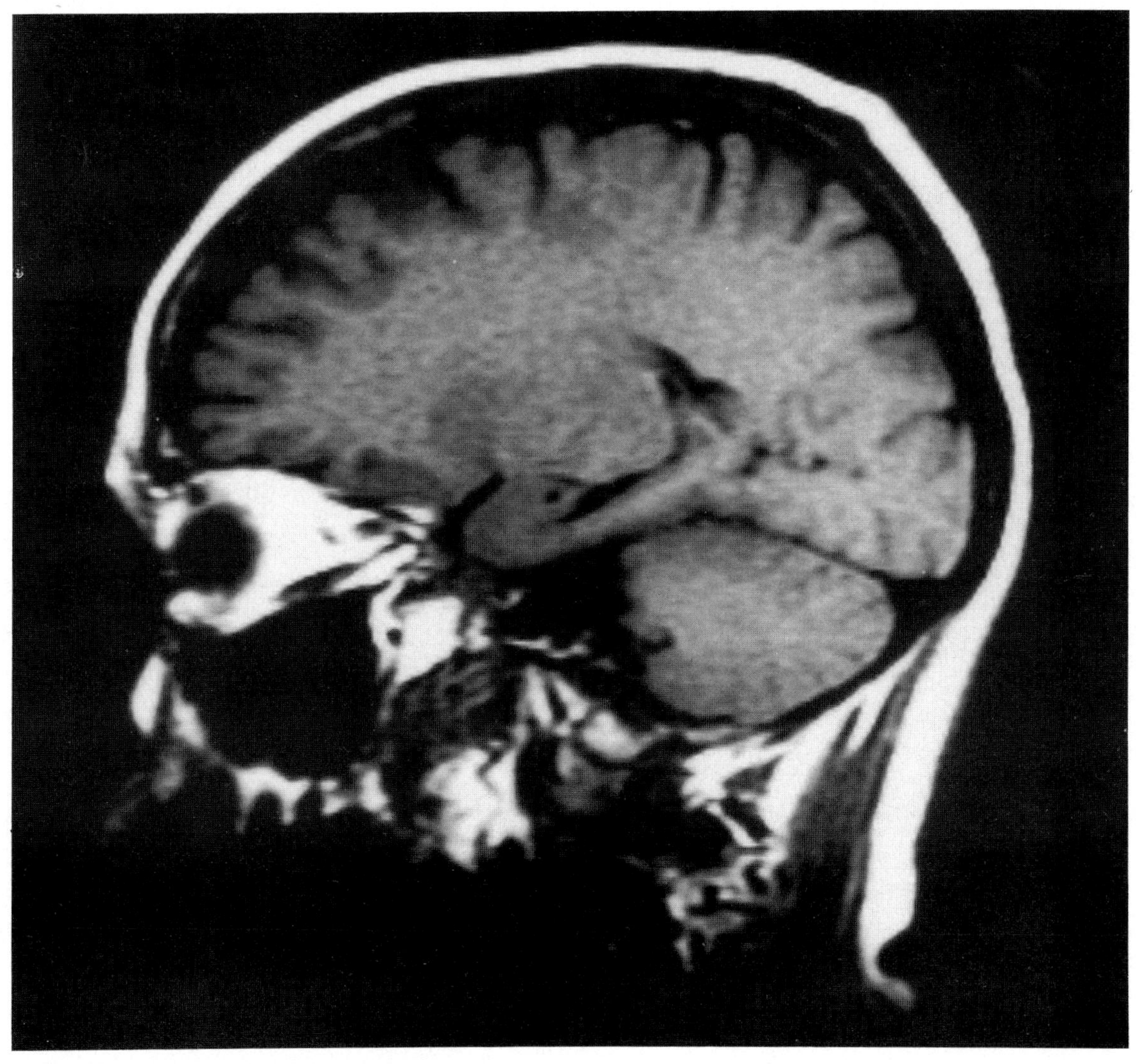

1-3 Head, sagittal view (TR 400; TE 20).

Head, Sagittal

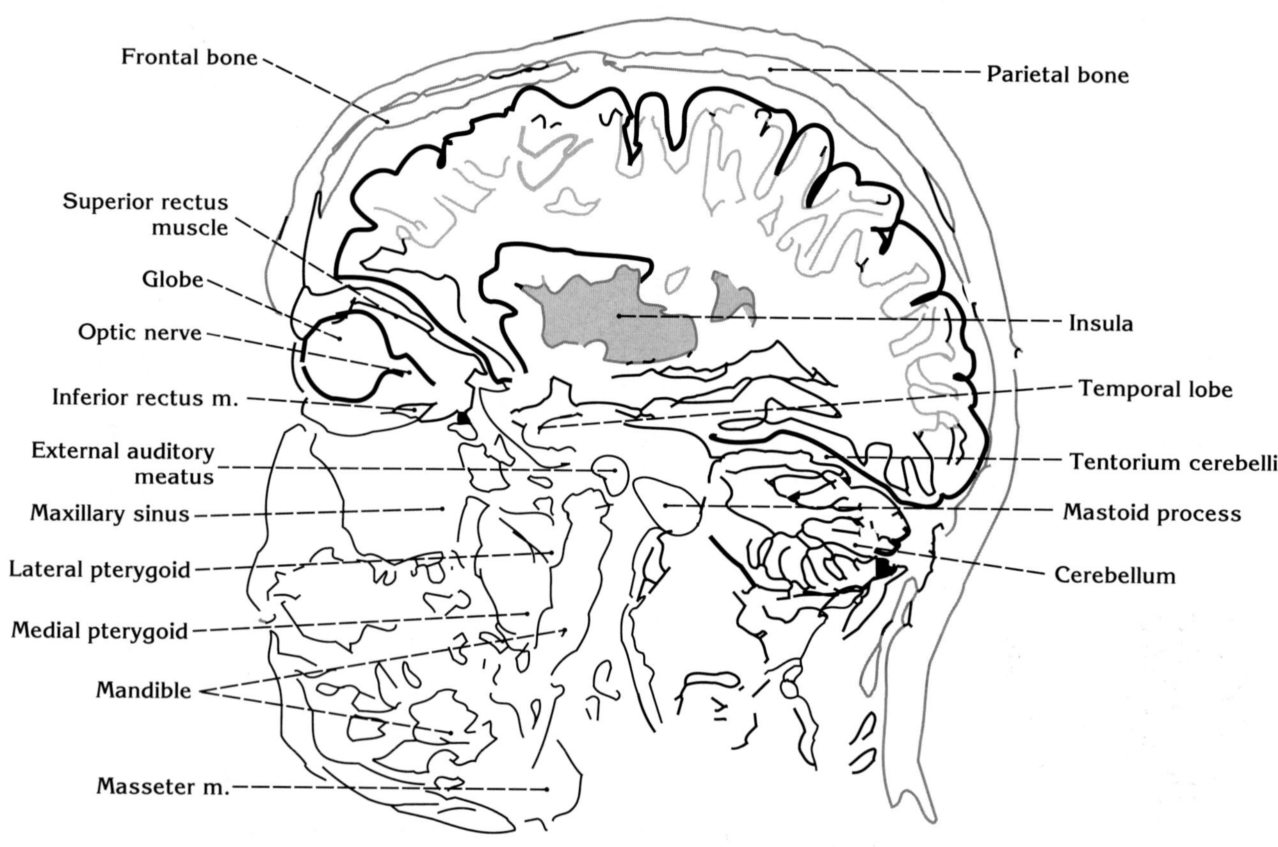

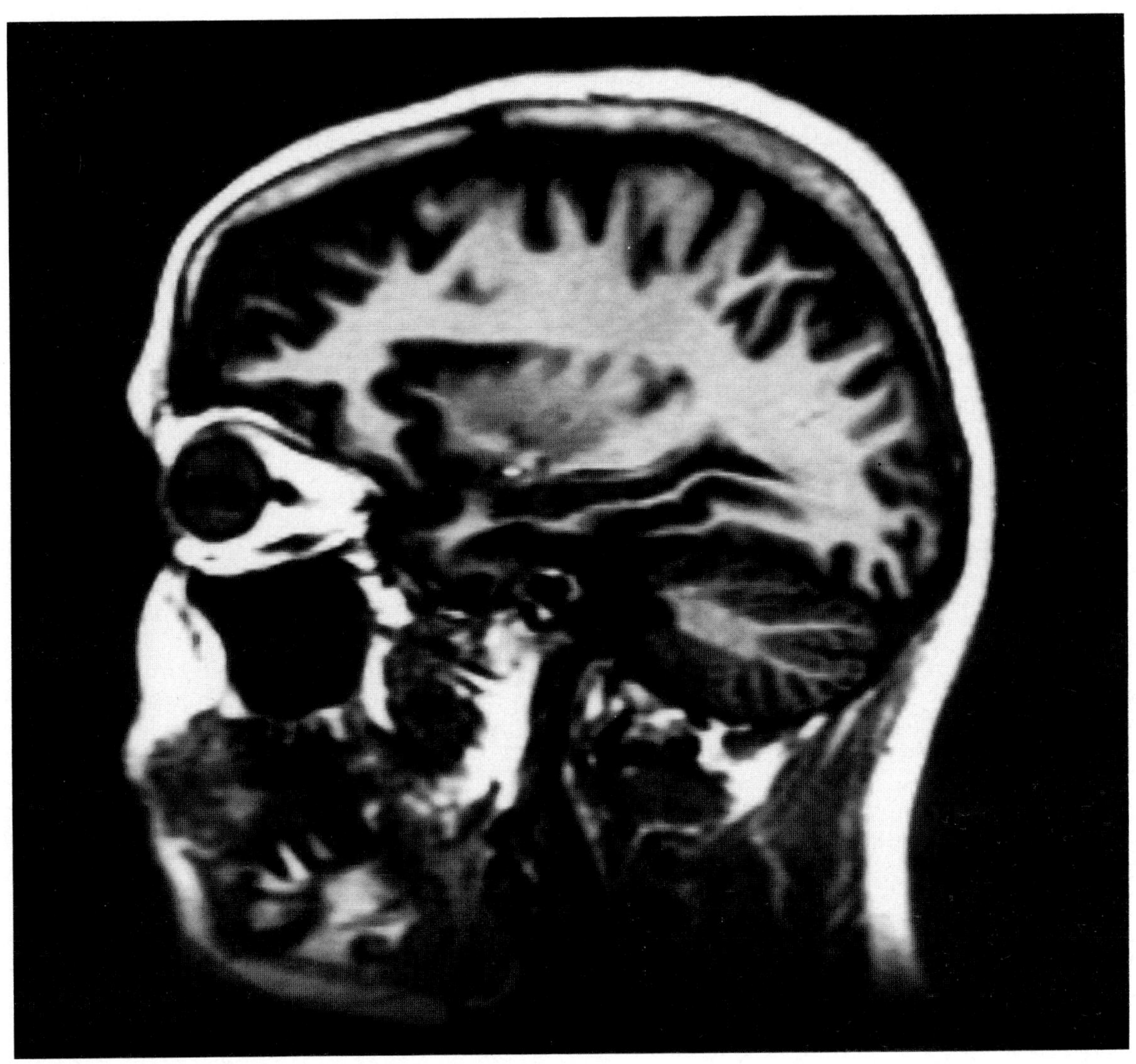

1-4 Head, sagittal view (inversion recovery).

Head, Sagittal

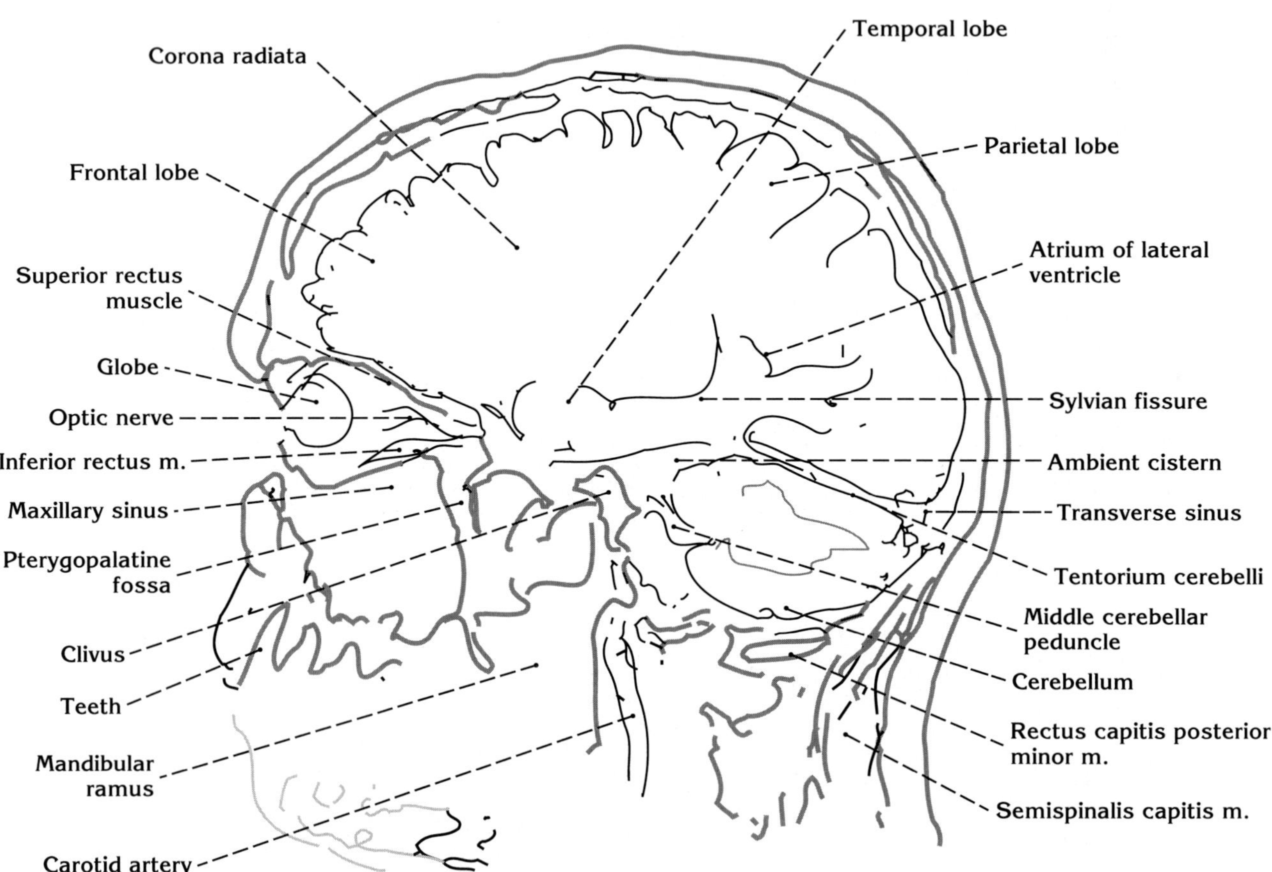

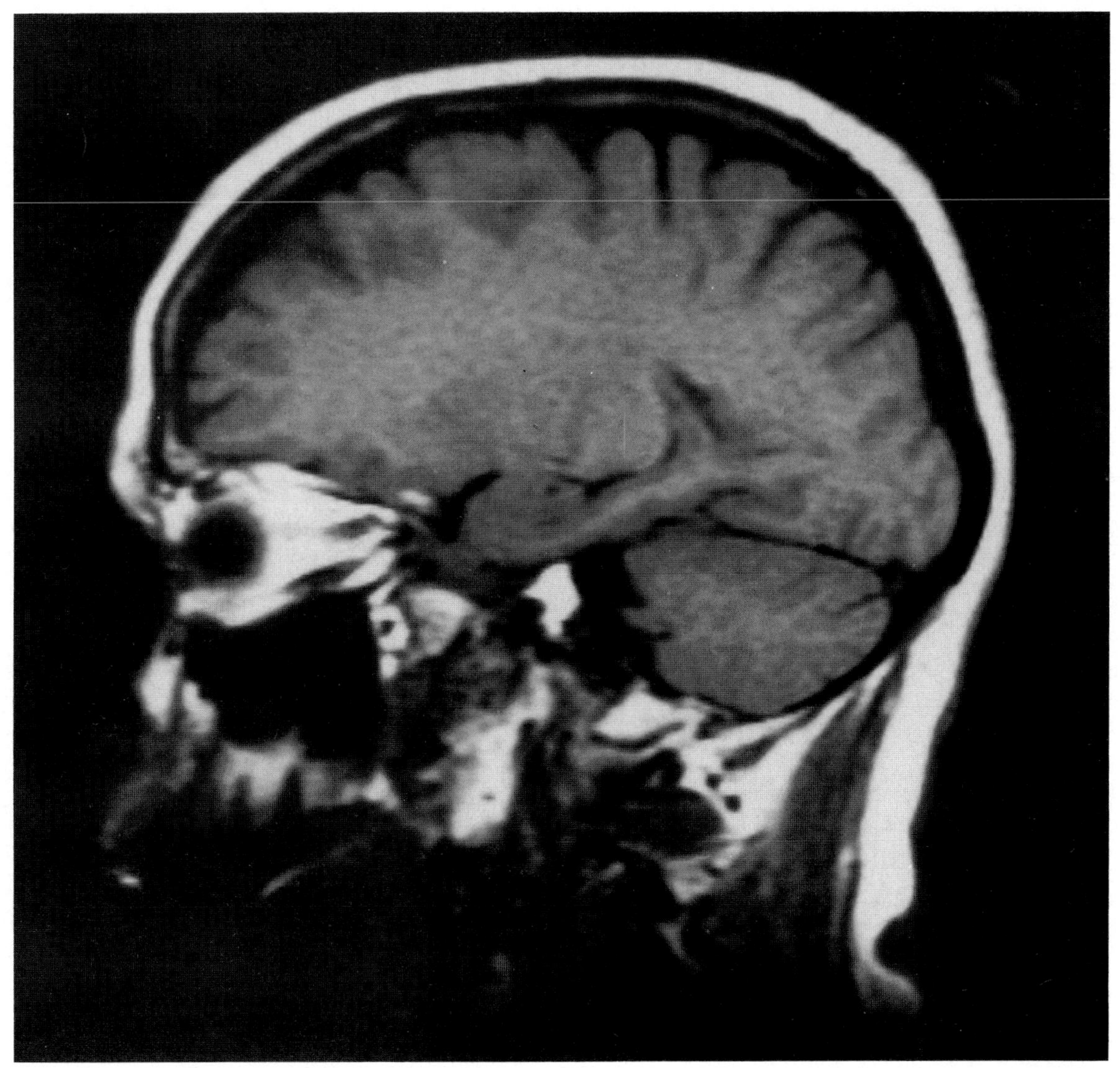

1-5 Head, sagittal view (TR 400; TE 20).

Head, Sagittal

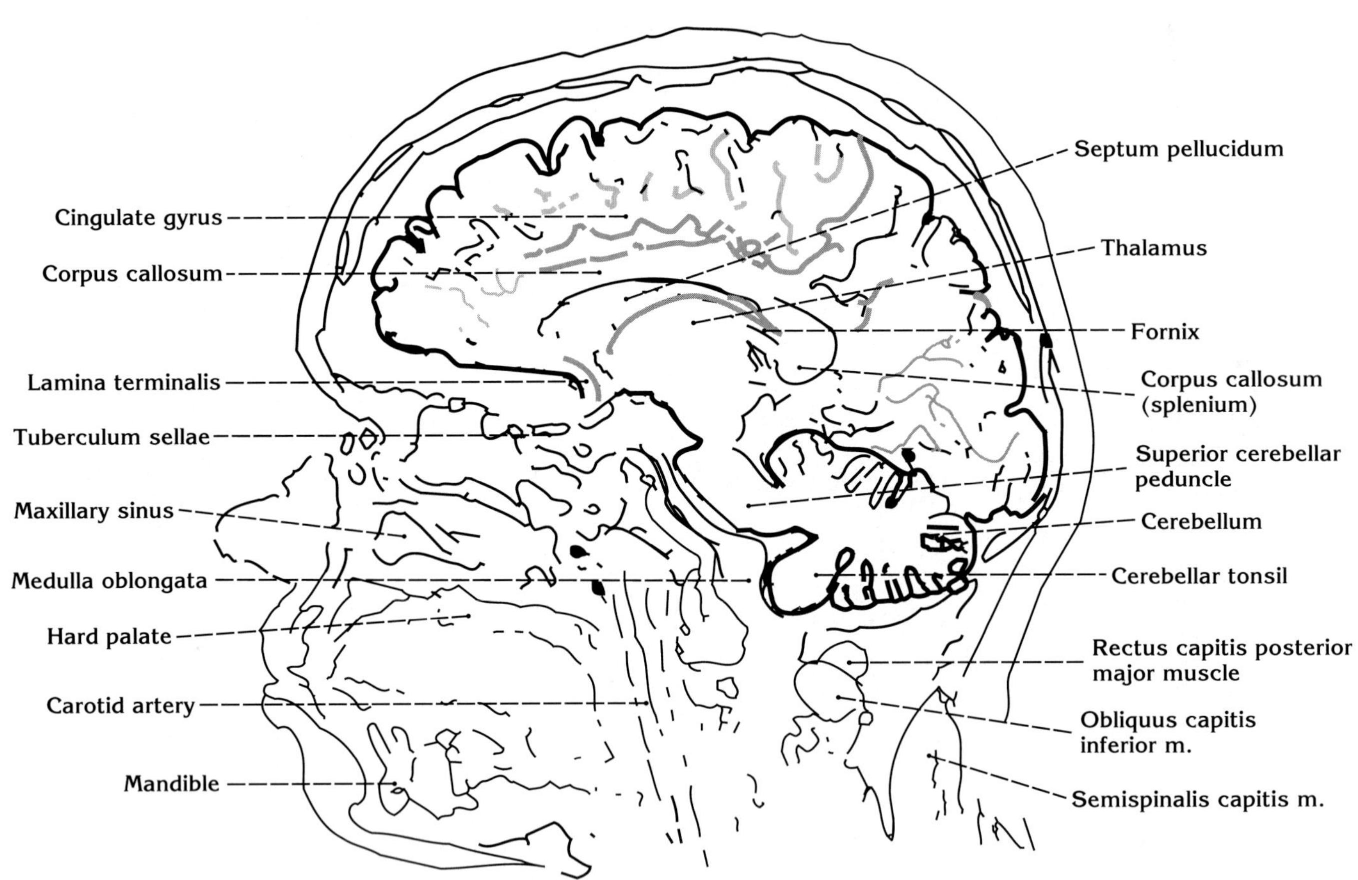

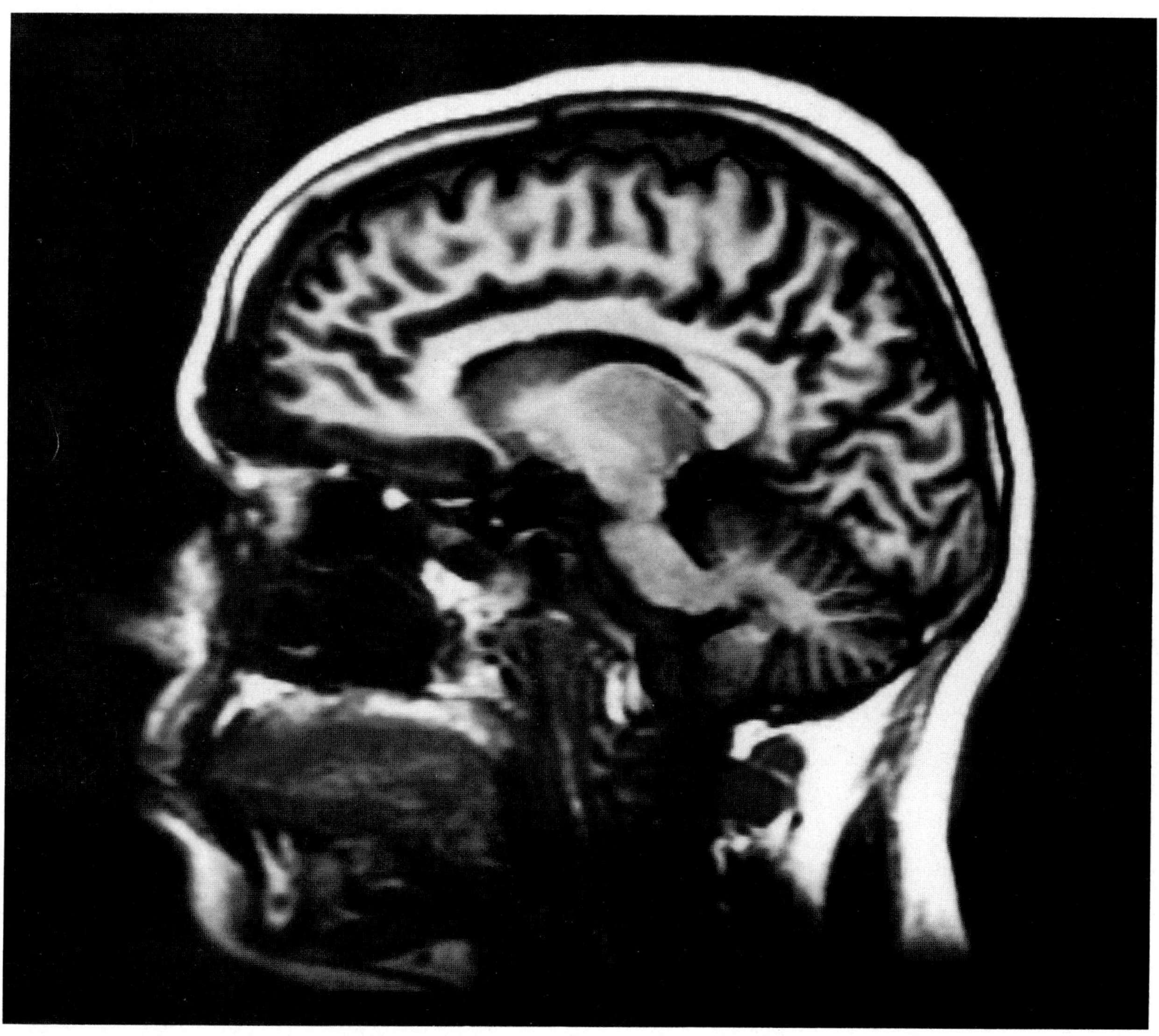

1-6 Head, sagittal view (TR 1800; TE 20).

Head, Sagittal

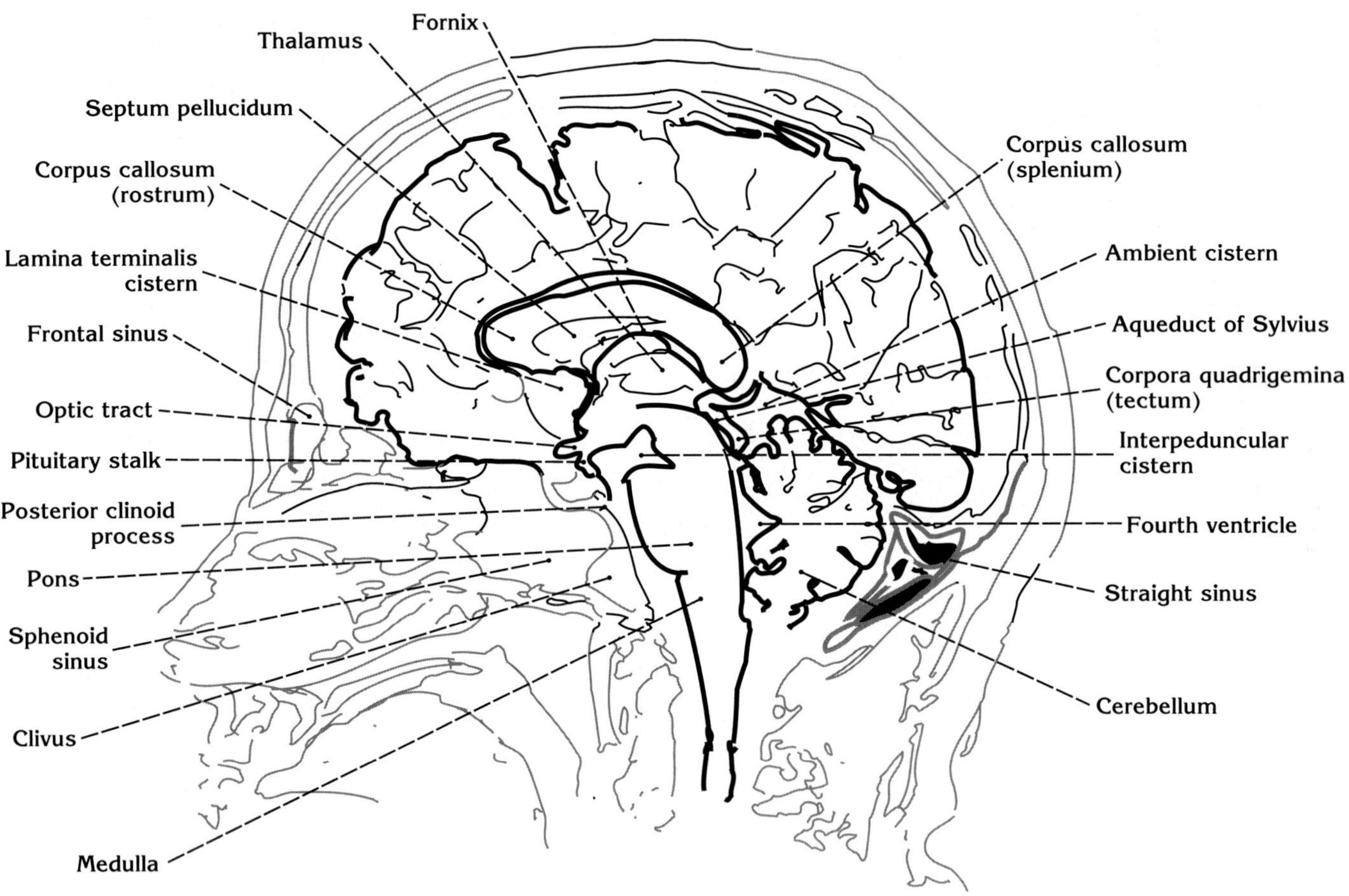

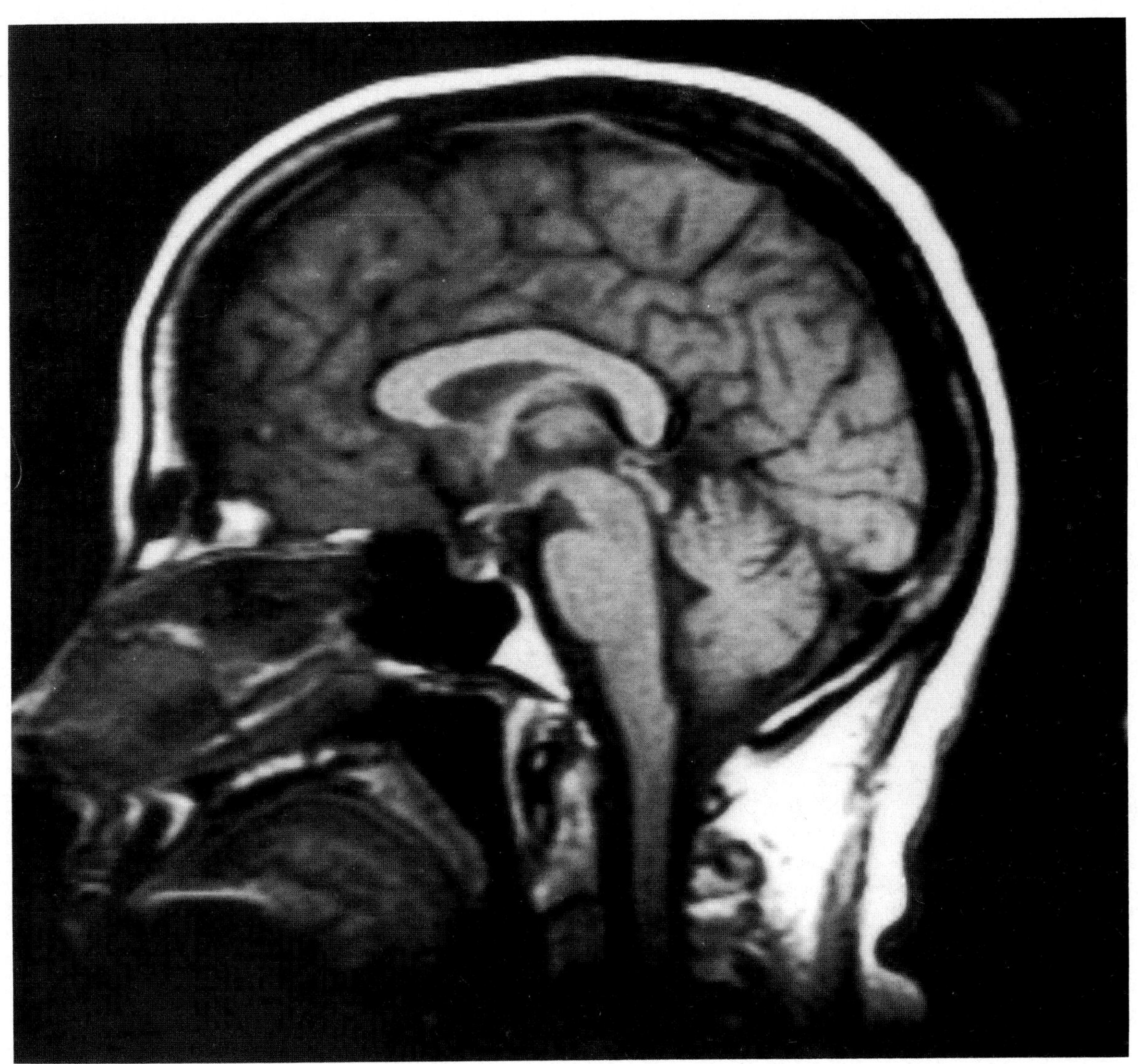

1-7 Head, sagittal view (TR 400; TE 20).

Head, Sagittal

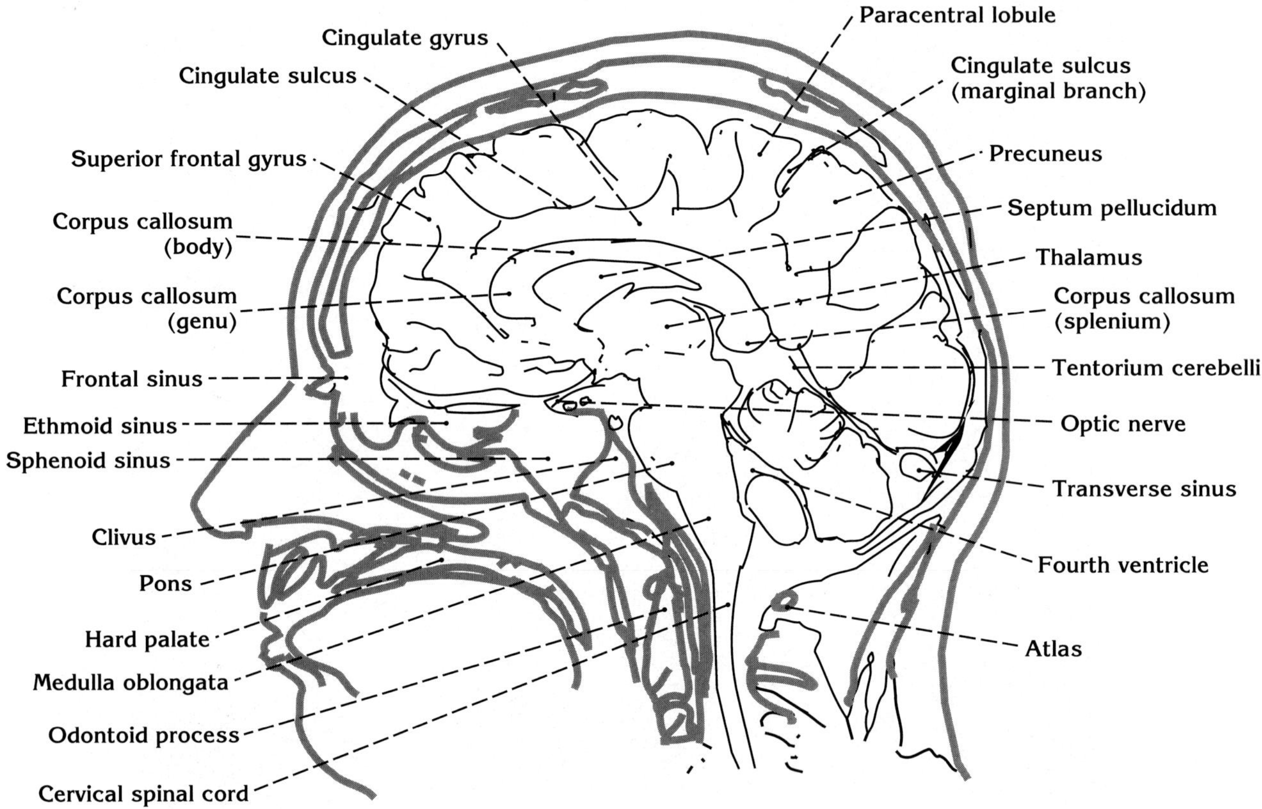

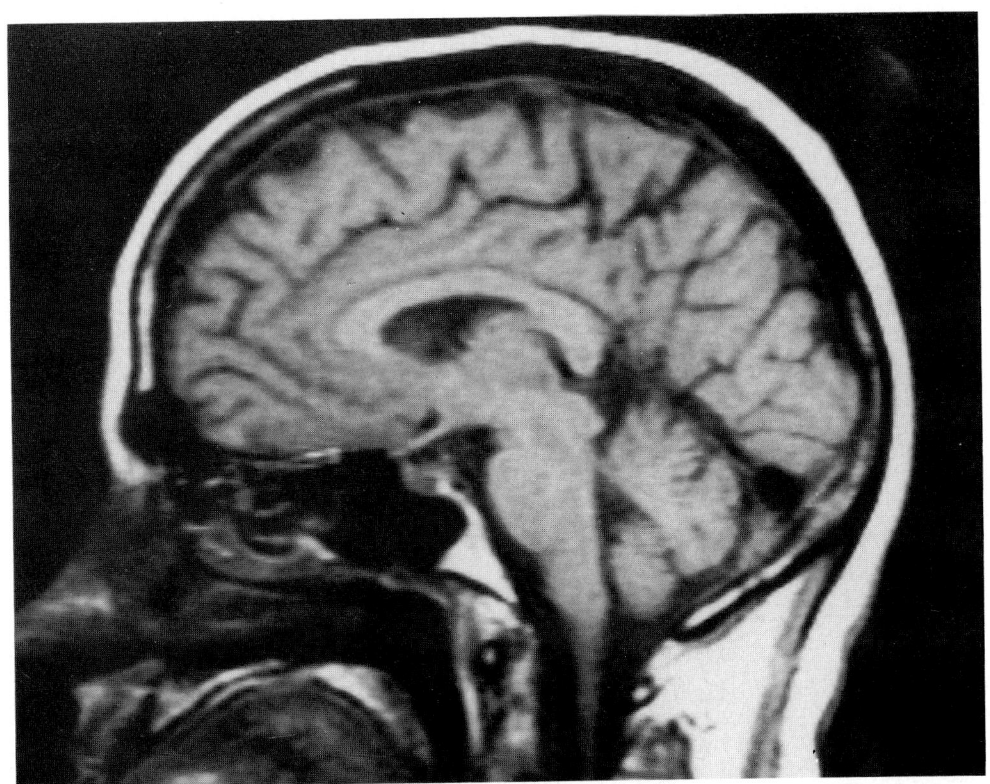

1-8a Head, sagittal view (TR 400; TE 20).

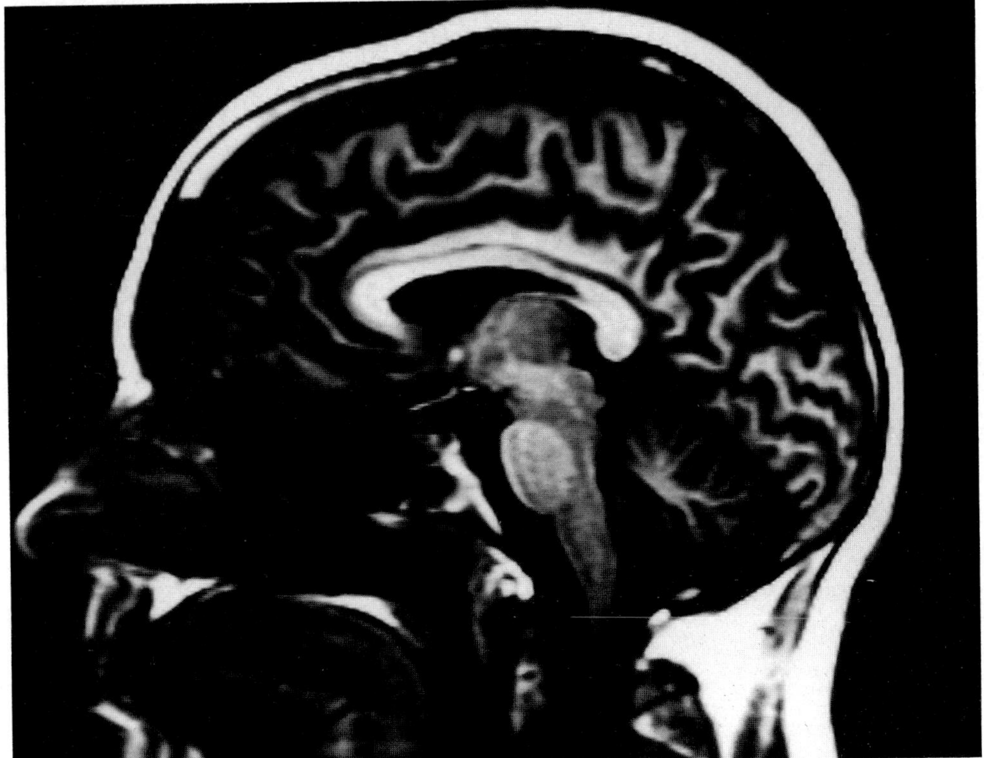

1-8b Head, sagittal view (inversion recovery).

Head, Coronal

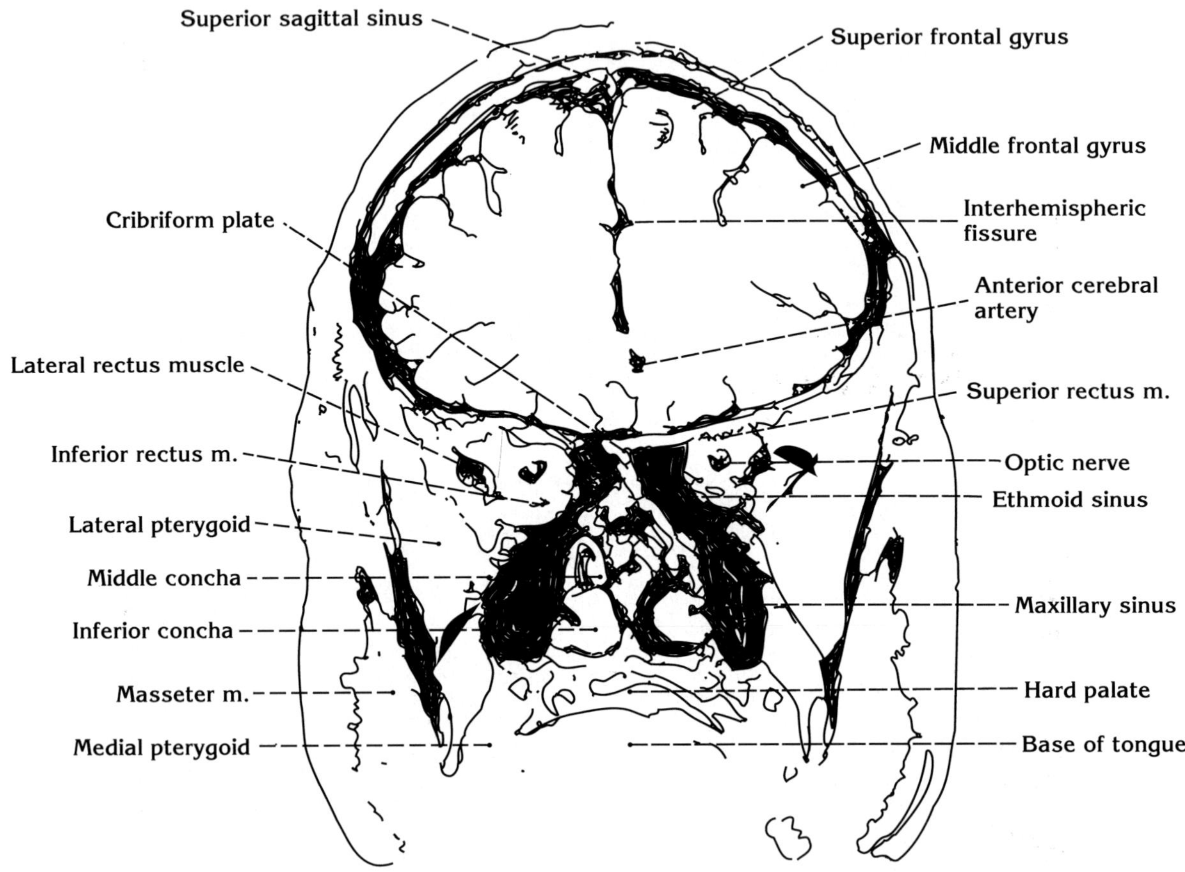

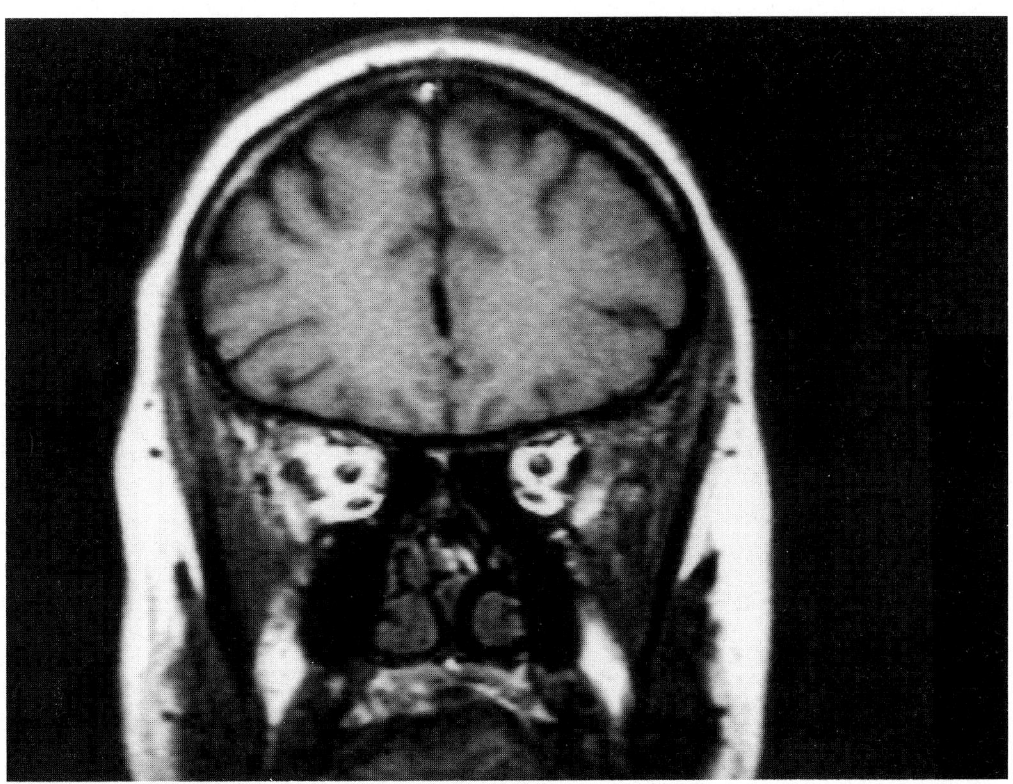

1-9a Head, coronal view (TR 800; TE 20).

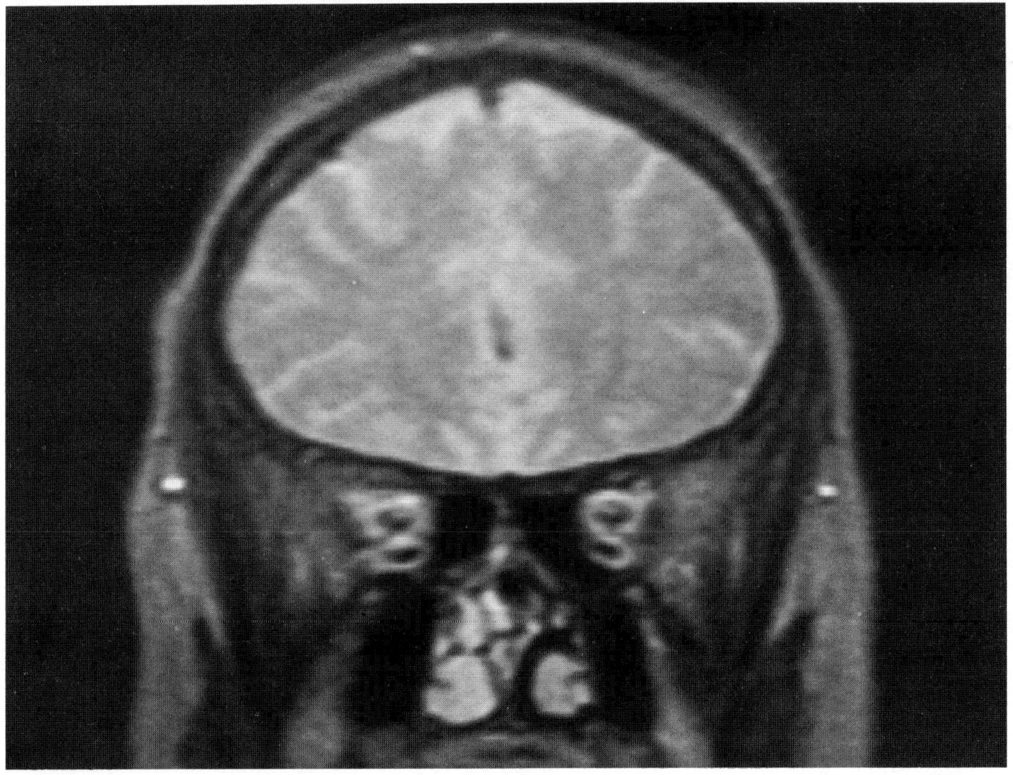

1-9b Head, coronal view (TR 2000; TE 80).

Head, Coronal

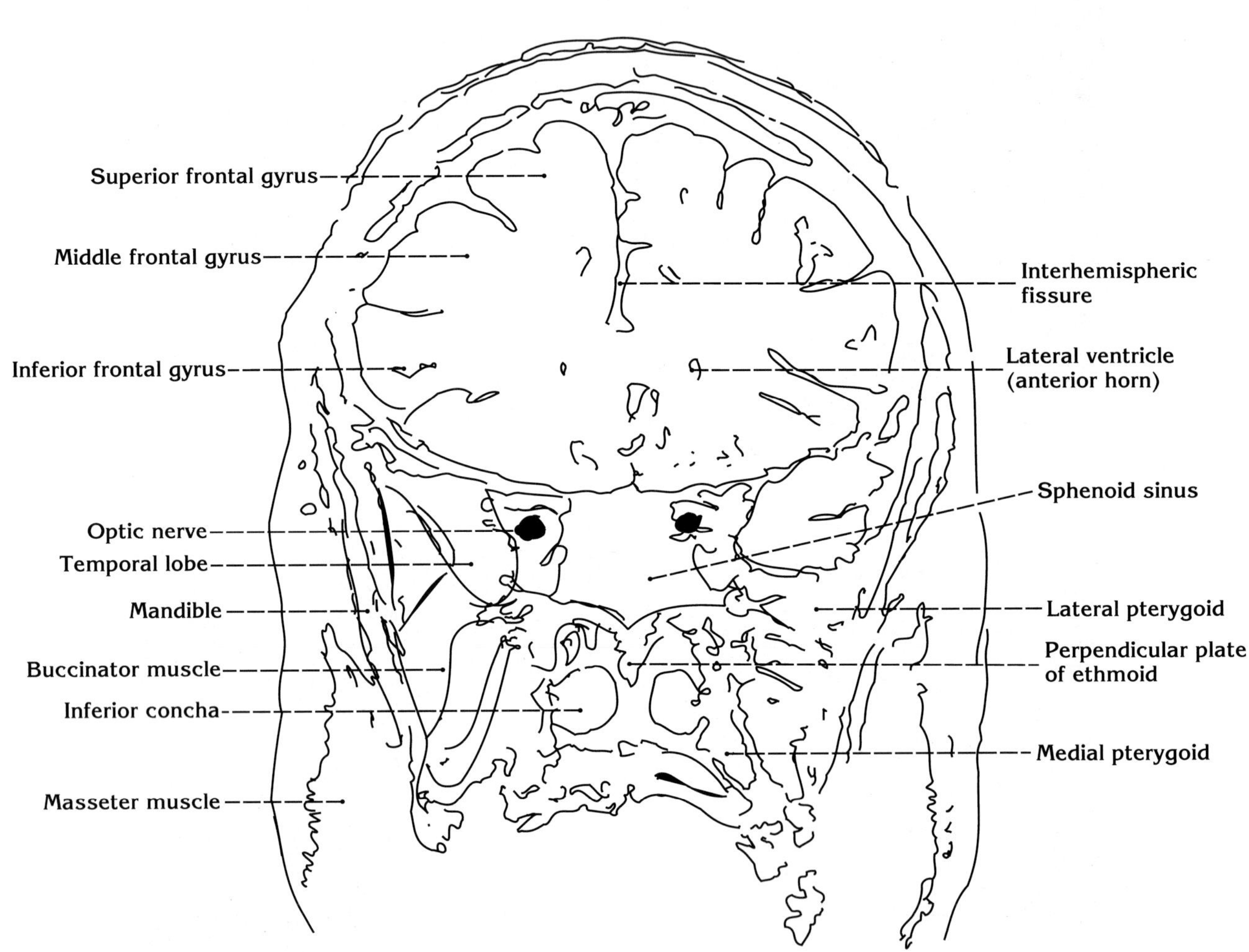

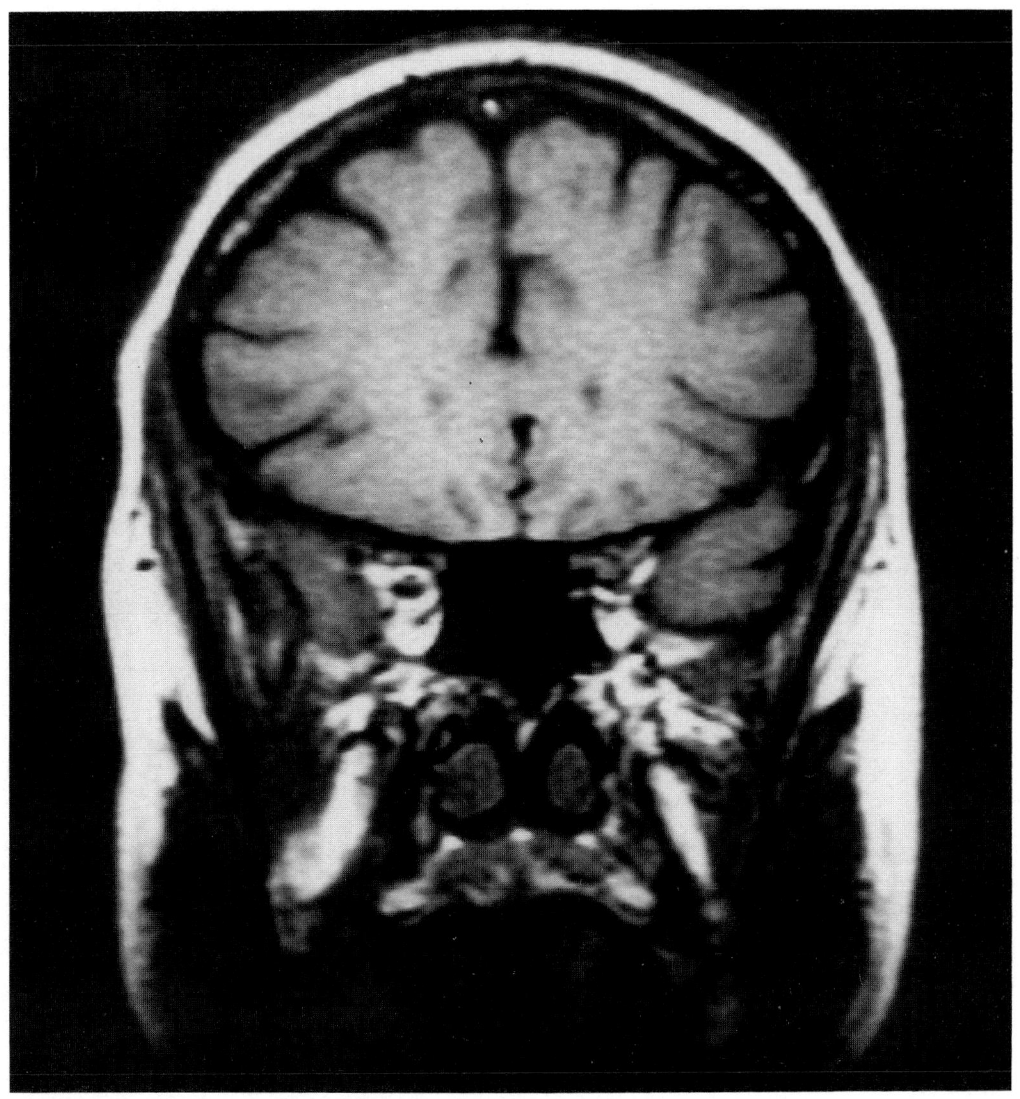

1-10 Head, coronal view (TR 800; TE 20).

Head, Coronal

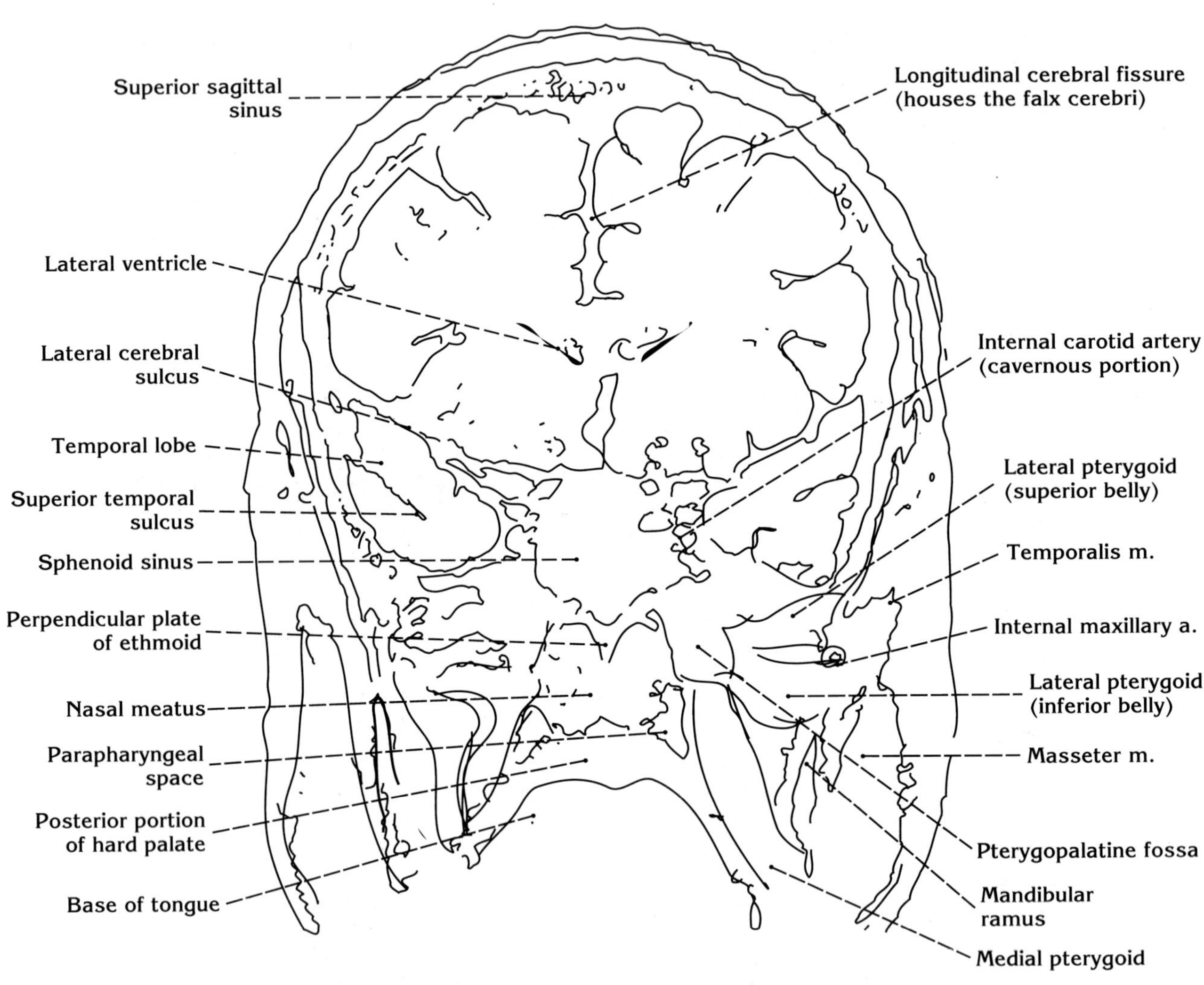

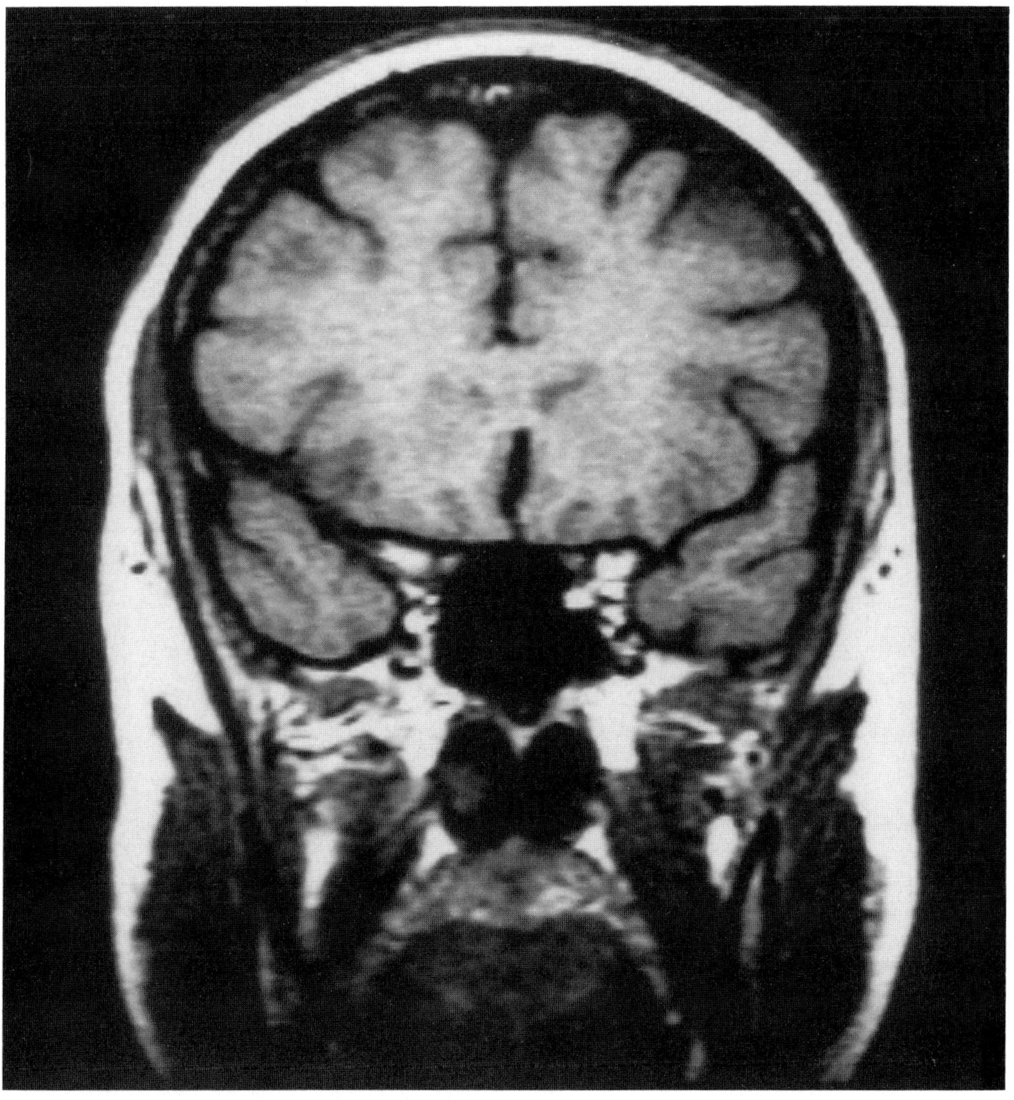

1-11 Head, coronal view (TR 800; TE 20).

Head, Coronal

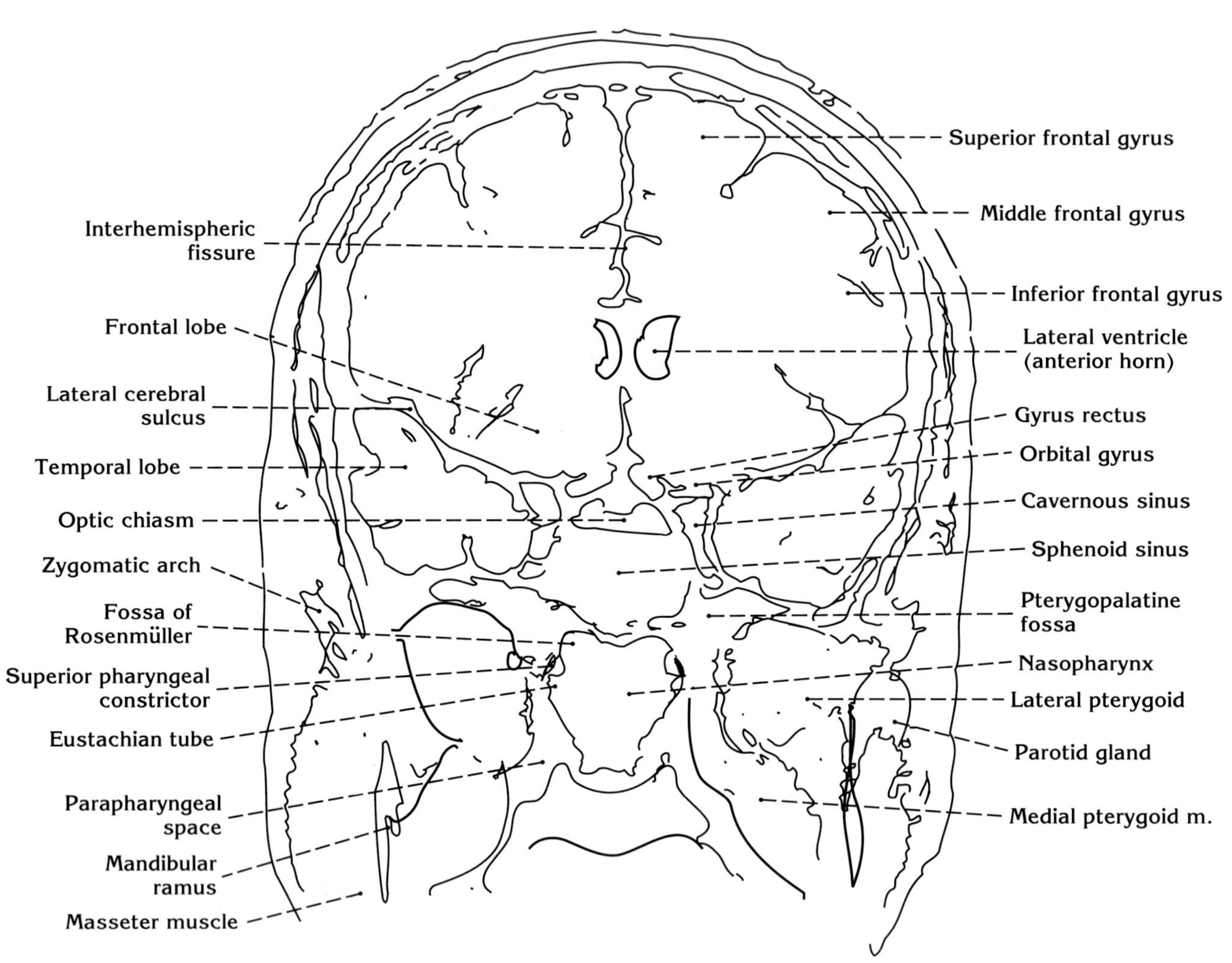

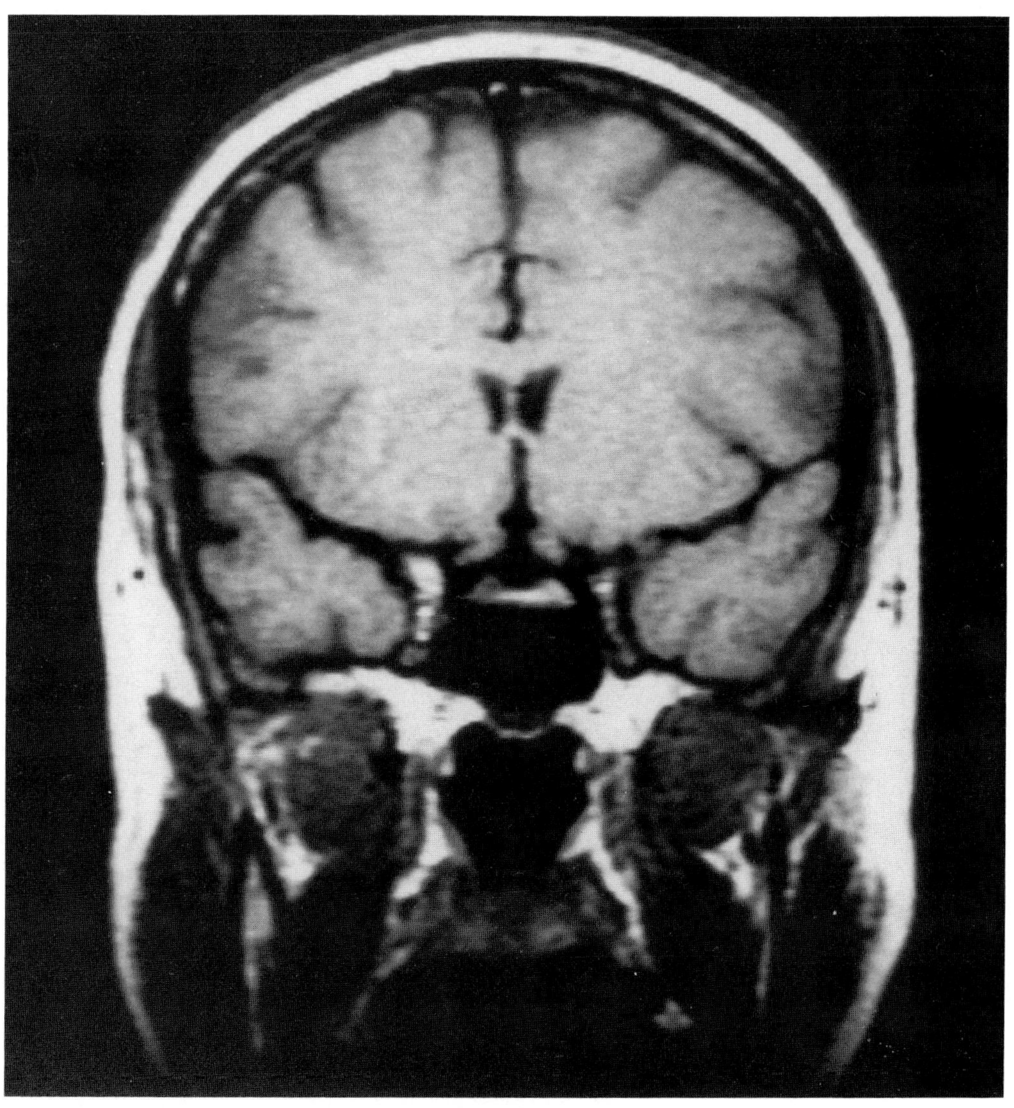

1-12 Head, coronal view (TR 800; TE 20).

Head, Coronal

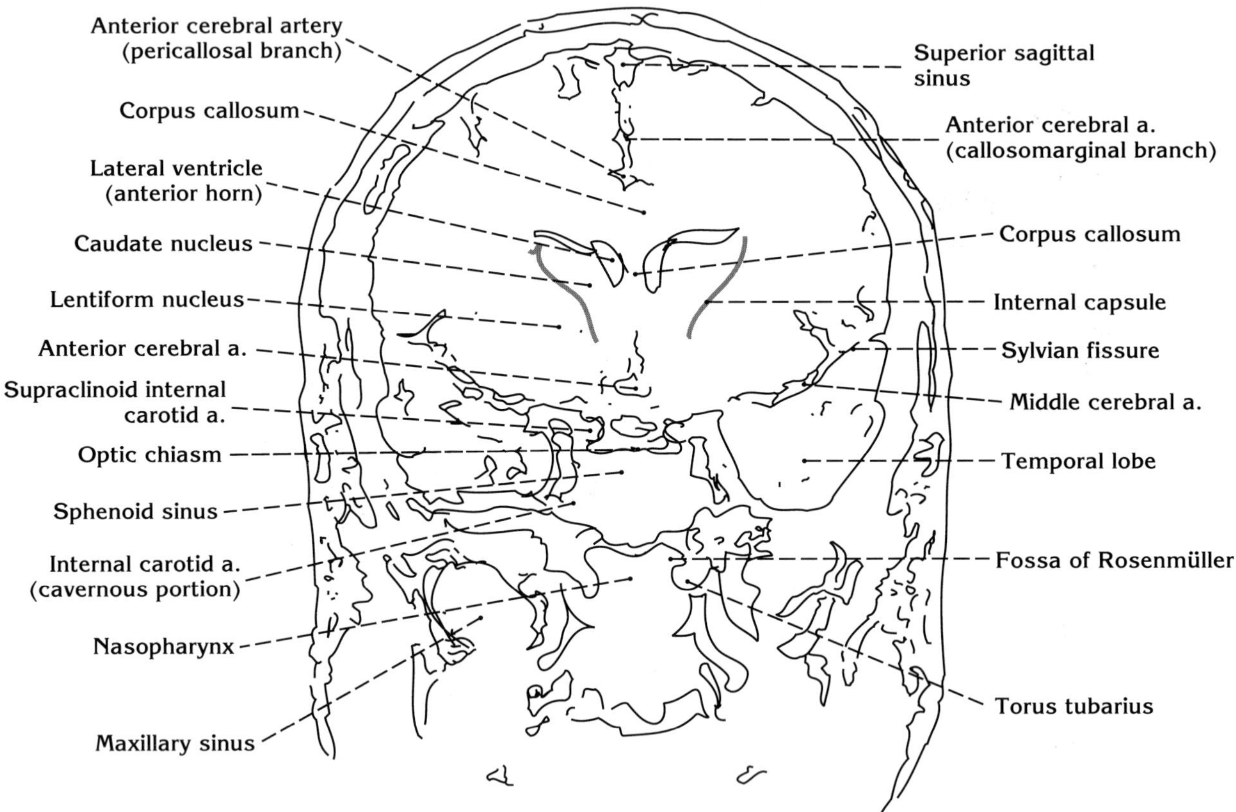

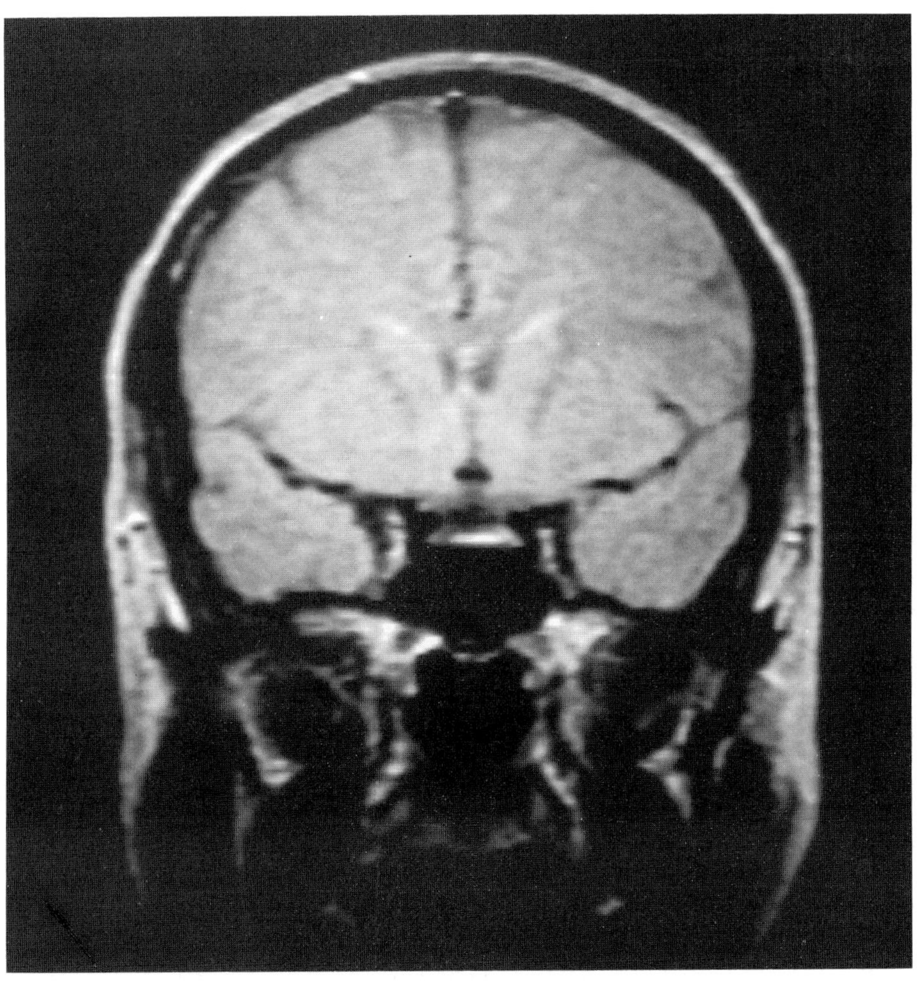

1-13 Head, coronal view (TR 2000; TE 40).

Head, Coronal

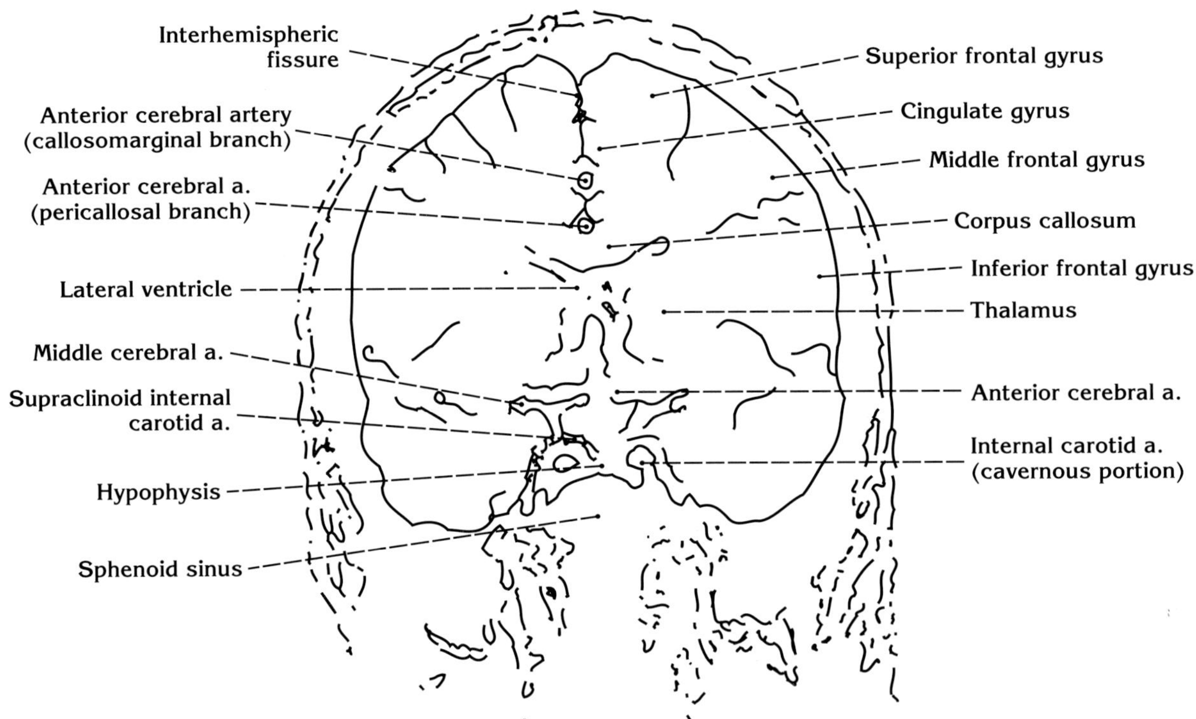

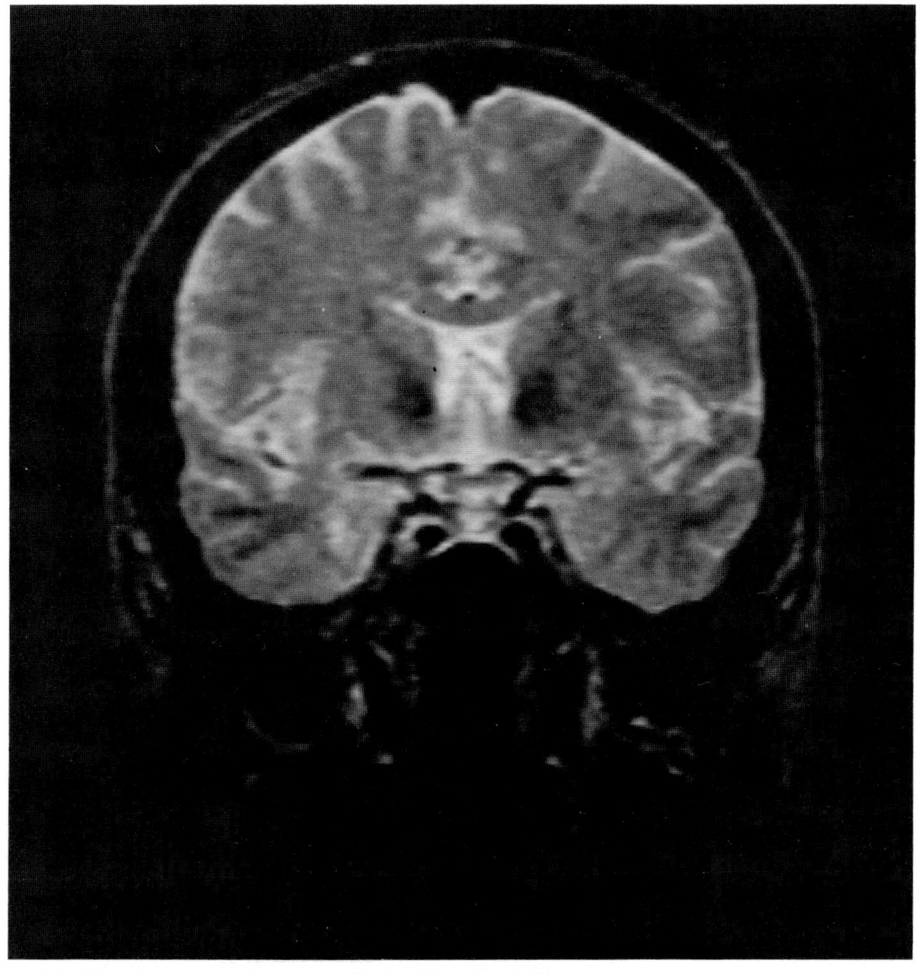

1-14 Head, coronal view (TR 2000; TE 80).

Head, Coronal

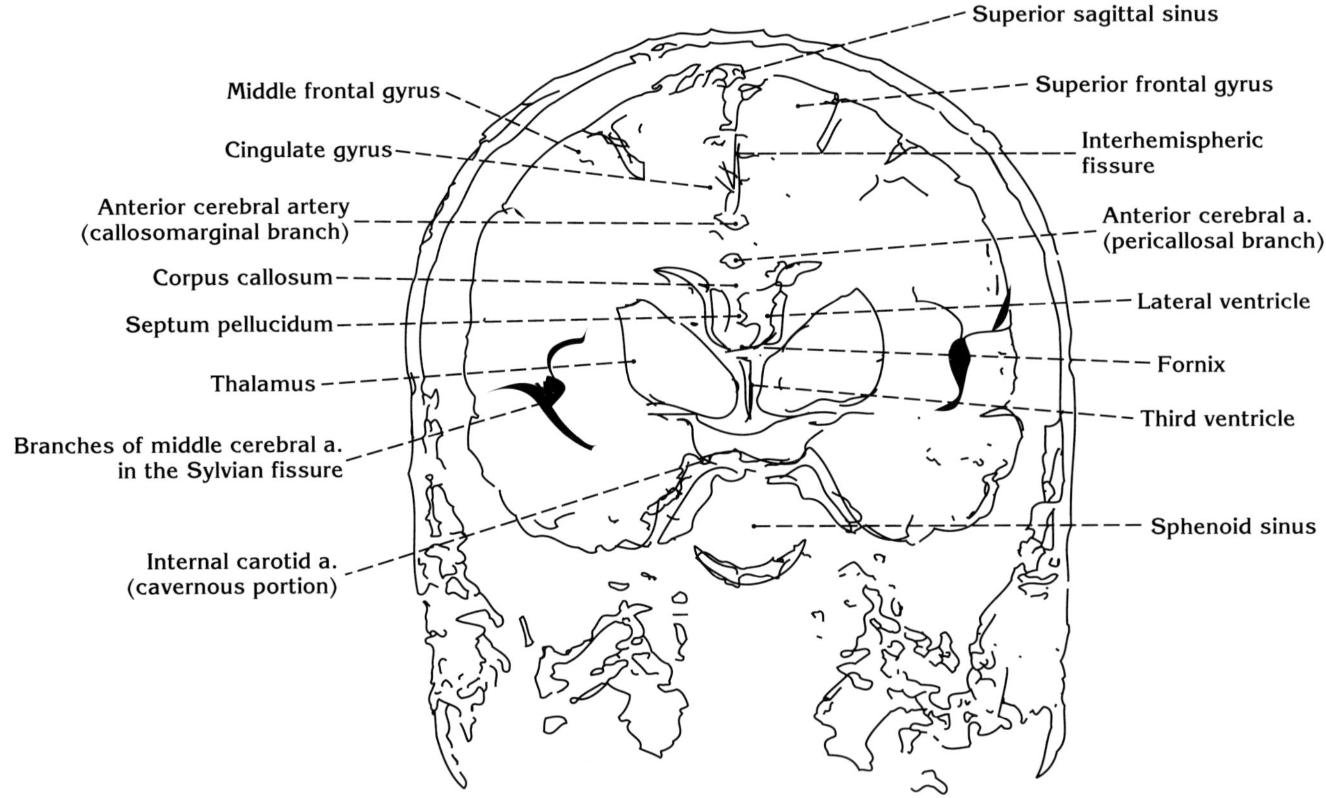

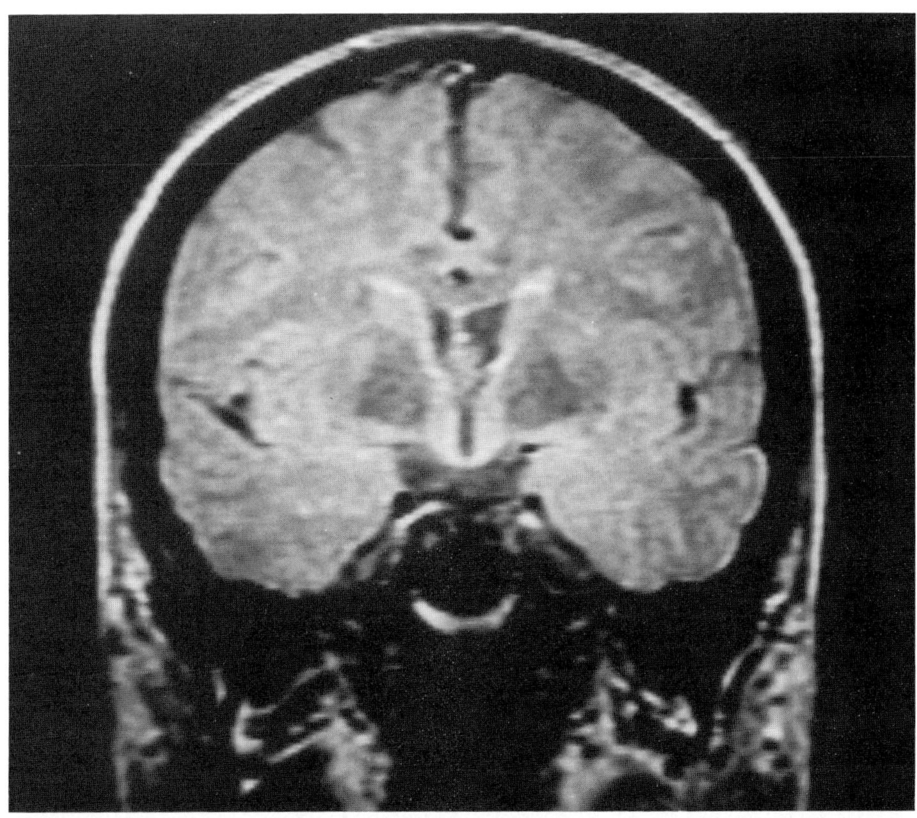

1-15a Head, coronal view (TR 2000; TE 40).

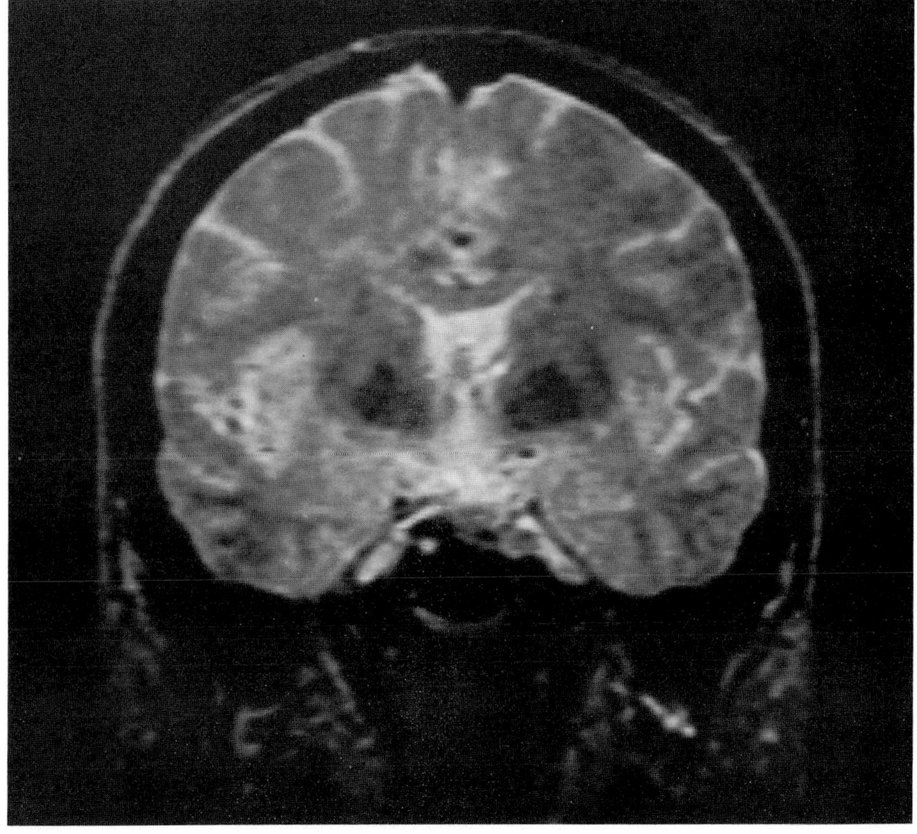

1-15b Head, coronal view (TR 2000; TE 80).

Head, Coronal

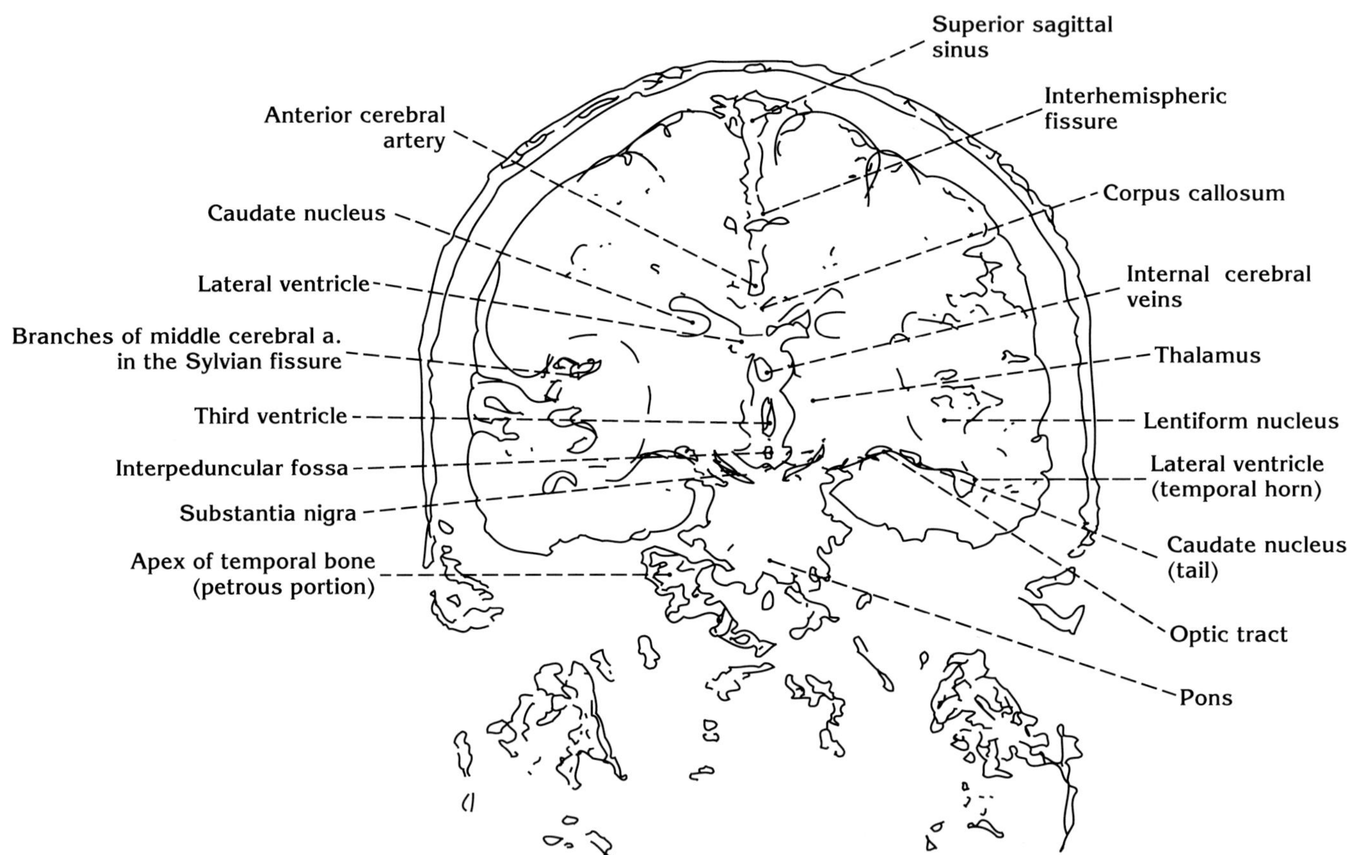

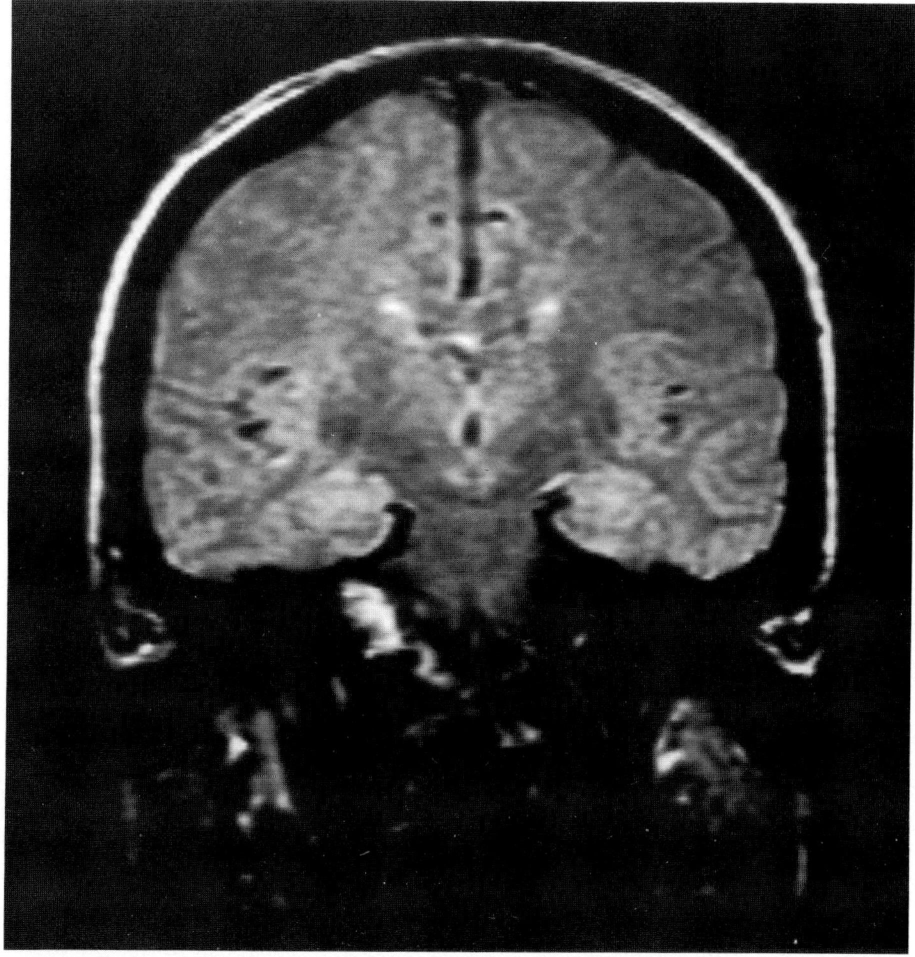

1-16 Head, coronal view (TR 2000; TE 40). *Note:* This image and Figs. 1-17a and 1-17b were selected for the purpose of demonstrating the relationship of the petrous portion of the temporal bone to the brain. The petrous temporal demonstrates high signal intensity secondary to changes produced by radiation. There is abnormally high signal in the tip of the right petrous temporal bone.

Head, Coronal

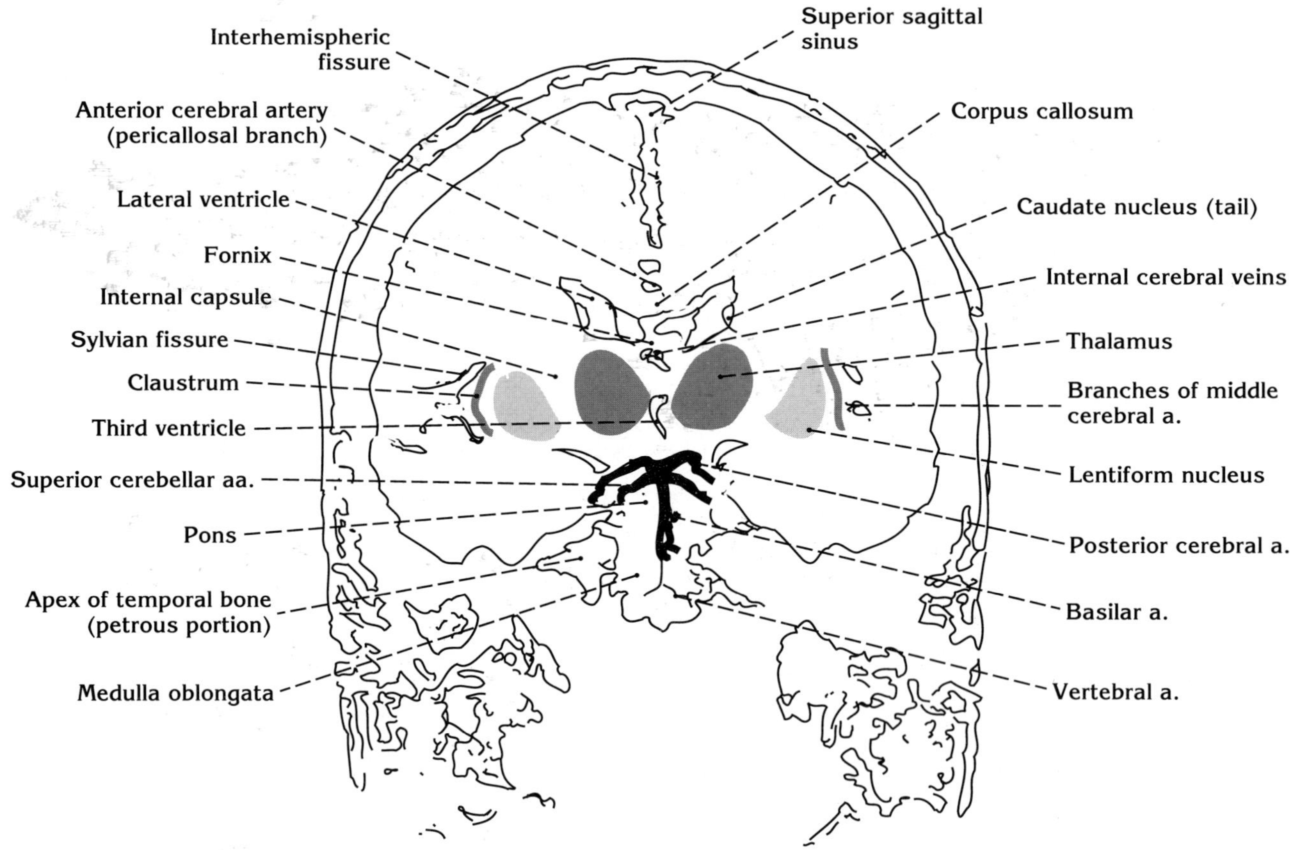

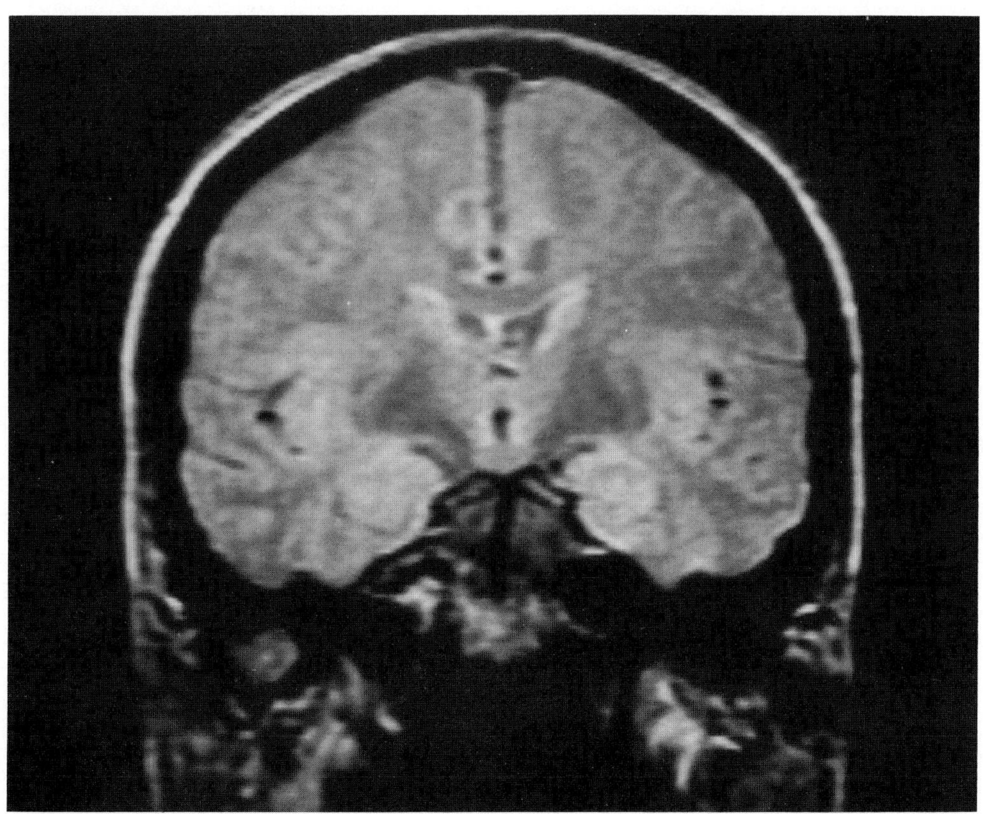

1-17a Head, coronal view (TR 2000; TE 40). (See note to Fig. 1-16.)

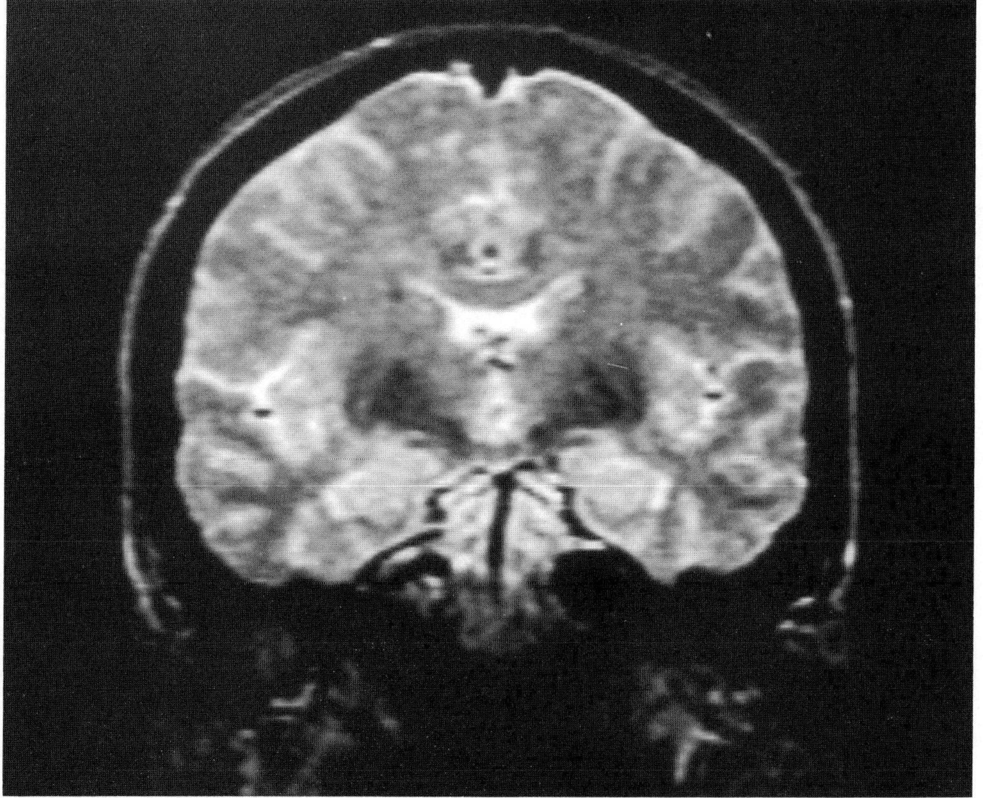

1-17b Head, coronal view (TR 2000; TE 80). (See note to Fig. 1-16.)

Head, Coronal

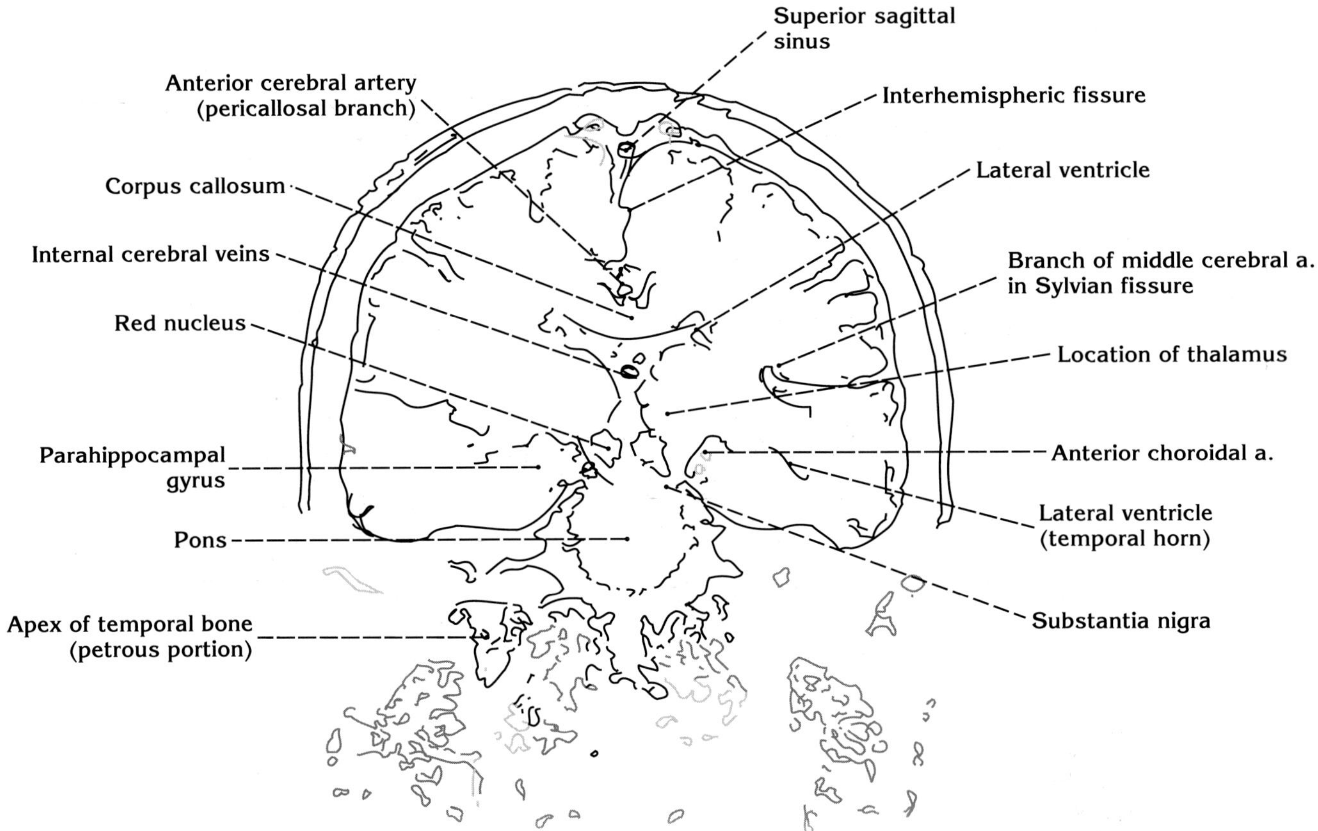

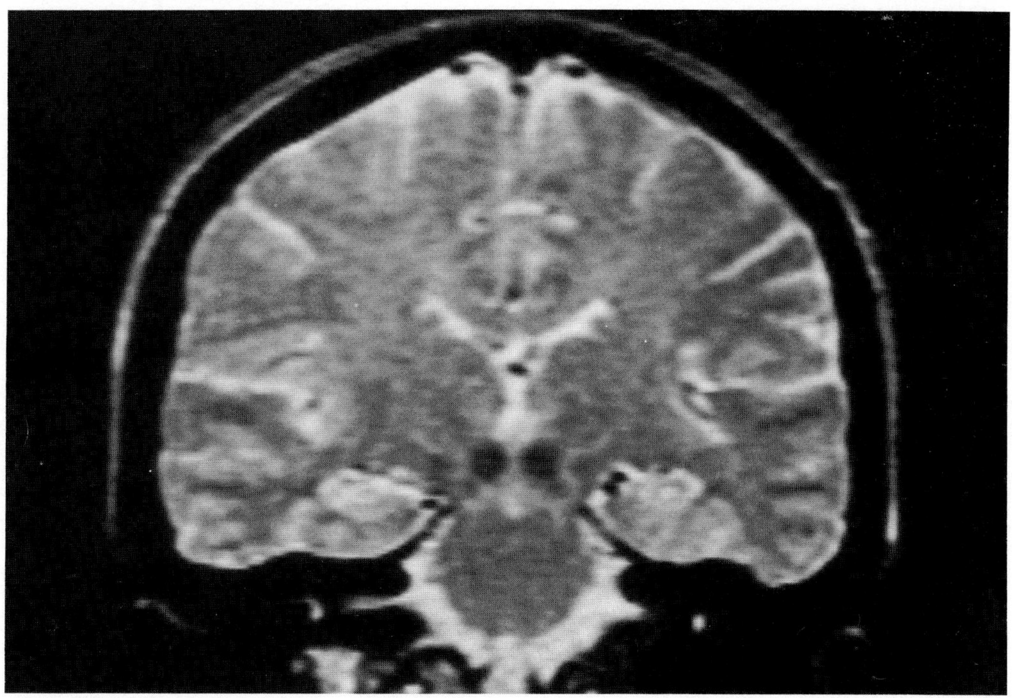

1-18a Head, coronal view (TR 2000; TE 80).

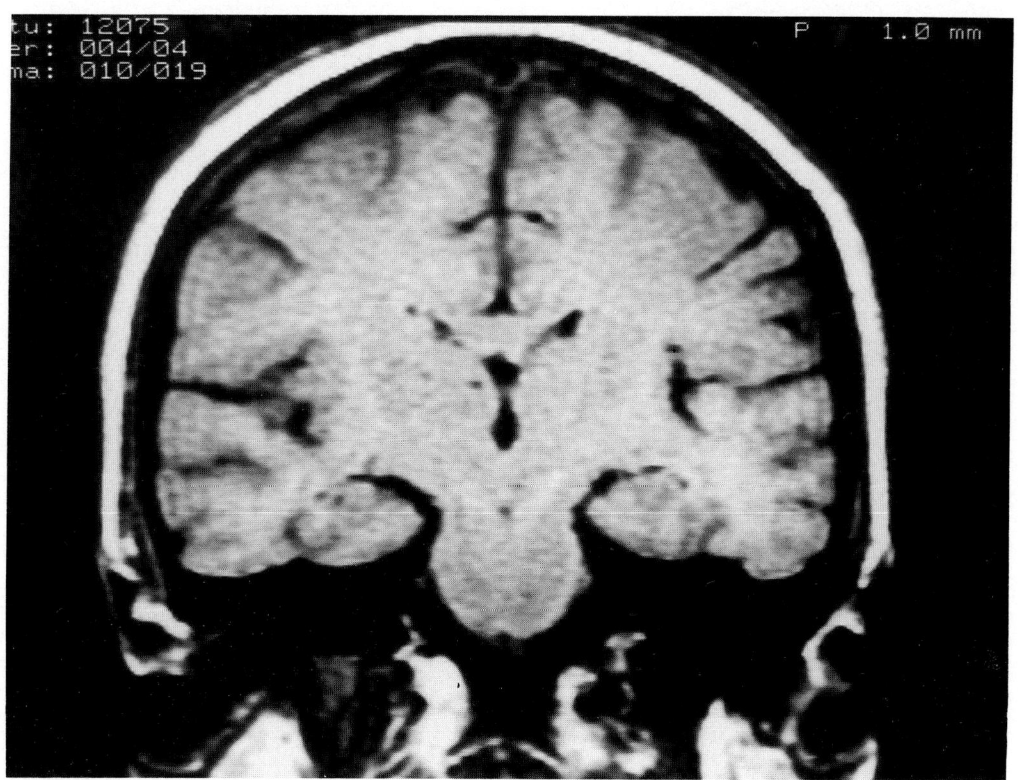

1-18b Head, coronal view (TR 800; TE 20).

Head, Coronal

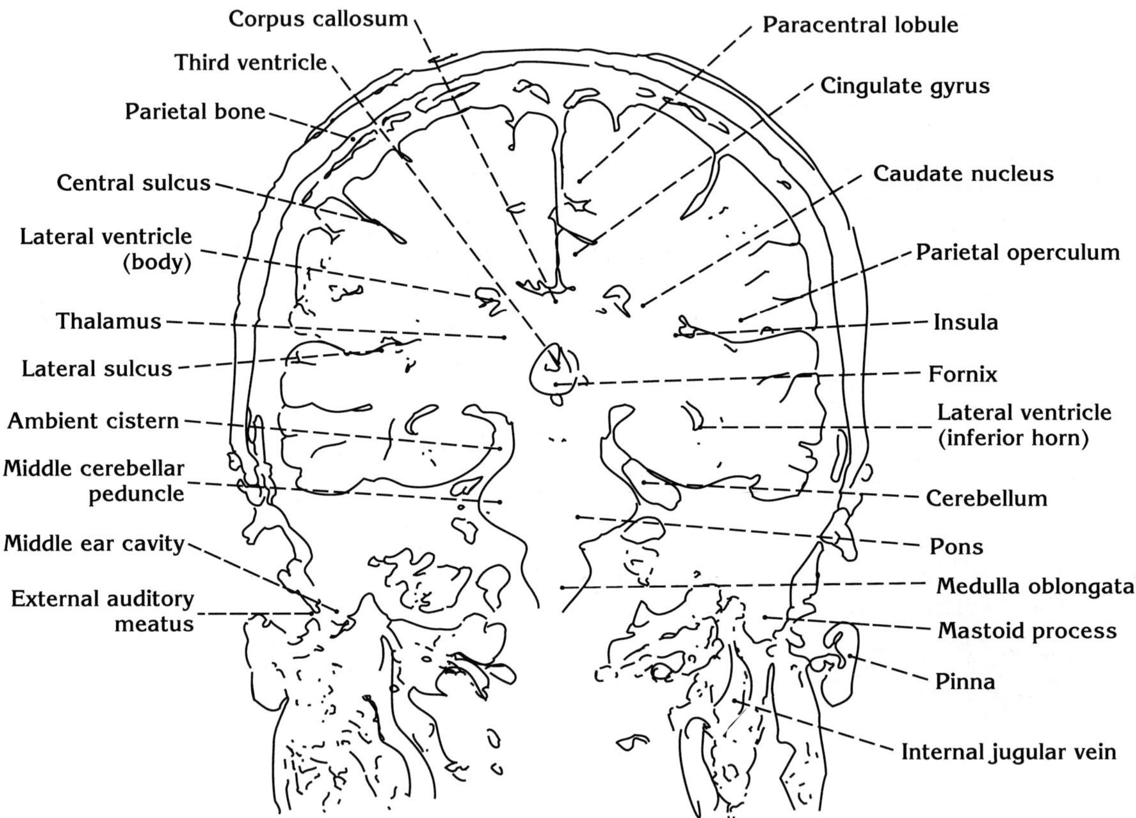

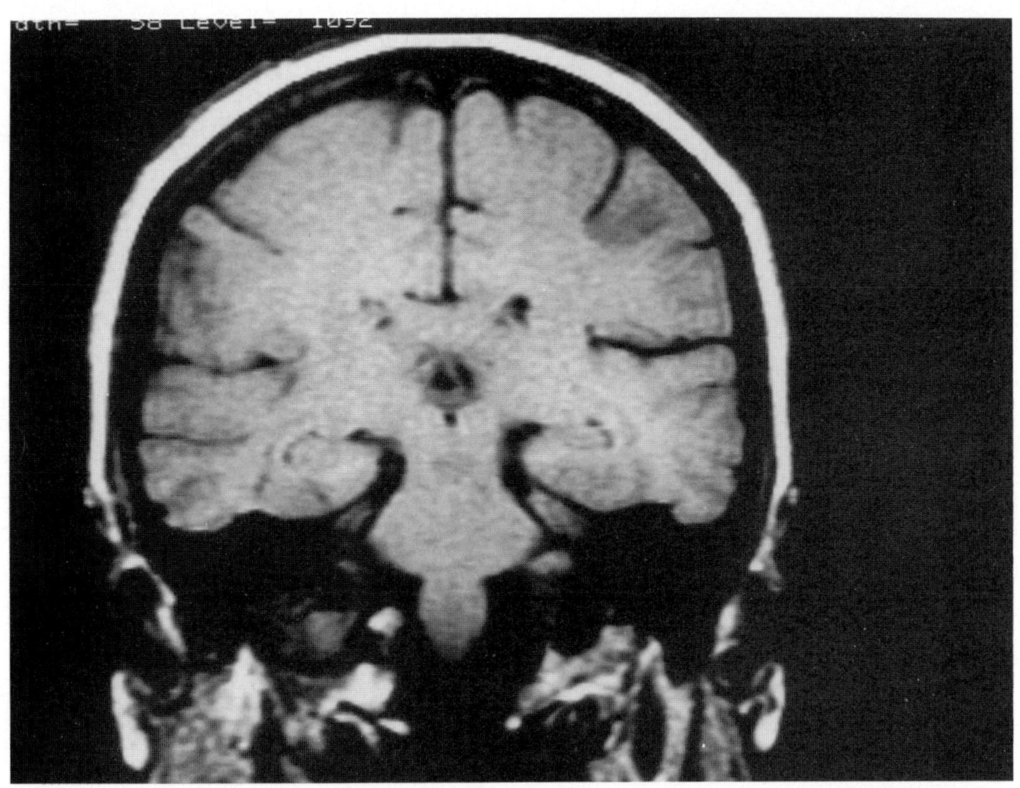

1-19a Head, coronal view (TR 800; TE 20).

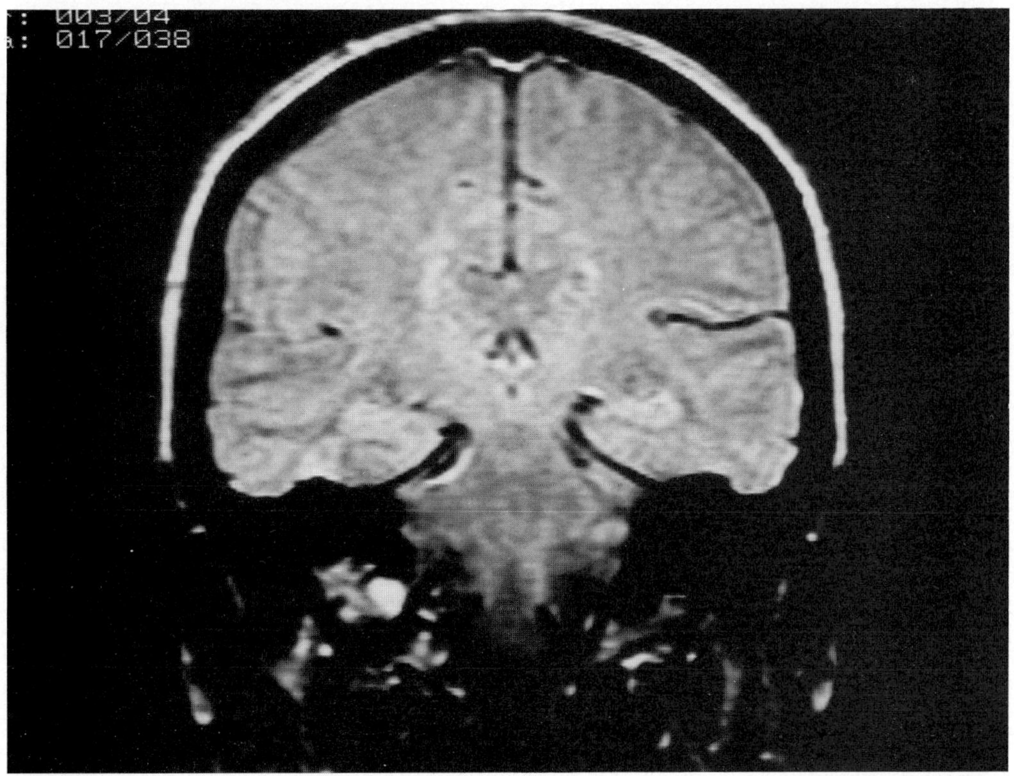

1-19b Head, coronal view (TR 2000; TE 40).

Head, Coronal

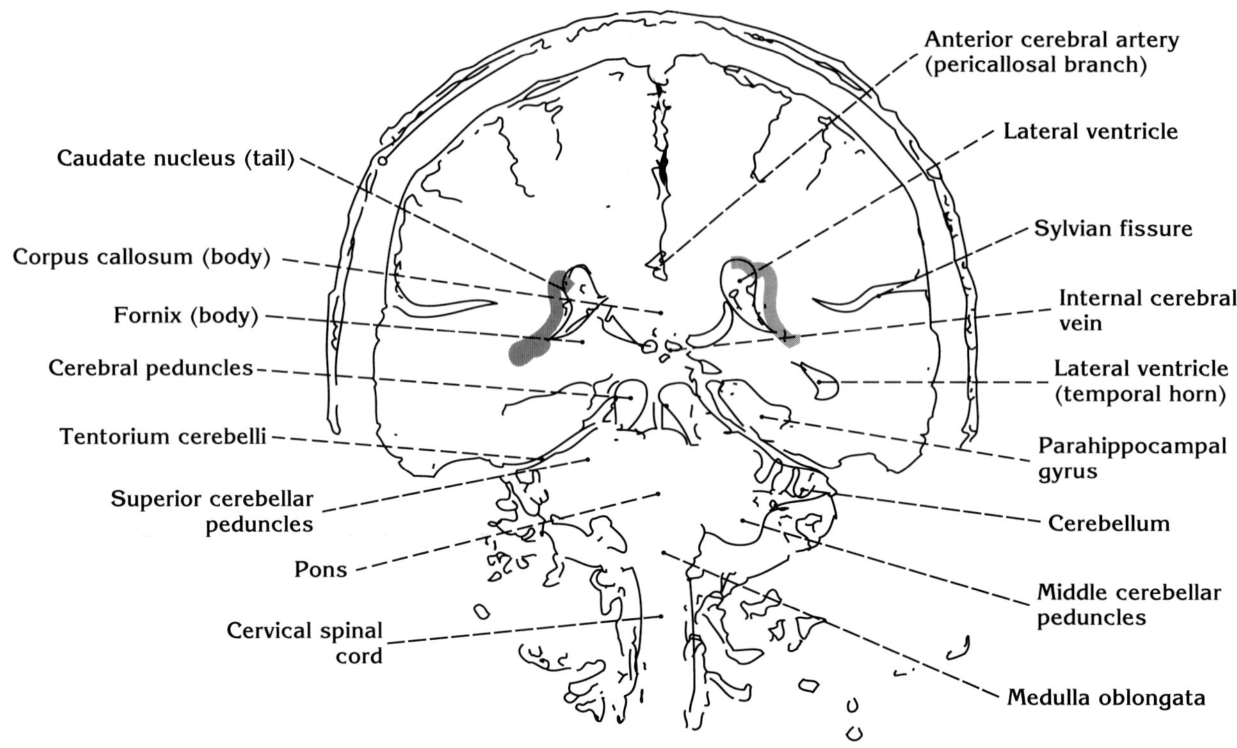

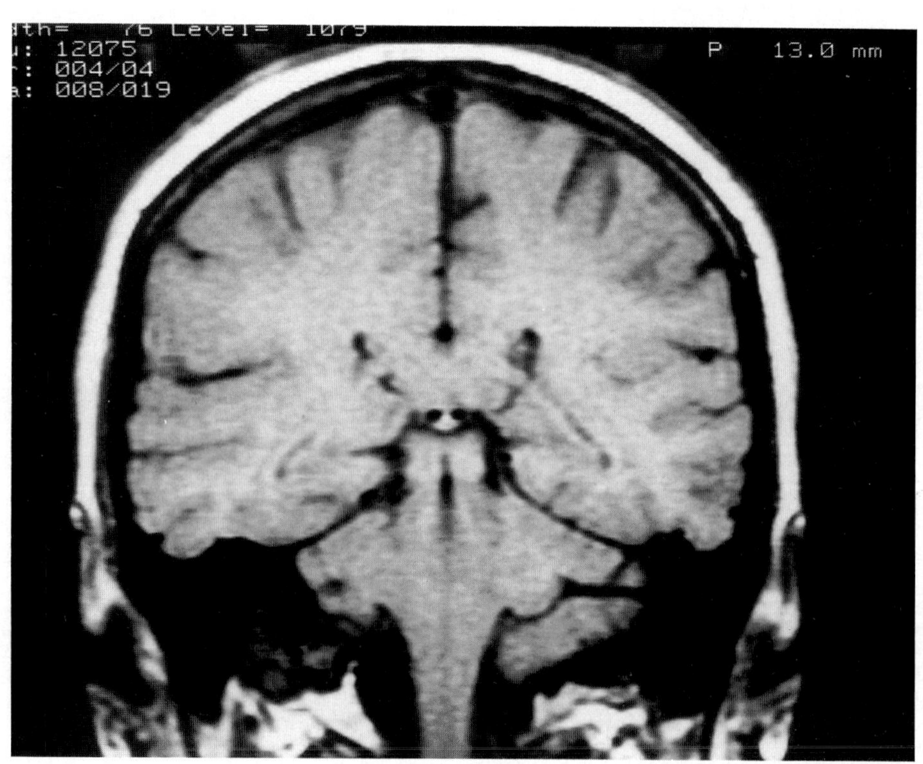

1-20c Head, coronal view (TR 800; TE 20).

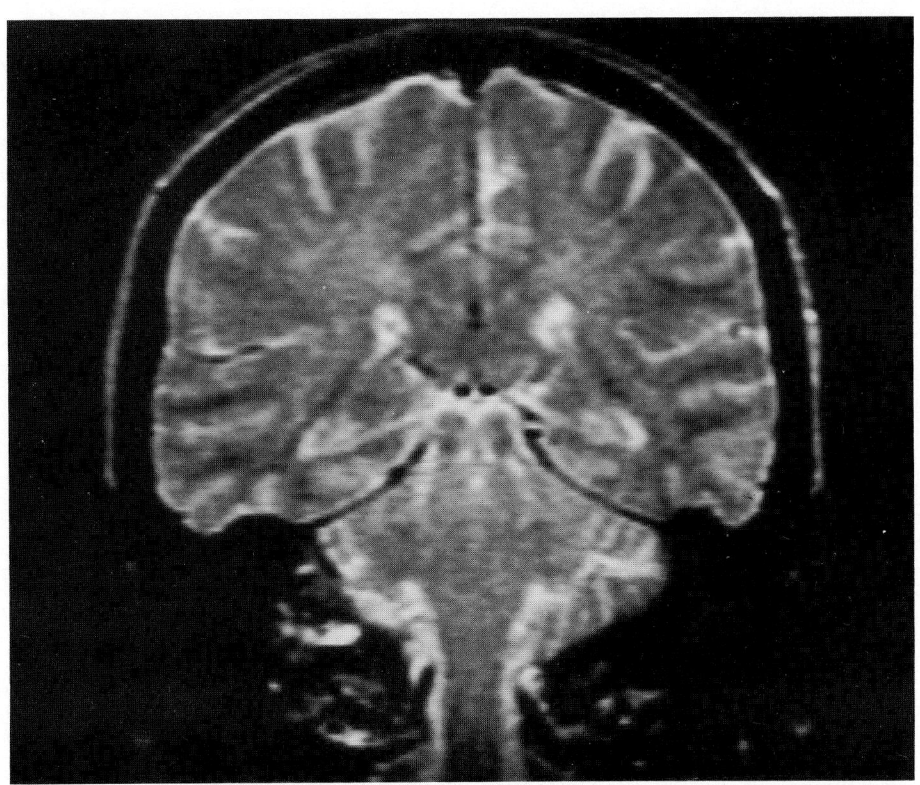

1-20a Head, coronal view (TR 2000; TE 80).

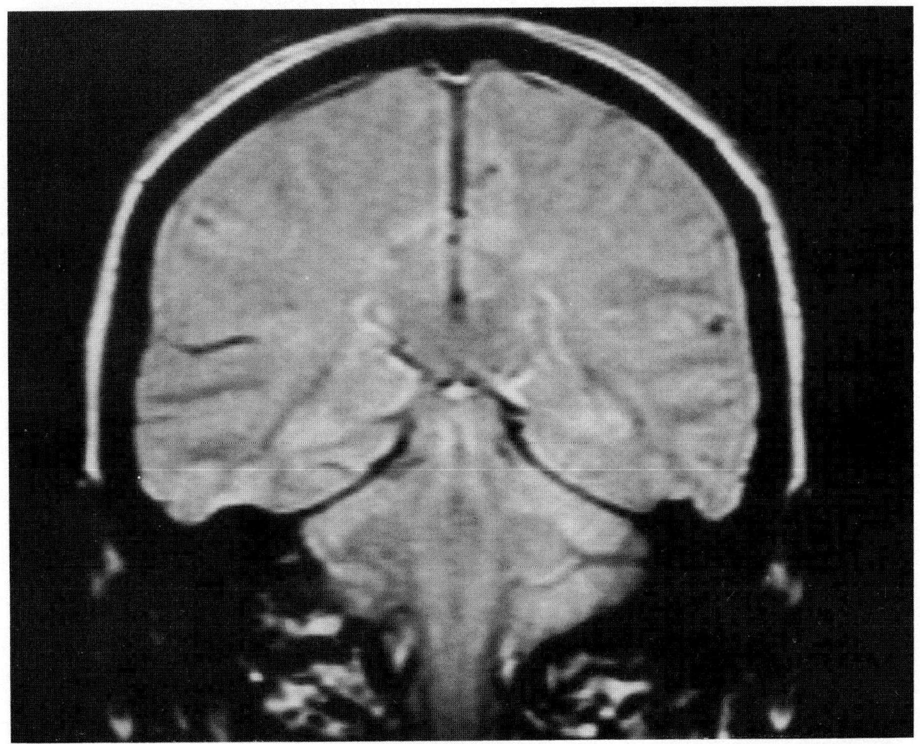

1-20b Head, coronal view (TR 2000; TE 40).

Head, Coronal

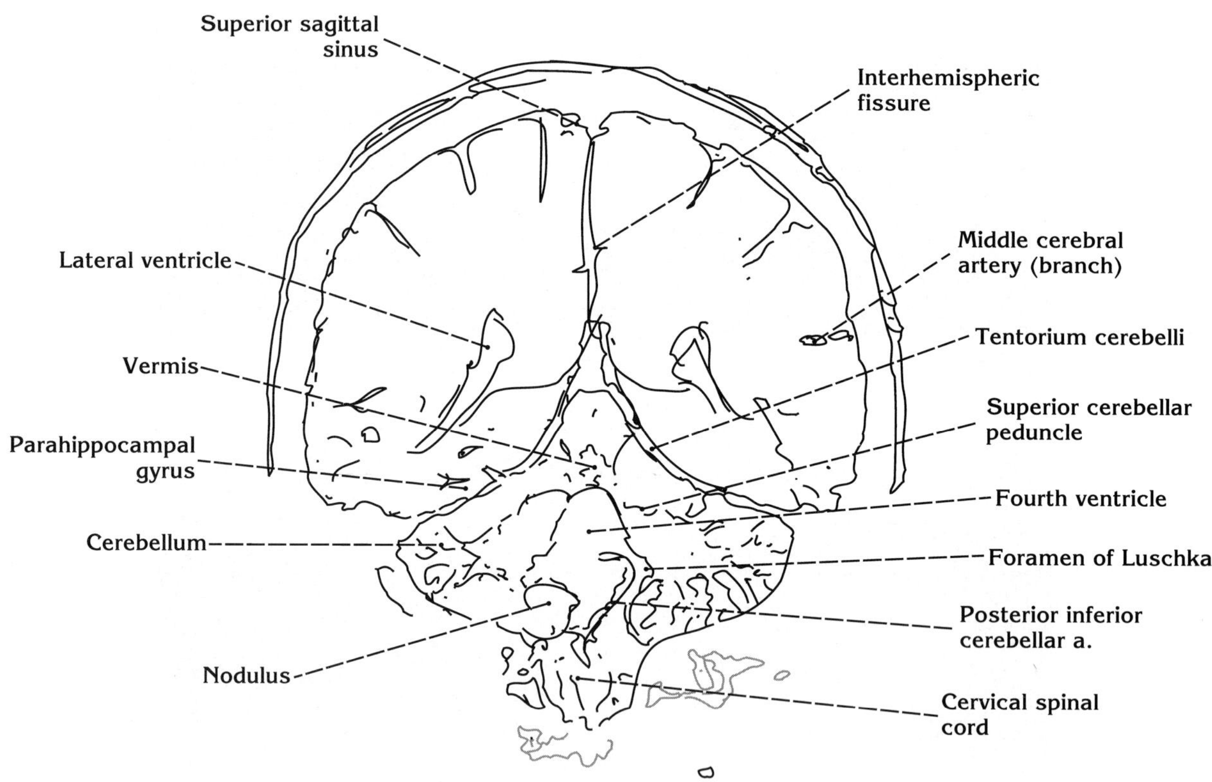

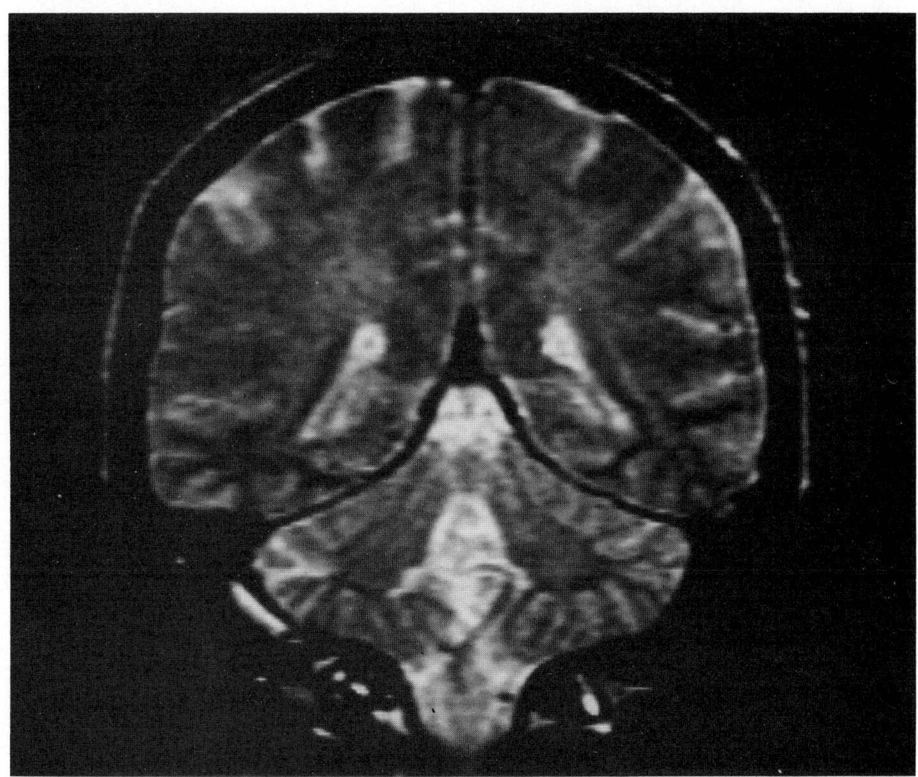

1-21a Head, coronal view (TR 2000; TE 40).

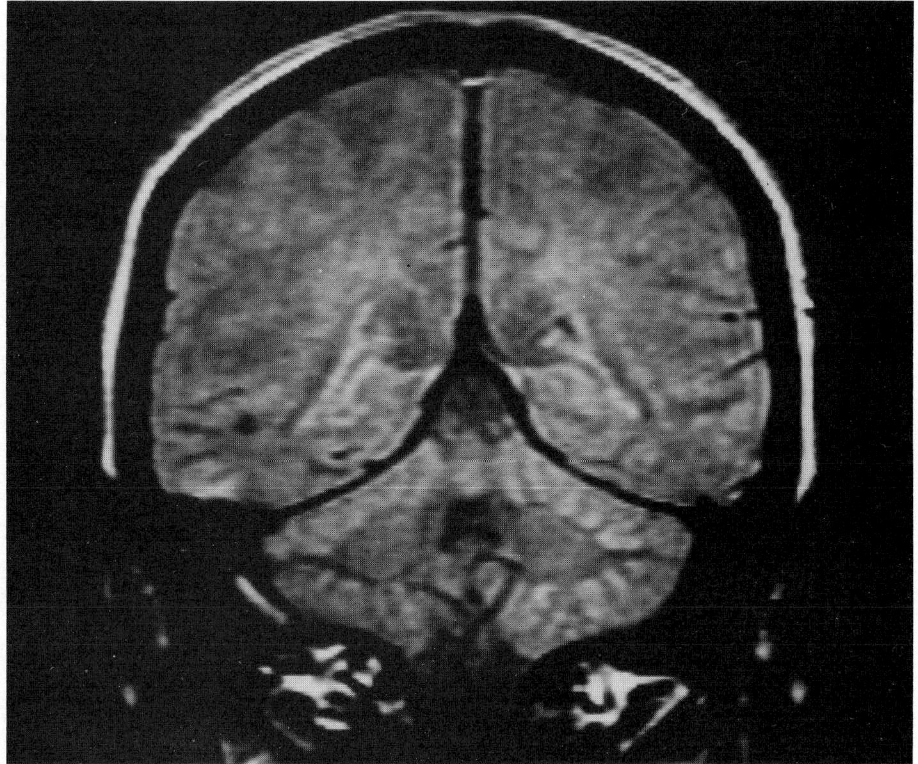

1-21b Head, coronal view (TR 2000; TE 80).

Head, Coronal

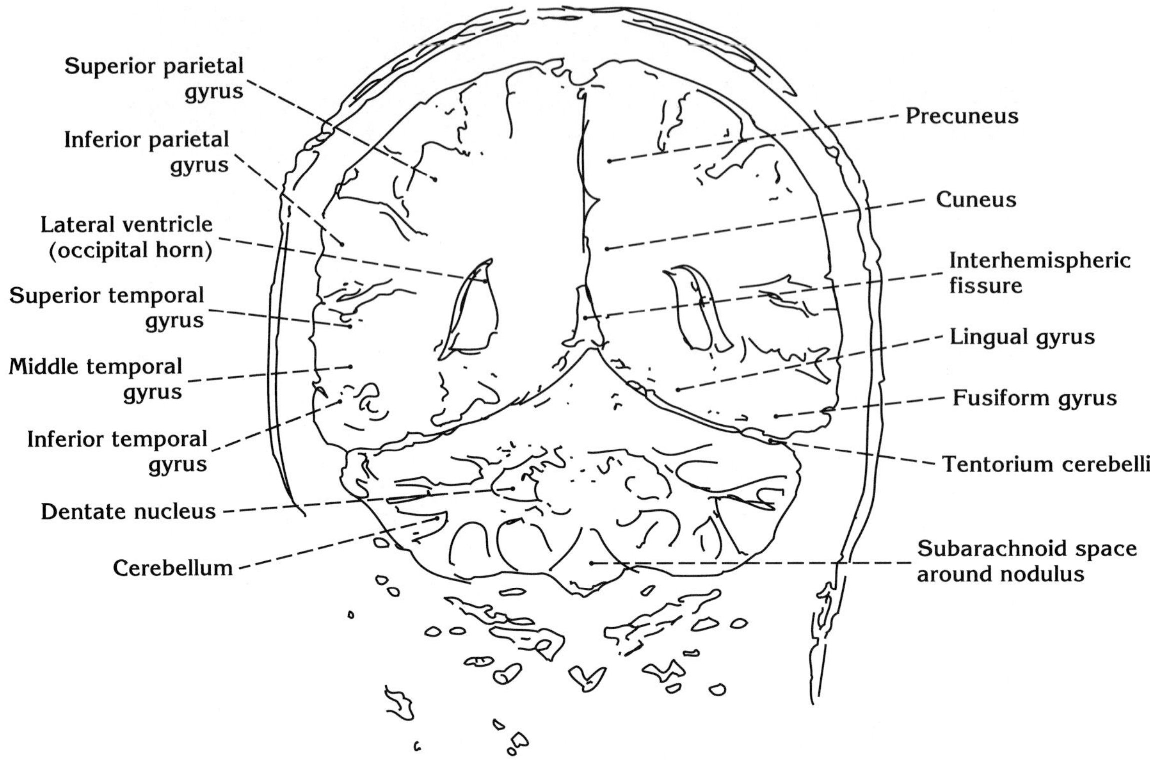

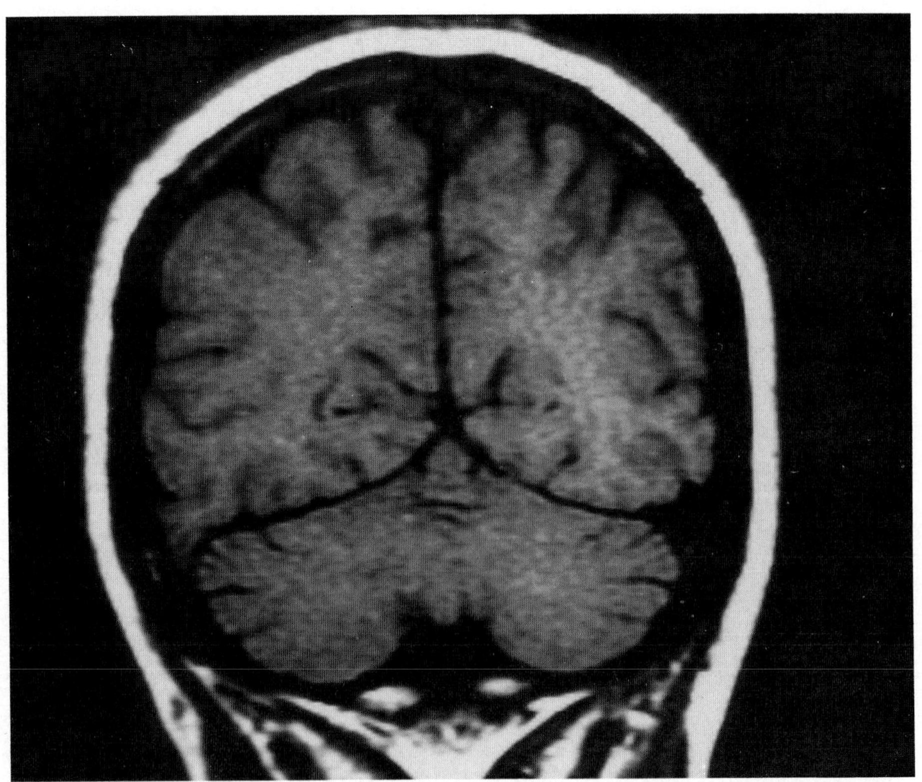

1-22c Head, coronal view (TR 800; TE 20).

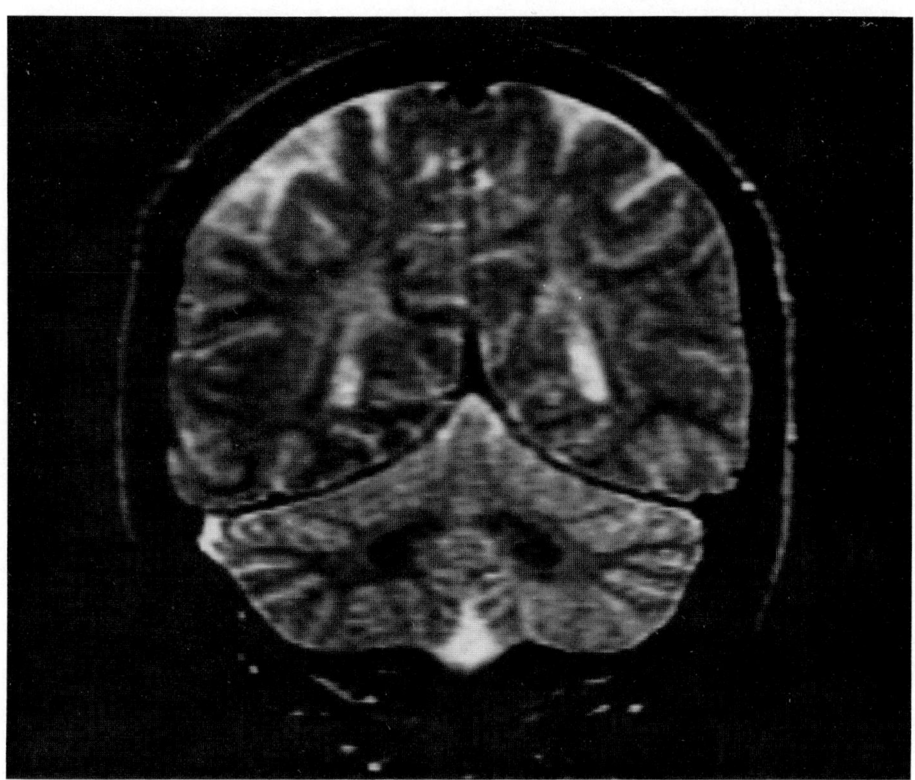

1-22a Head, coronal view (TR 2000; TE 80).

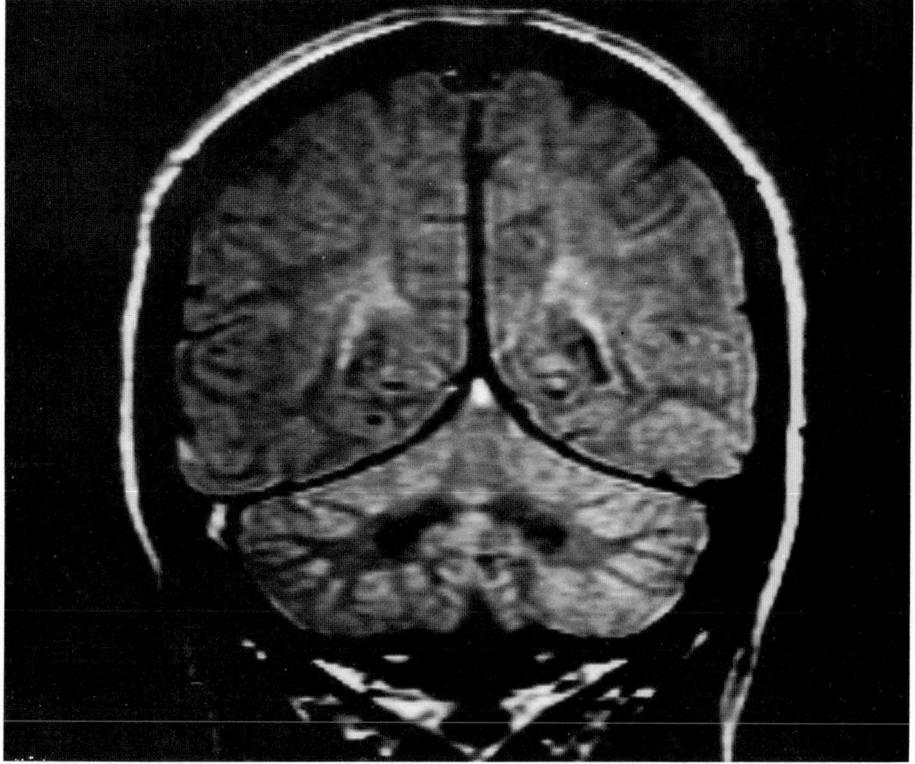

1-22b Head, coronal view (TR 2000; TE 40).

Head, Coronal

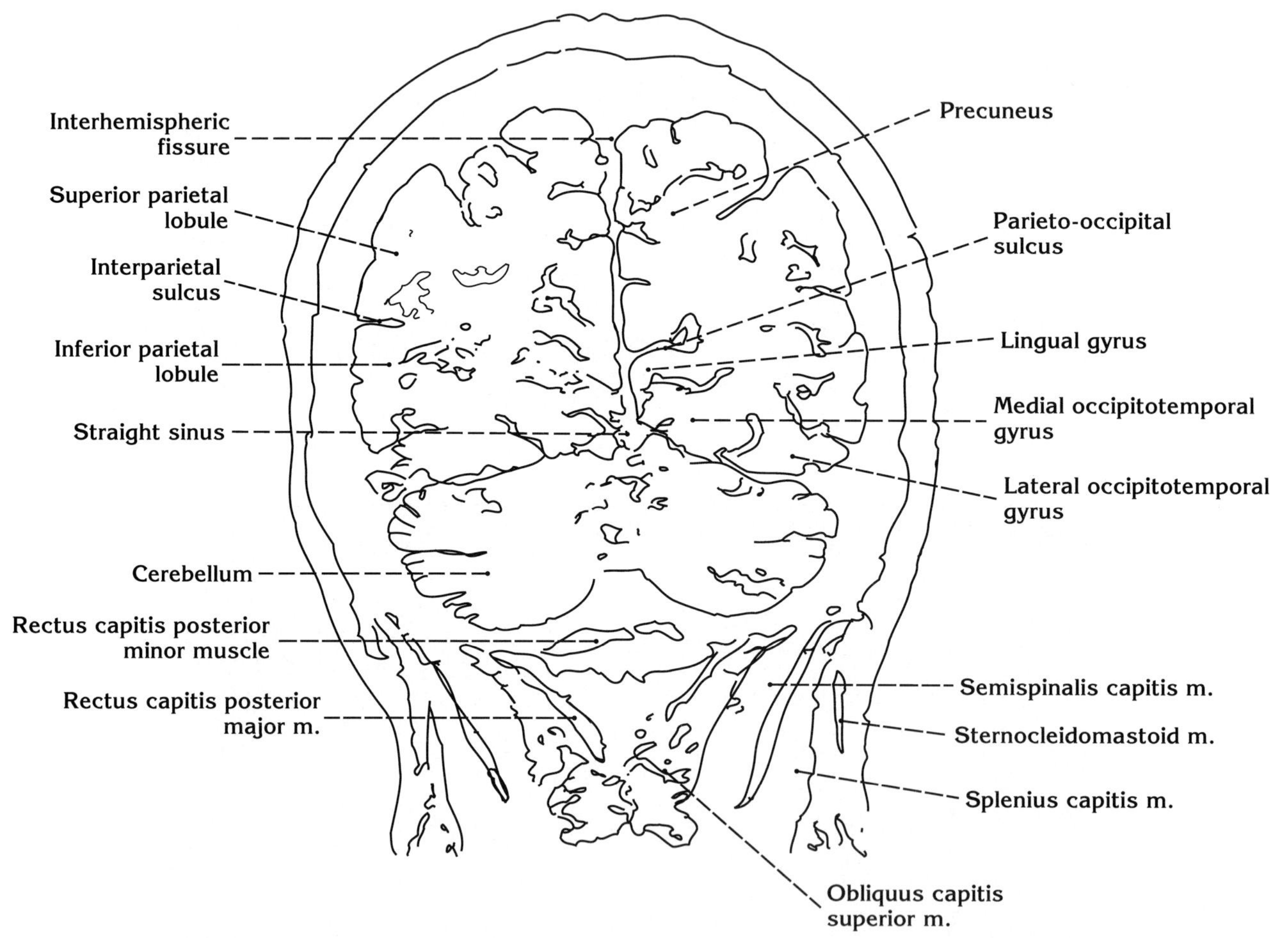

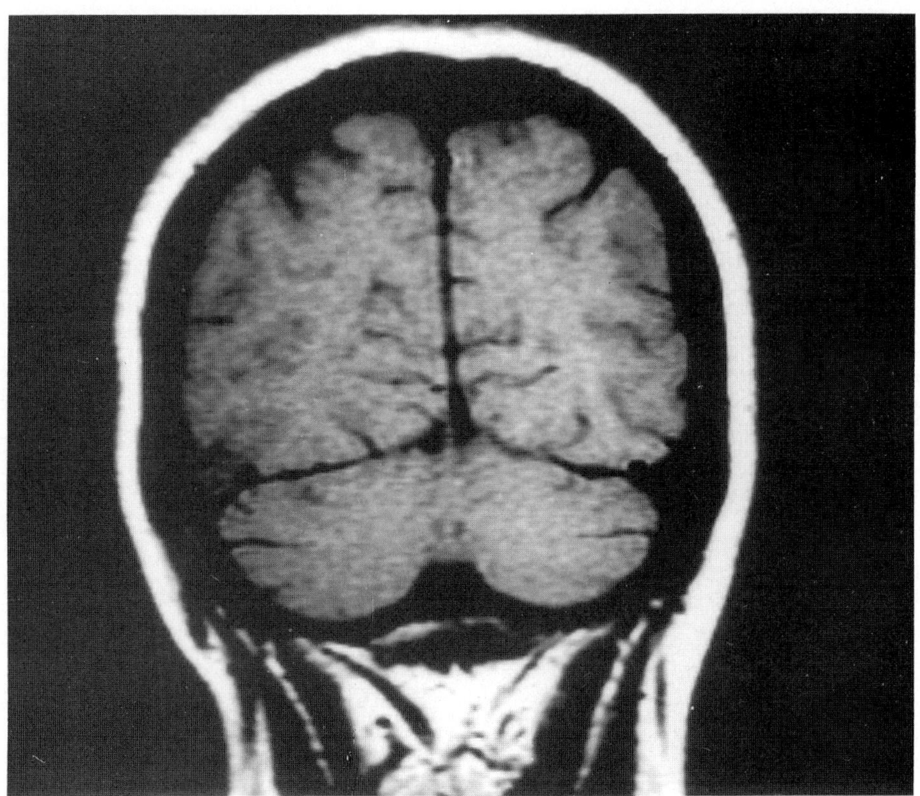

1-23a Head, coronal view (TR 800; TE 20).

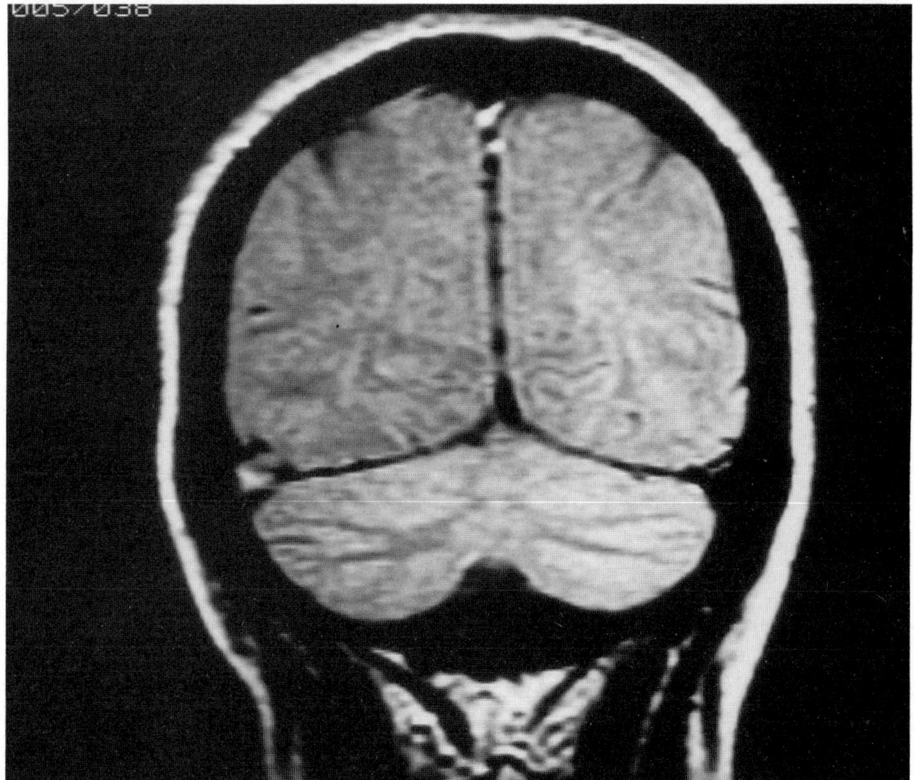

1-23b Head, coronal view (TR 2000; TE 40).

Head, Coronal

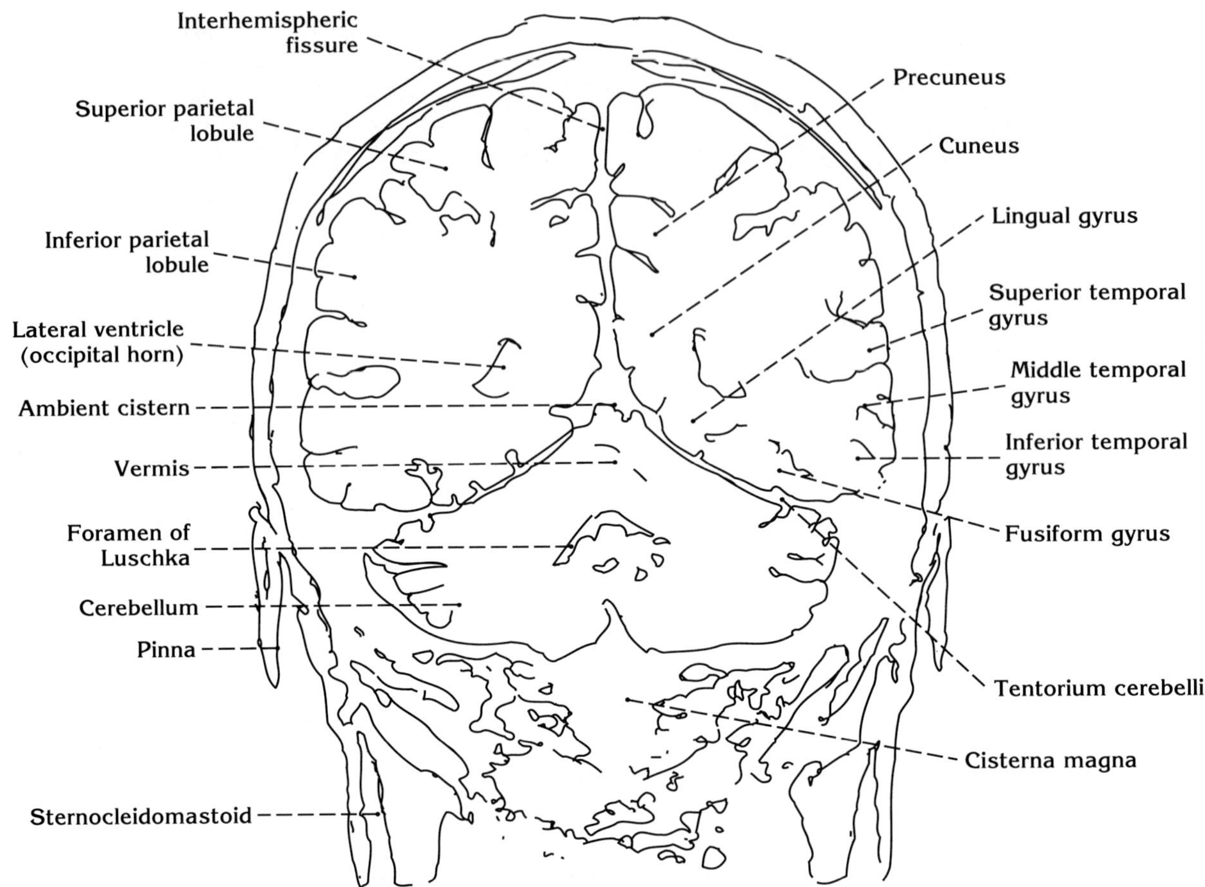

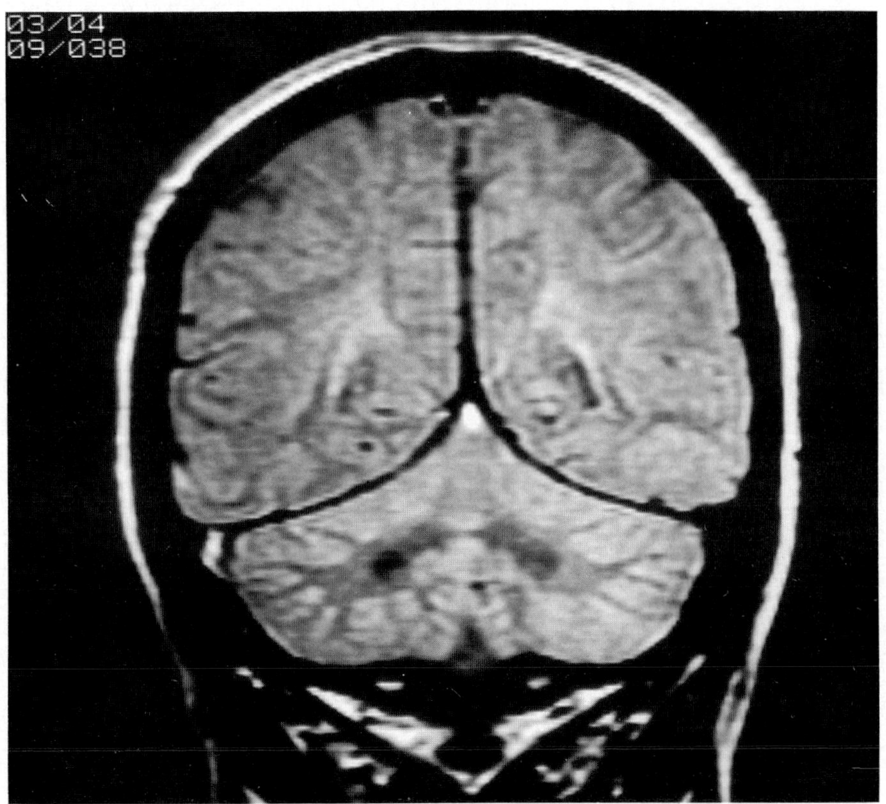

1-24c Head, coronal view (TR 2000; TE 40).

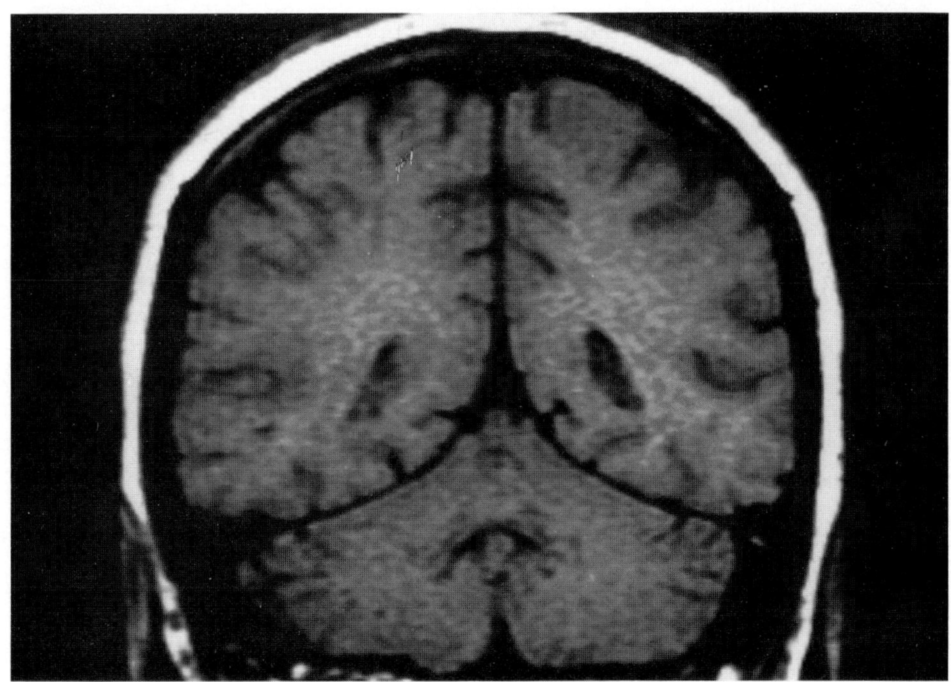

1-24a Head, coronal view (TR 800; TE 20).

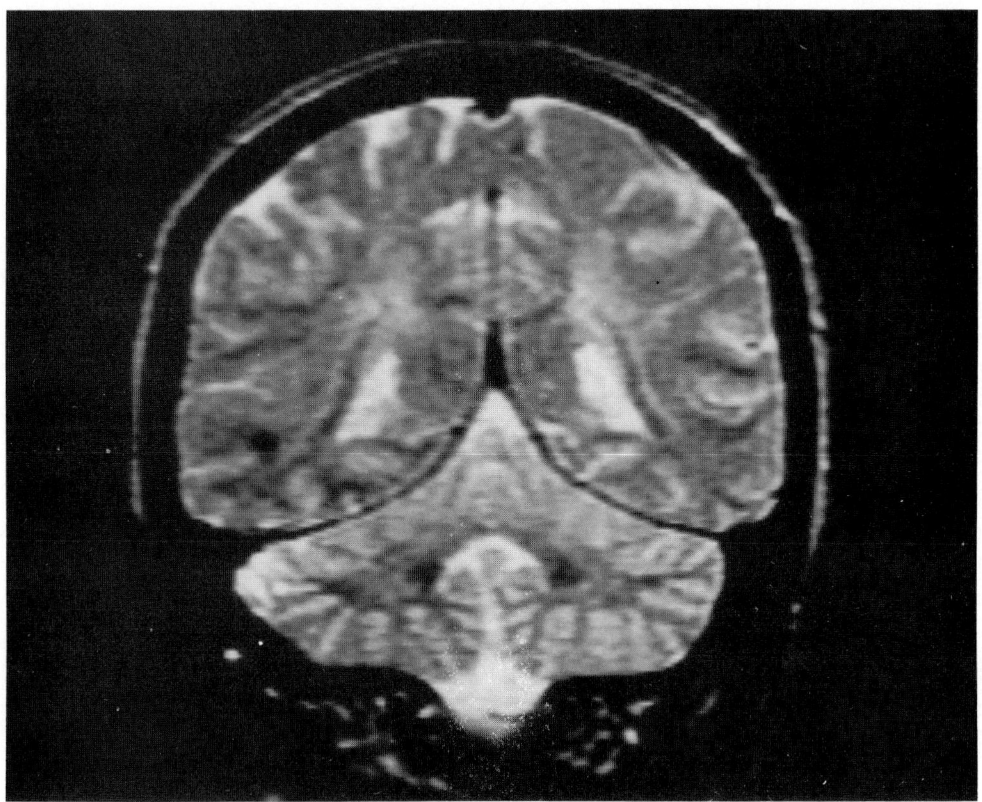

1-24b Head, coronal view (TR 2000; TE 80).

Head, Coronal

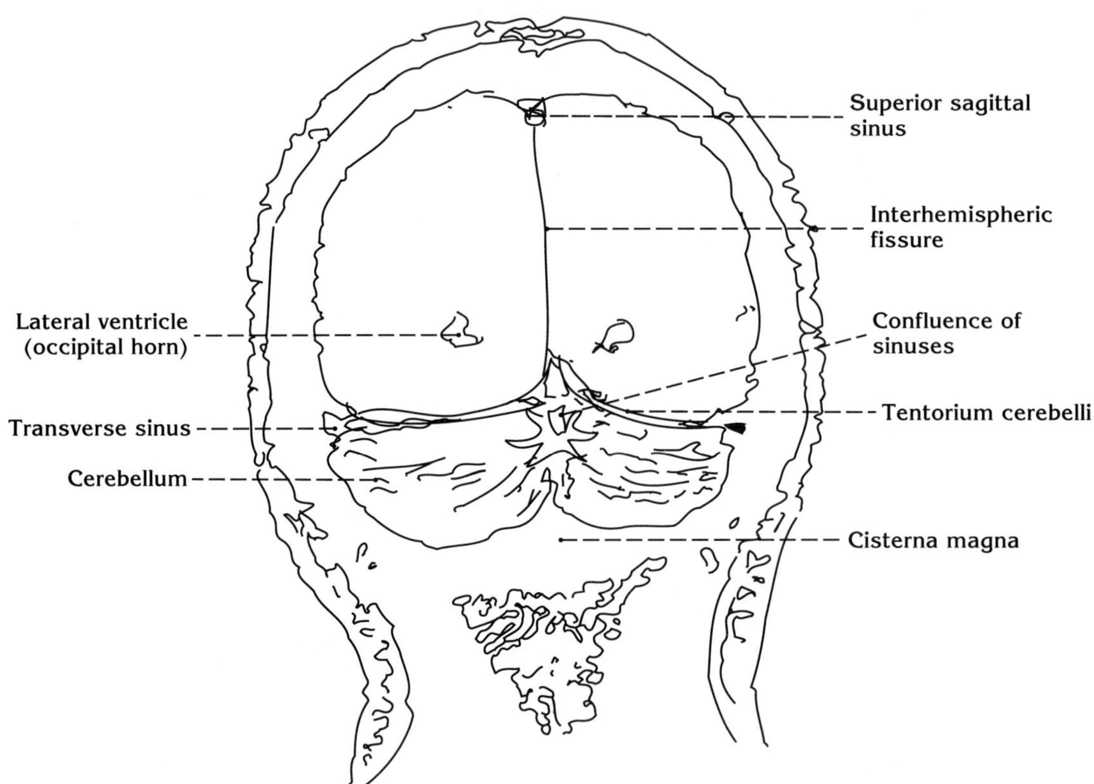

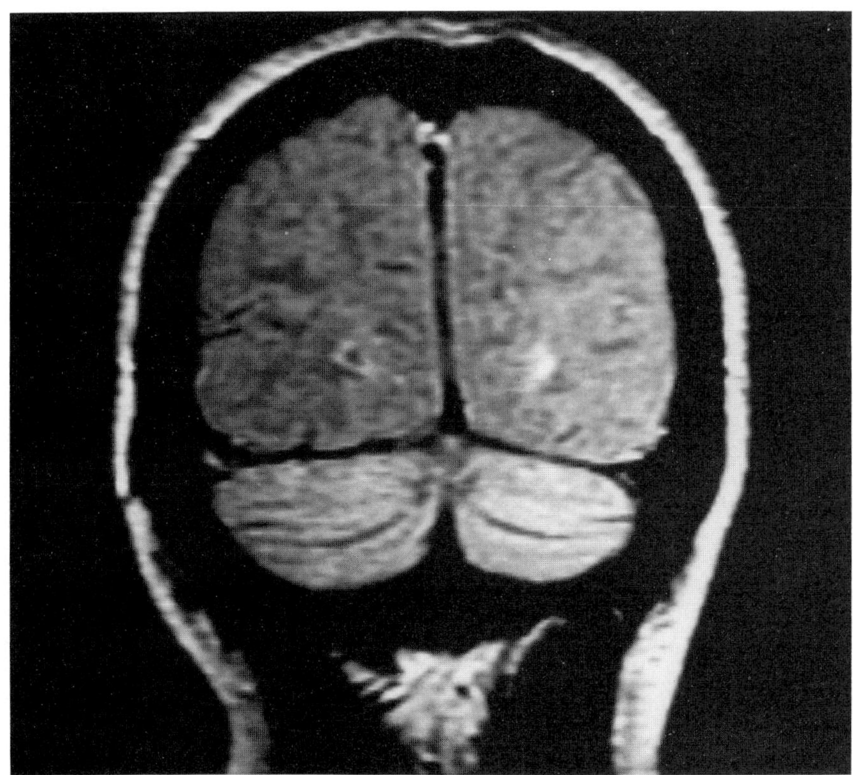

1-25a Head, coronal view (TR 2000; TE 40).

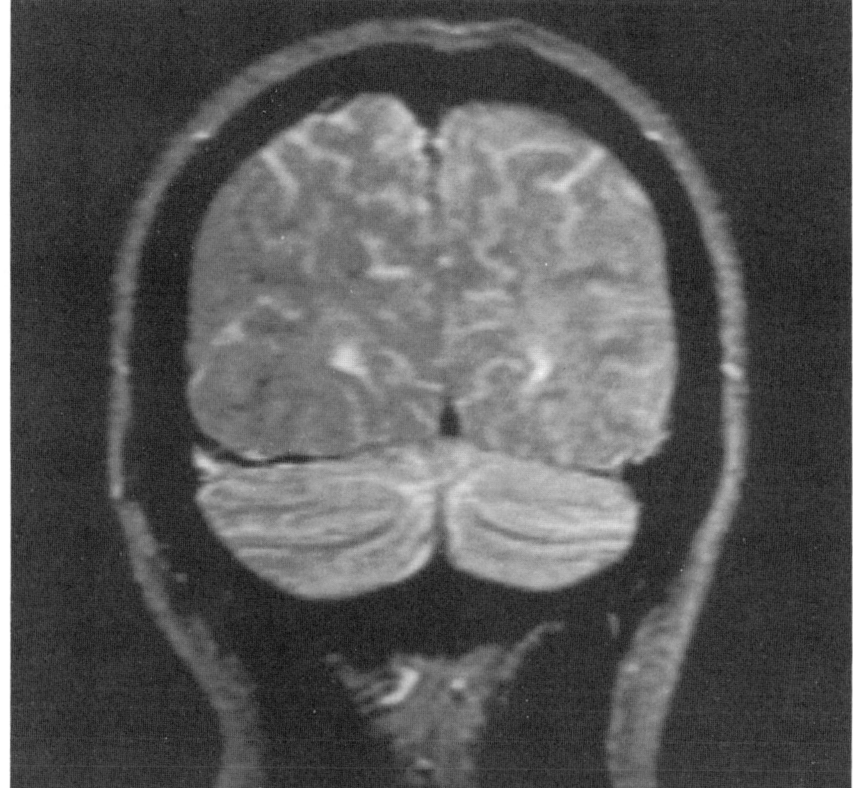

1-25b Head, coronal view (TR 2000; TE 80).

Head, Axial

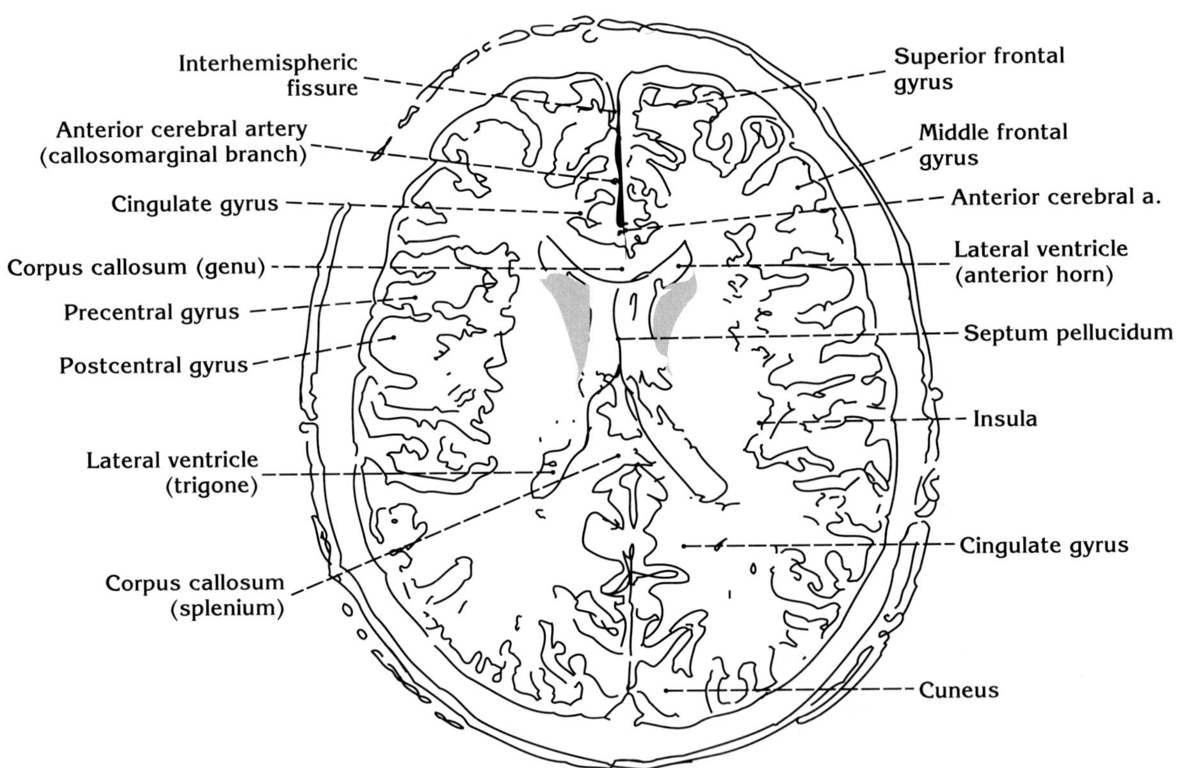
Interhemispheric fissure
Anterior cerebral artery (callosomarginal branch)
Cingulate gyrus
Corpus callosum (genu)
Precentral gyrus
Postcentral gyrus
Lateral ventricle (trigone)
Corpus callosum (splenium)
Superior frontal gyrus
Middle frontal gyrus
Anterior cerebral a.
Lateral ventricle (anterior horn)
Septum pellucidum
Insula
Cingulate gyrus
Cuneus

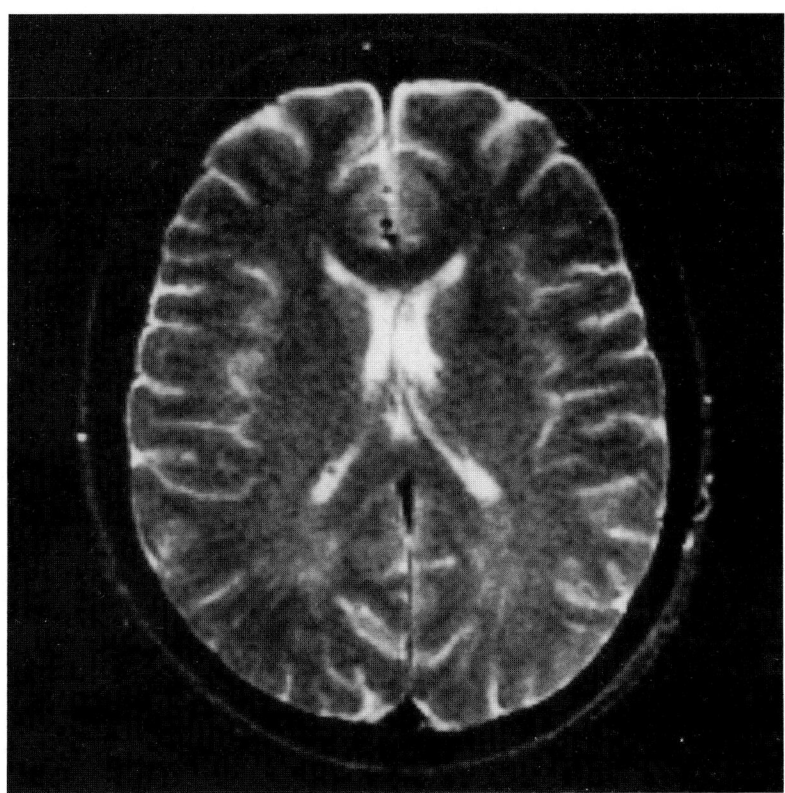

1-26a Head, coronal view (TR 2000; TE 90).

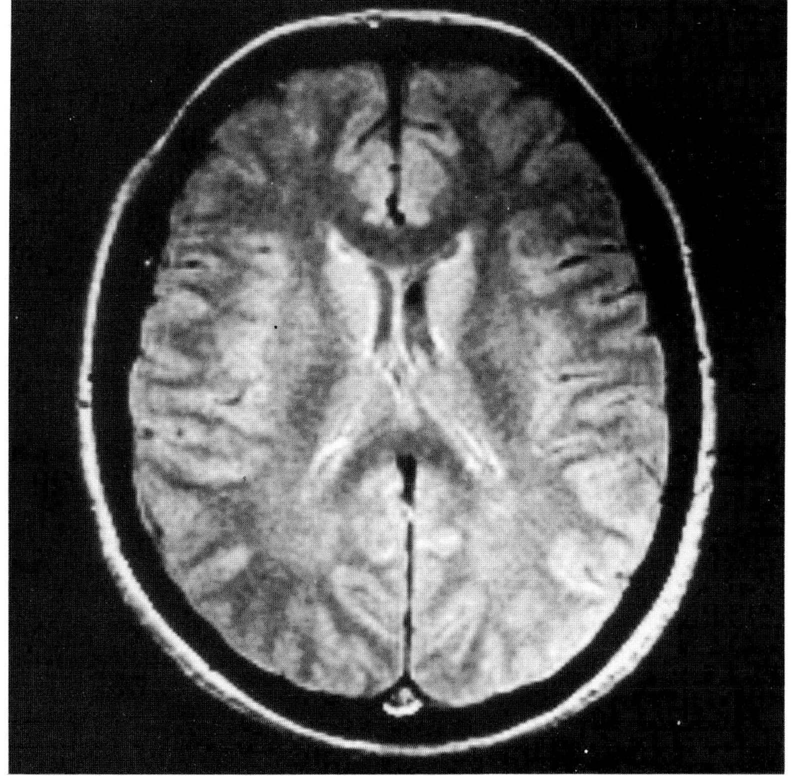

1-26b Head, coronal view (TR 2000; TE 30).

Head, Axial

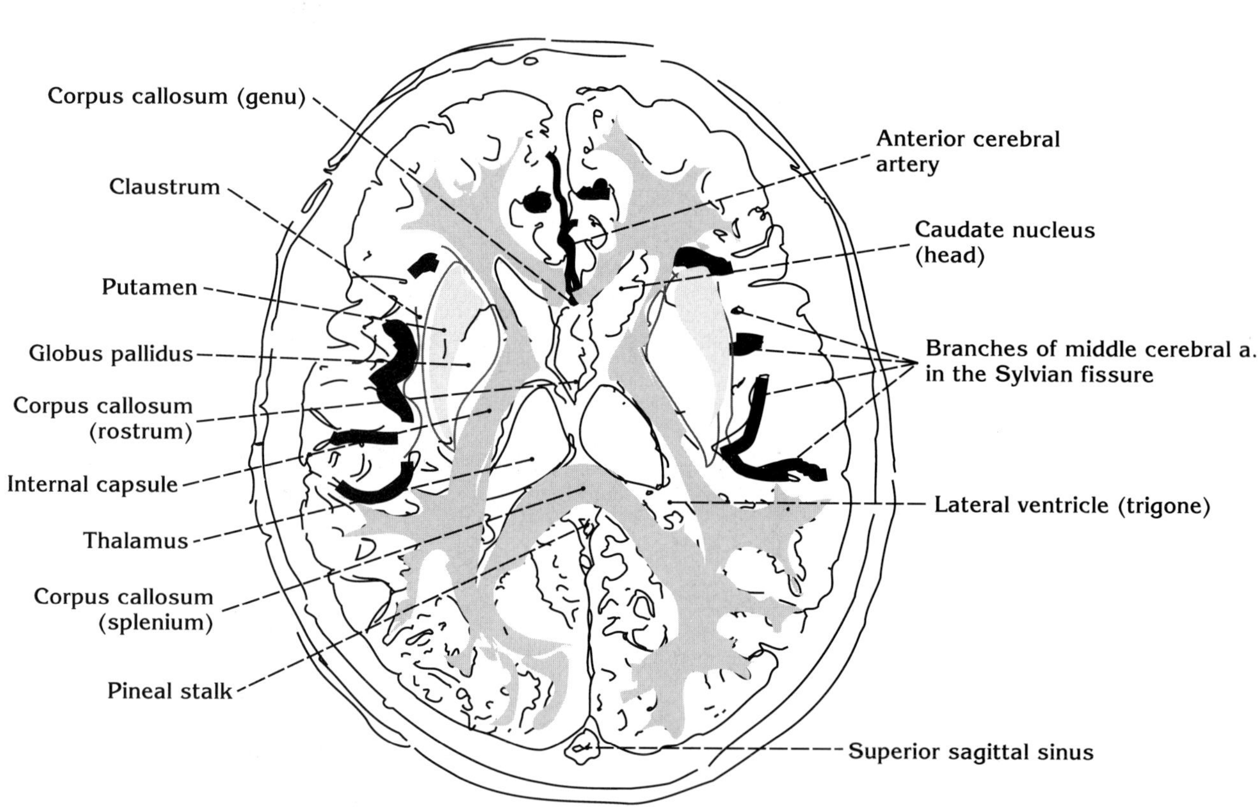
Corpus callosum (genu)
Claustrum
Putamen
Globus pallidus
Corpus callosum (rostrum)
Internal capsule
Thalamus
Corpus callosum (splenium)
Pineal stalk
Anterior cerebral artery
Caudate nucleus (head)
Branches of middle cerebral a. in the Sylvian fissure
Lateral ventricle (trigone)
Superior sagittal sinus

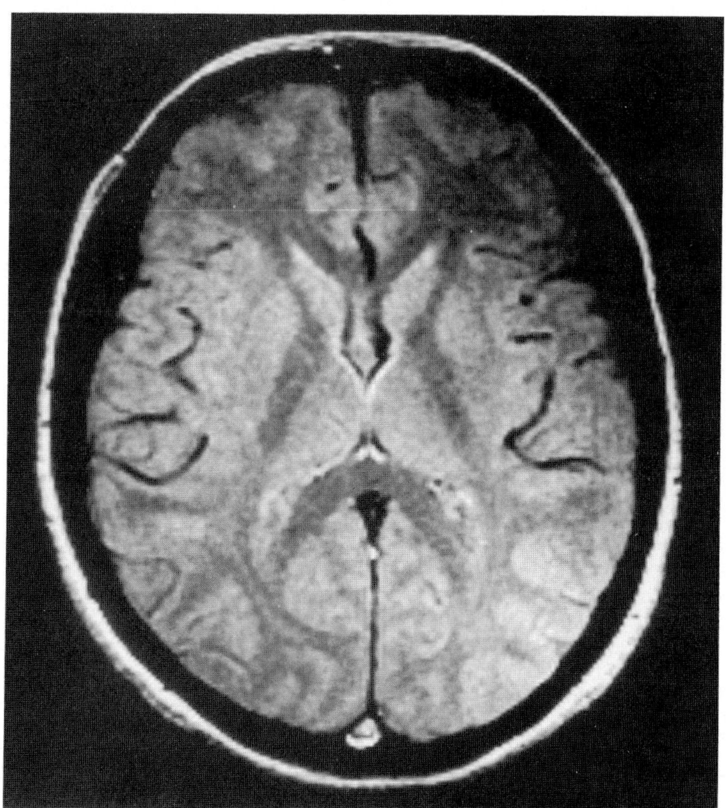

1-27a Head, axial view (TR 2000; TE 30).

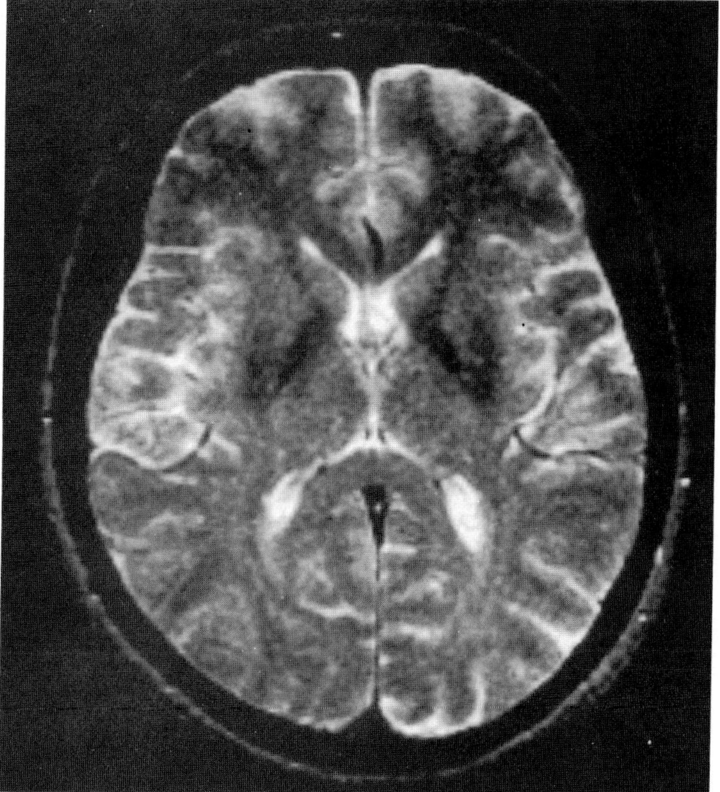

1-27b Head, axial view (TR 2000; TE 90).

Head, Axial

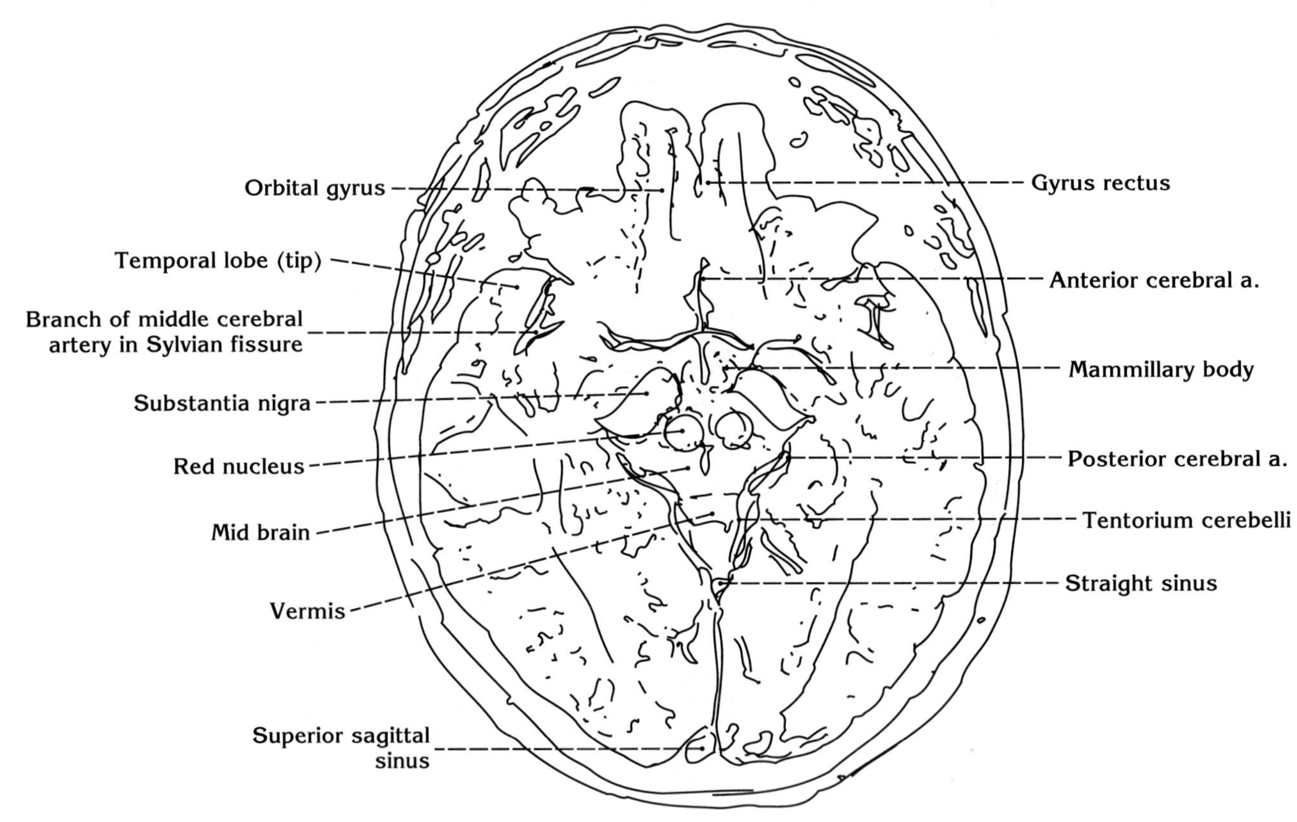
Orbital gyrus
Temporal lobe (tip)
Branch of middle cerebral artery in Sylvian fissure
Substantia nigra
Red nucleus
Mid brain
Vermis
Superior sagittal sinus
Gyrus rectus
Anterior cerebral a.
Mammillary body
Posterior cerebral a.
Tentorium cerebelli
Straight sinus

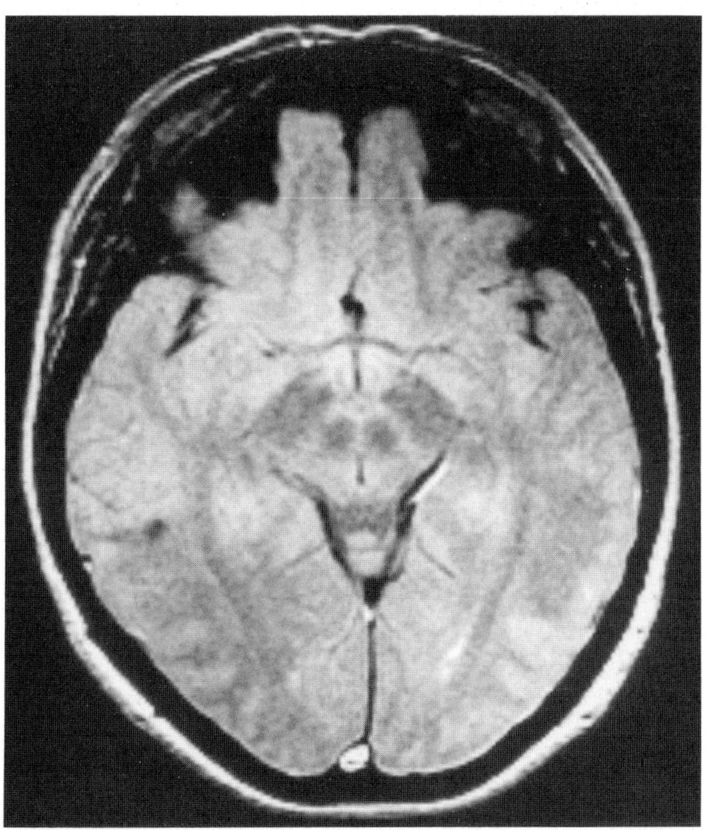

1-28a Head, axial view (TR 2000; TE 30).

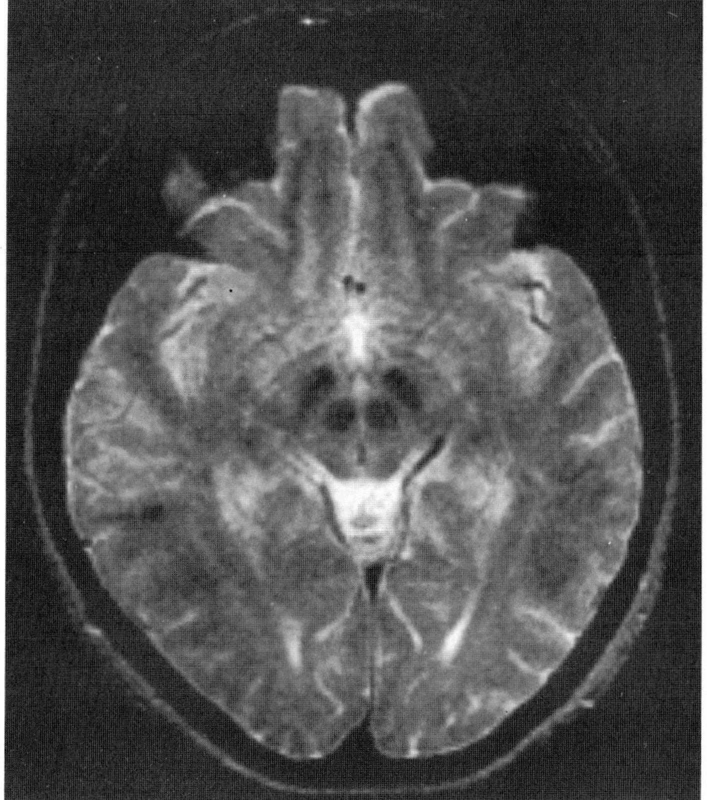

1-28b Head, axial view (TR 2000; TE 90).

Head, Axial

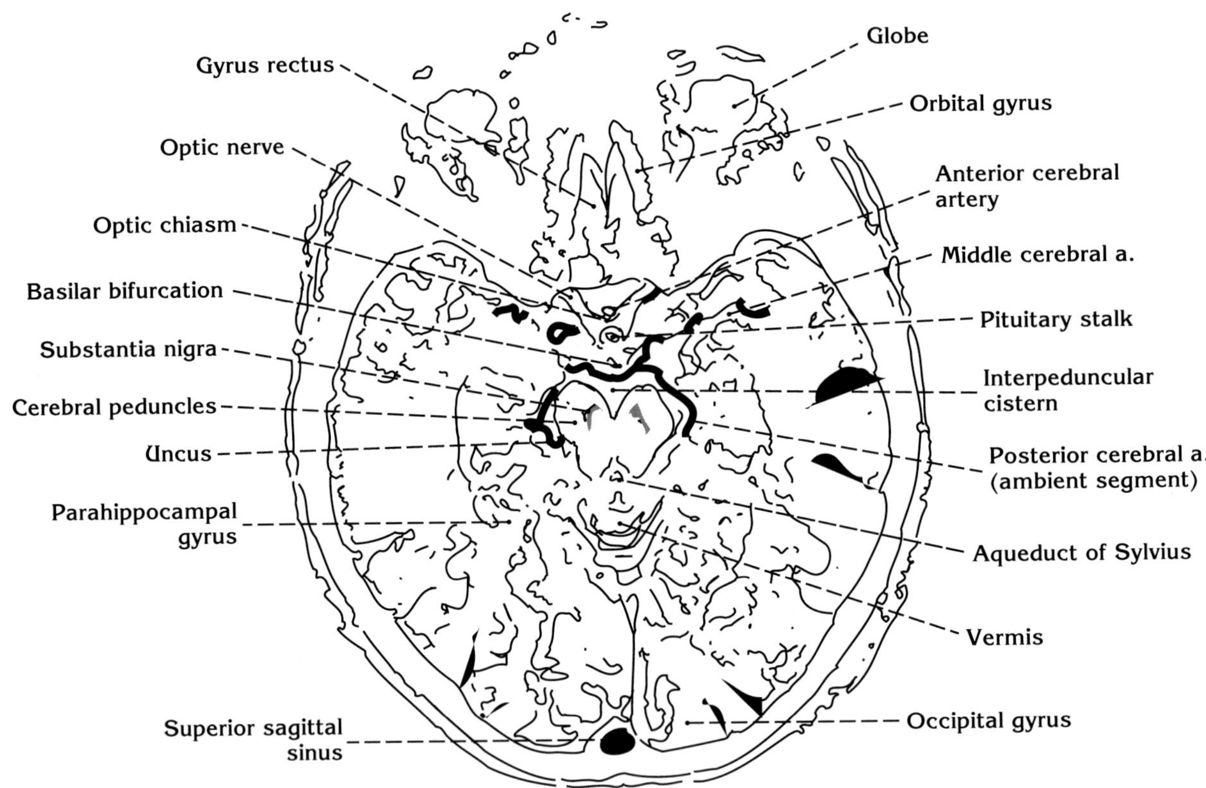
Gyrus rectus
Optic nerve
Optic chiasm
Basilar bifurcation
Substantia nigra
Cerebral peduncles
Uncus
Parahippocampal gyrus
Superior sagittal sinus
Globe
Orbital gyrus
Anterior cerebral artery
Middle cerebral a.
Pituitary stalk
Interpeduncular cistern
Posterior cerebral a. (ambient segment)
Aqueduct of Sylvius
Vermis
Occipital gyrus

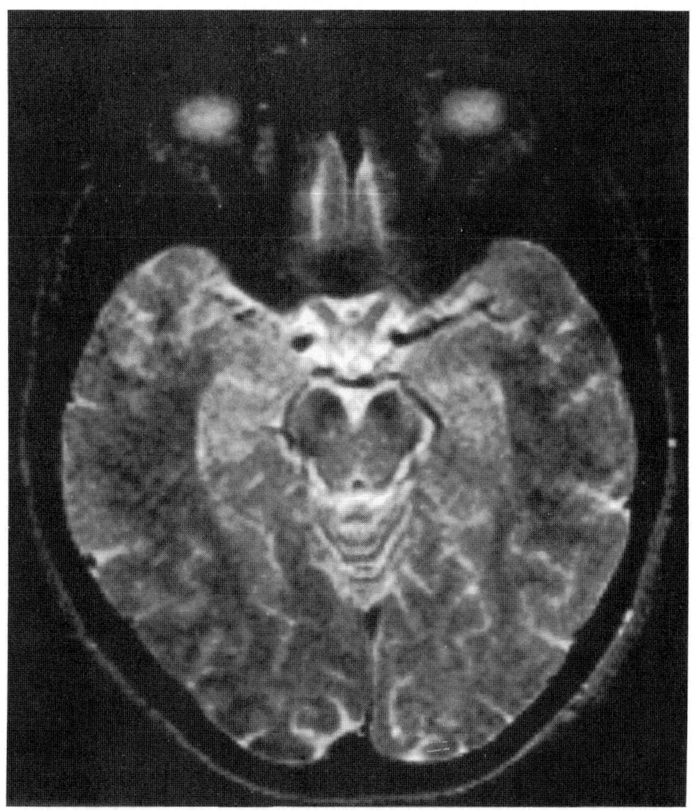

1-29a Head, axial view (TR 2000; TE 90).

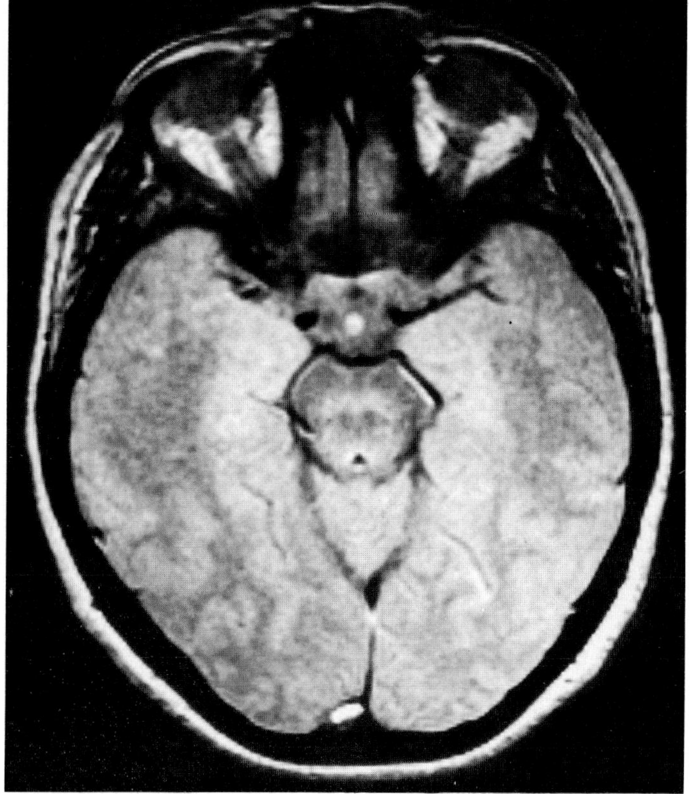

1-29b Head, axial view (TR 2000; TE 30).

Head, Axial

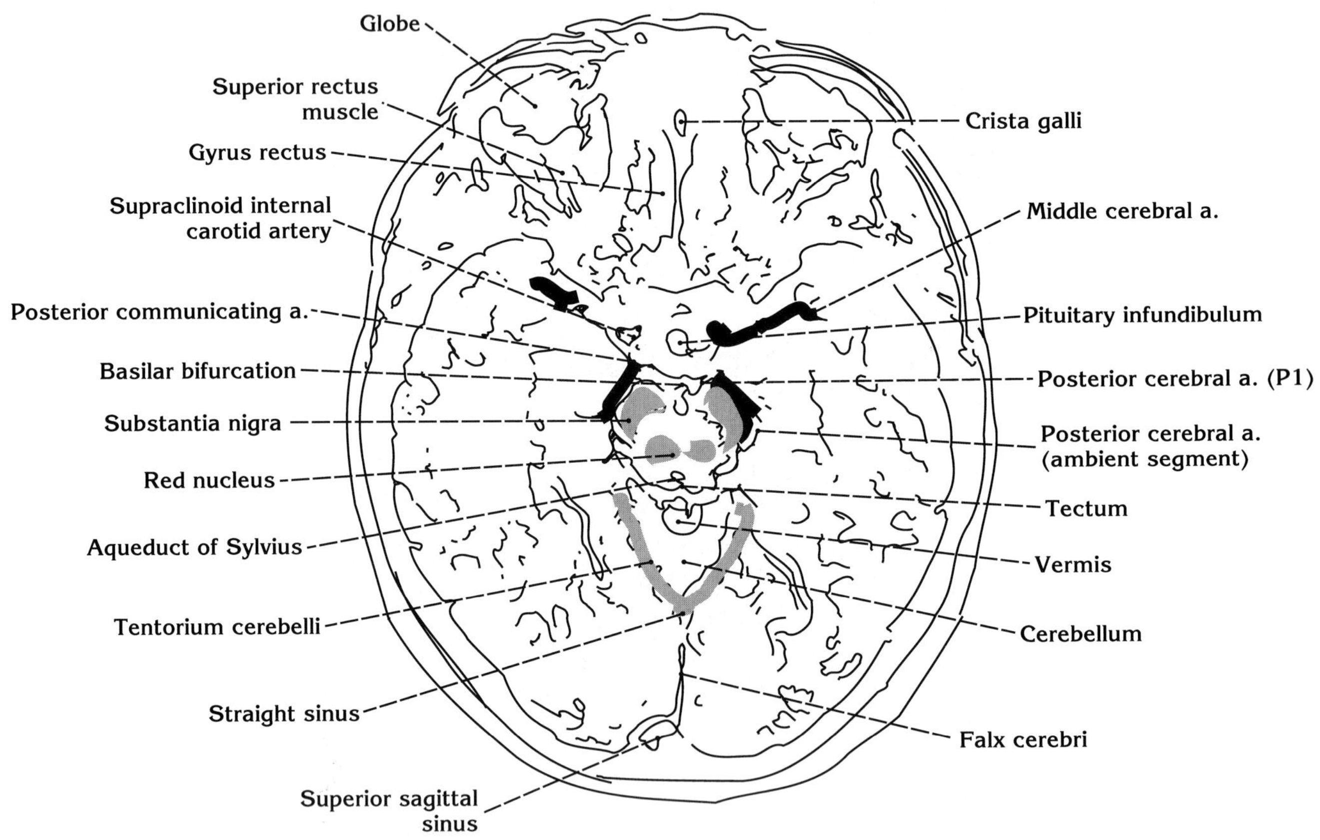
Globe
Superior rectus muscle
Gyrus rectus
Supraclinoid internal carotid artery
Posterior communicating a.
Basilar bifurcation
Substantia nigra
Red nucleus
Aqueduct of Sylvius
Tentorium cerebelli
Straight sinus
Superior sagittal sinus
Crista galli
Middle cerebral a.
Pituitary infundibulum
Posterior cerebral a. (P1)
Posterior cerebral a. (ambient segment)
Tectum
Vermis
Cerebellum
Falx cerebri

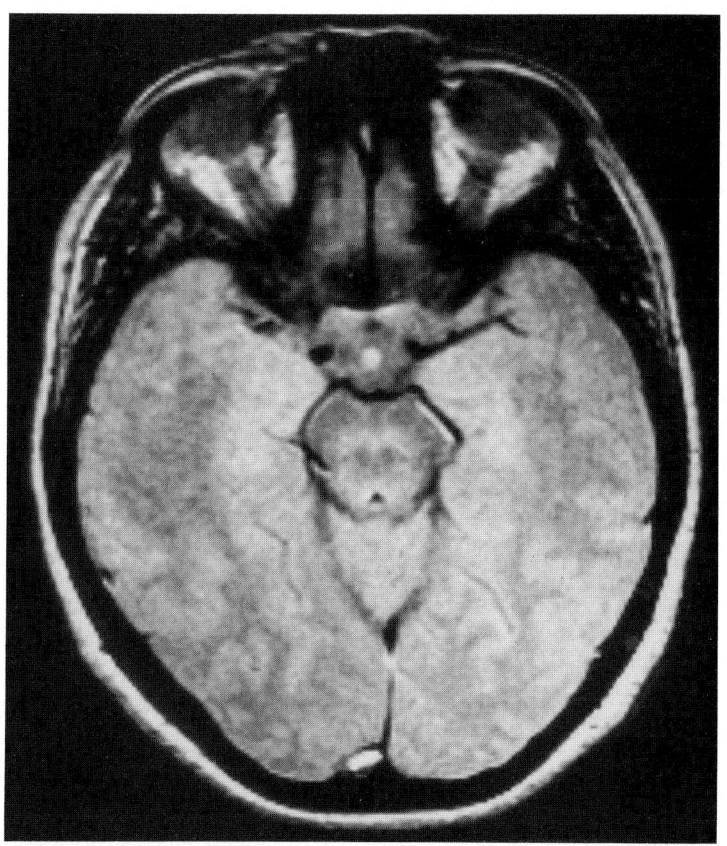

1-30a Head, axial view (TR 2000; TE 30).

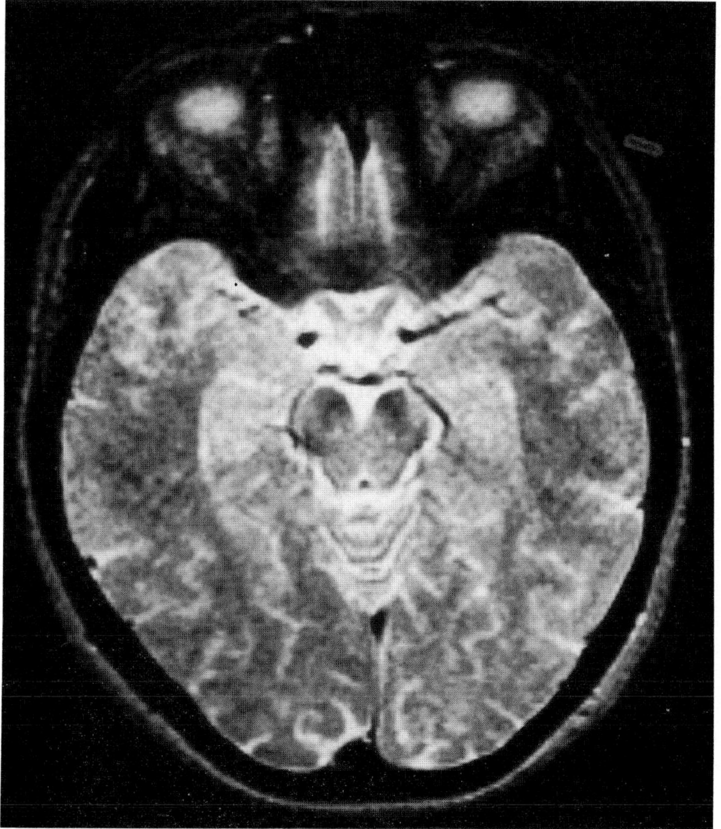

1-30b Head, axial view (TR 2000; TE 90).

Head, Axial

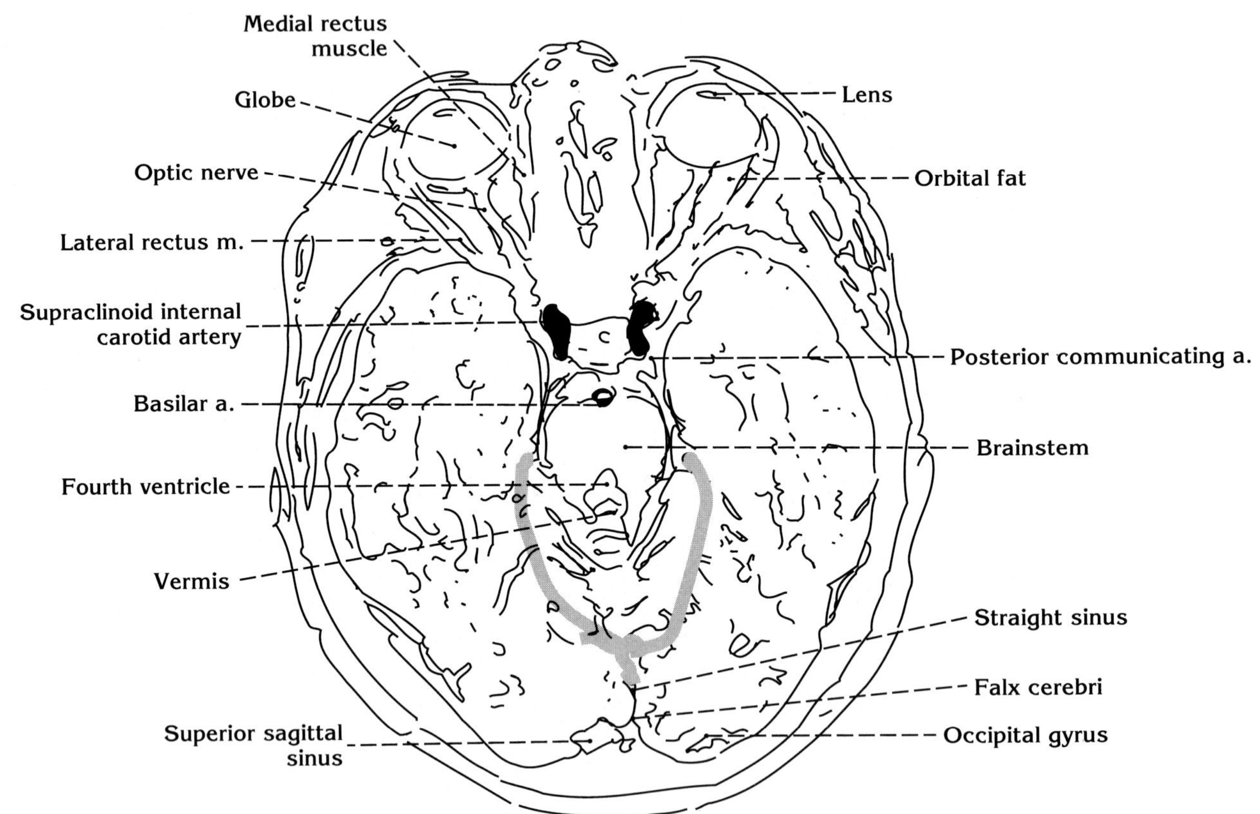
Medial rectus muscle
Globe
Optic nerve
Lateral rectus m.
Supraclinoid internal carotid artery
Basilar a.
Fourth ventricle
Vermis
Superior sagittal sinus
Lens
Orbital fat
Posterior communicating a.
Brainstem
Straight sinus
Falx cerebri
Occipital gyrus

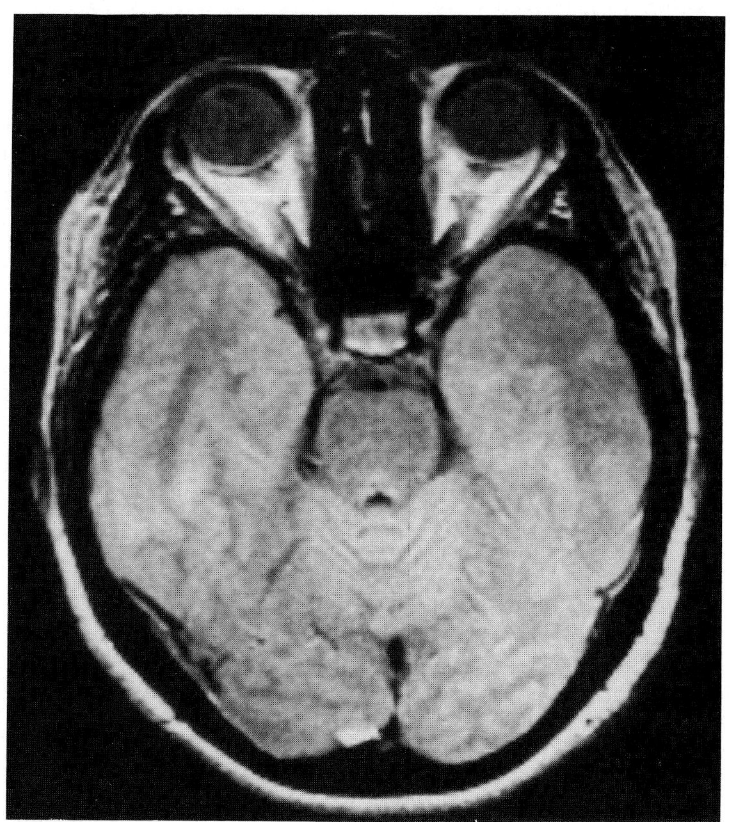

1-31a Head, axial view (TR 2000; TE 30).

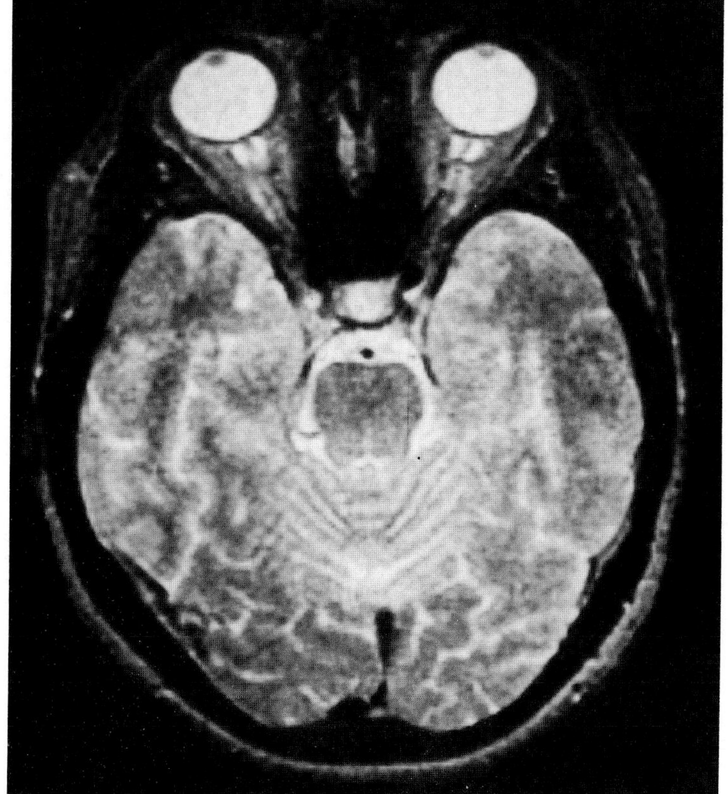

1-31b Head, axial view (TR 2000; TE 90).

Head, Axial

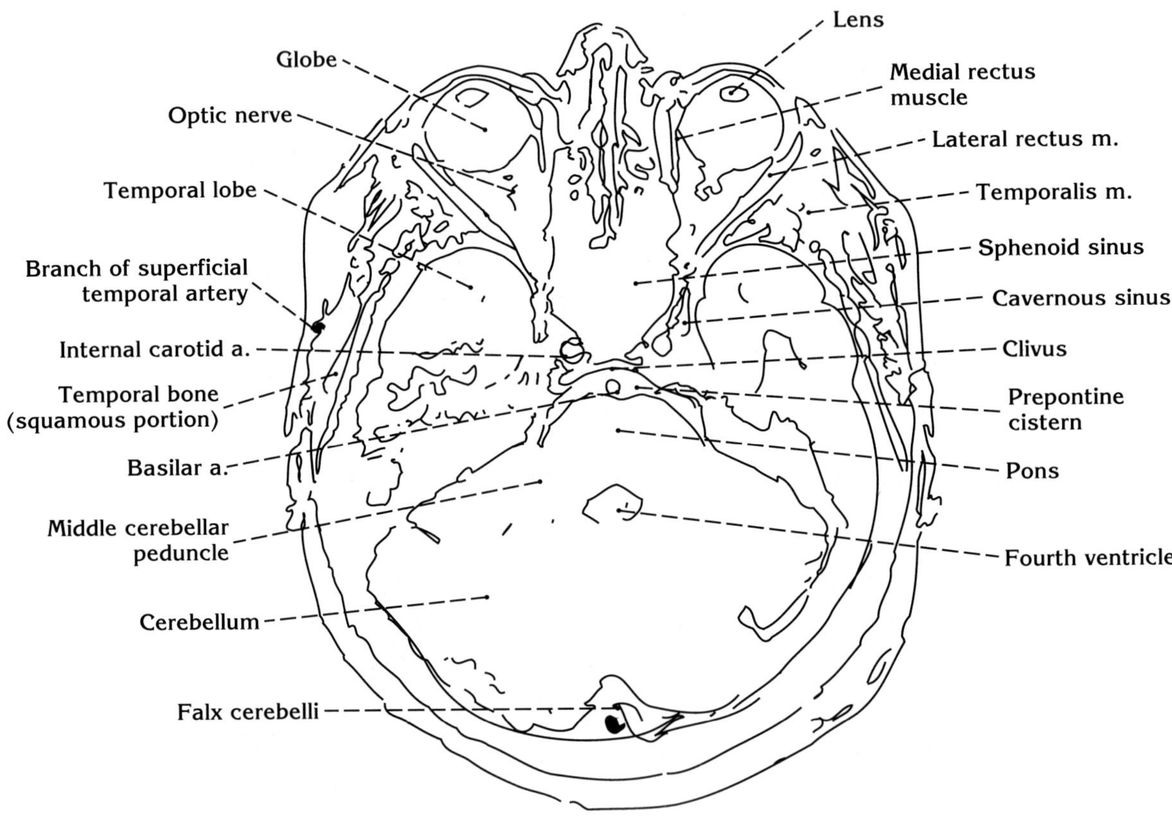
Lens
Globe
Medial rectus muscle
Optic nerve
Lateral rectus m.
Temporal lobe
Temporalis m.
Sphenoid sinus
Branch of superficial temporal artery
Cavernous sinus
Internal carotid a.
Clivus
Temporal bone (squamous portion)
Prepontine cistern
Basilar a.
Pons
Middle cerebellar peduncle
Fourth ventricle
Cerebellum
Falx cerebelli

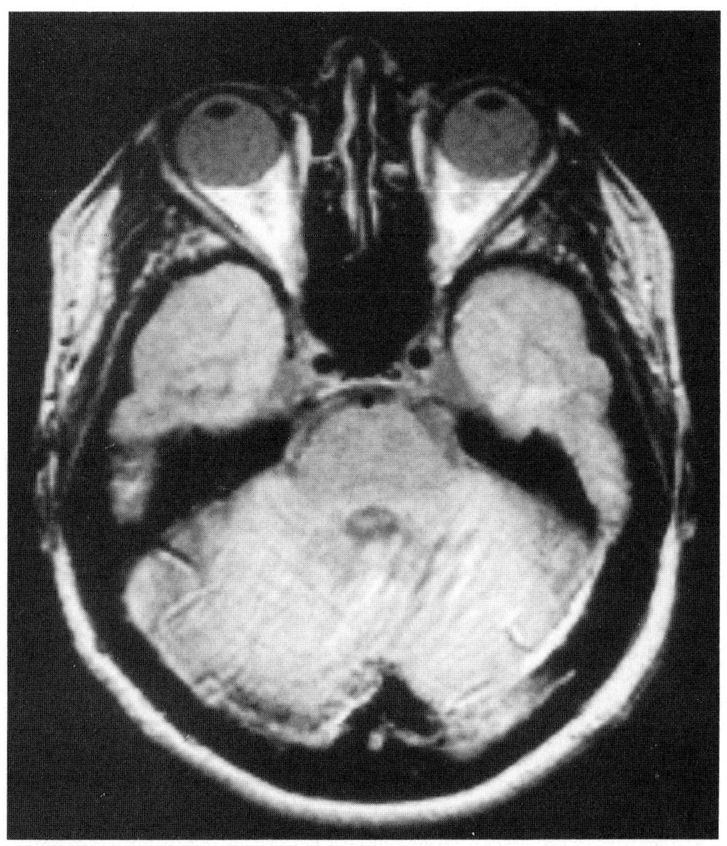

1-32a Head, axial view (TR 2000; TE 30).

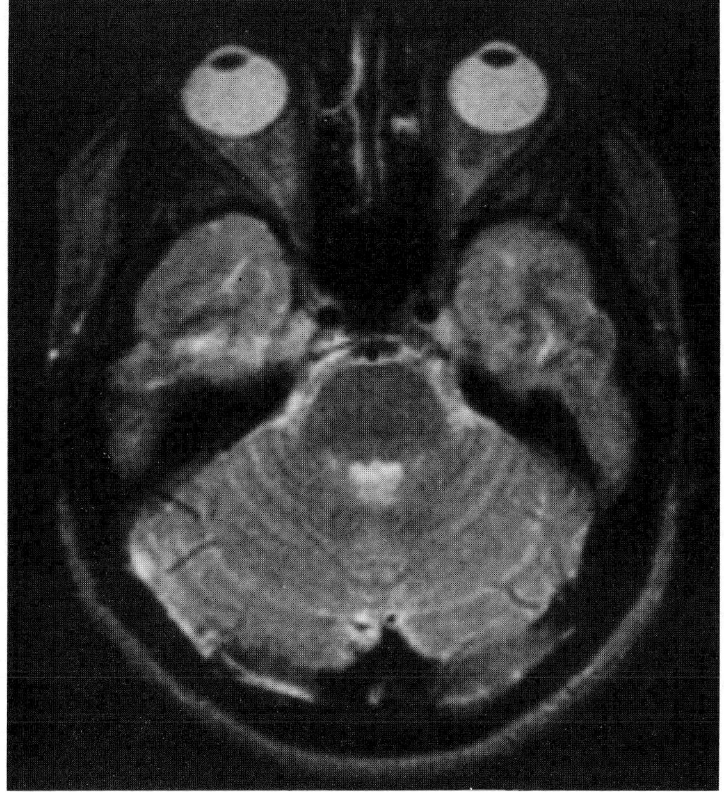

1-32b Head, axial view (TR 2000; TE 90).

Head, Axial

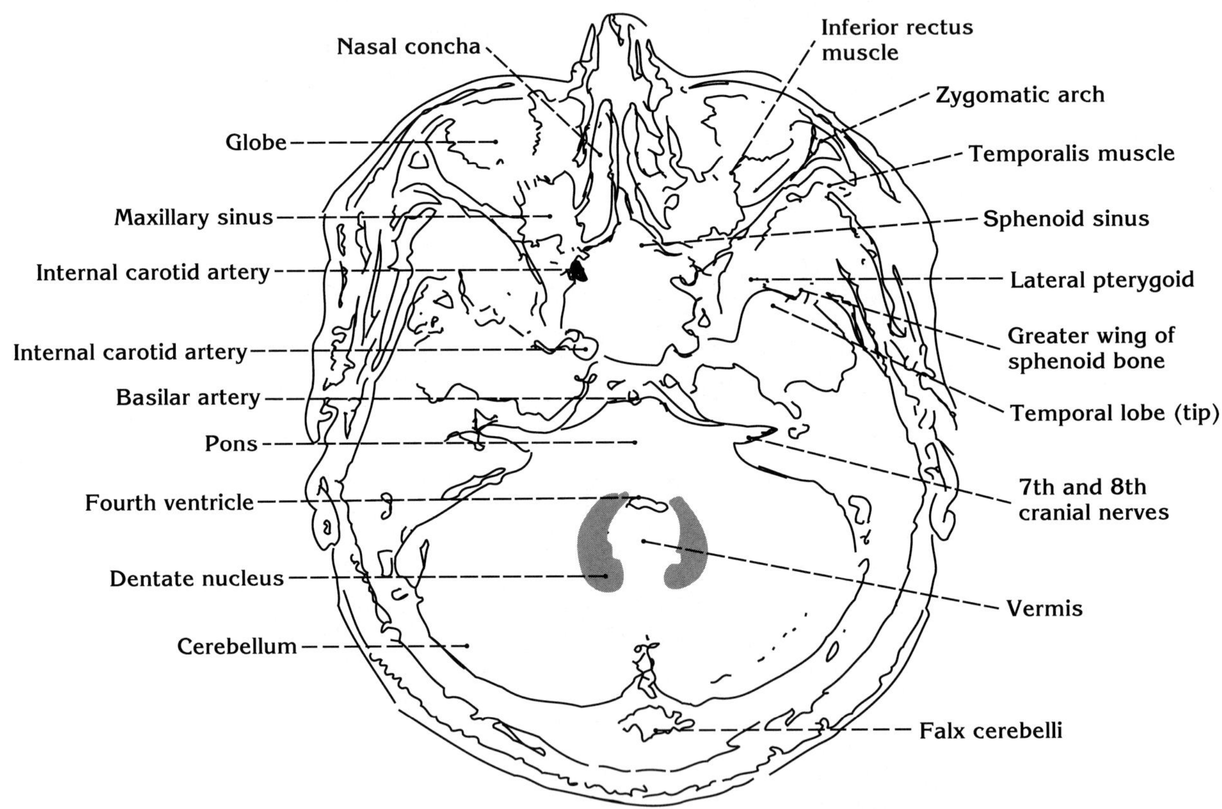
Nasal concha
Inferior rectus muscle
Zygomatic arch
Globe
Temporalis muscle
Maxillary sinus
Sphenoid sinus
Internal carotid artery
Lateral pterygoid
Internal carotid artery
Greater wing of sphenoid bone
Basilar artery
Temporal lobe (tip)
Pons
7th and 8th cranial nerves
Fourth ventricle
Dentate nucleus
Vermis
Cerebellum
Falx cerebelli

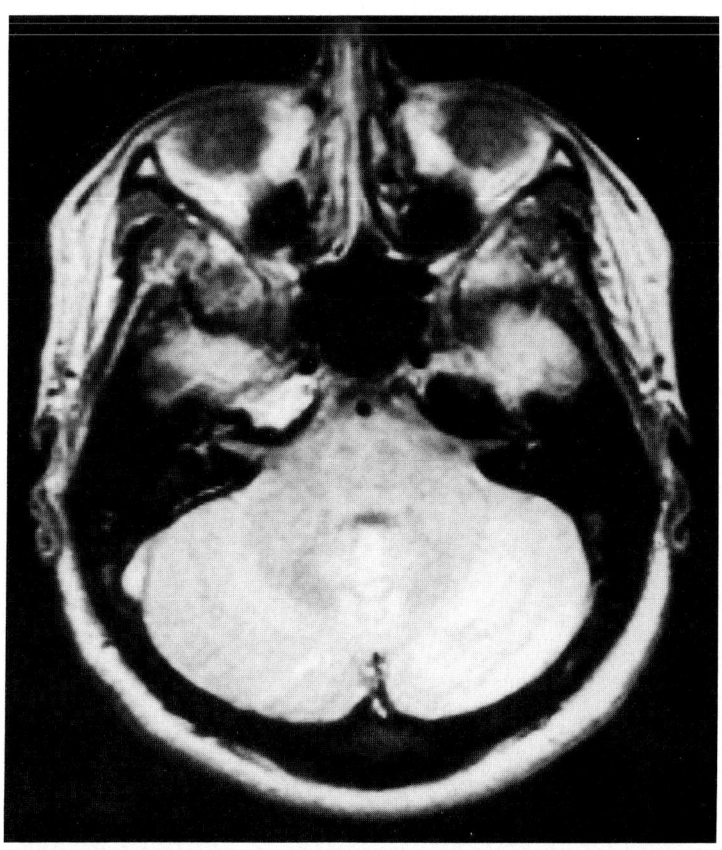

1-33a Head, axial view (TR 2000; TE 30).

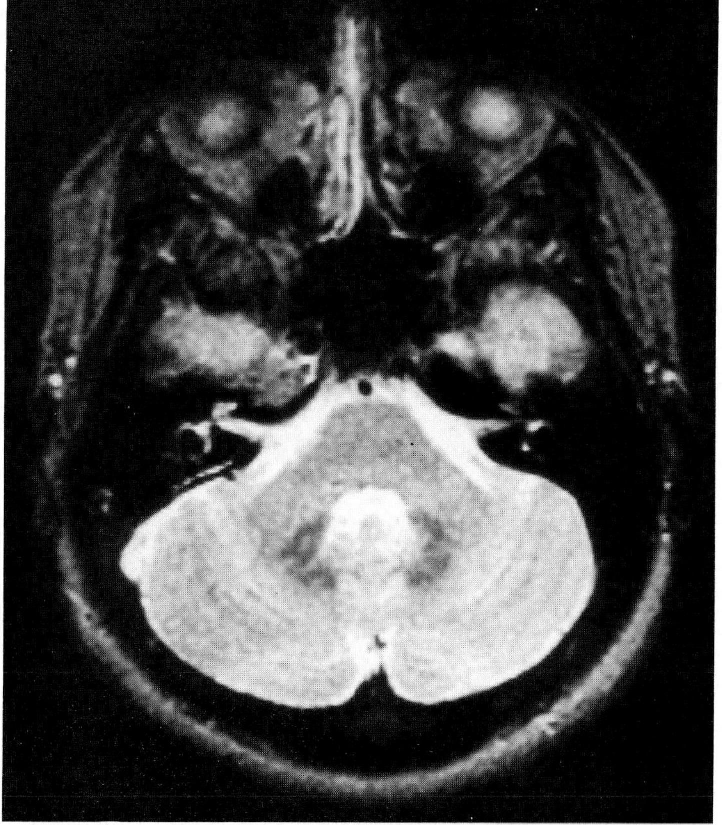

1-33b Head, axial view (TR 2000; TE 90).

Head, Axial

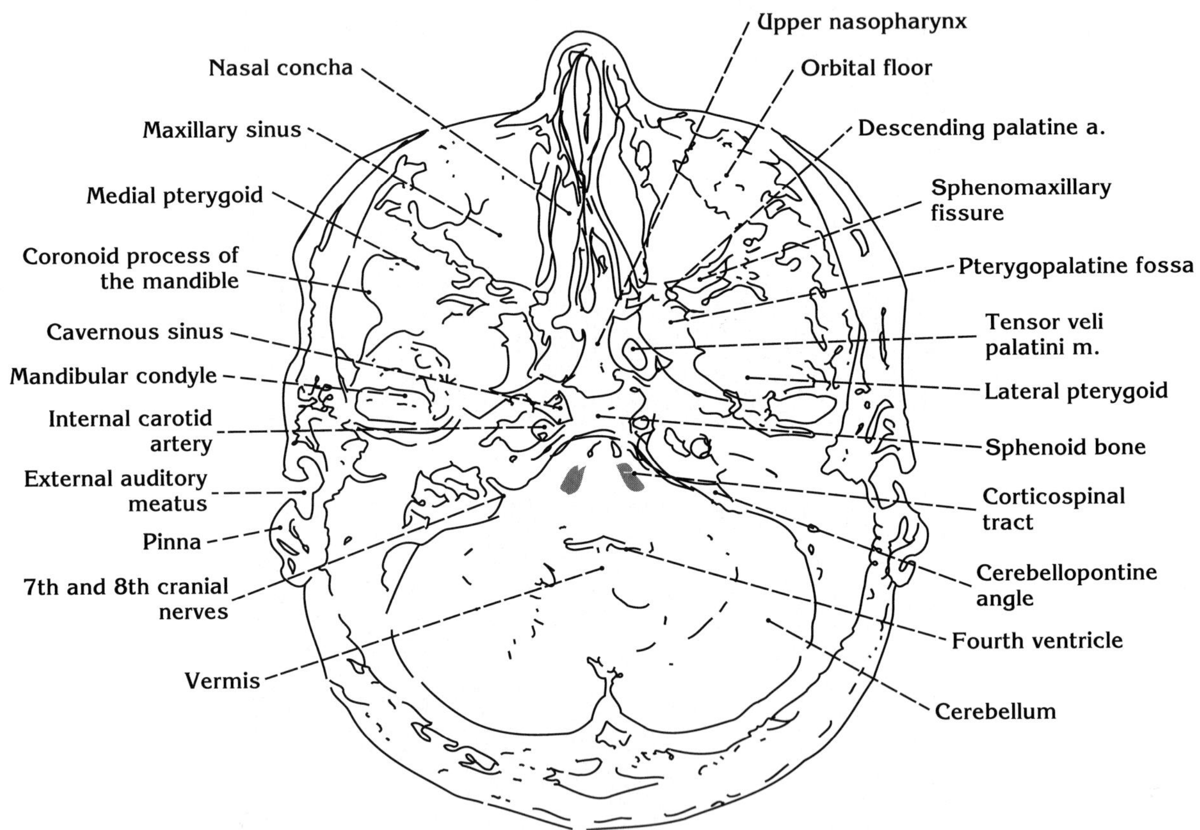

Upper nasopharynx
Nasal concha
Orbital floor
Maxillary sinus
Descending palatine a.
Medial pterygoid
Sphenomaxillary fissure
Coronoid process of the mandible
Pterygopalatine fossa
Cavernous sinus
Tensor veli palatini m.
Mandibular condyle
Lateral pterygoid
Internal carotid artery
Sphenoid bone
External auditory meatus
Corticospinal tract
Pinna
Cerebellopontine angle
7th and 8th cranial nerves
Fourth ventricle
Vermis
Cerebellum

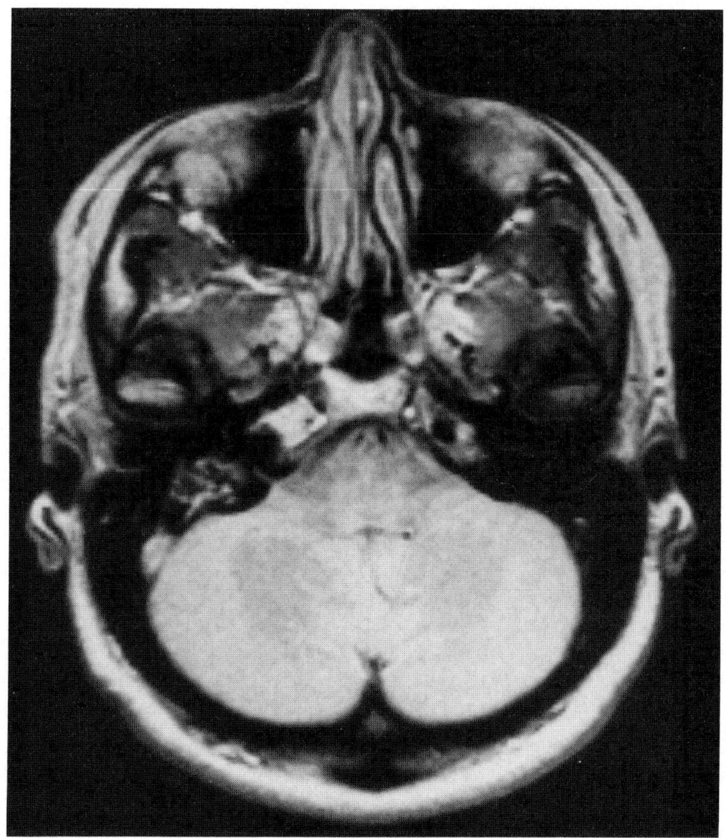

1-34a Head, axial view (TR 2000; TE 30).

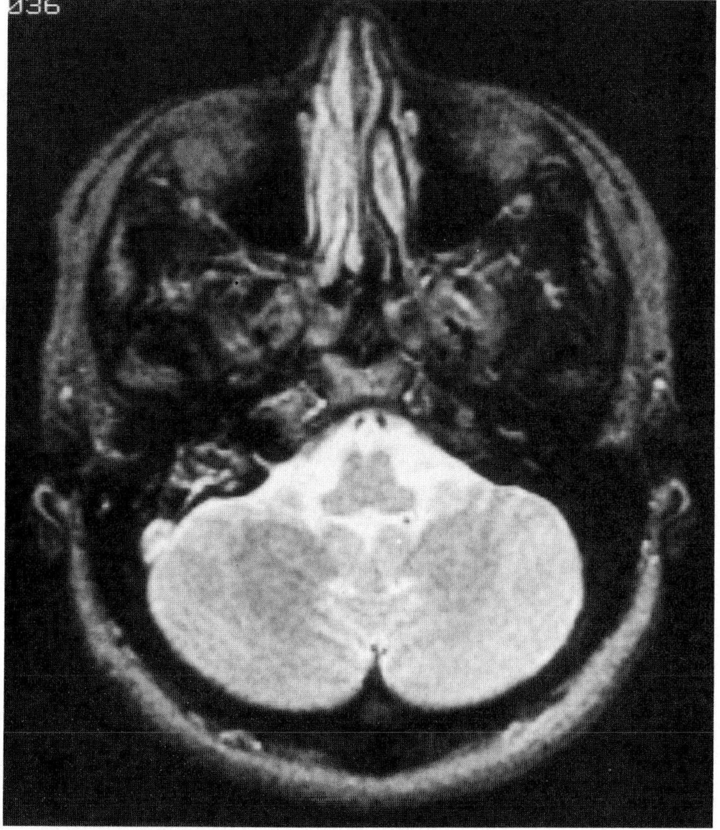

1-34b Head, axial view (TR 2000; TE 90).

Head, Axial

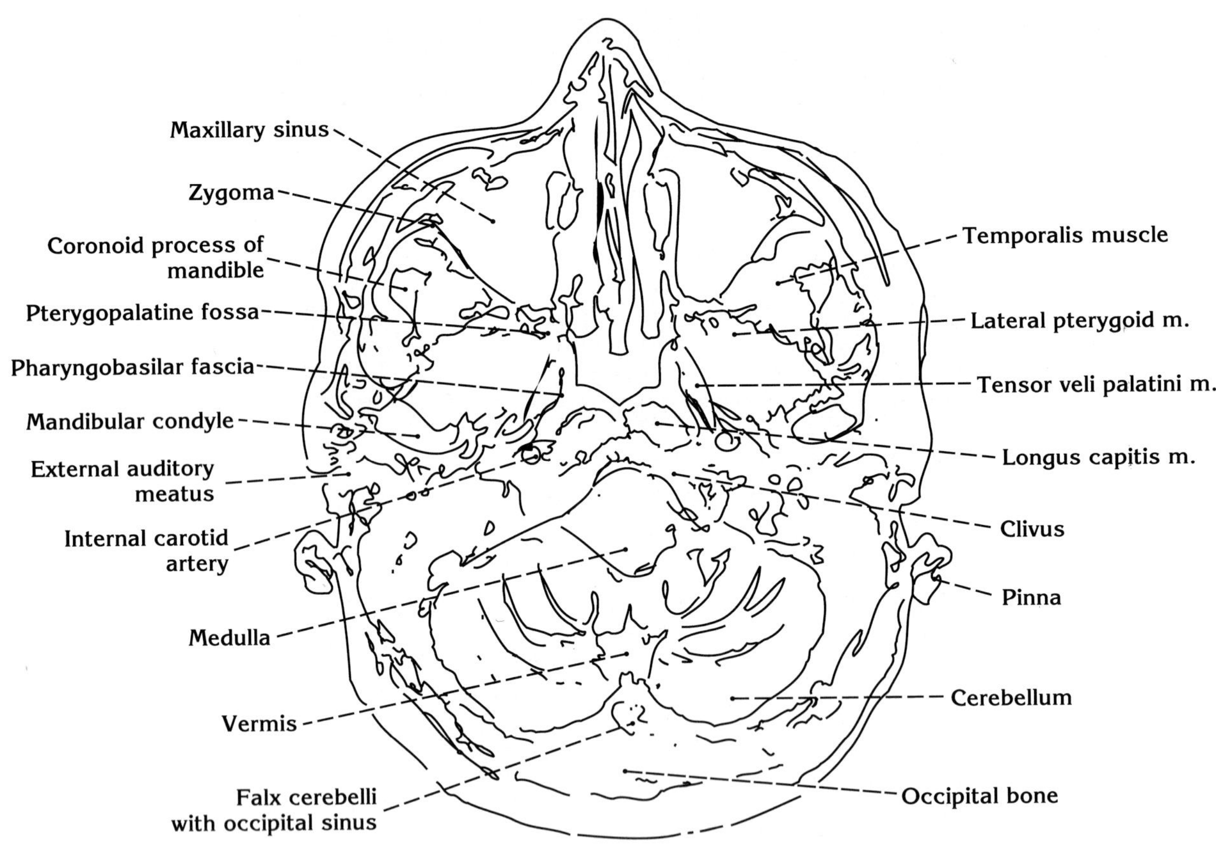
Maxillary sinus
Zygoma
Coronoid process of mandible
Pterygopalatine fossa
Pharyngobasilar fascia
Mandibular condyle
External auditory meatus
Internal carotid artery
Medulla
Vermis
Falx cerebelli with occipital sinus
Temporalis muscle
Lateral pterygoid m.
Tensor veli palatini m.
Longus capitis m.
Clivus
Pinna
Cerebellum
Occipital bone

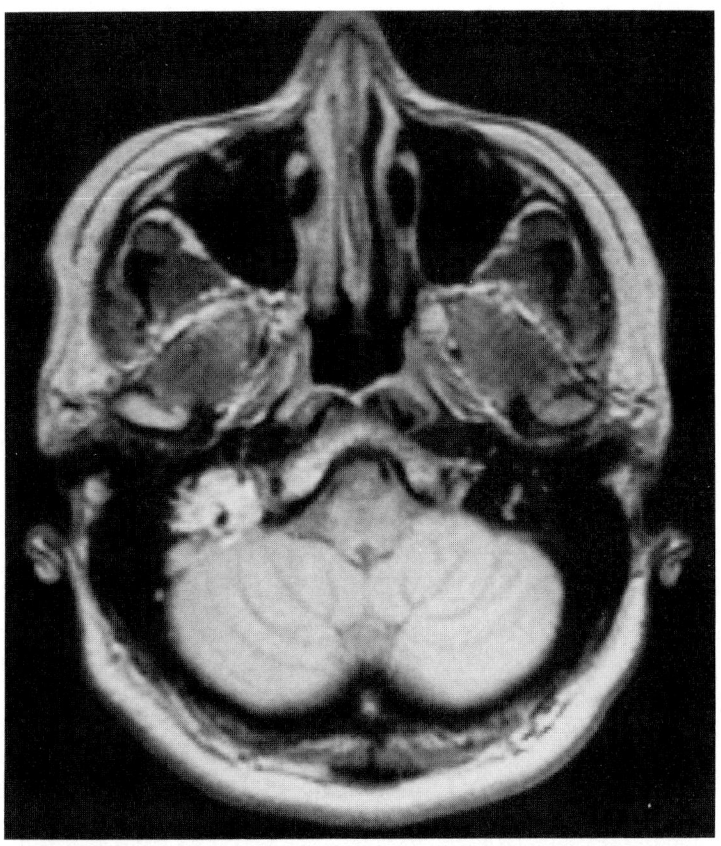

1-35a Head, axial view (TR 2000; TE 30).

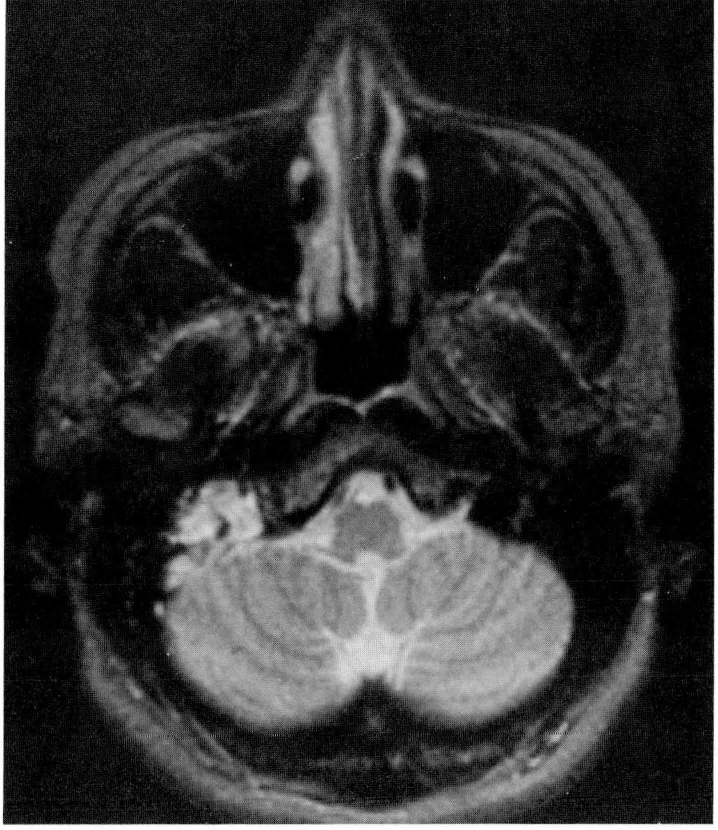

1-35b Head, axial view (TR 2000; TE 90).

Head, Axial

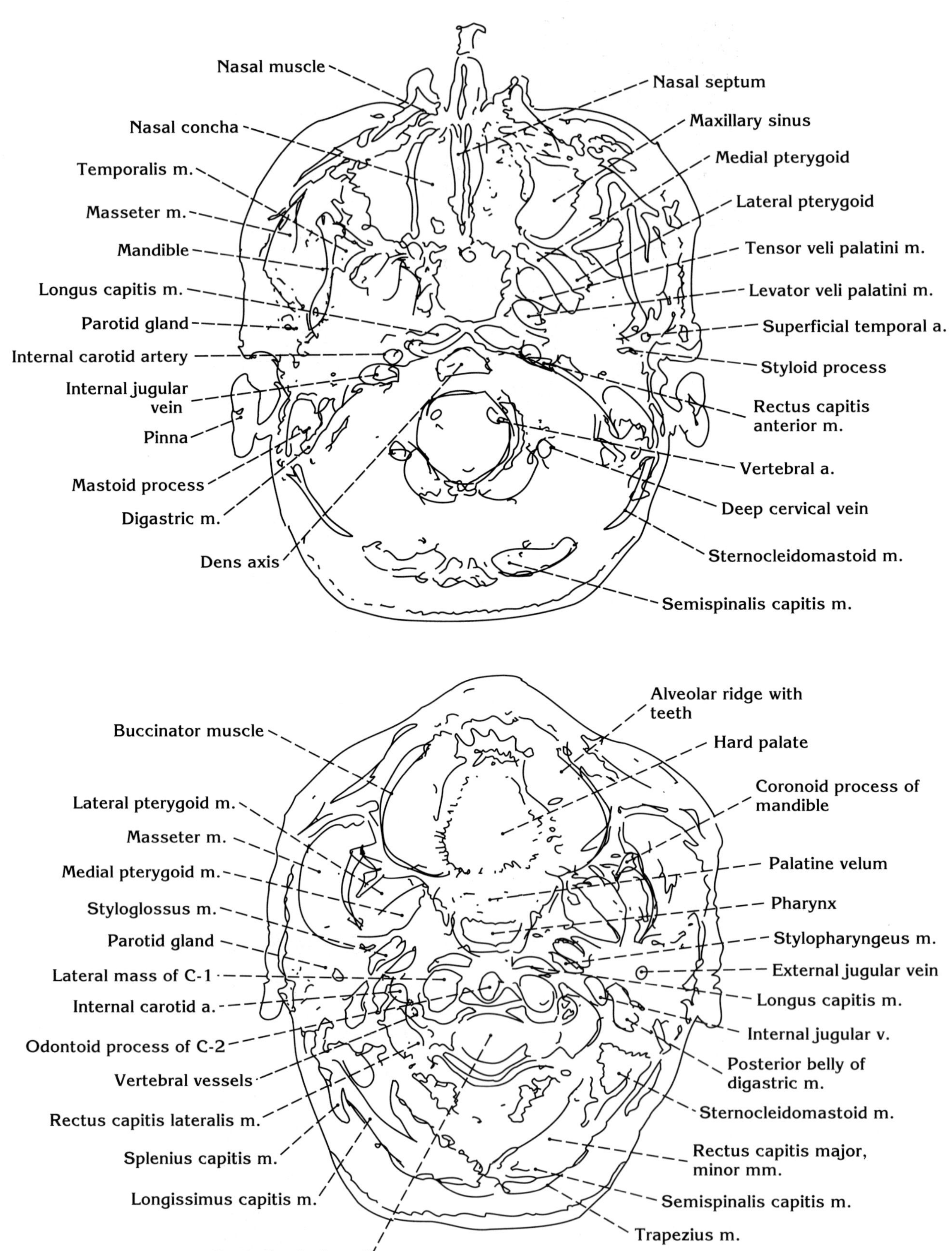
Nasal muscle
Nasal septum
Nasal concha
Maxillary sinus
Temporalis m.
Medial pterygoid
Masseter m.
Lateral pterygoid
Mandible
Tensor veli palatini m.
Longus capitis m.
Levator veli palatini m.
Parotid gland
Superficial temporal a.
Internal carotid artery
Styloid process
Internal jugular vein
Rectus capitis anterior m.
Pinna
Vertebral a.
Mastoid process
Deep cervical vein
Digastric m.
Sternocleidomastoid m.
Dens axis
Semispinalis capitis m.
Buccinator muscle
Alveolar ridge with teeth
Hard palate
Lateral pterygoid m.
Coronoid process of mandible
Masseter m.
Palatine velum
Medial pterygoid m.
Pharynx
Styloglossus m.
Stylopharyngeus m.
Parotid gland
External jugular vein
Lateral mass of C-1
Longus capitis m.
Internal carotid a.
Internal jugular v.
Odontoid process of C-2
Posterior belly of digastric m.
Vertebral vessels
Sternocleidomastoid m.
Rectus capitis lateralis m.
Rectus capitis major, minor mm.
Splenius capitis m.
Semispinalis capitis m.
Longissimus capitis m.
Trapezius m.
Cervical spinal cord

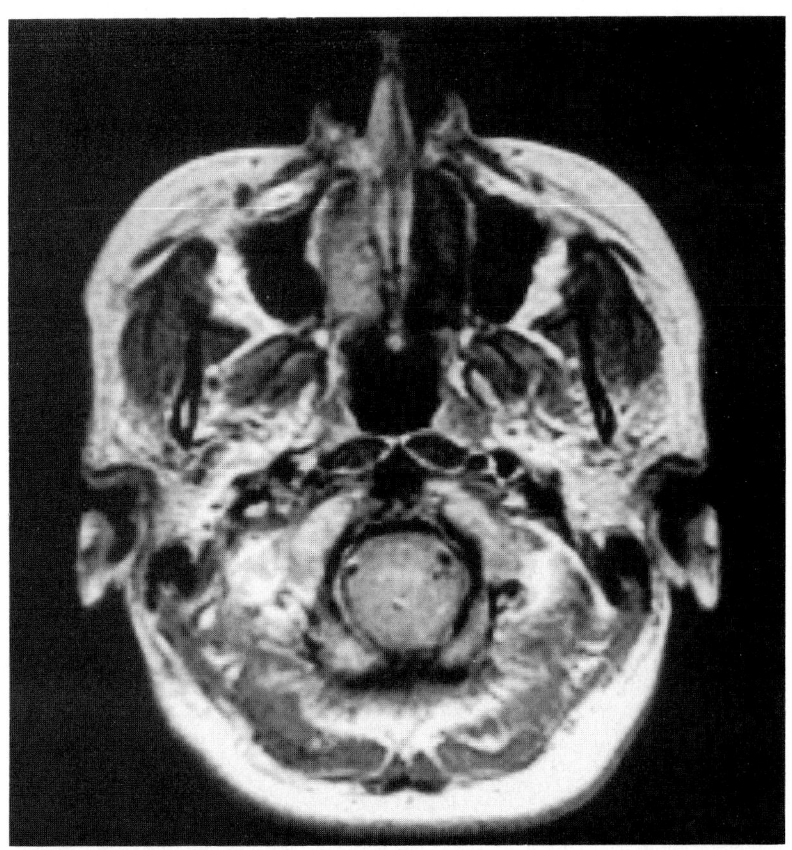

1-36 Head, axial view (TR 2000; TE 30).

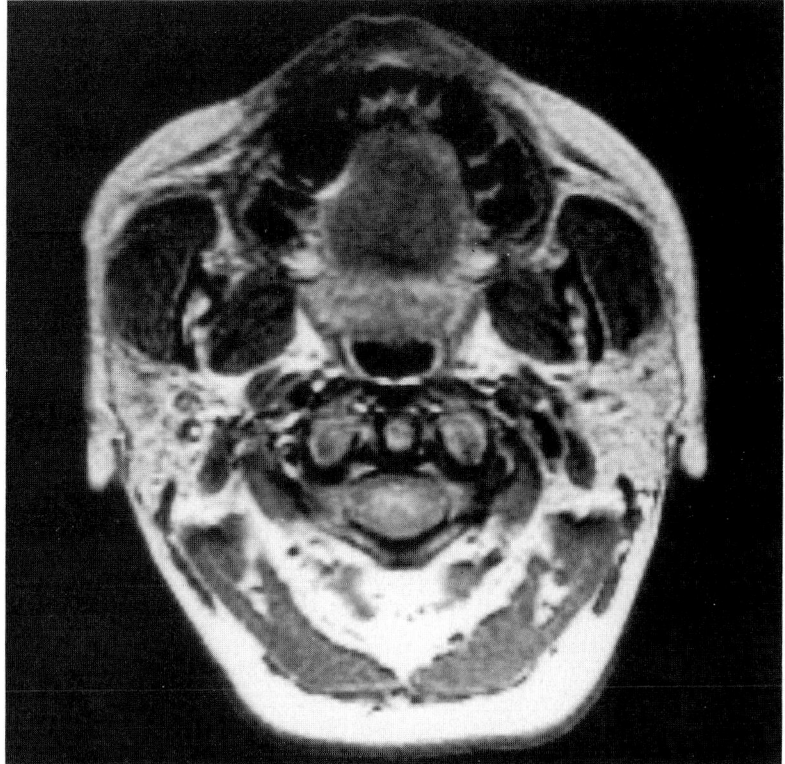

1-37 Head, axial view (TR 2000; TE 30).

Head and Neck, Sagittal

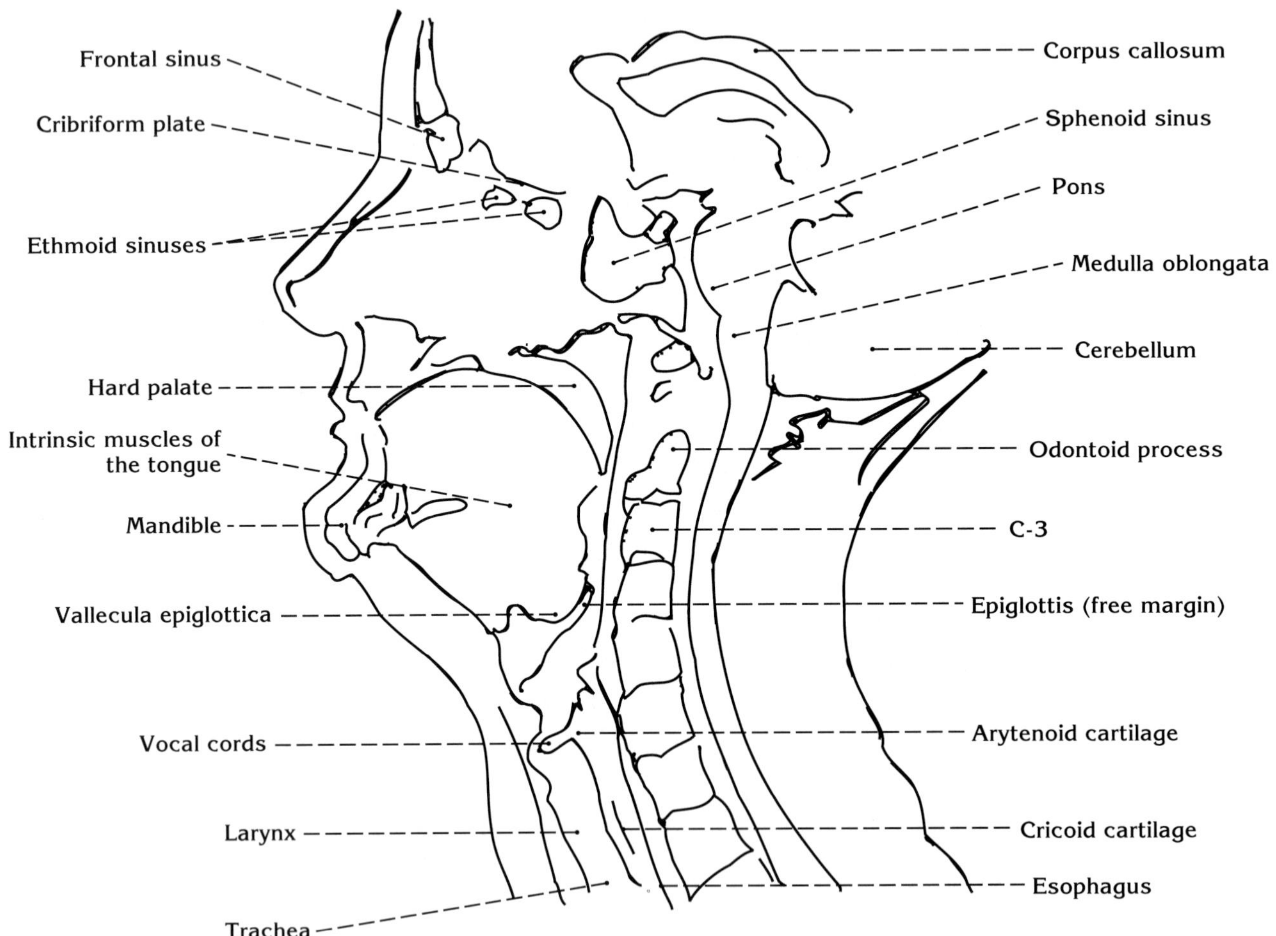

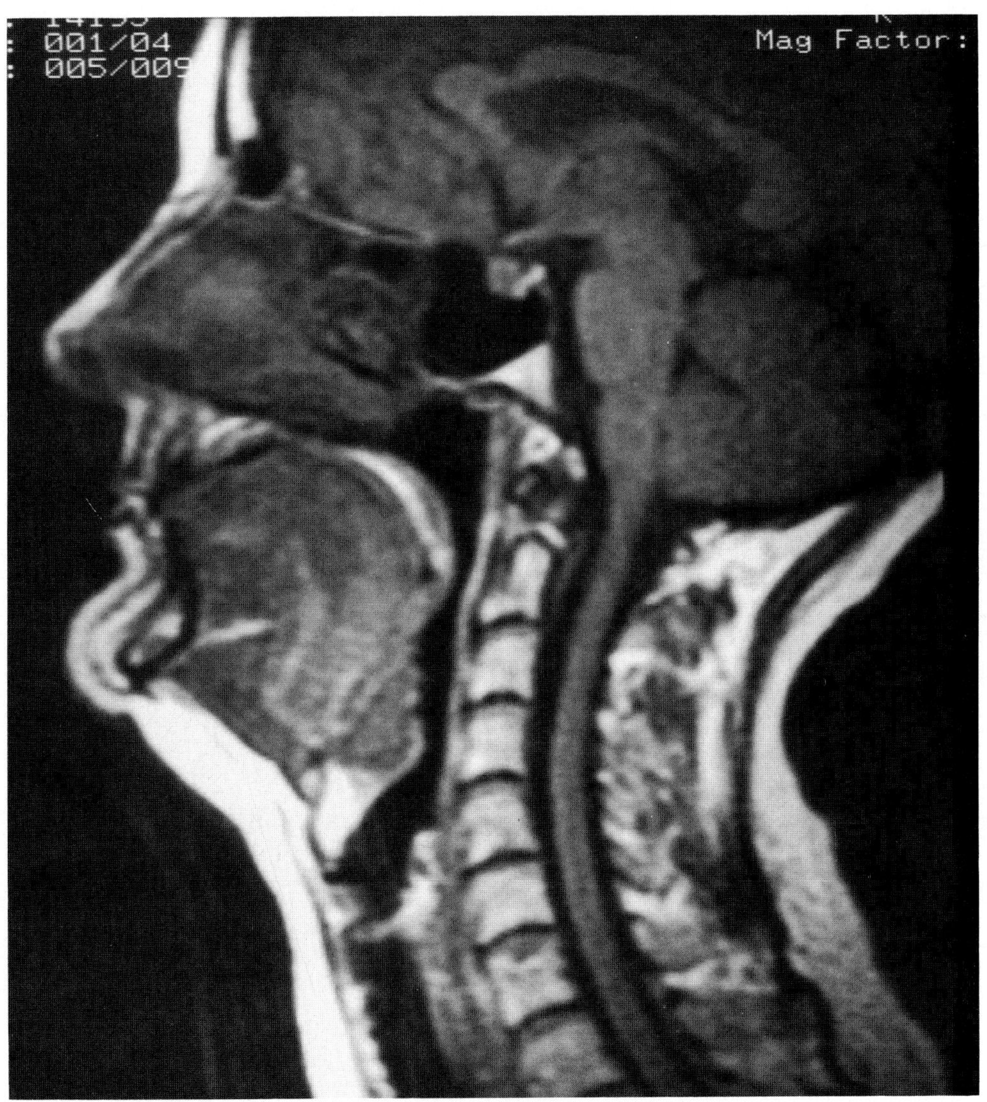

1-38 Head and neck, sagittal view (TR 400; TE 20).

Head and Neck, Sagittal

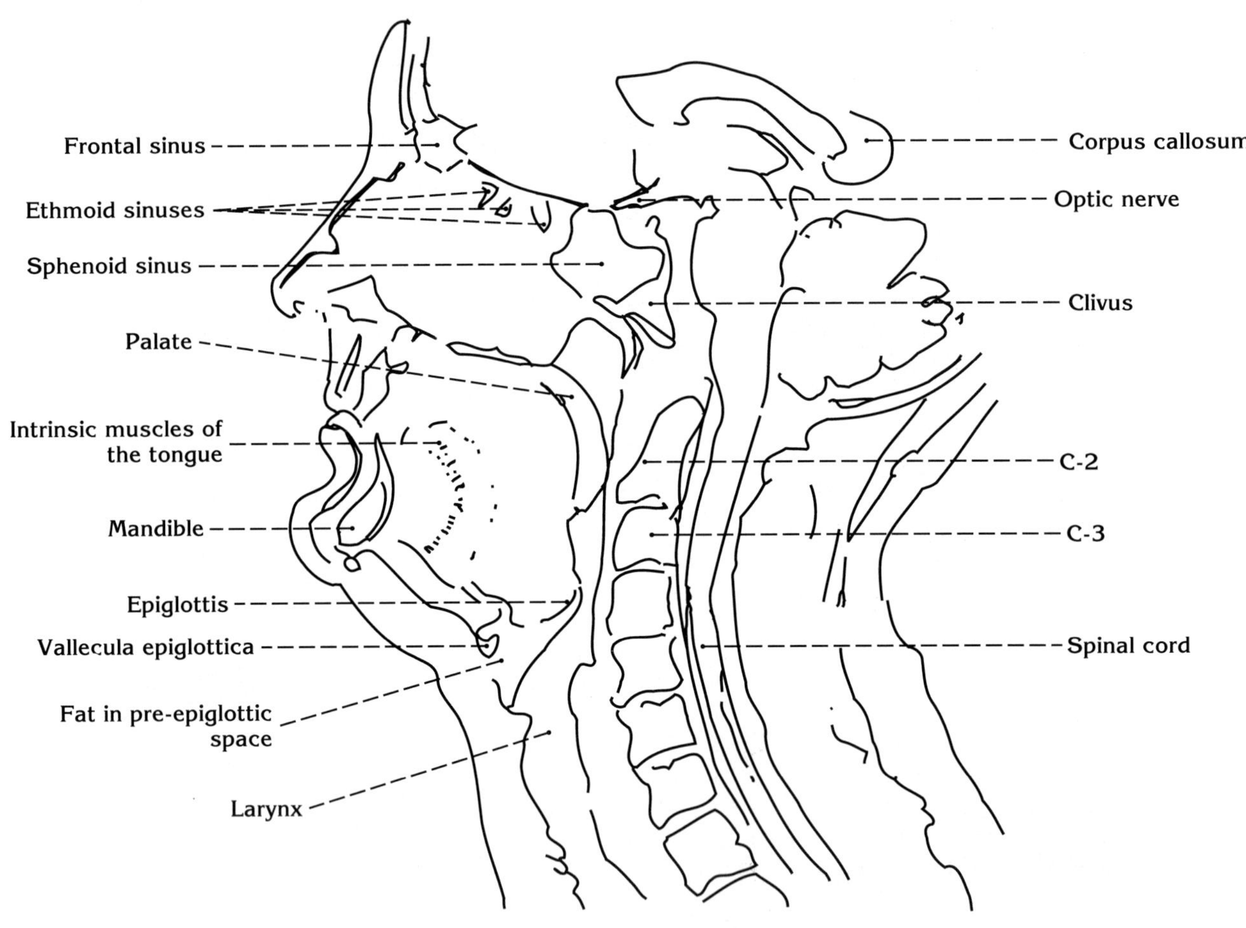

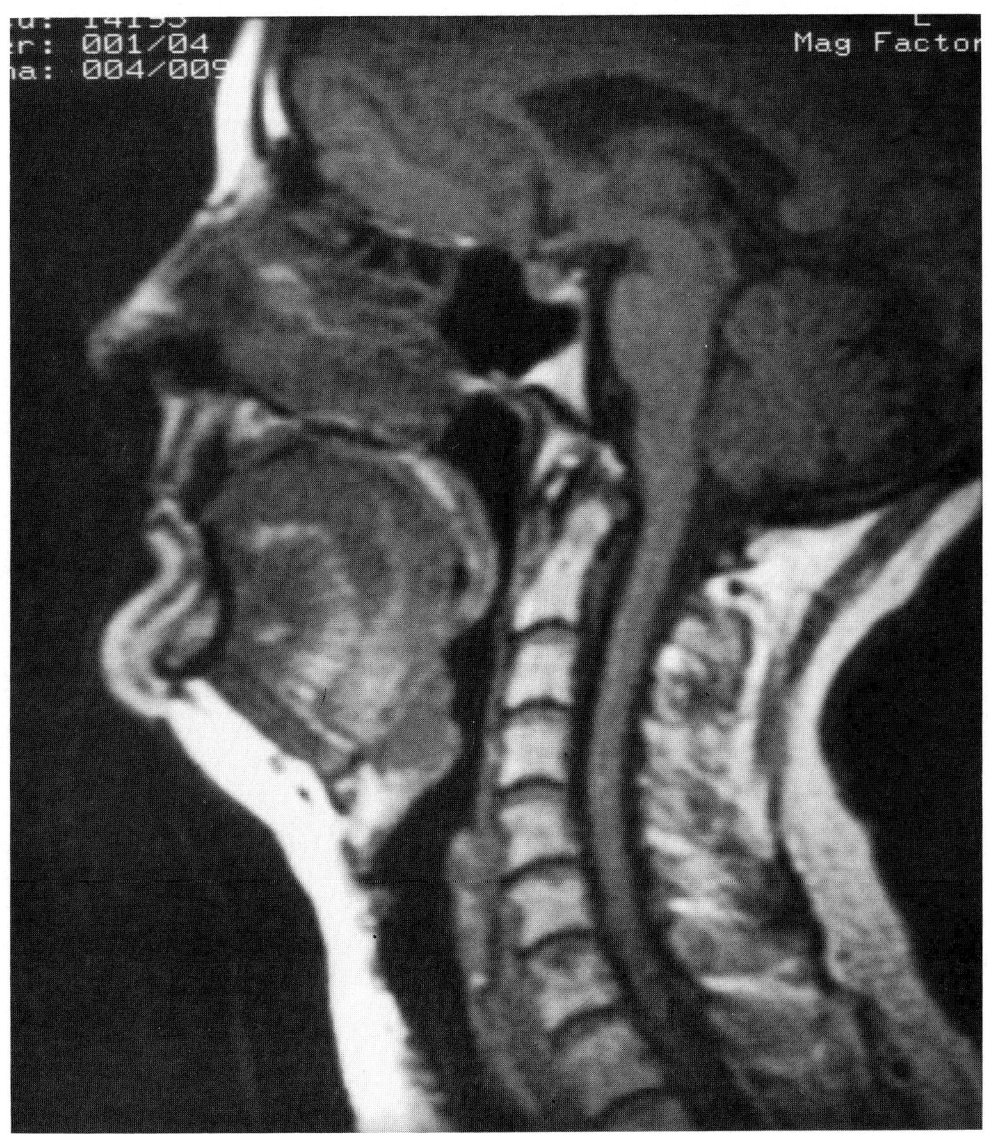

1-39 Head and neck, sagittal view (TR 400; TE 20).

Head and Neck, Sagittal

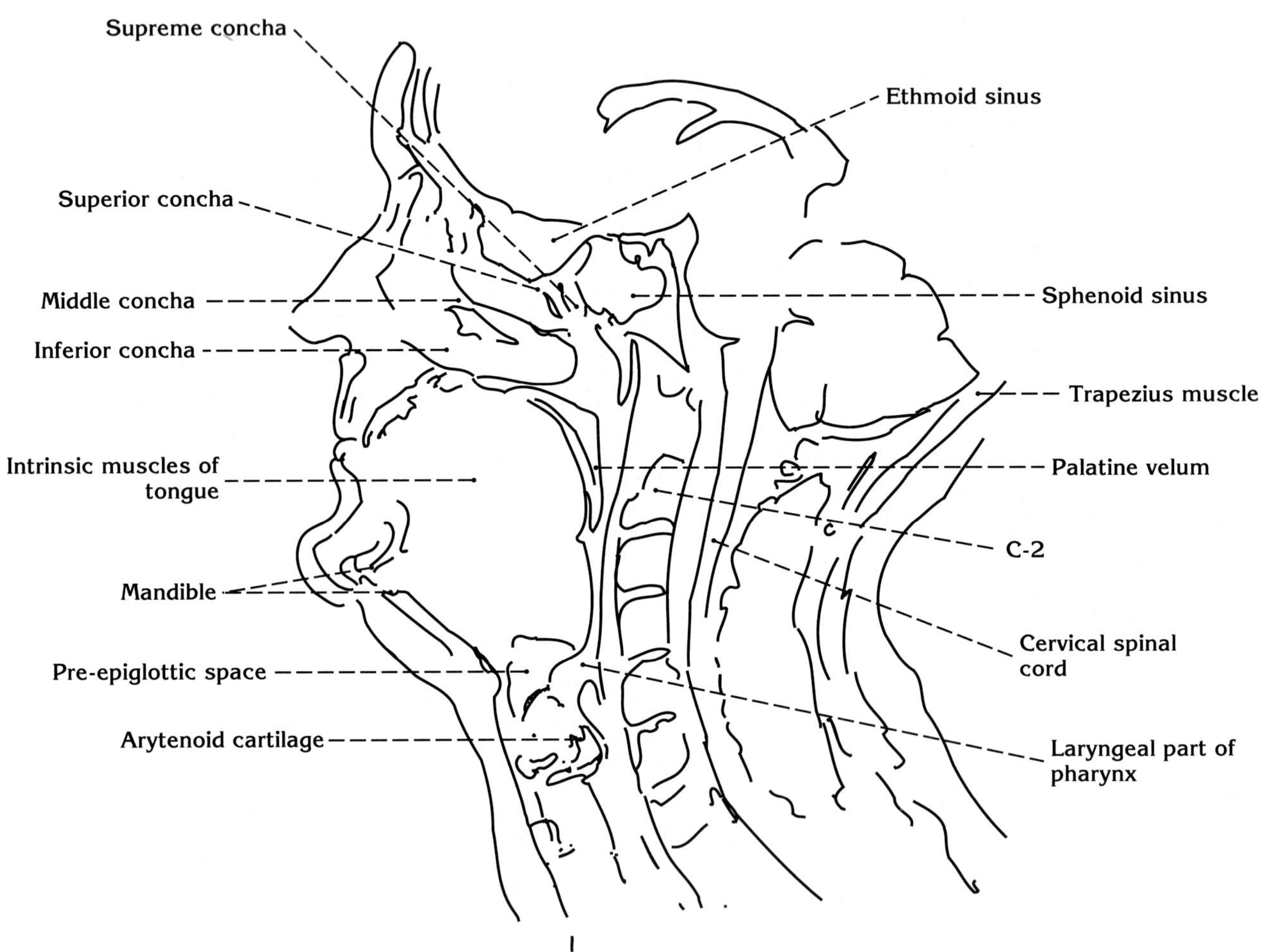

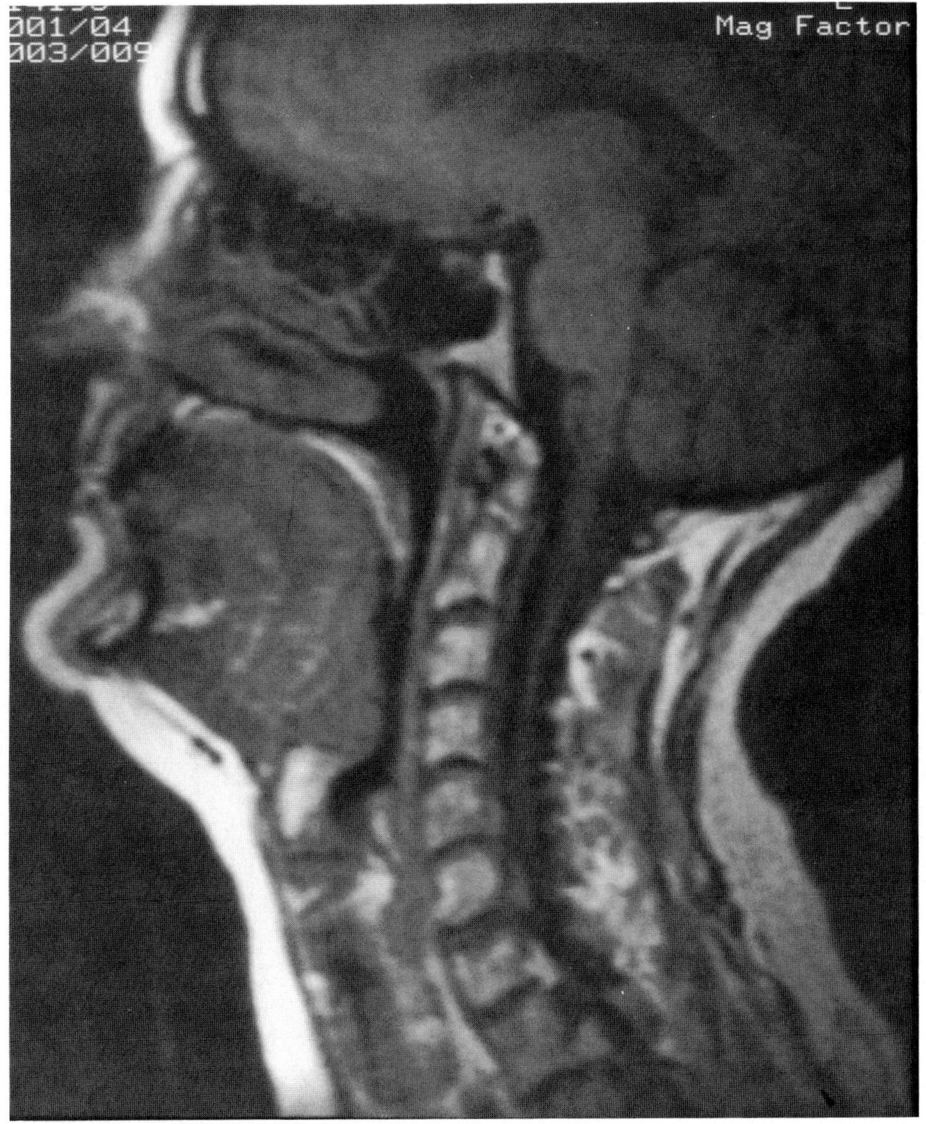

1-40 Head and neck, sagittal view (TR 400; TE 20).

Head and Neck, Sagittal

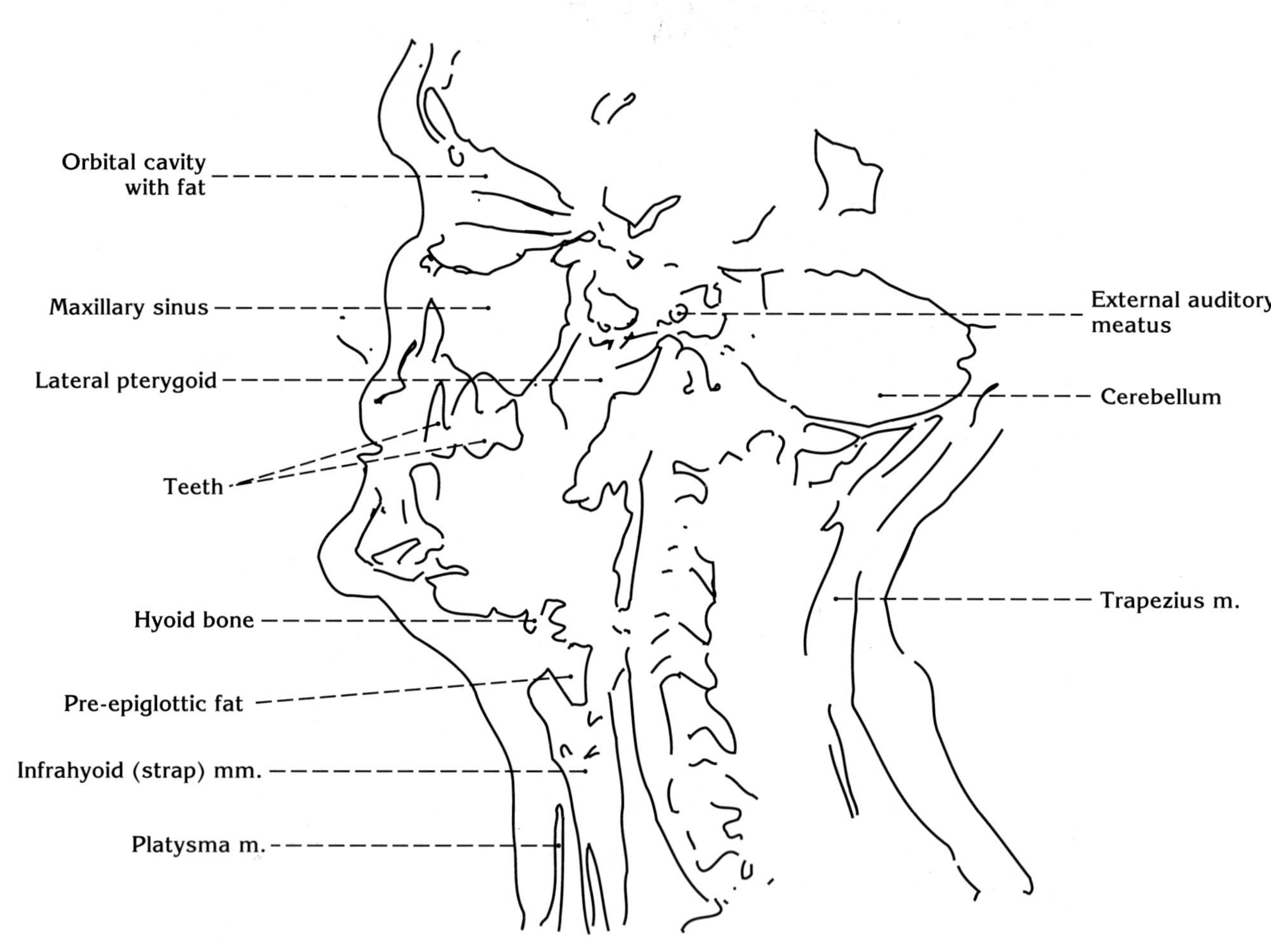

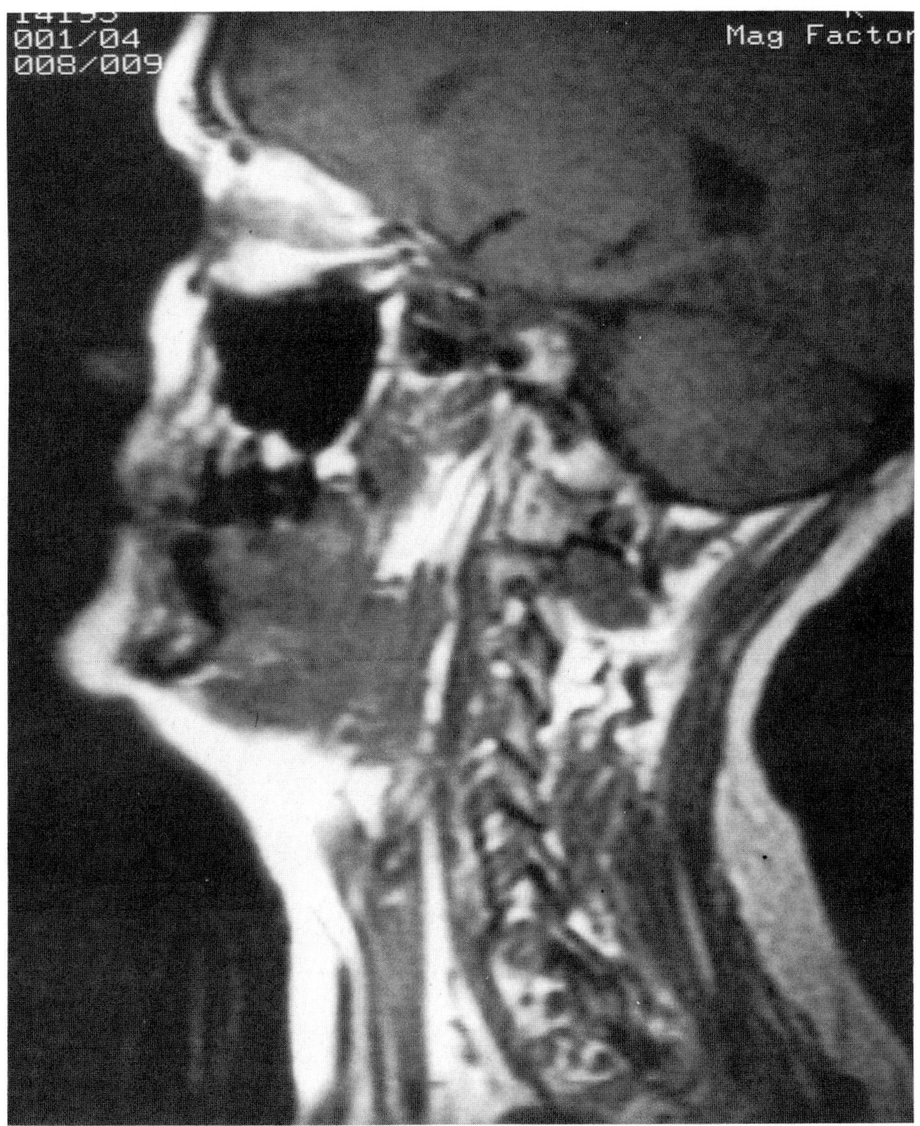

1-41 Head and neck, sagittal view (TR 400; TE 20).

Head and Neck, Sagittal

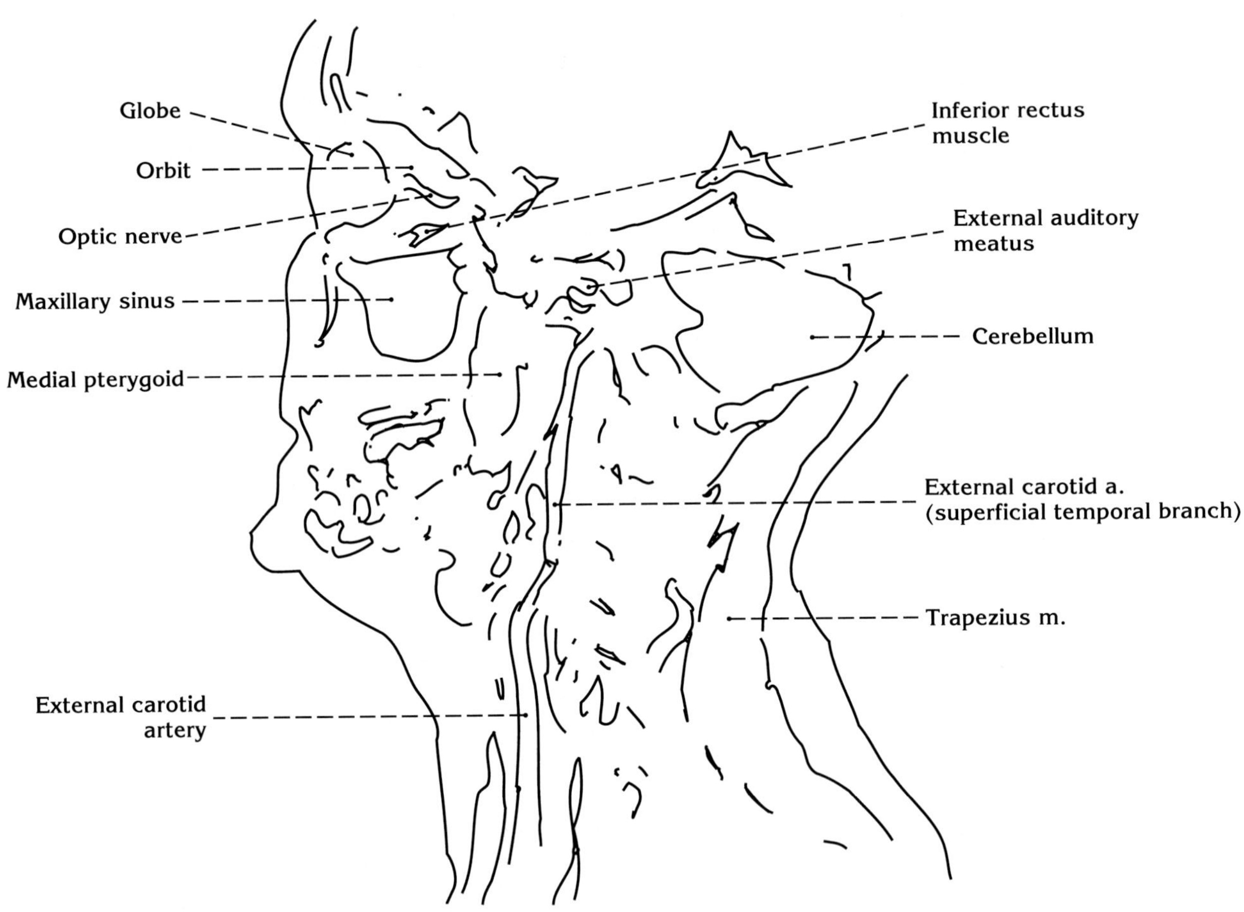

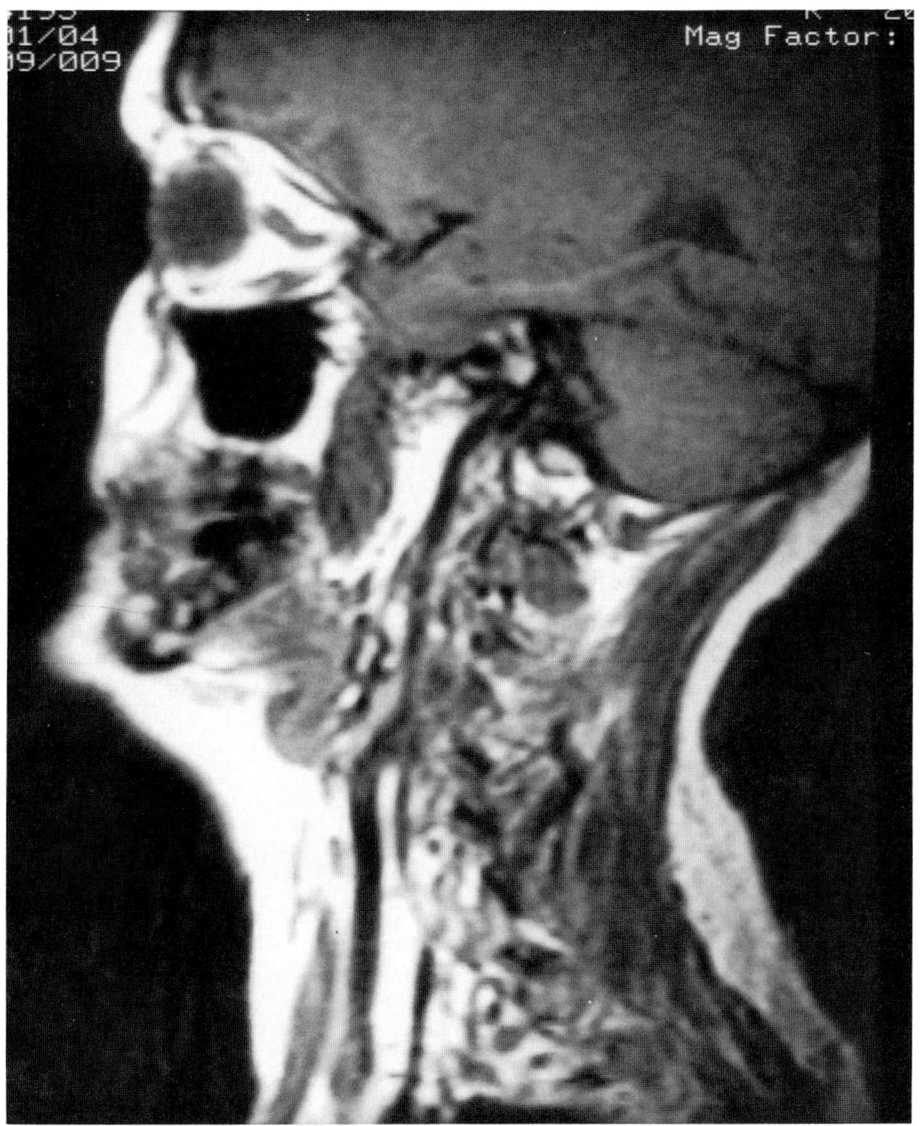

1-42 Head and neck, sagittal view (TR 400; TE 20).

Head and Neck, Axial

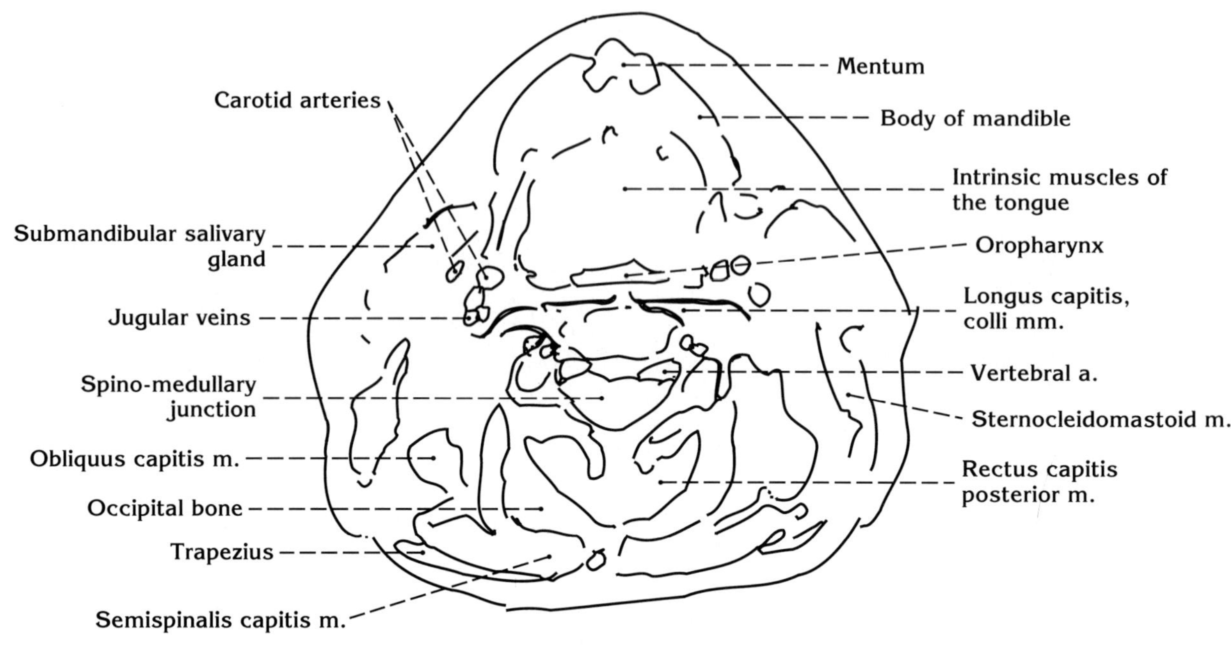

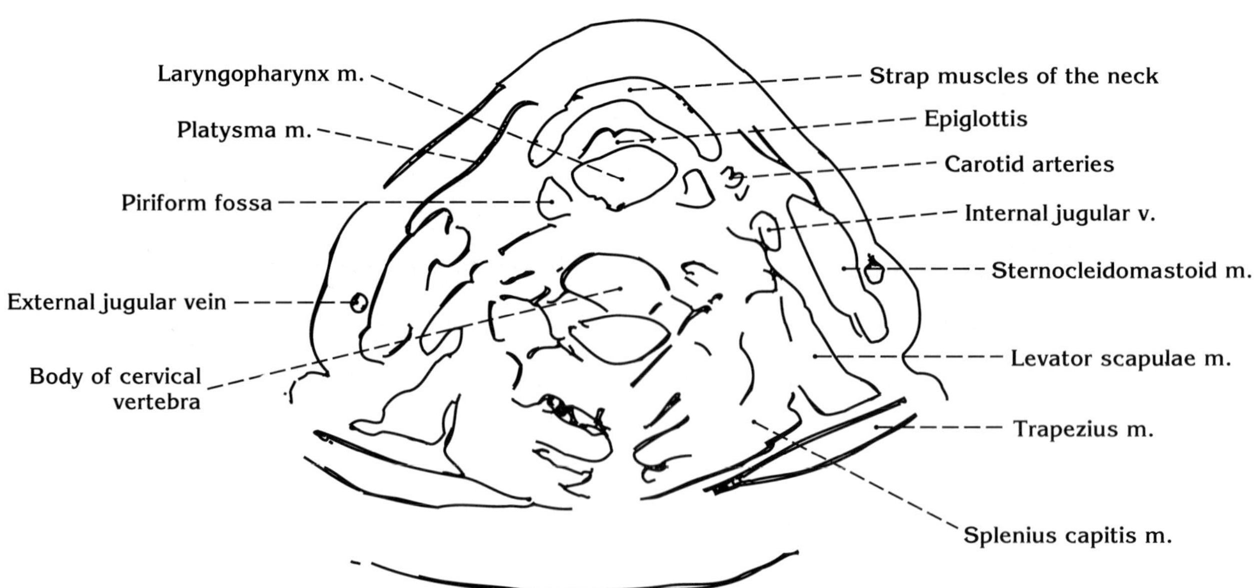

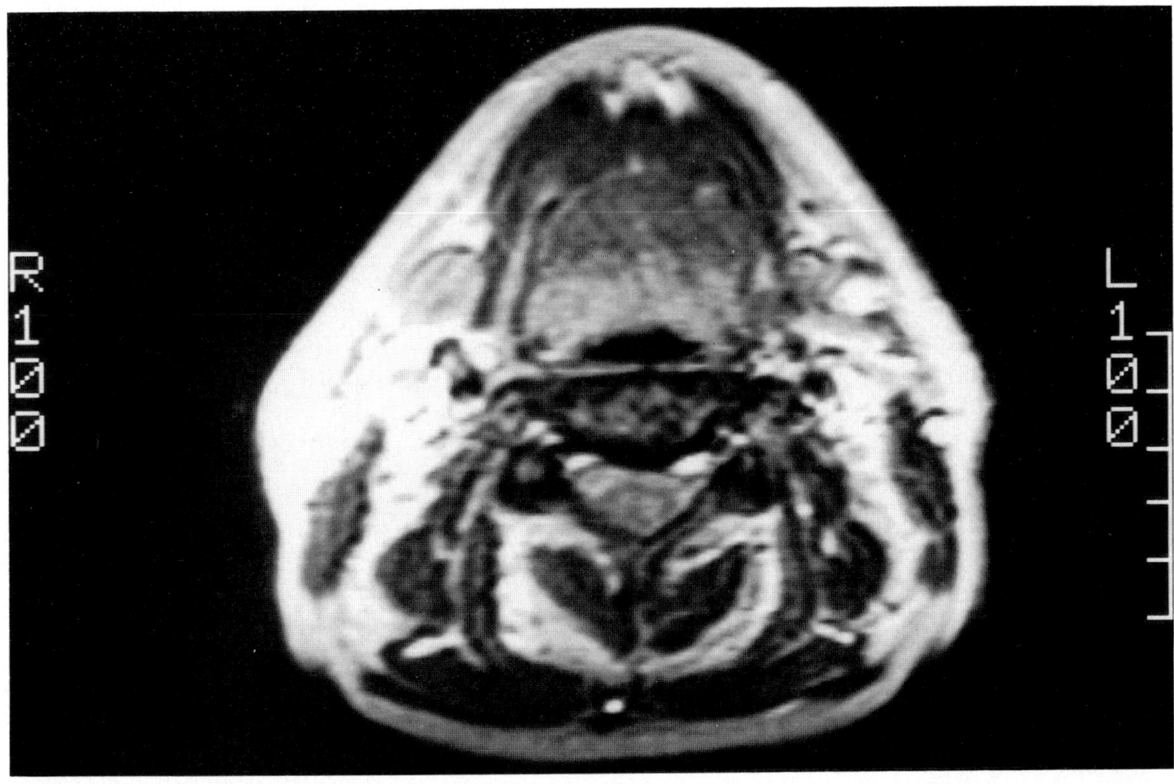

1-43 Head and neck, axial view (TR 2000; TE 30).

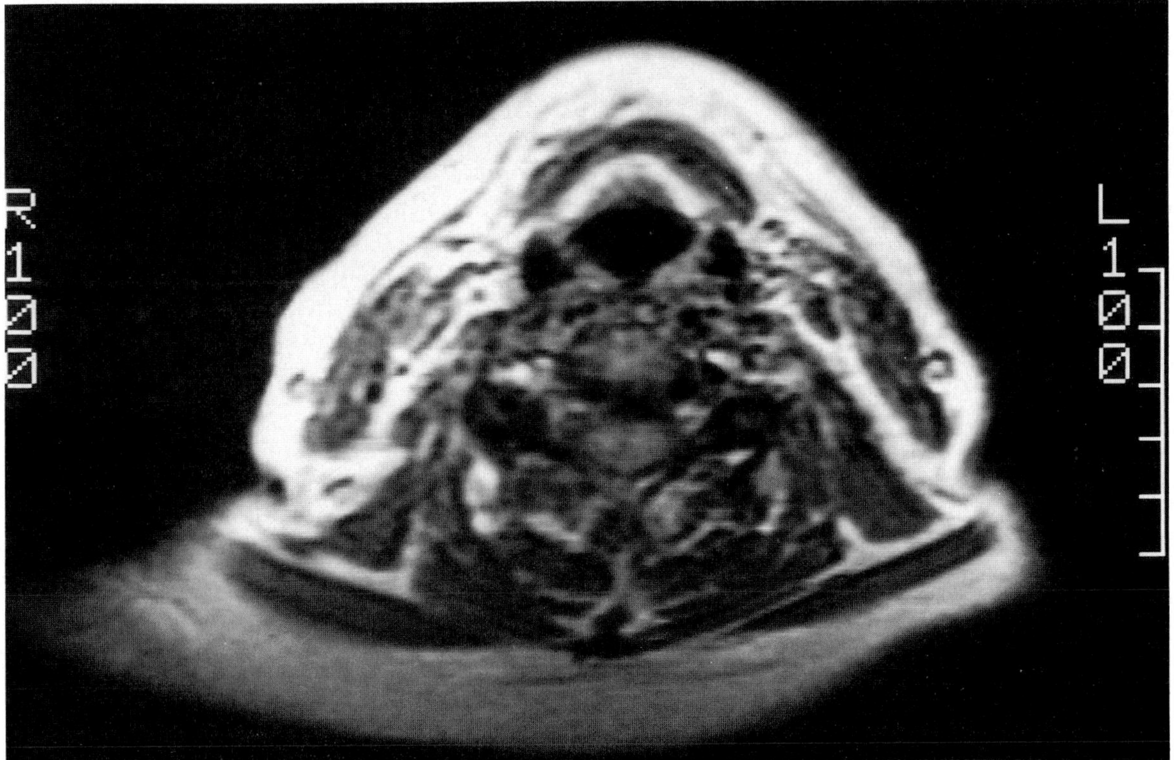

1-44 Head and neck, axial view (TR 2000; TE 30).

Head and Neck, Axial

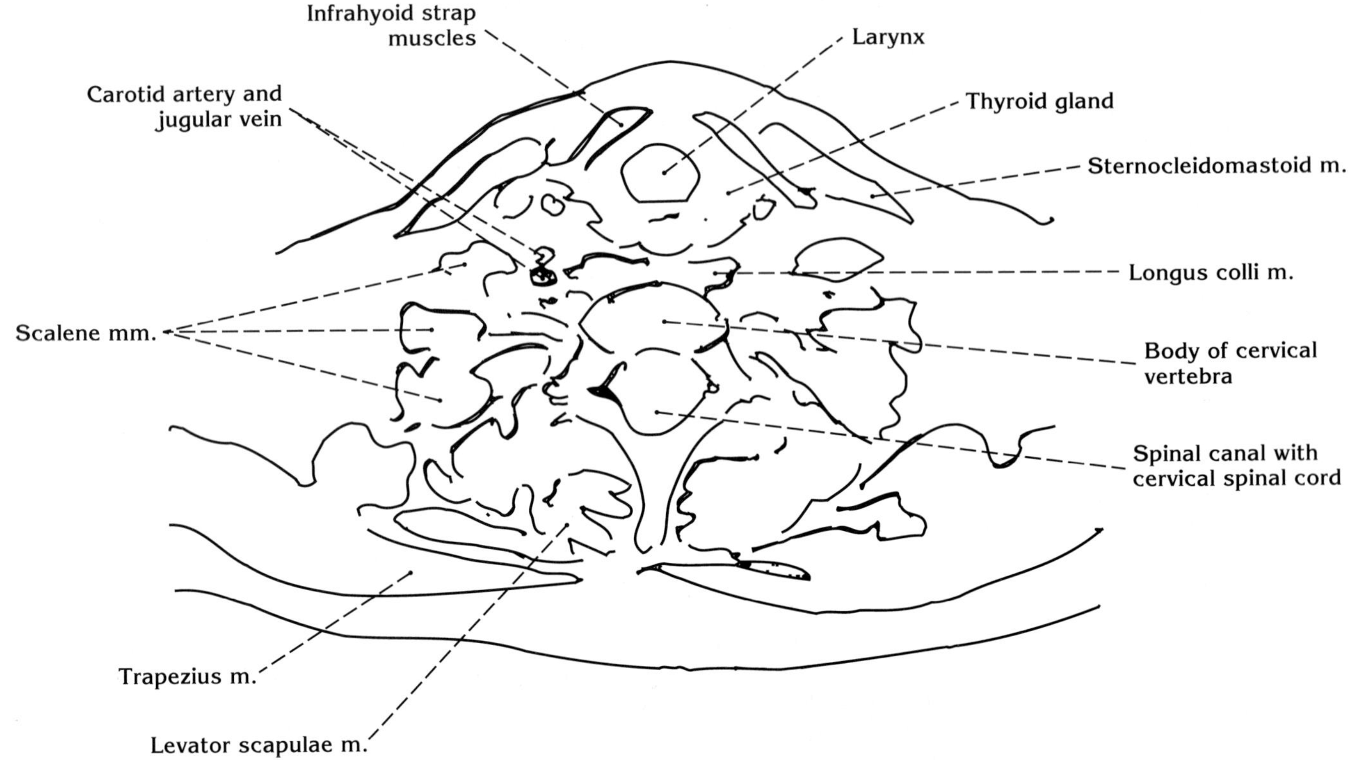

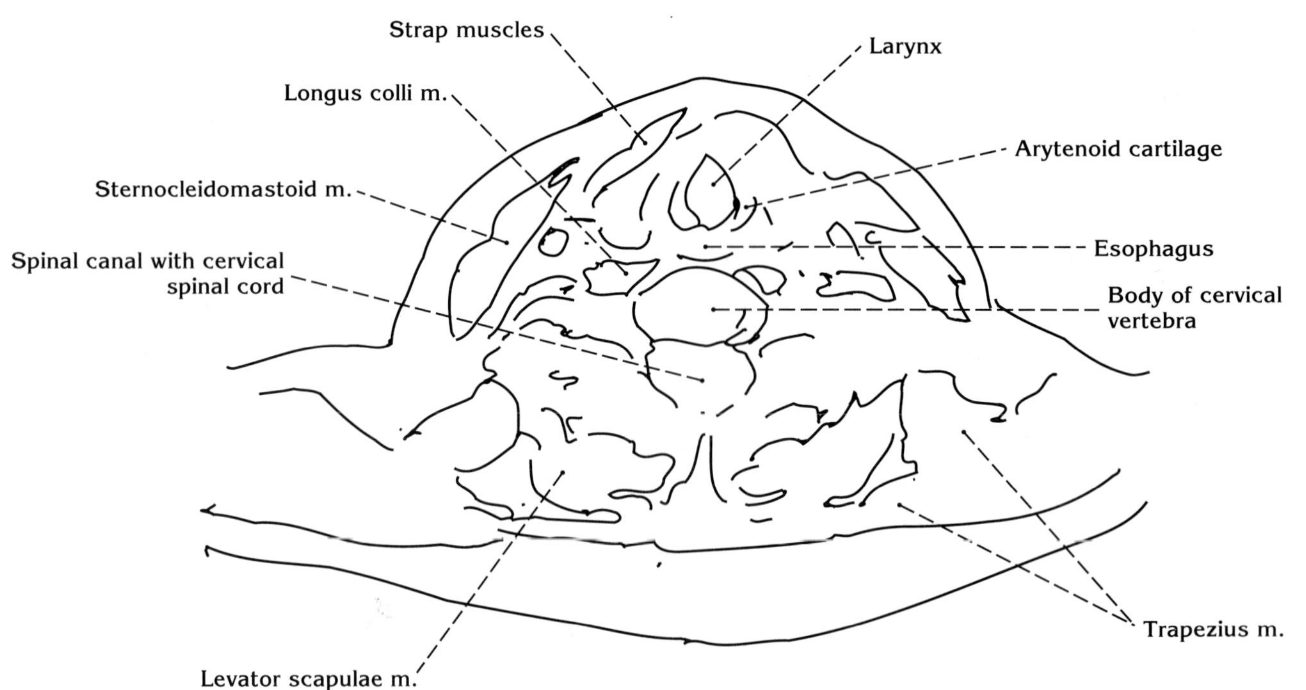

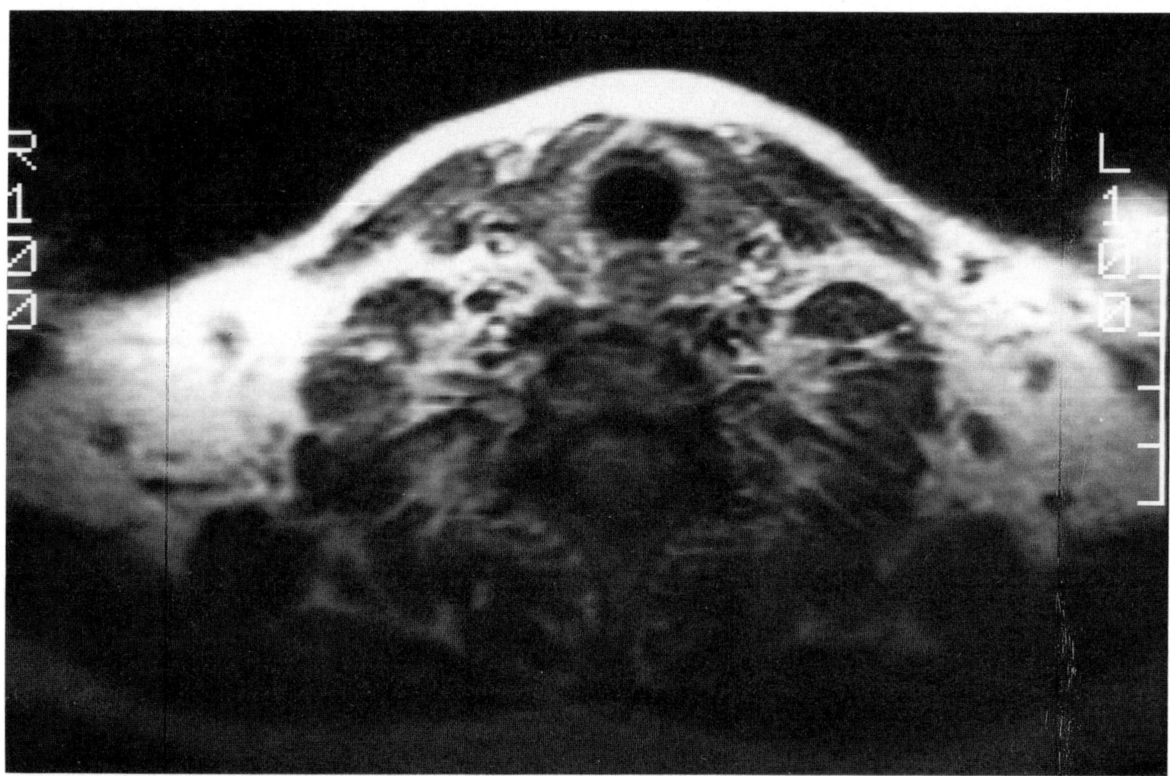

1-45 Head and neck, axial view (TR 2000; TE 30).

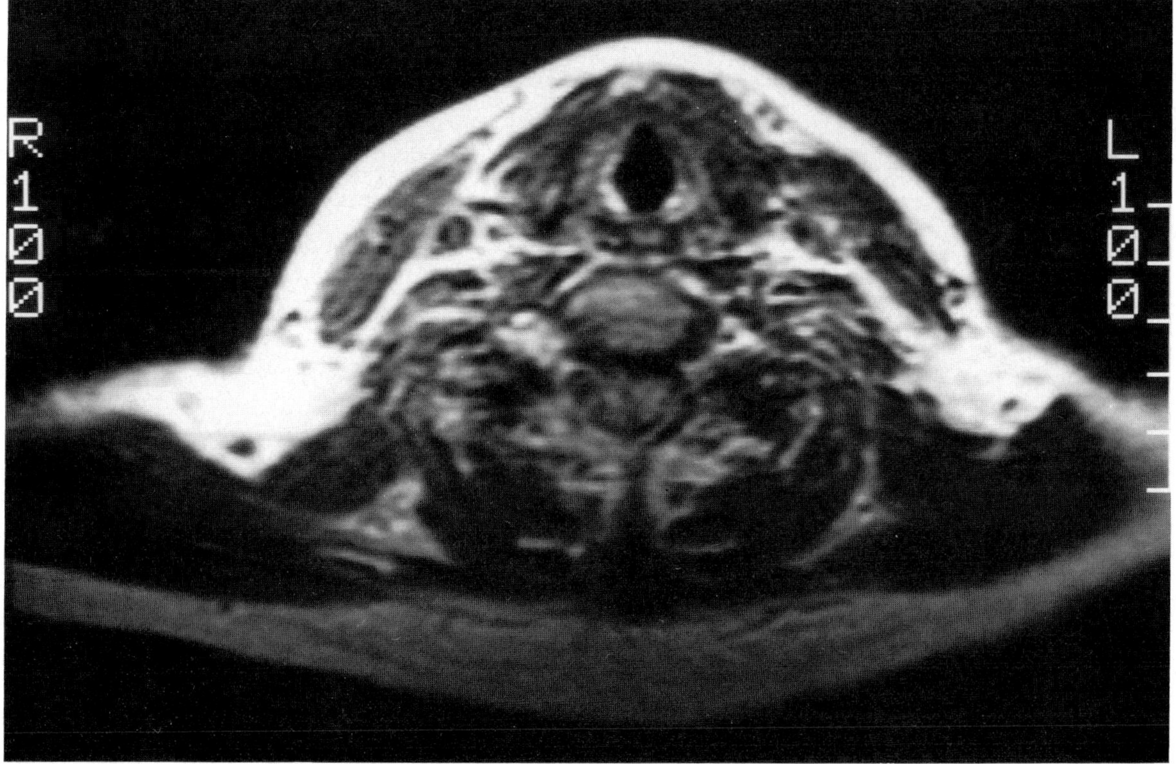

1-46 Head and neck, axial view (TR 2000; TE 30).

Cervical Spine, Lateral

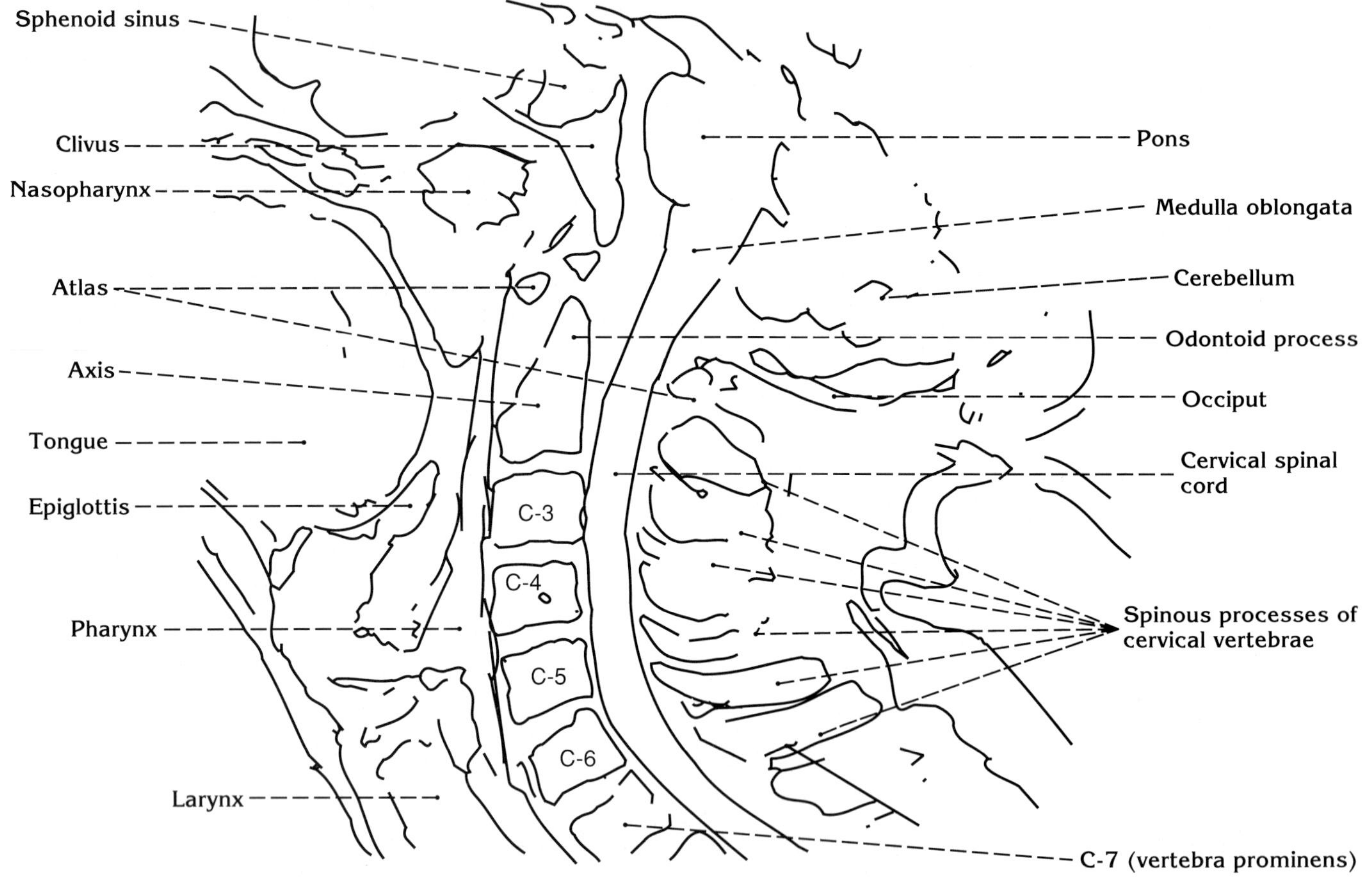

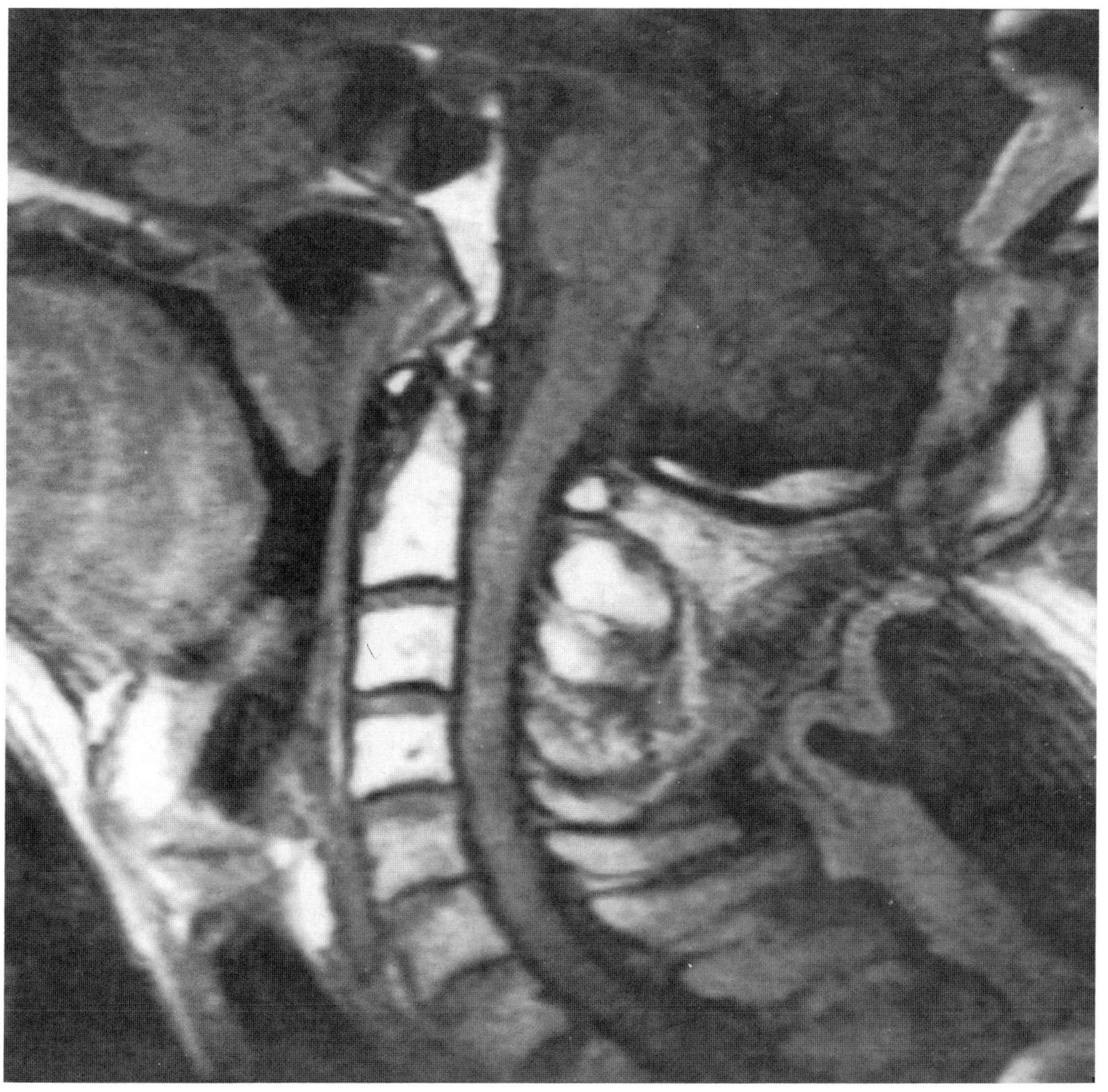

1-47 Cervical spine, lateral view.

Cervical Spine, Coronal

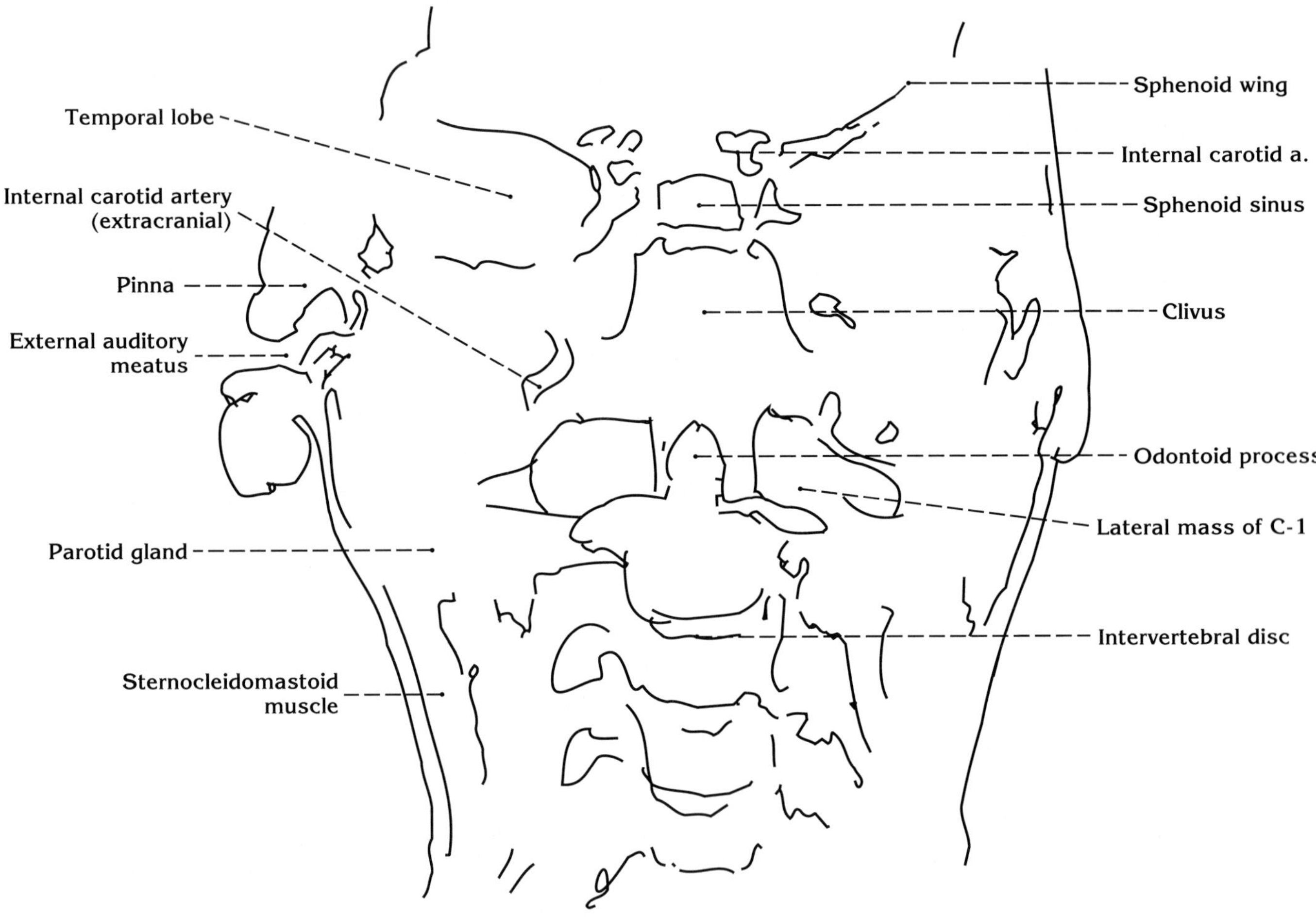

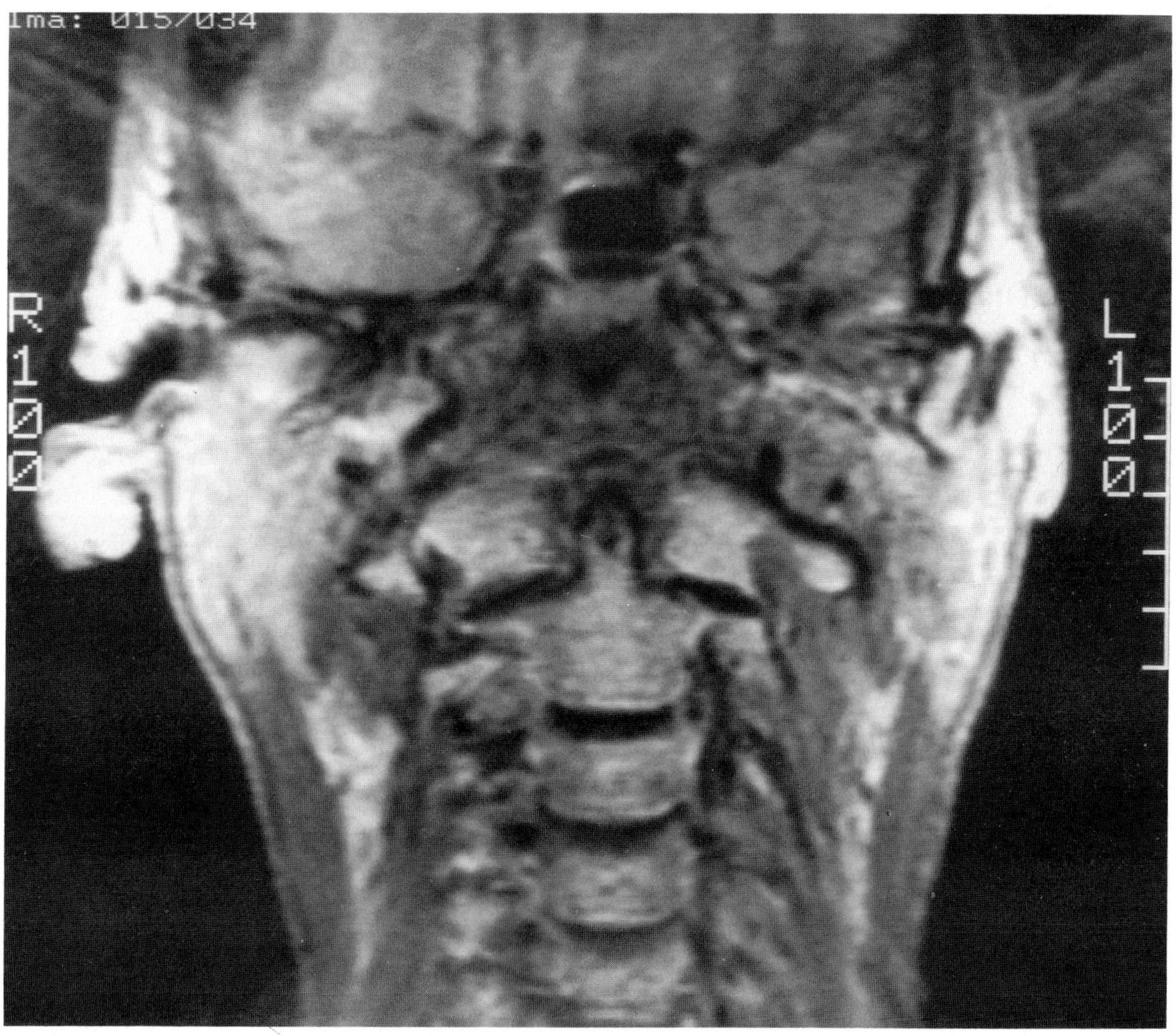

1-48 Cervical spine, coronal view.

Thoracic Spine, Sagittal

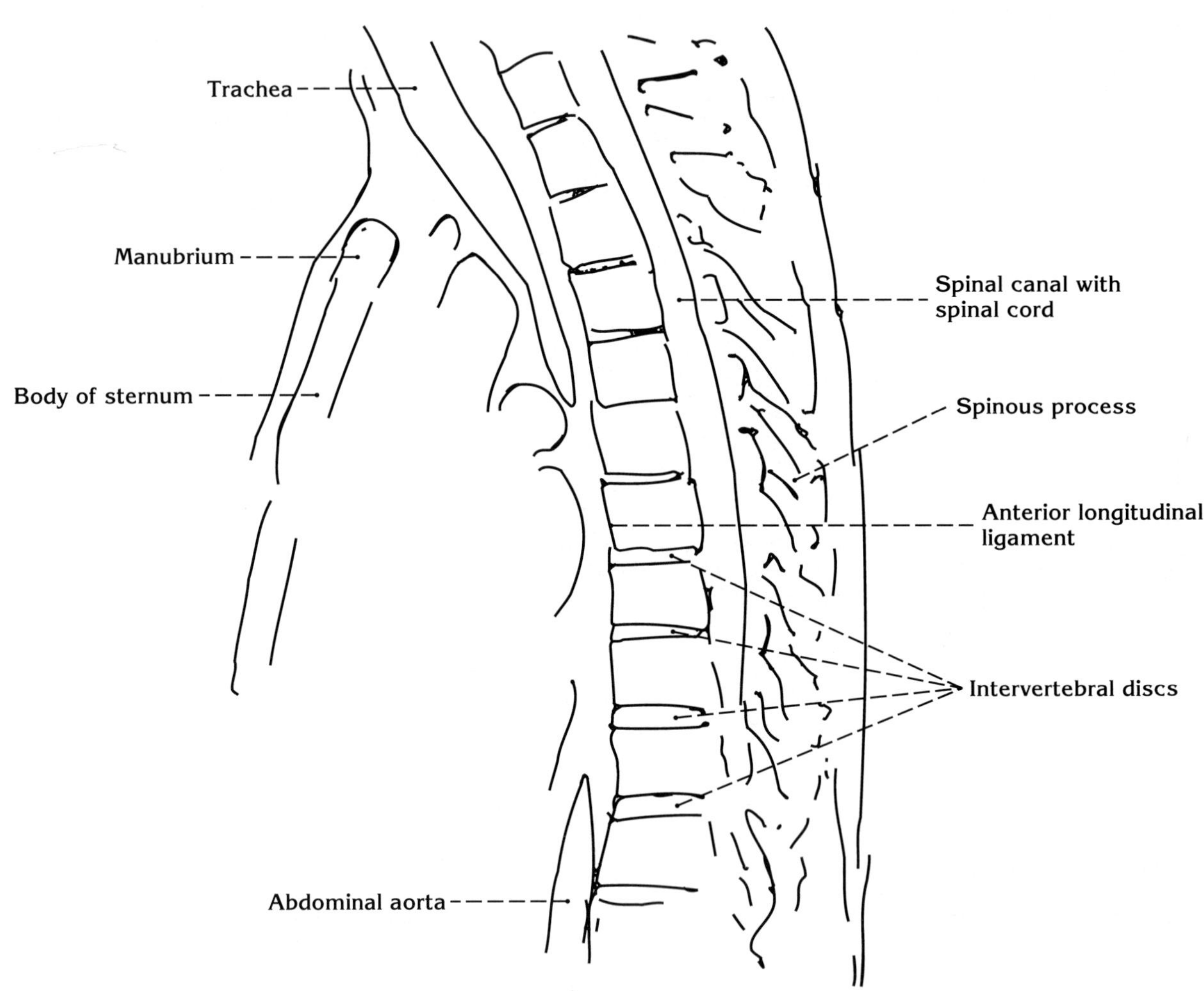

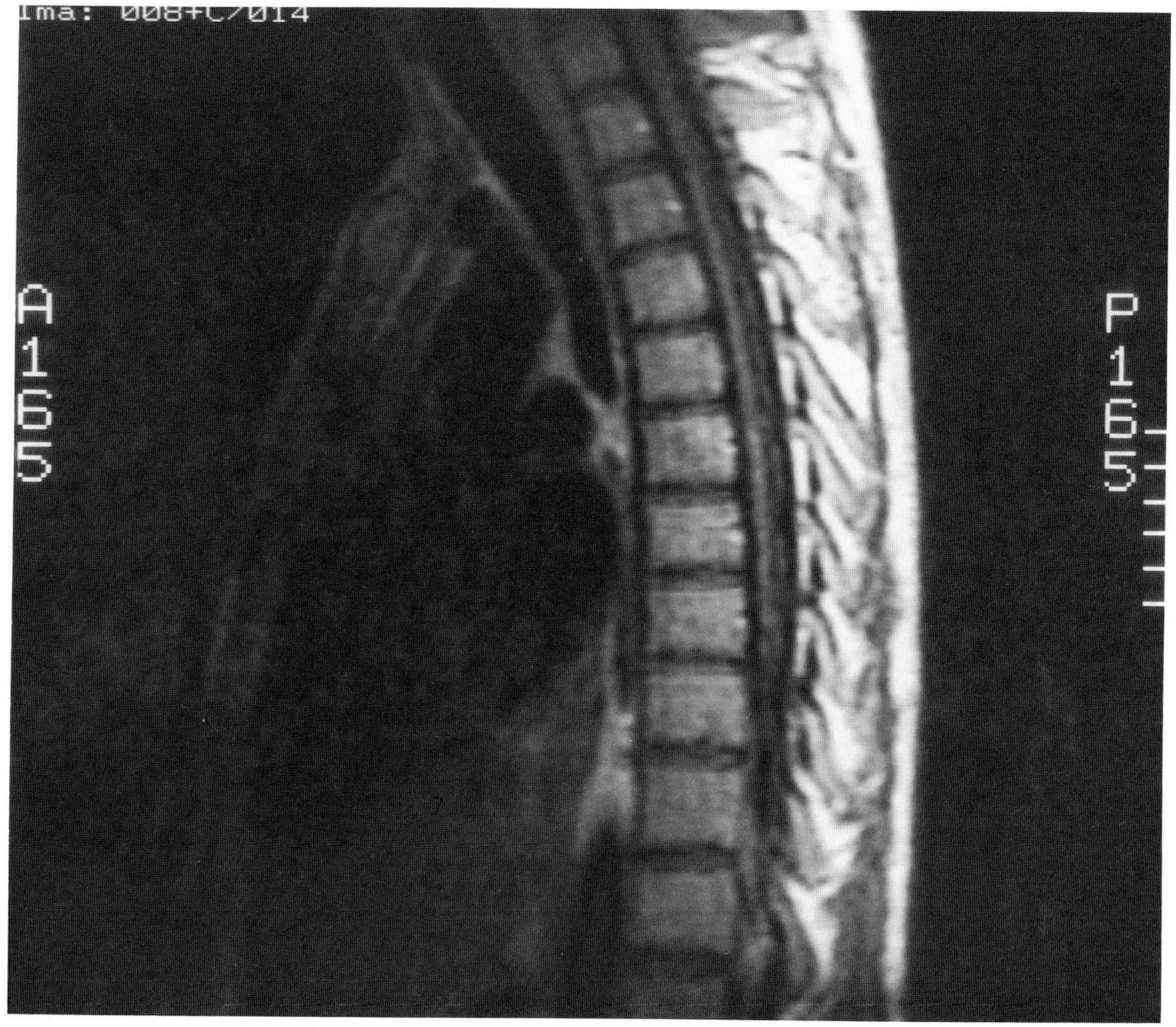

1-49 Thoracic spine, sagittal view (TR 600; TE 15).

Lumbosacral Spine, Midsagittal

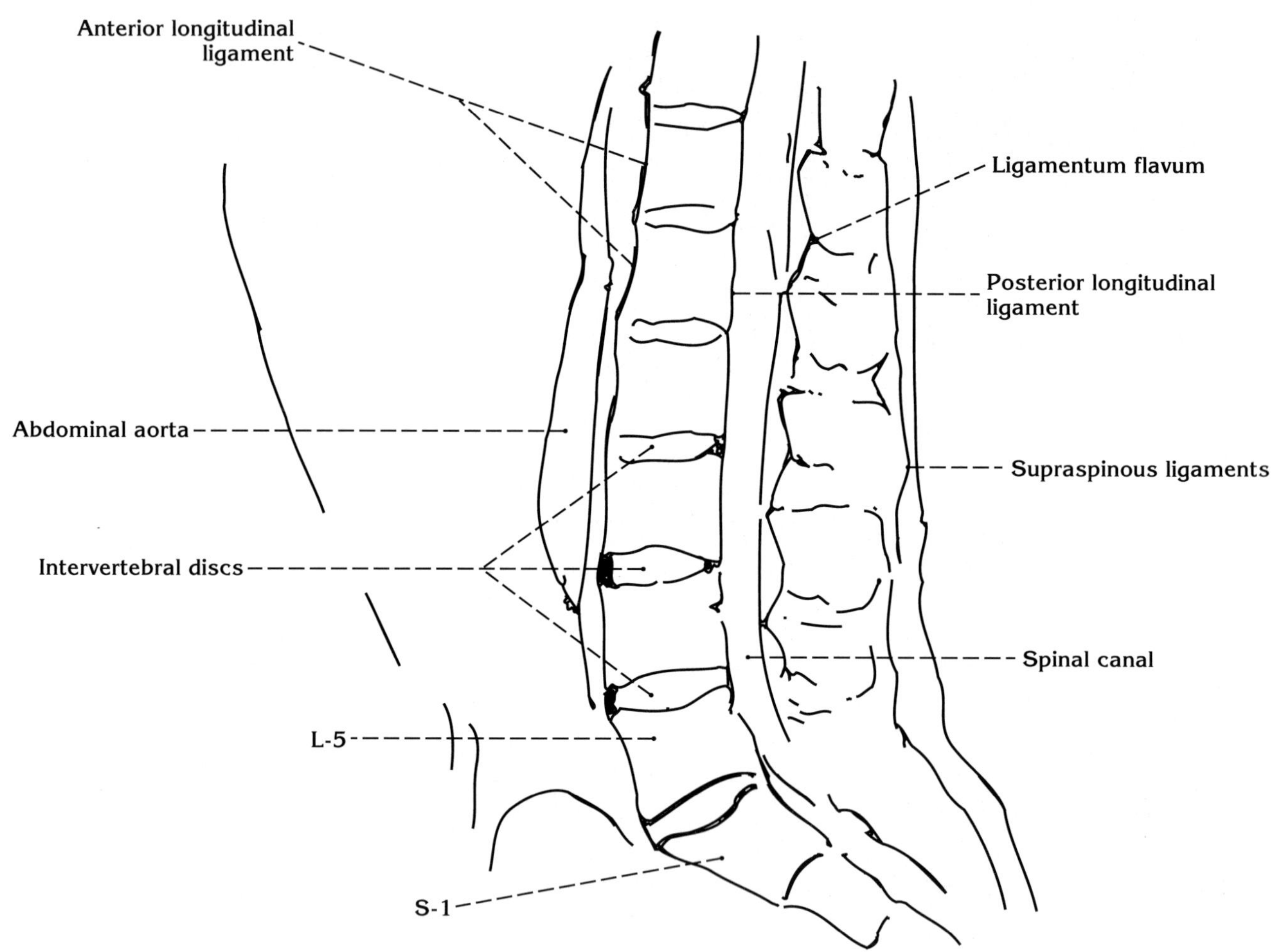

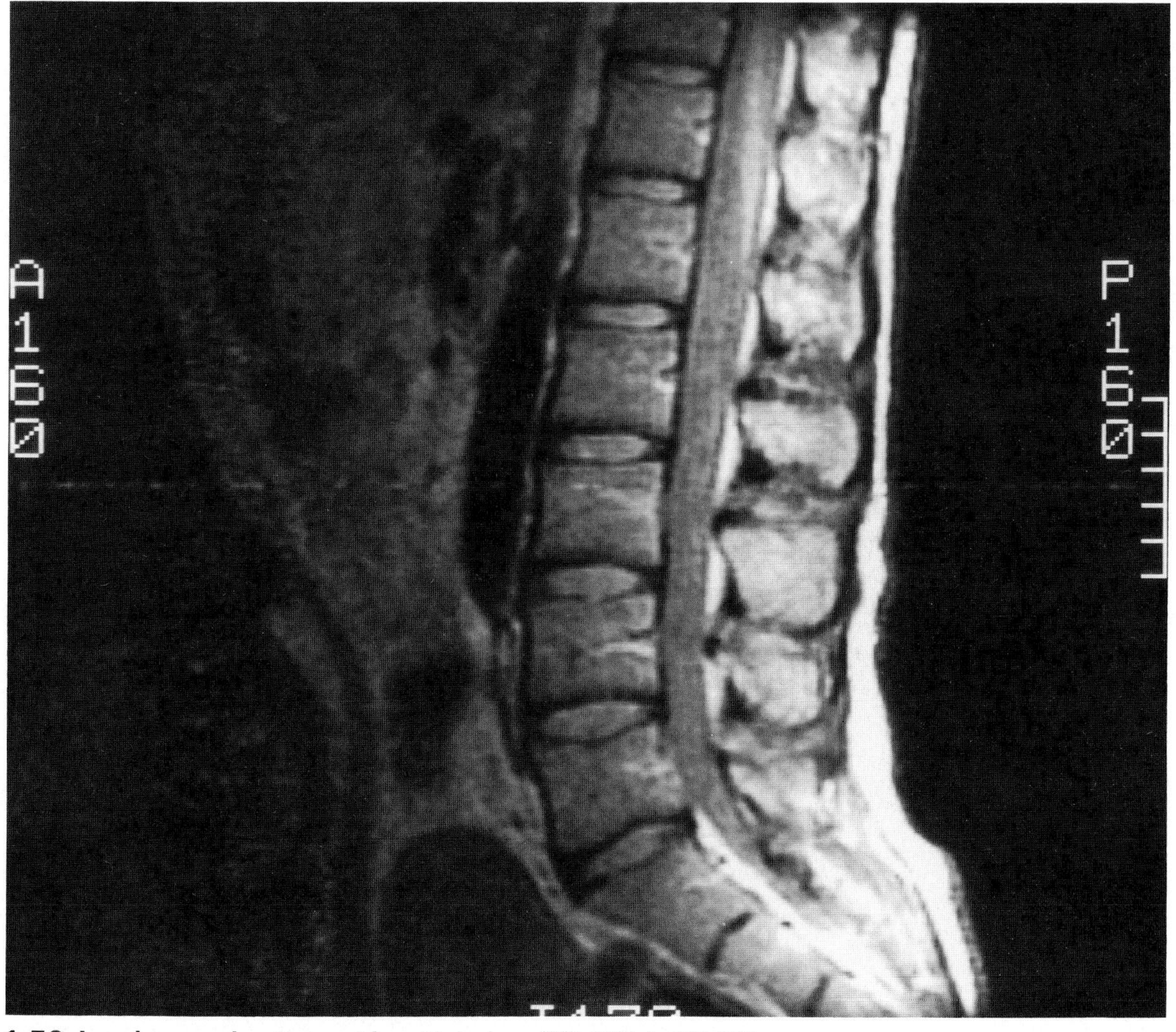

1-50 Lumbosacral spine, midsagittal view (TR 1714; TE 30).

Lumbosacral Spine, Parasagittal

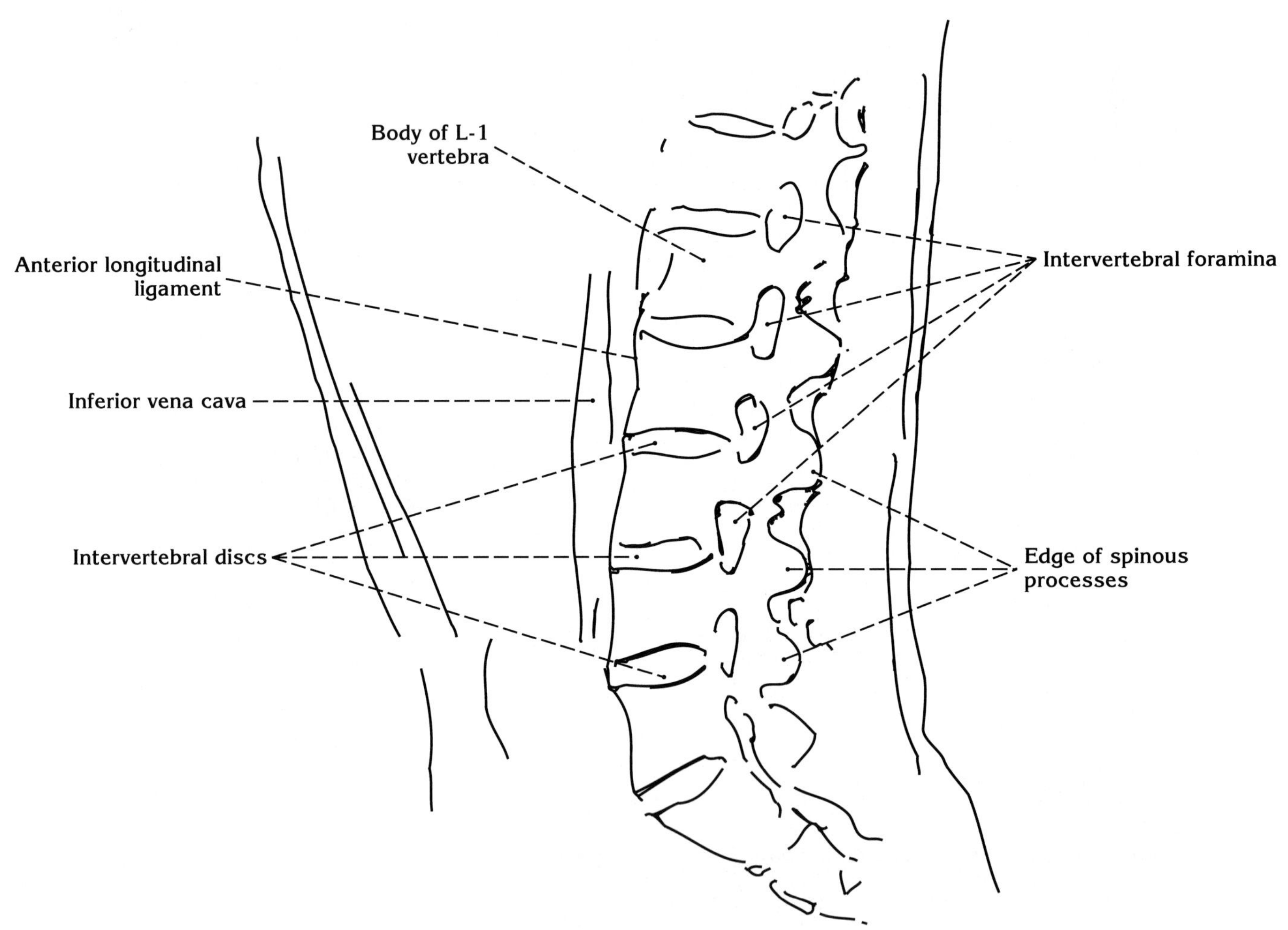

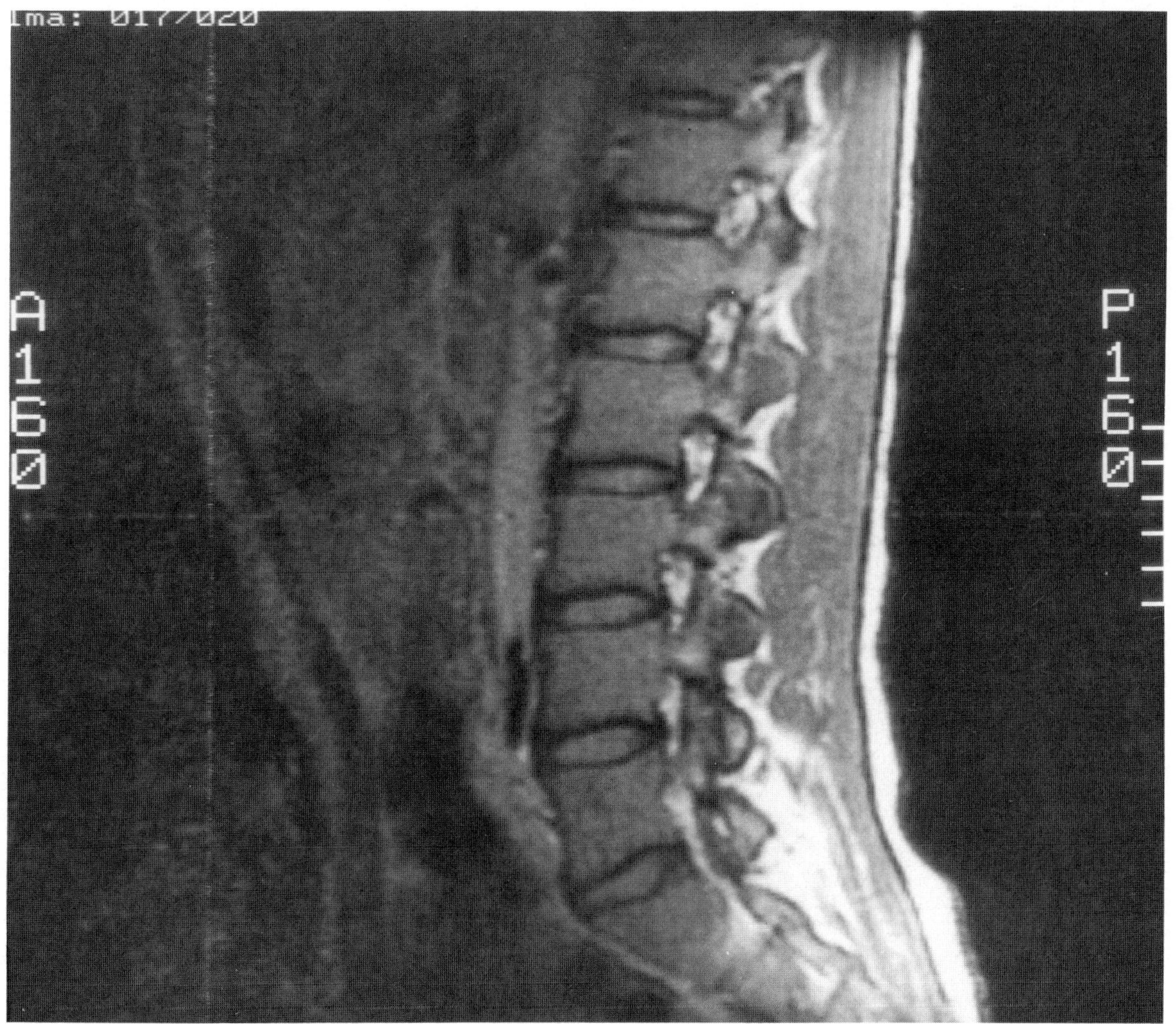

1-51 Lumbosacral spine, parasagittal view (TR 1714; TE 30).

TMJ (Closed), Sagittal

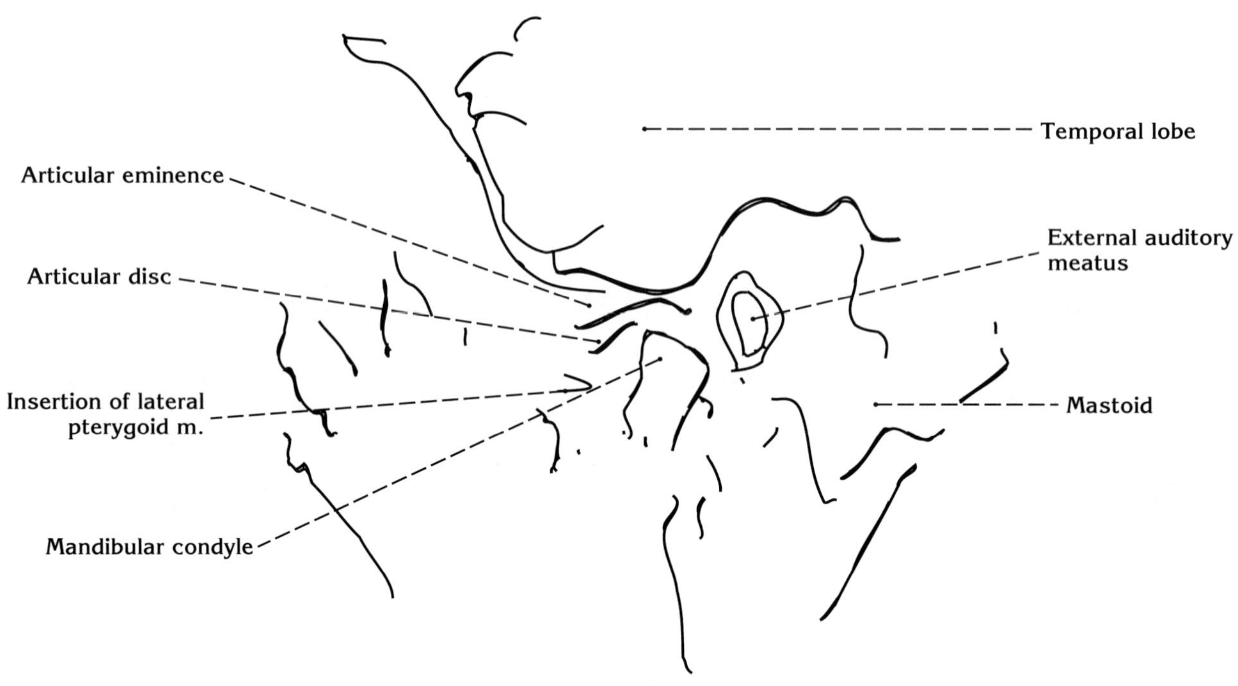

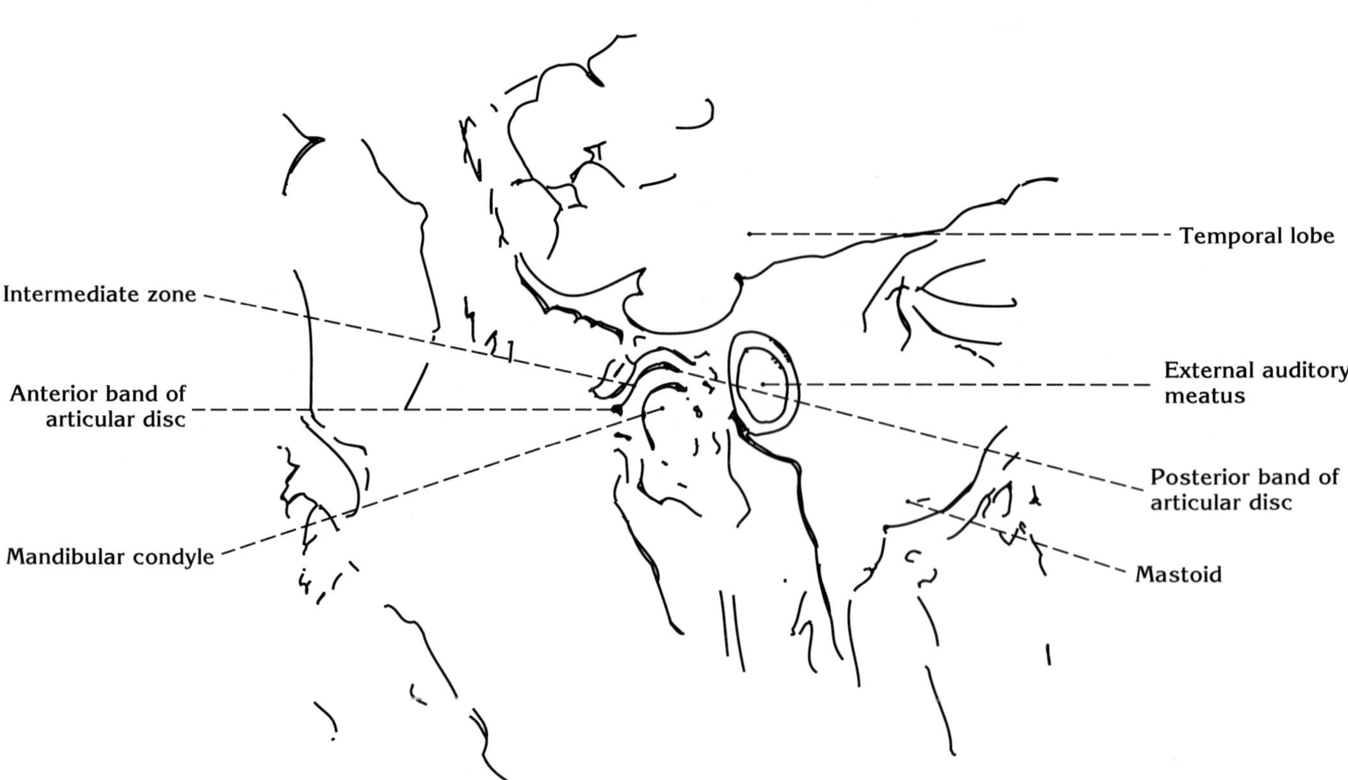

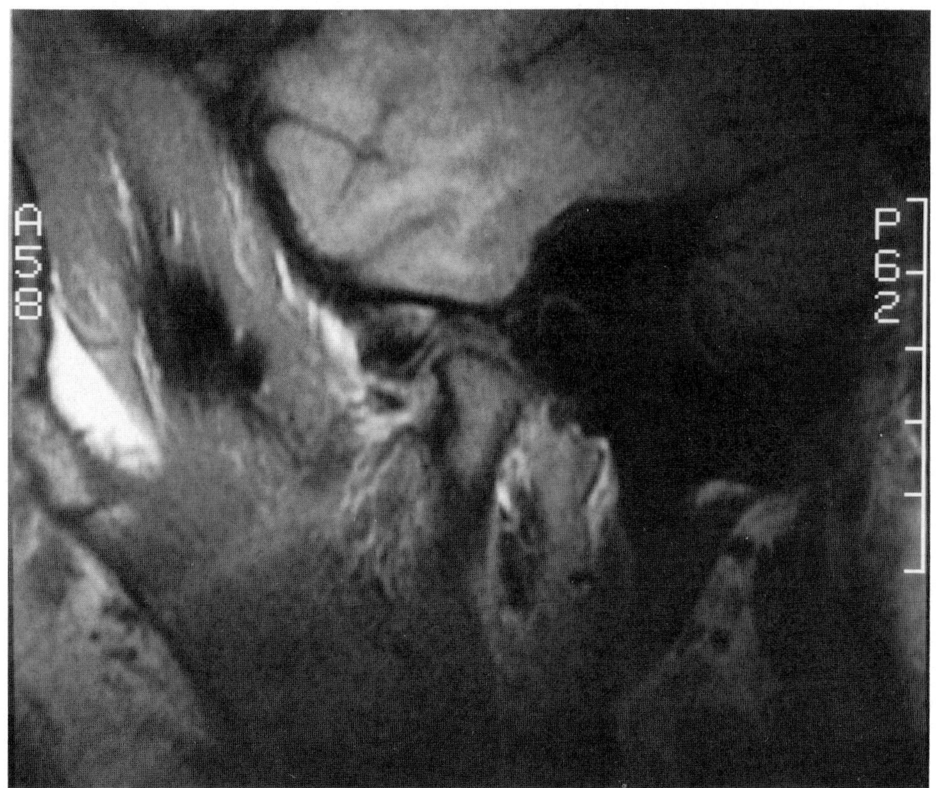

1-52 Temporomandibular joint (closed), sagittal view (TR 1000; TE 20).

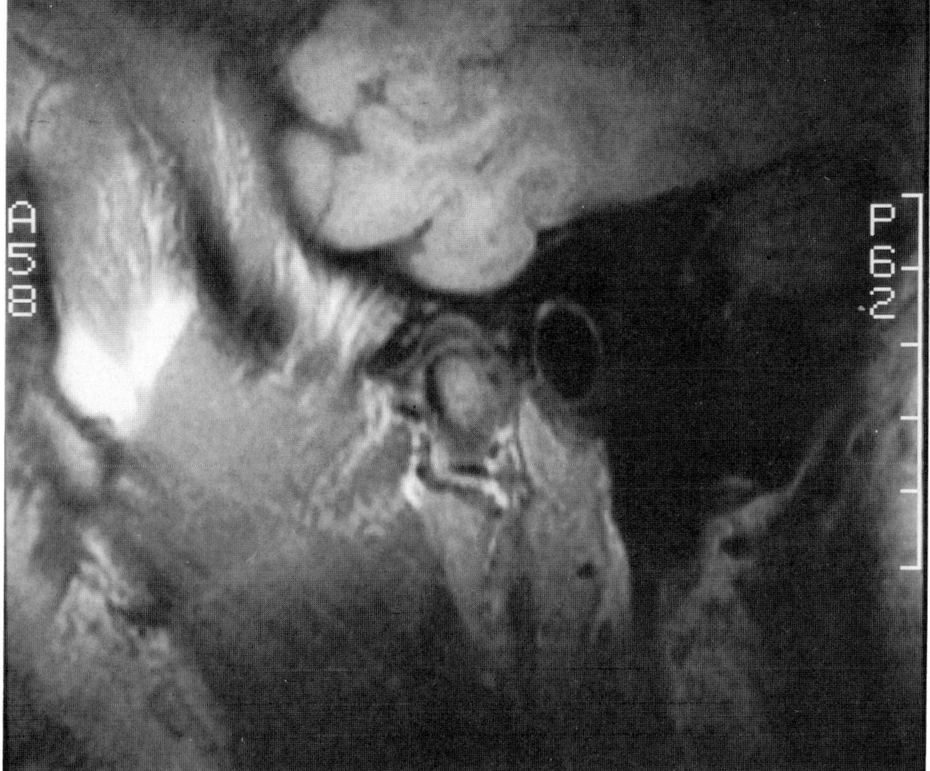

1-53 Temporomandibular joint (closed), sagittal view (TR 1000; TE 20).

Chest, Coronal

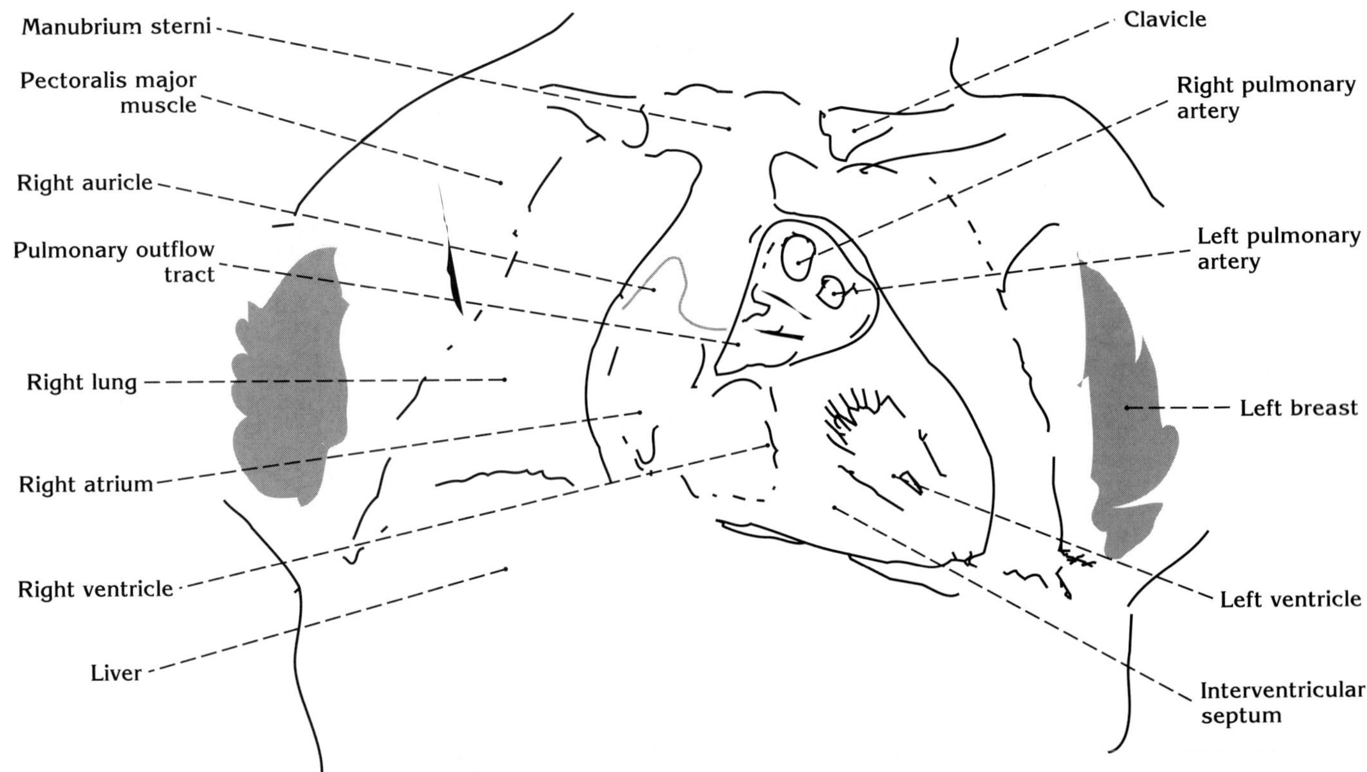

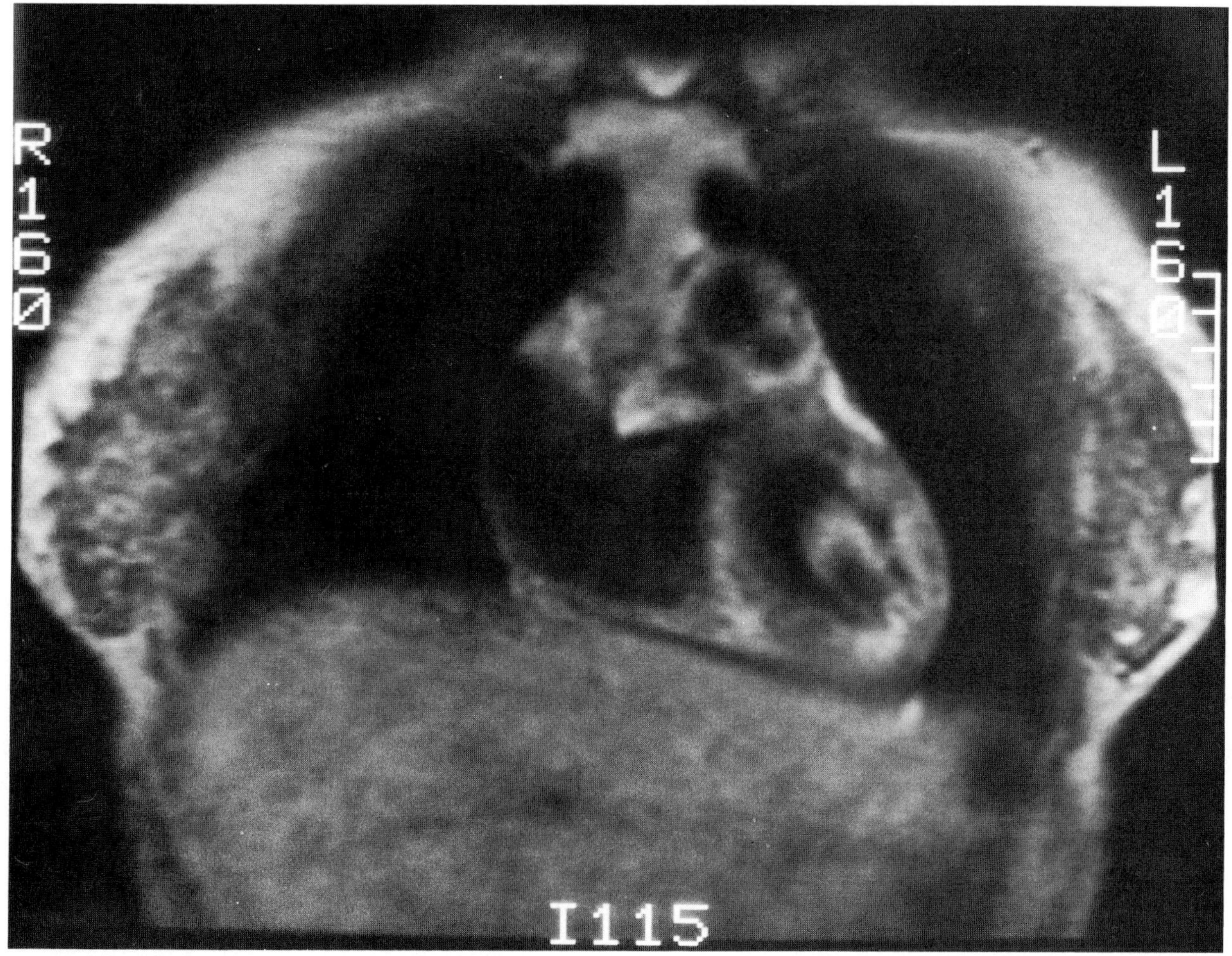

2-1 Chest, coronal view (TR 1333; TE 30).

Chest, Coronal

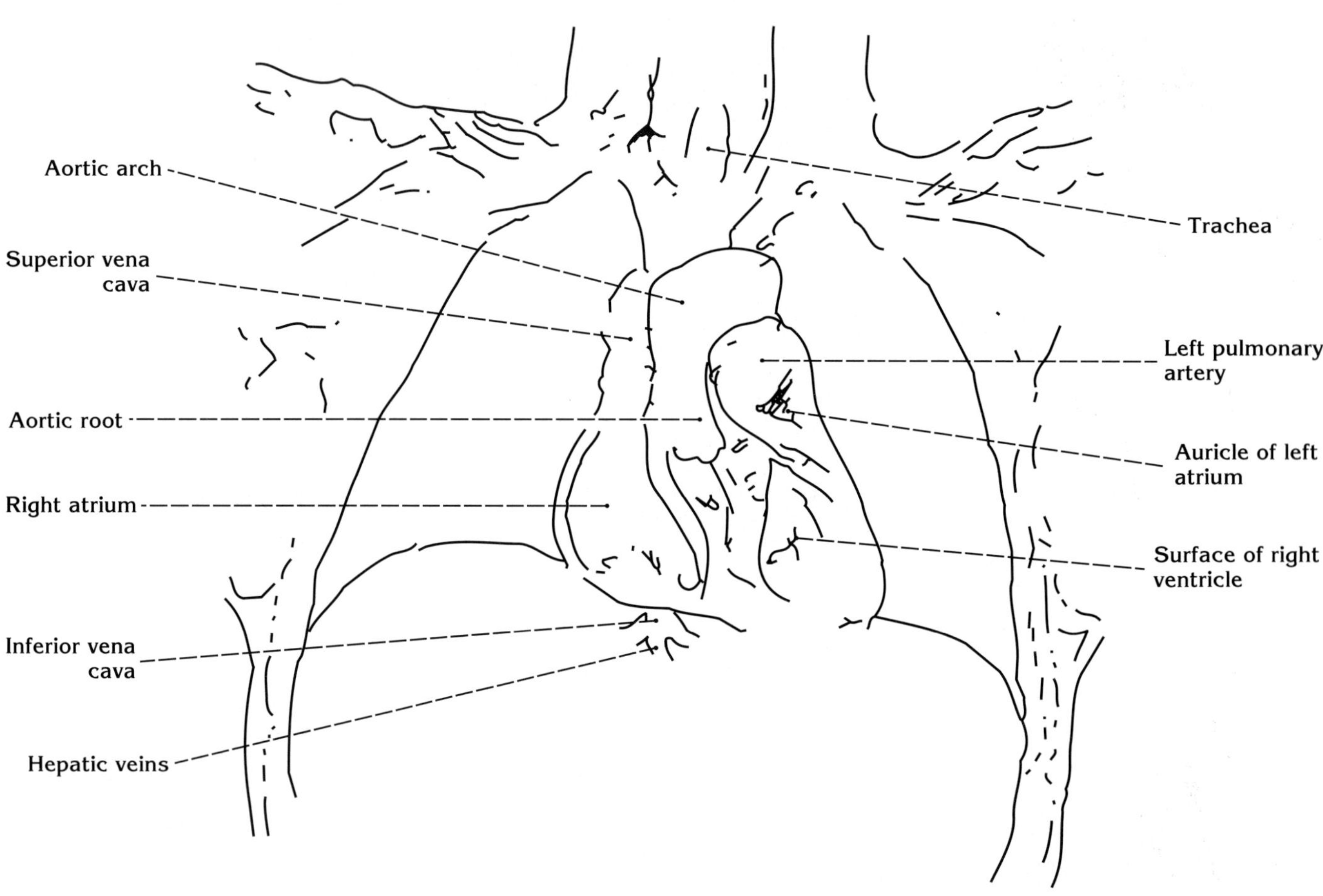

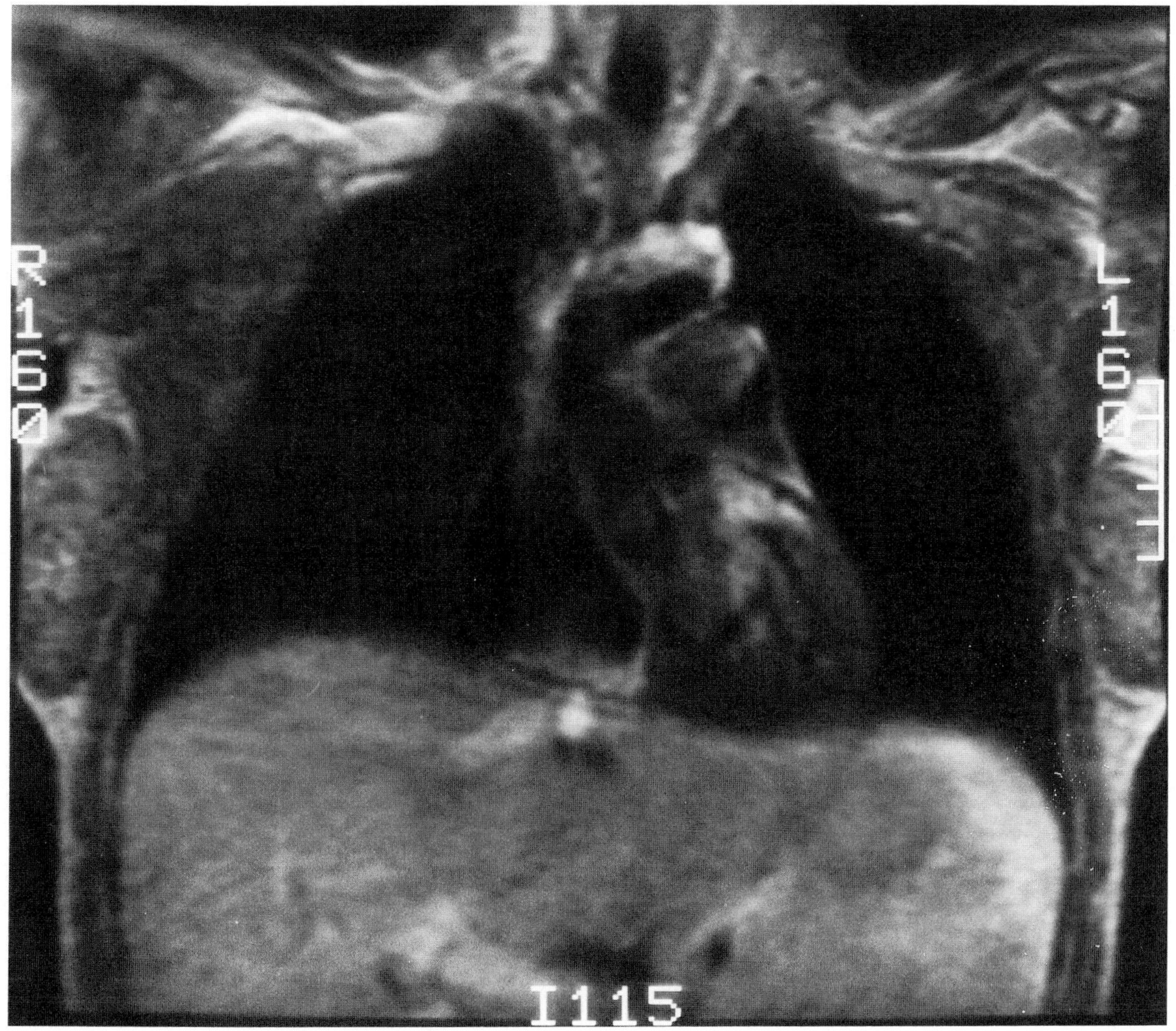

2-2 Chest, coronal view (TR 1333; TE 30).

Chest, Coronal

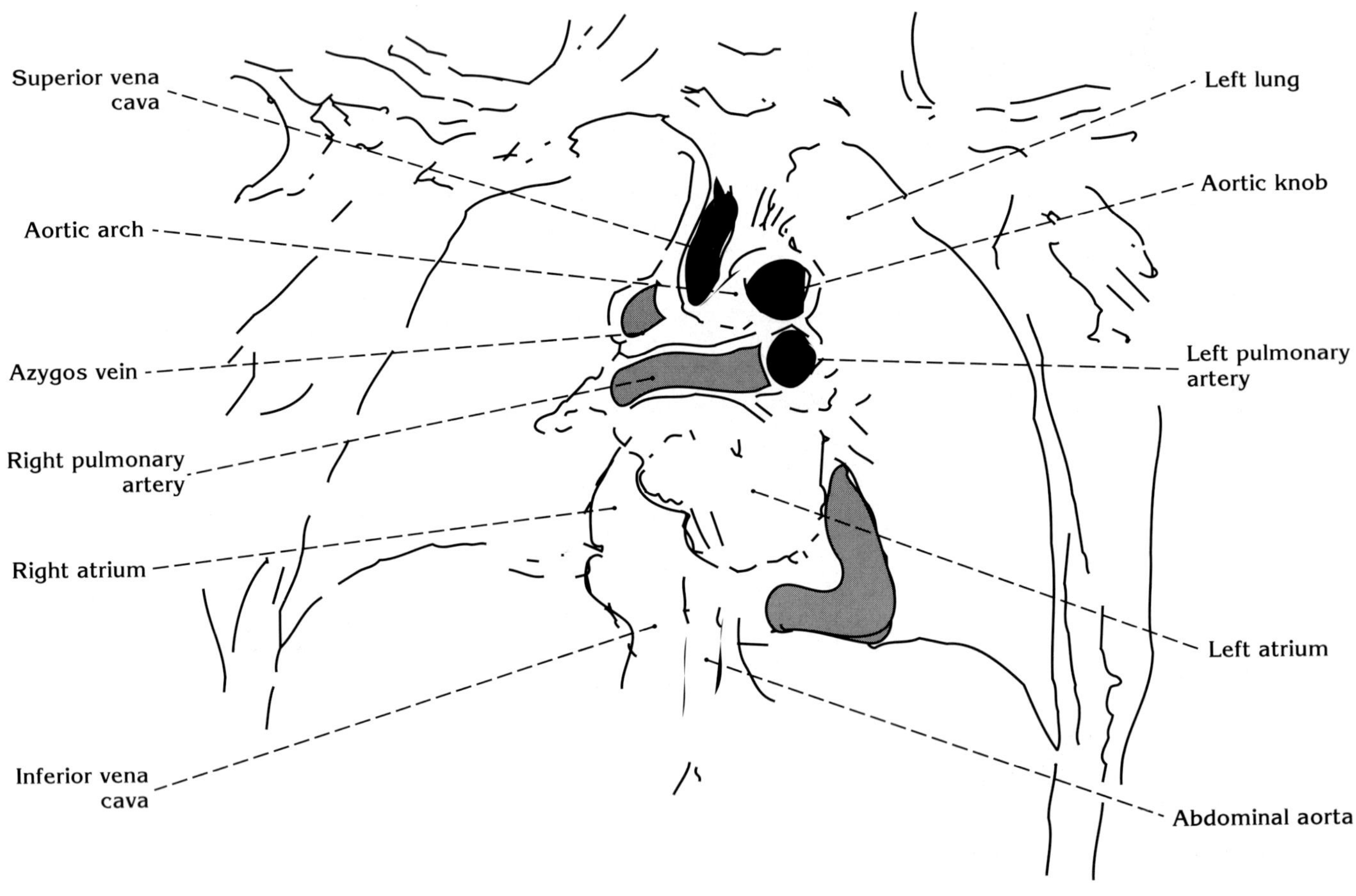

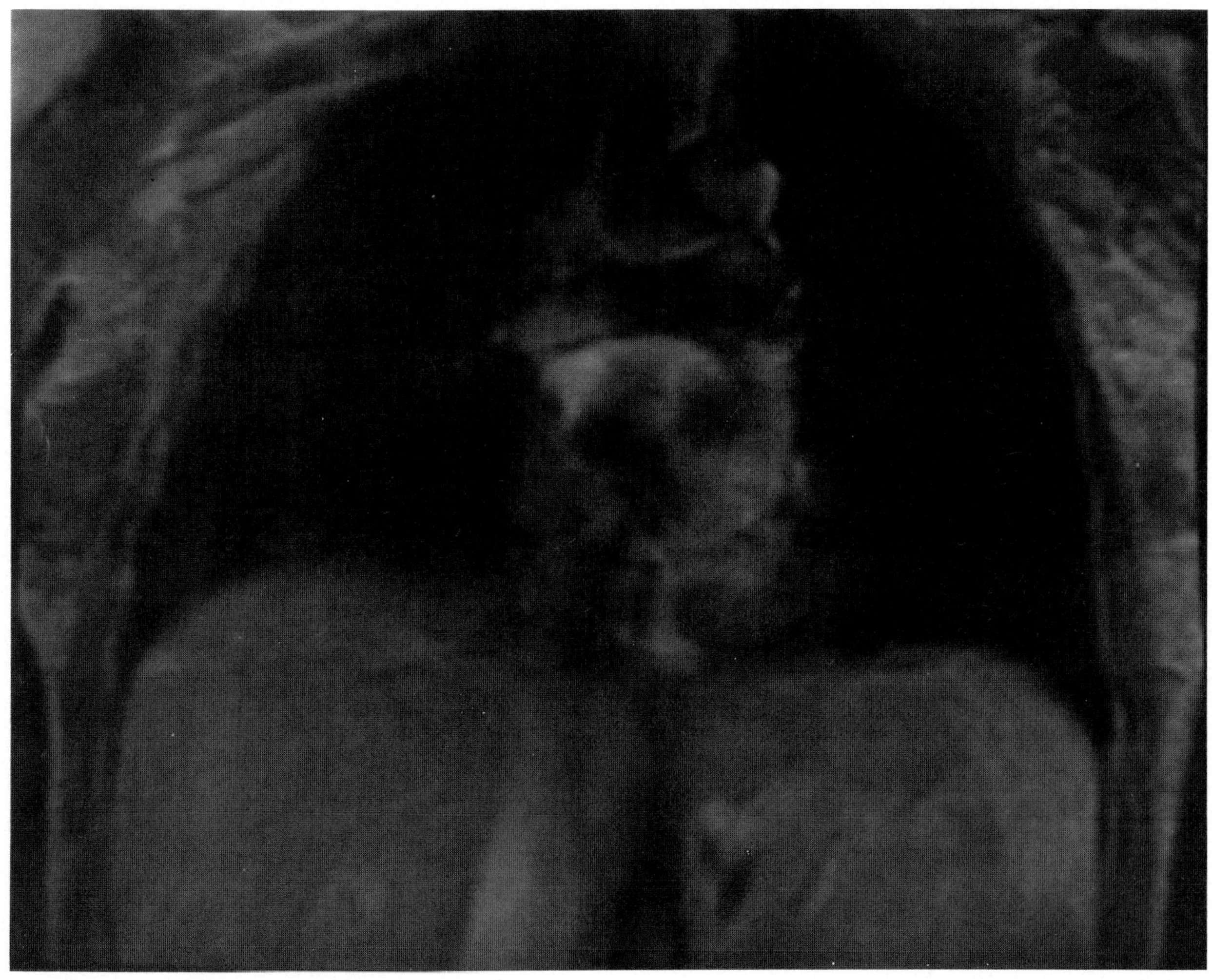

2-3 Chest, coronal view (TR 1333; TE 30).

Chest, Coronal

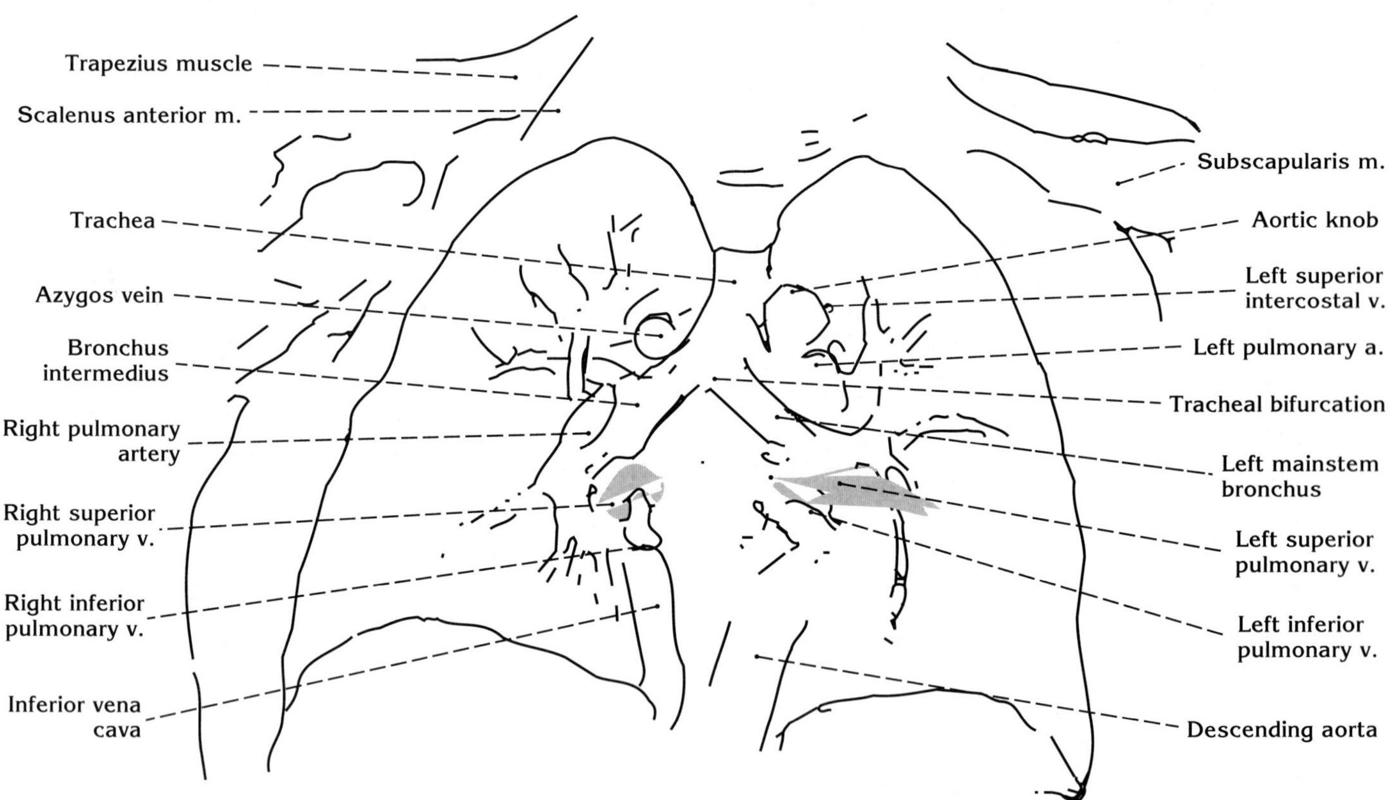

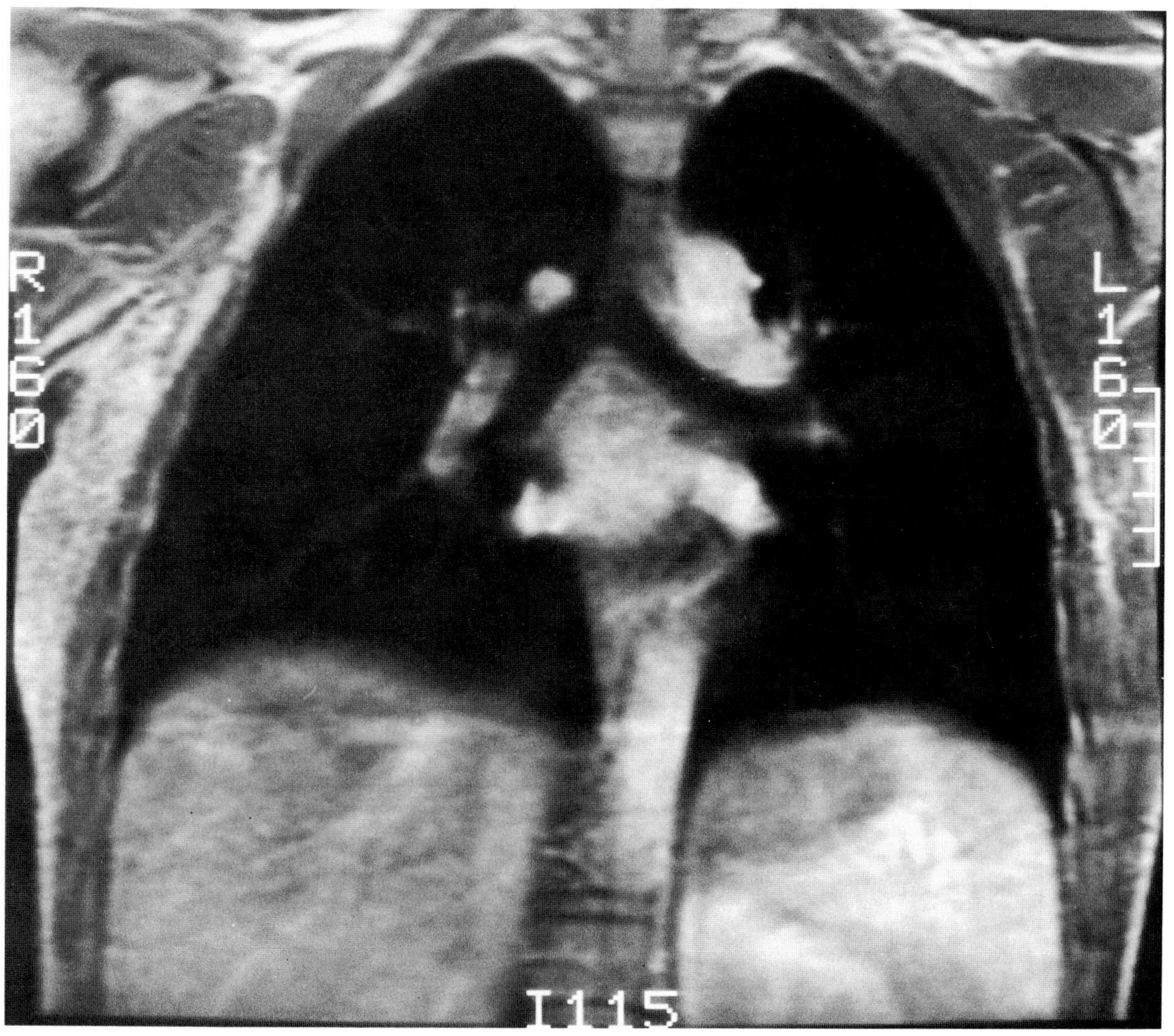

2-4 Chest, coronal view (TR 1333; TE 30).

Chest, Axial

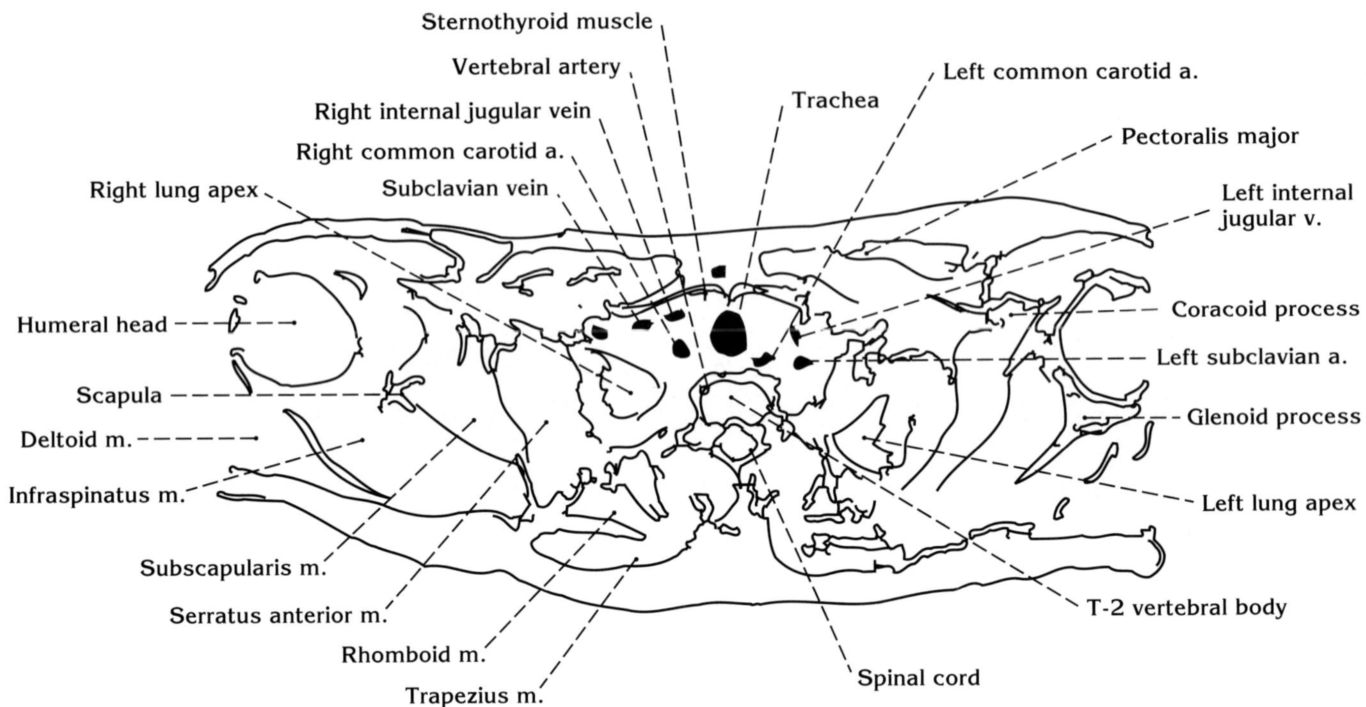
Sternothyroid muscle
Vertebral artery
Right internal jugular vein
Right common carotid a.
Subclavian vein
Right lung apex
Trachea
Left common carotid a.
Pectoralis major
Left internal jugular v.
Humeral head
Coracoid process
Left subclavian a.
Scapula
Glenoid process
Deltoid m.
Infraspinatus m.
Left lung apex
Subscapularis m.
Serratus anterior m.
T-2 vertebral body
Rhomboid m.
Trapezius m.
Spinal cord

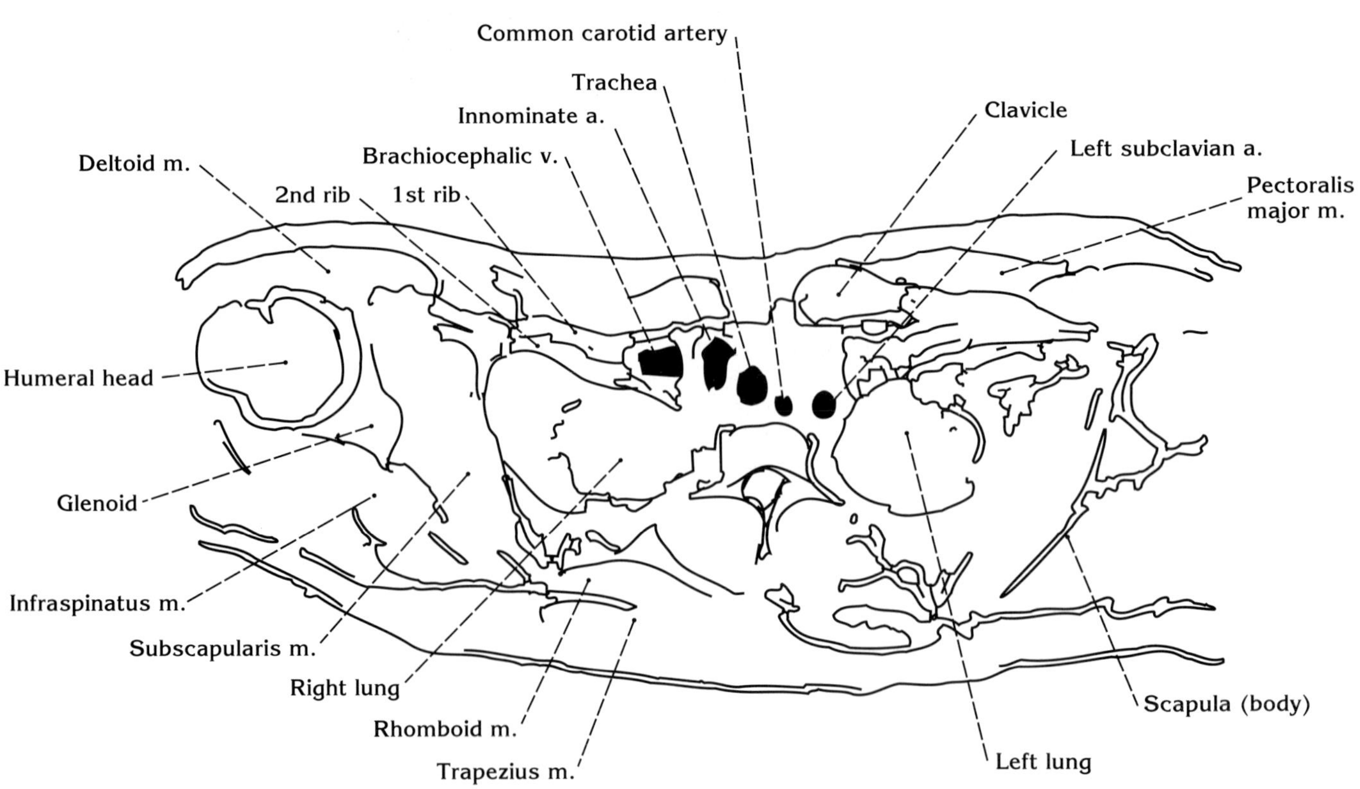
Common carotid artery
Trachea
Innominate a.
Clavicle
Left subclavian a.
Brachiocephalic v.
Deltoid m.
2nd rib
1st rib
Pectoralis major m.
Humeral head
Glenoid
Infraspinatus m.
Subscapularis m.
Right lung
Rhomboid m.
Trapezius m.
Scapula (body)
Left lung

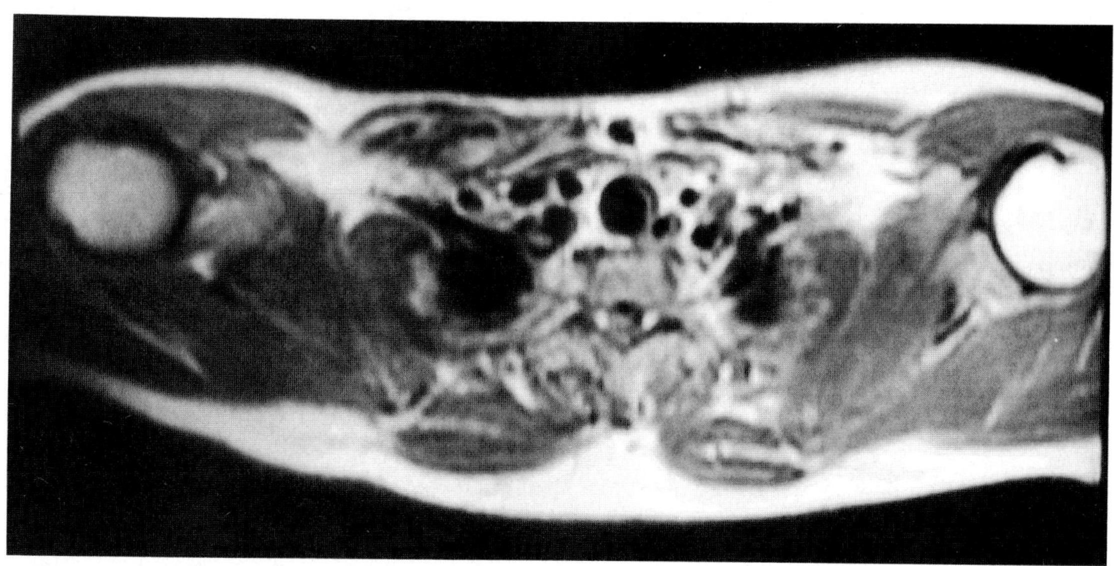

2-5 Chest, axial view (TR 1667; TE 20).

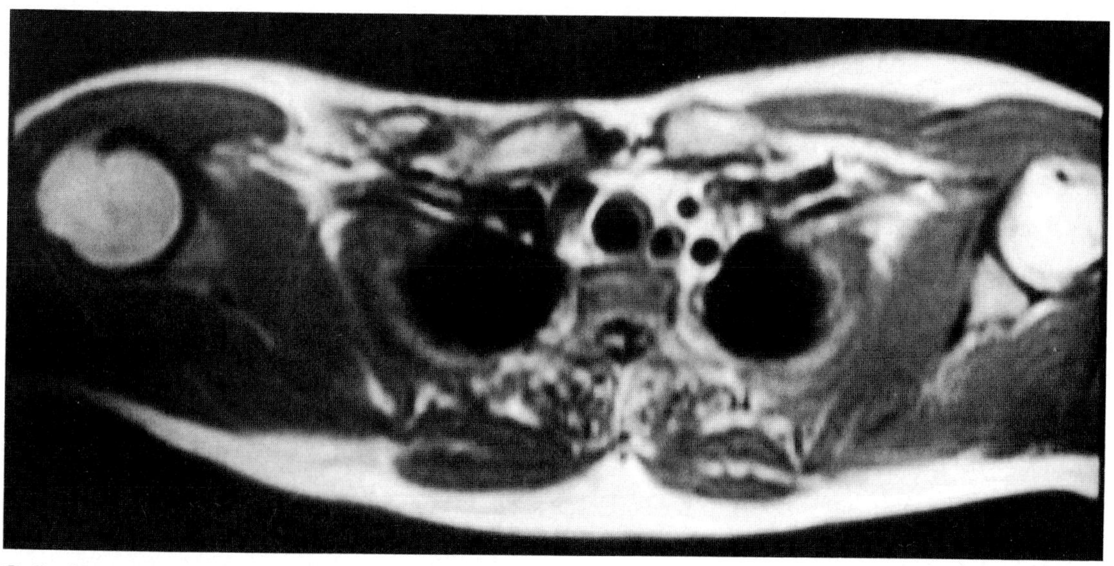

2-6 Chest, axial view (TR 1667; TE 20).

Chest, Axial

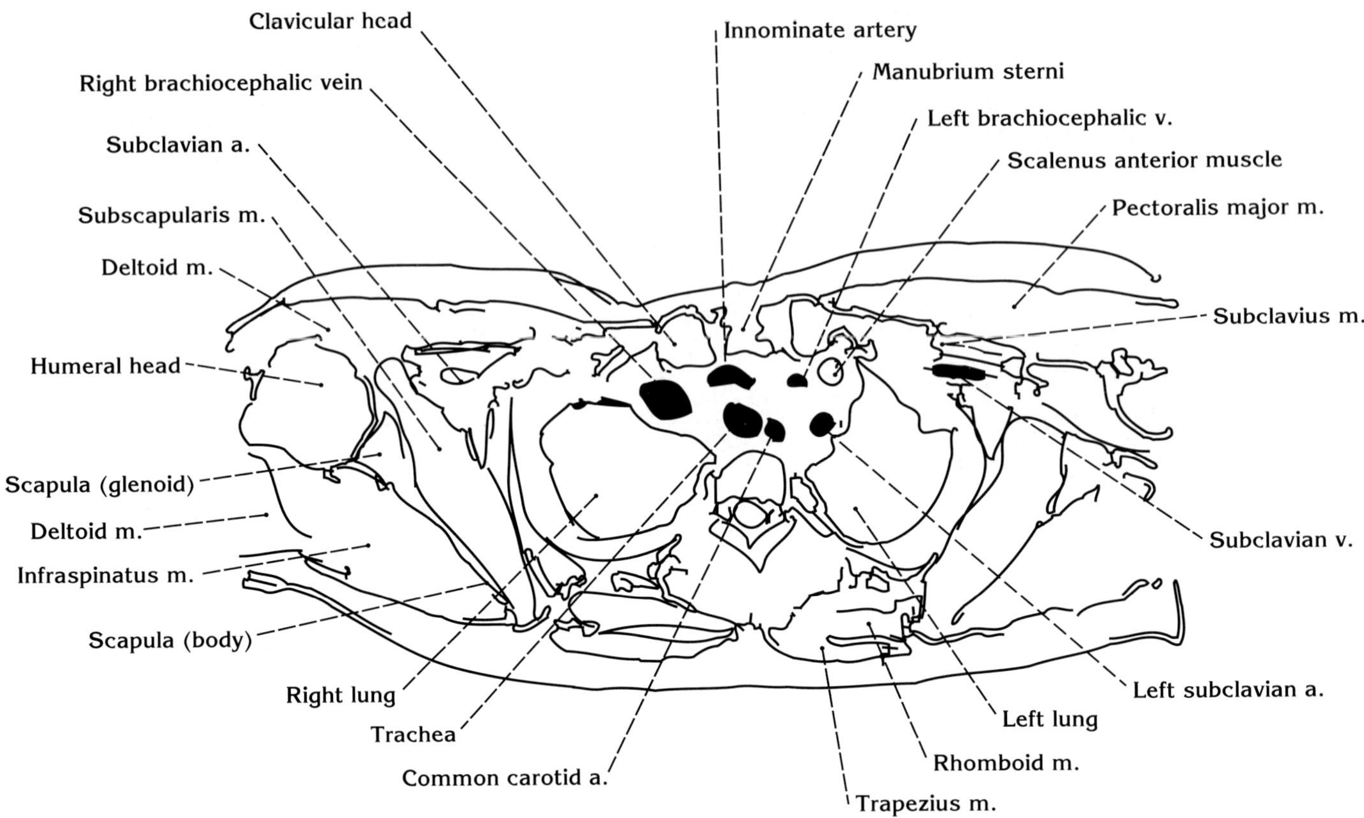
Clavicular head
Innominate artery
Right brachiocephalic vein
Manubrium sterni
Left brachiocephalic v.
Subclavian a.
Scalenus anterior muscle
Subscapularis m.
Pectoralis major m.
Deltoid m.
Subclavius m.
Humeral head
Scapula (glenoid)
Deltoid m.
Subclavian v.
Infraspinatus m.
Scapula (body)
Left subclavian a.
Right lung
Left lung
Trachea
Rhomboid m.
Common carotid a.
Trapezius m.

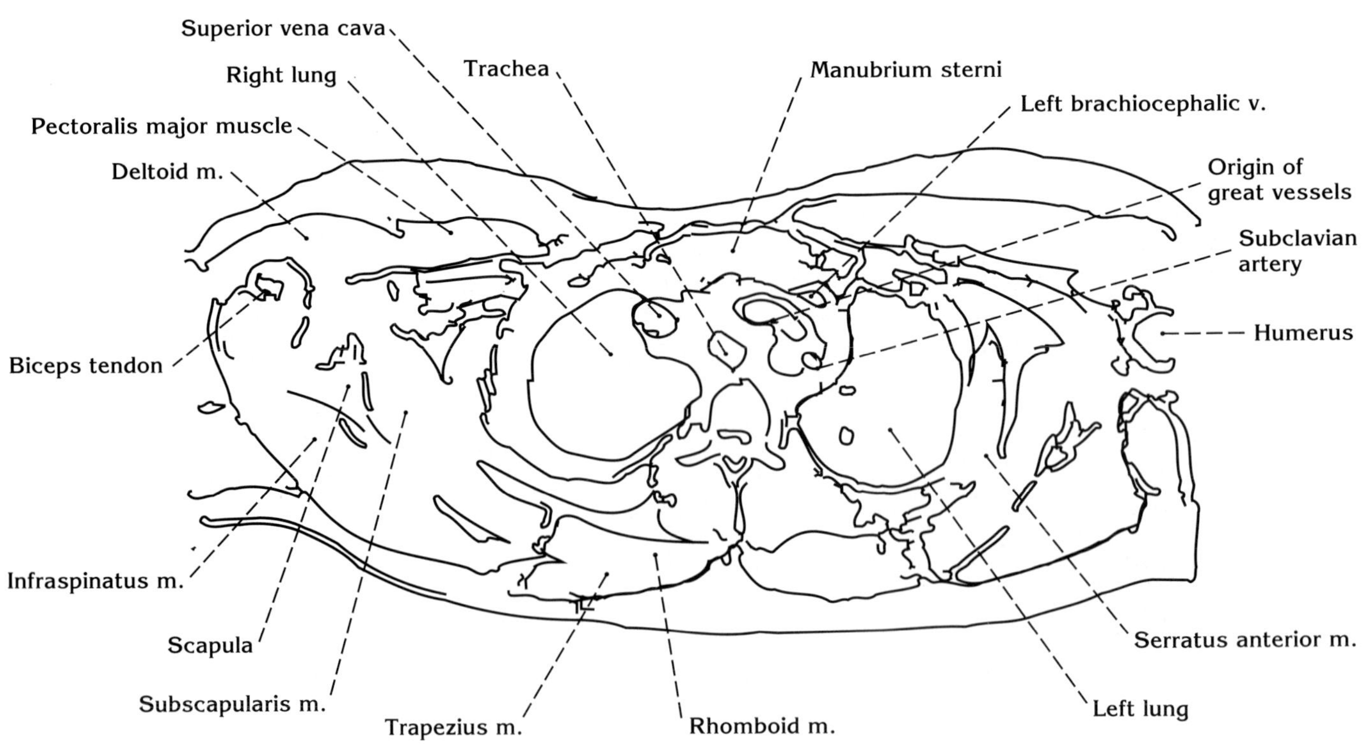
Superior vena cava
Right lung
Trachea
Manubrium sterni
Left brachiocephalic v.
Pectoralis major muscle
Origin of great vessels
Deltoid m.
Subclavian artery
Humerus
Biceps tendon
Infraspinatus m.
Serratus anterior m.
Scapula
Left lung
Subscapularis m.
Trapezius m.
Rhomboid m.

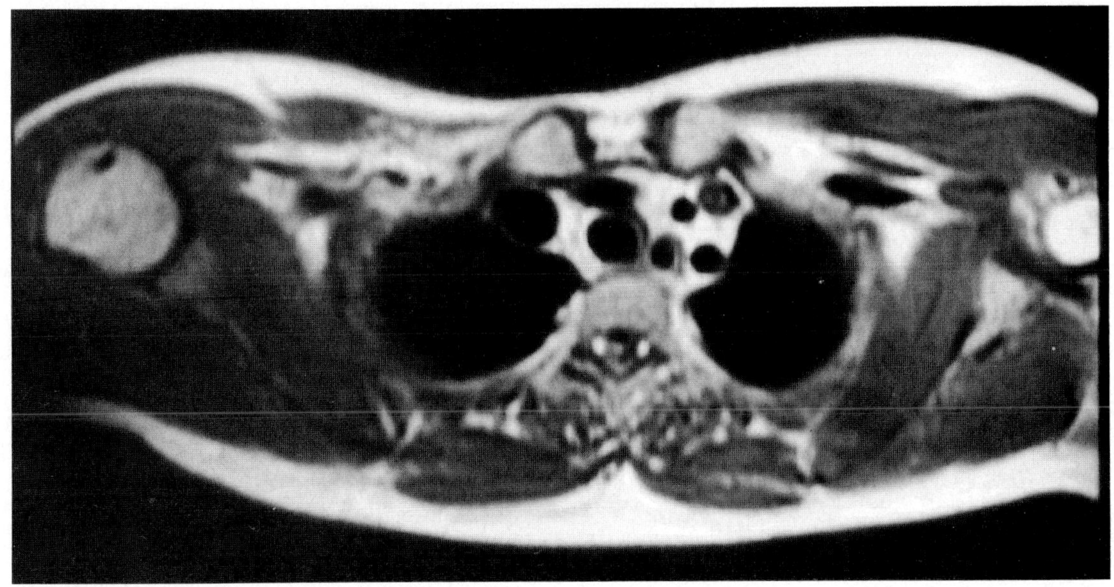

2-7 Chest, axial view (TR 1667; TE 20).

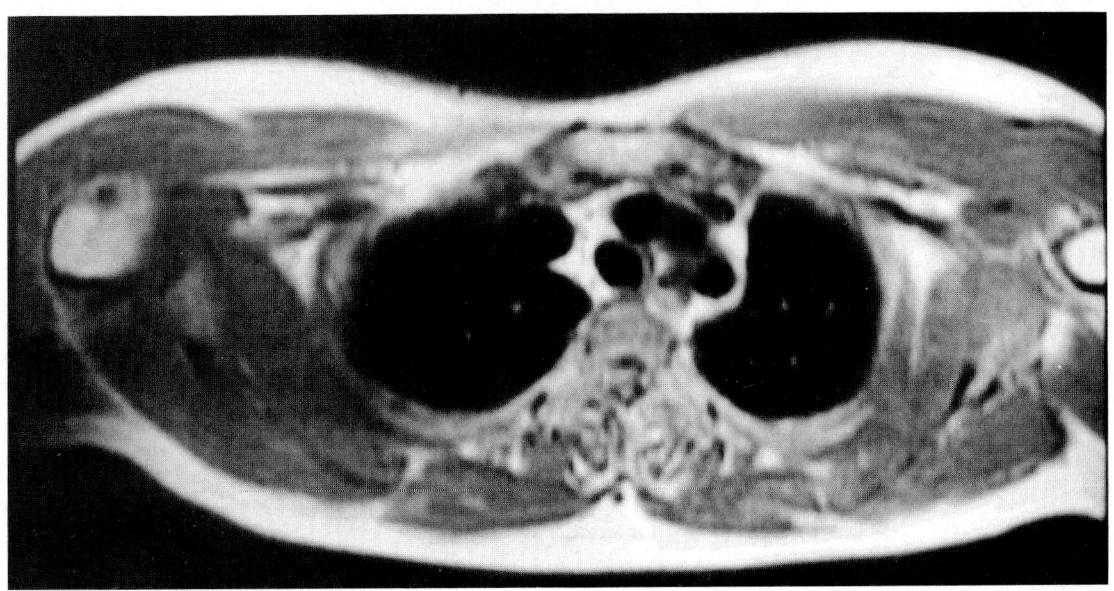

2-8 Chest, axial view (TR 1667; TE 20).

Chest, Axial

Superior vena cava
Right lung
Trachea
Aortic arch
Accessory hemiazygos v.
Deltoid m.
Biceps tendon
Humerus
Infraspinatus m.
Scapula
Subscapularis m.
Trapezius m.
Rhomboid m.
Serratus anterior m.
Left lung

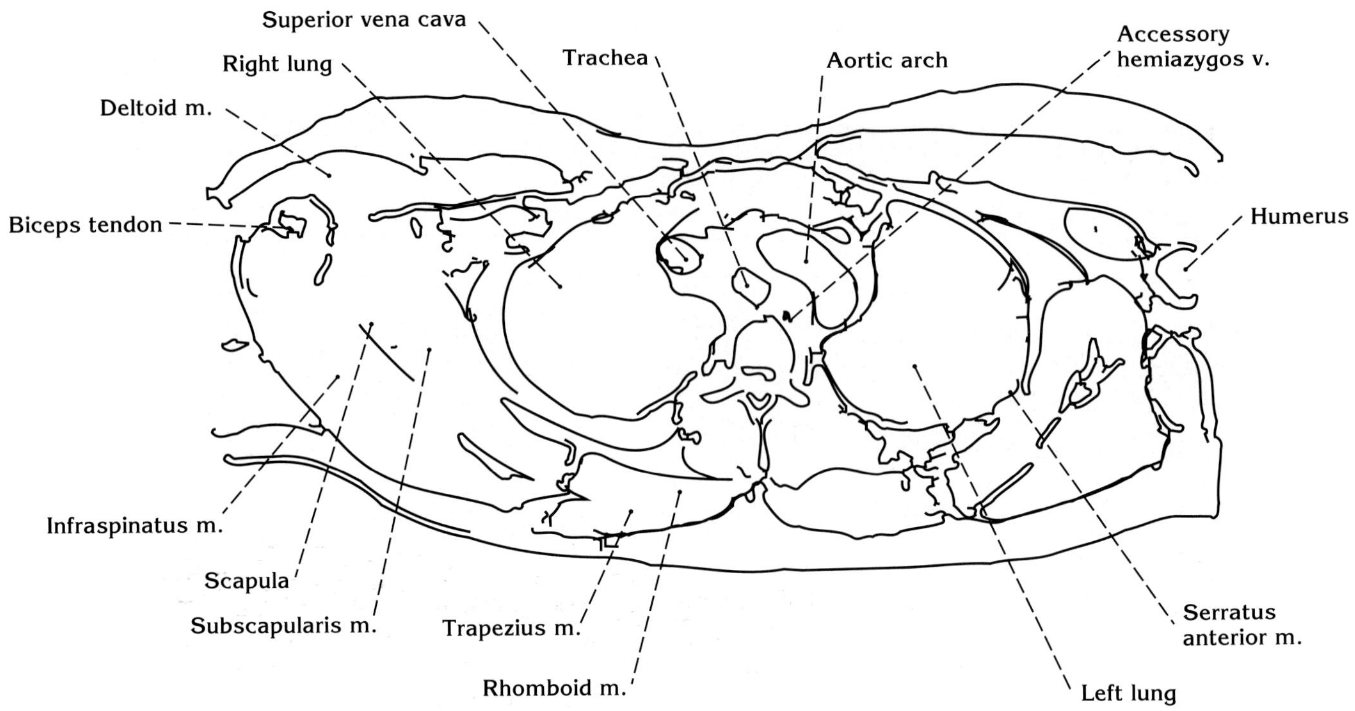

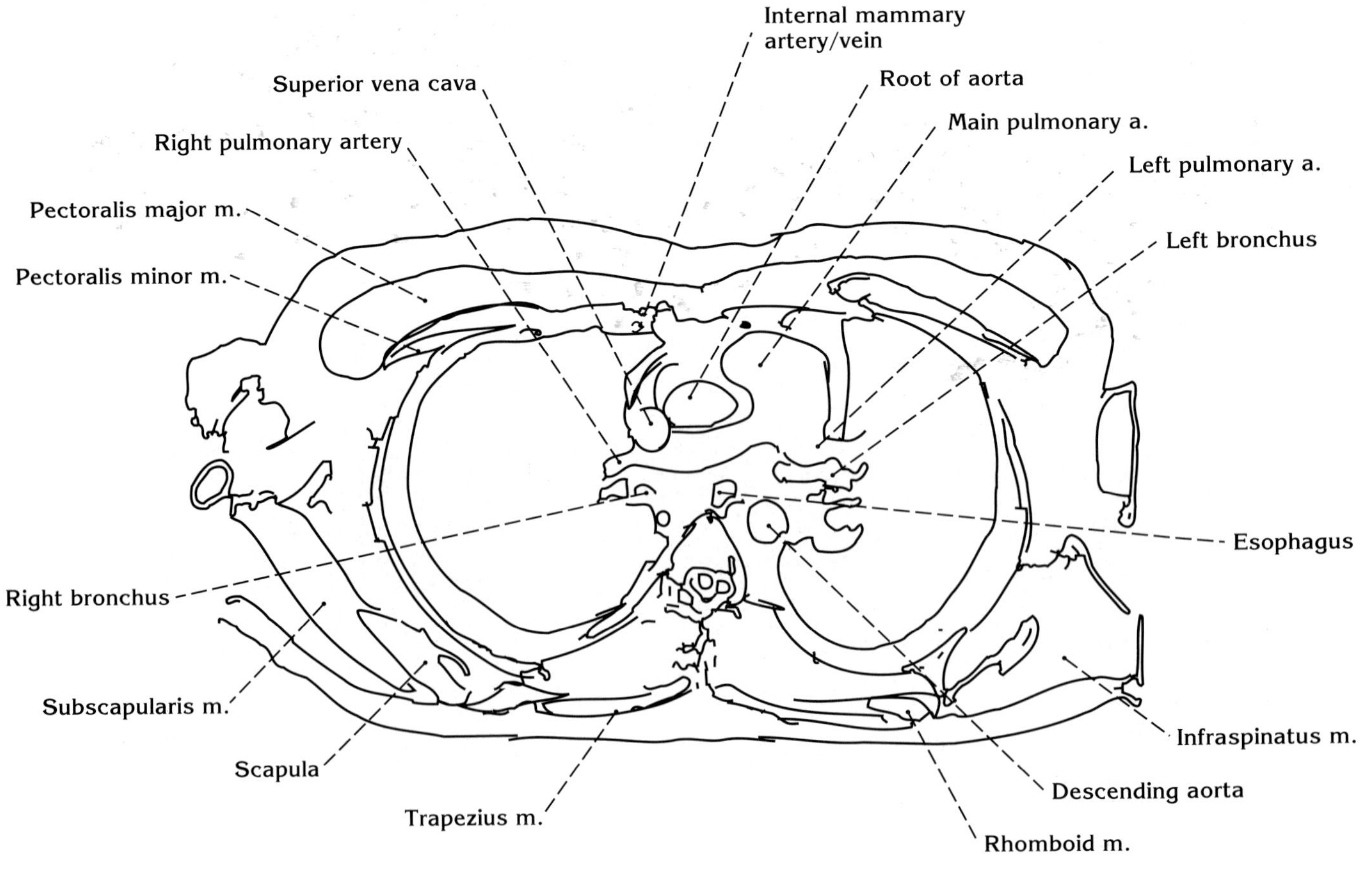

Internal mammary artery/vein
Superior vena cava
Root of aorta
Main pulmonary a.
Right pulmonary artery
Left pulmonary a.
Pectoralis major m.
Left bronchus
Pectoralis minor m.
Esophagus
Right bronchus
Subscapularis m.
Infraspinatus m.
Scapula
Descending aorta
Trapezius m.
Rhomboid m.

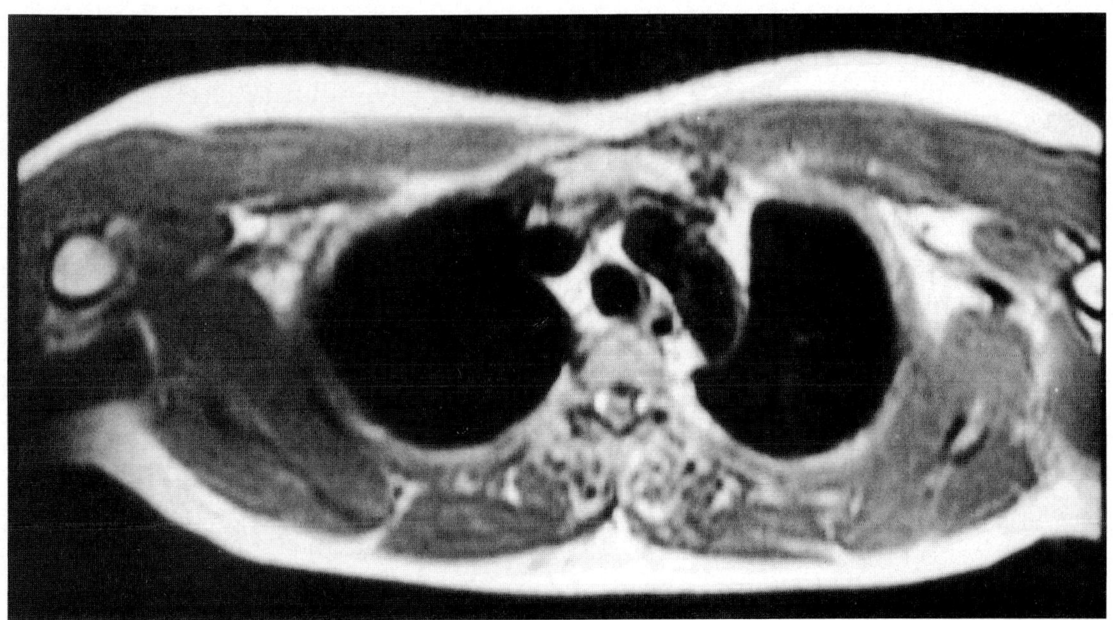

2-9 Chest, axial view (TR 1667; TE 20).

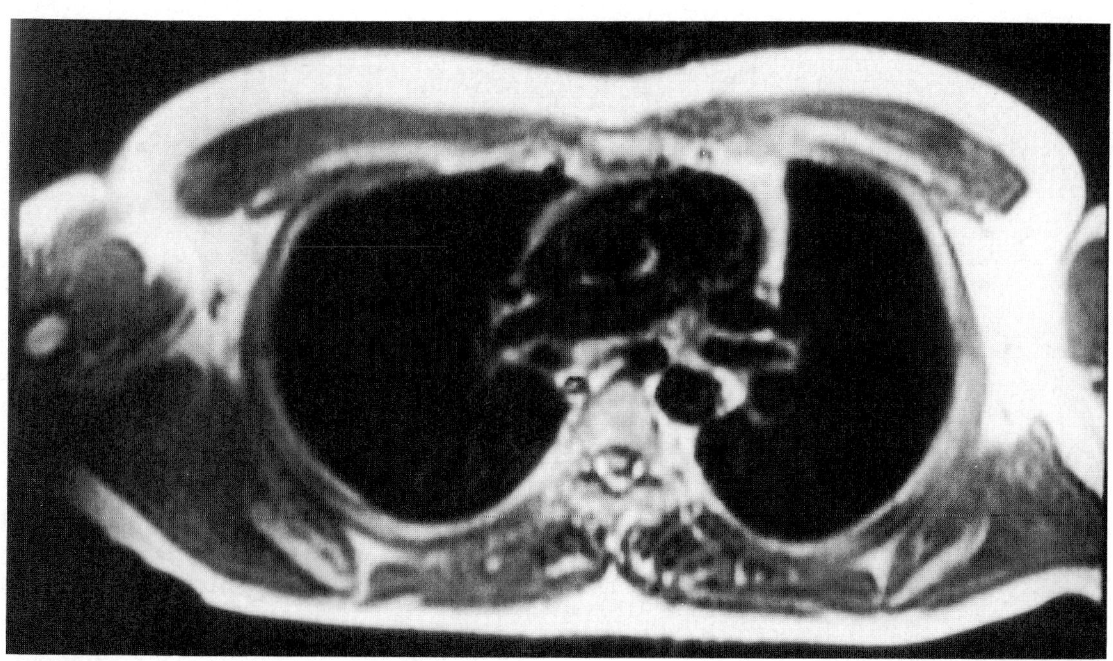

2-10 Chest, axial view (TR 1667; TE 20).

Chest, Axial

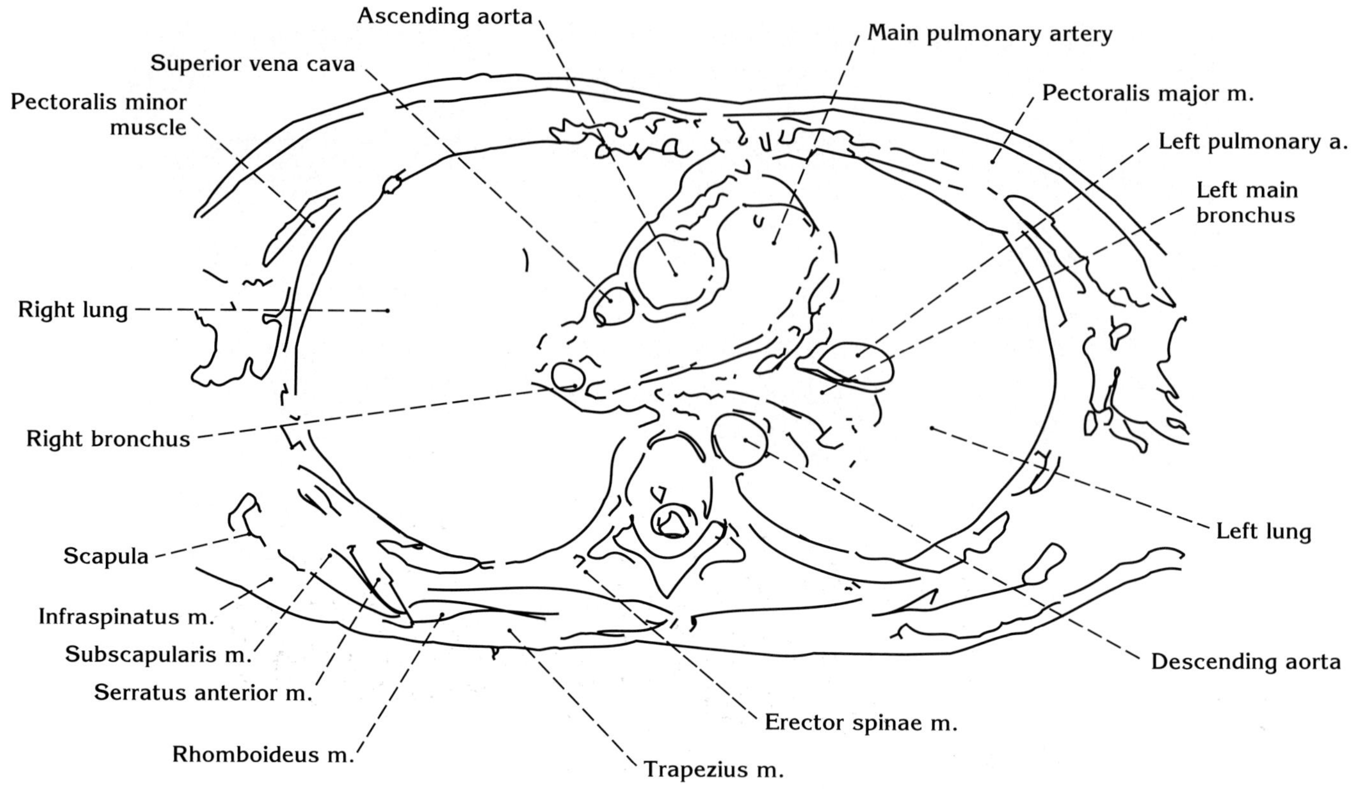
Ascending aorta
Main pulmonary artery
Superior vena cava
Pectoralis minor muscle
Pectoralis major m.
Left pulmonary a.
Left main bronchus
Right lung
Right bronchus
Left lung
Scapula
Infraspinatus m.
Subscapularis m.
Serratus anterior m.
Rhomboideus m.
Descending aorta
Erector spinae m.
Trapezius m.

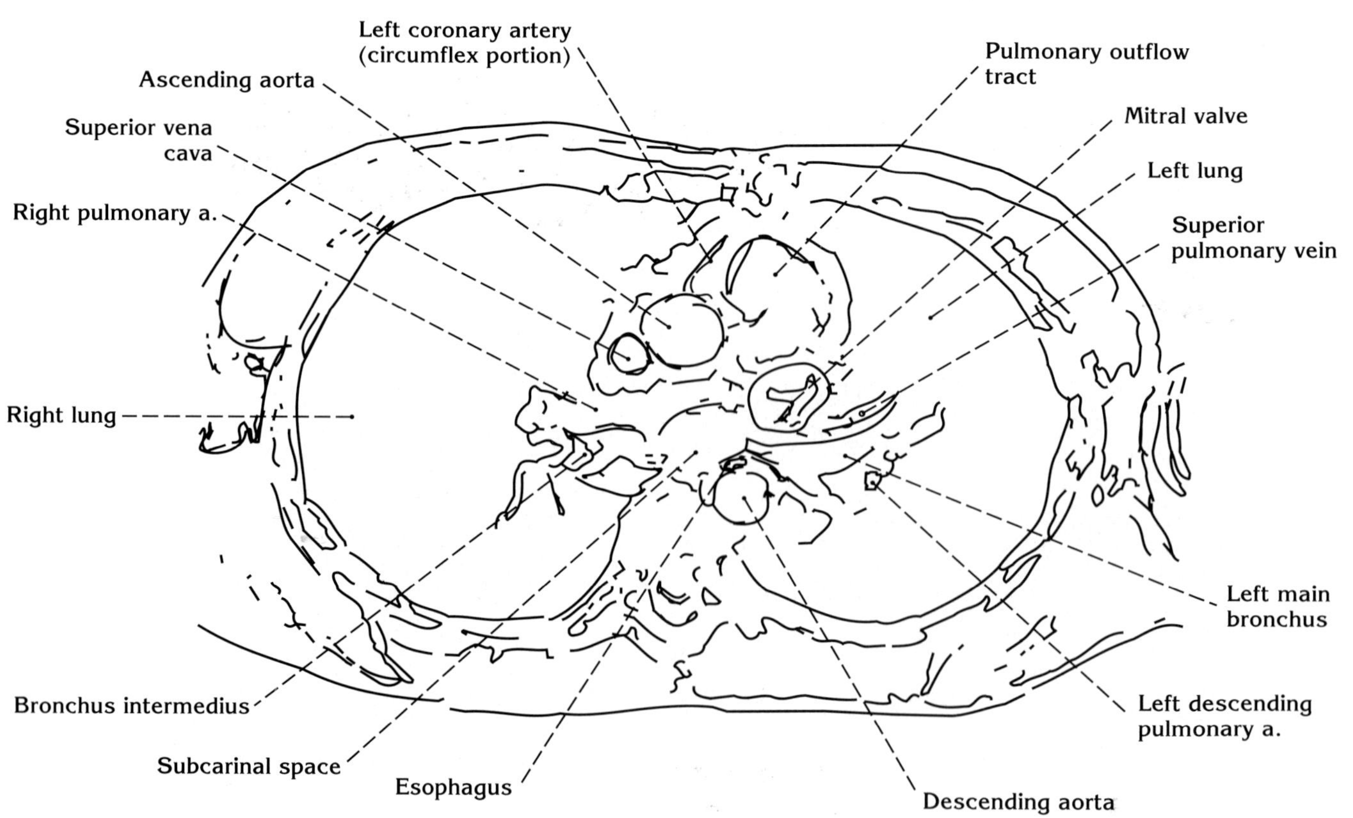
Left coronary artery (circumflex portion)
Ascending aorta
Pulmonary outflow tract
Superior vena cava
Mitral valve
Left lung
Right pulmonary a.
Superior pulmonary vein
Right lung
Left main bronchus
Bronchus intermedius
Left descending pulmonary a.
Subcarinal space
Esophagus
Descending aorta

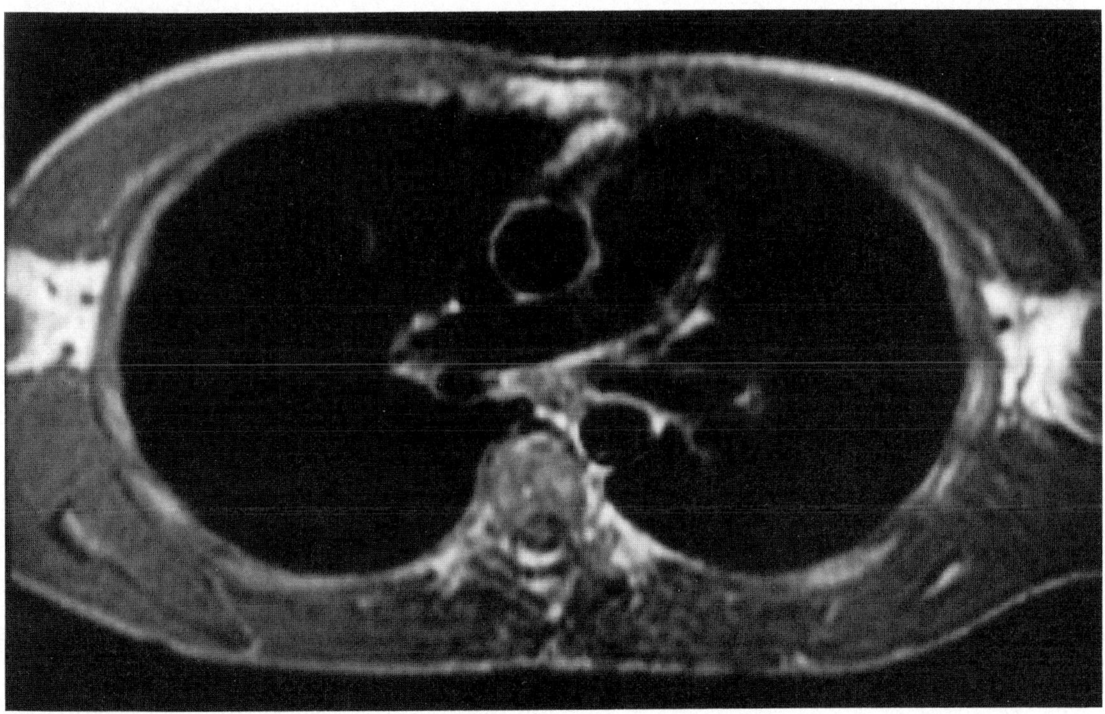

2-11 Chest, axial view (TR 1667; TE 20).

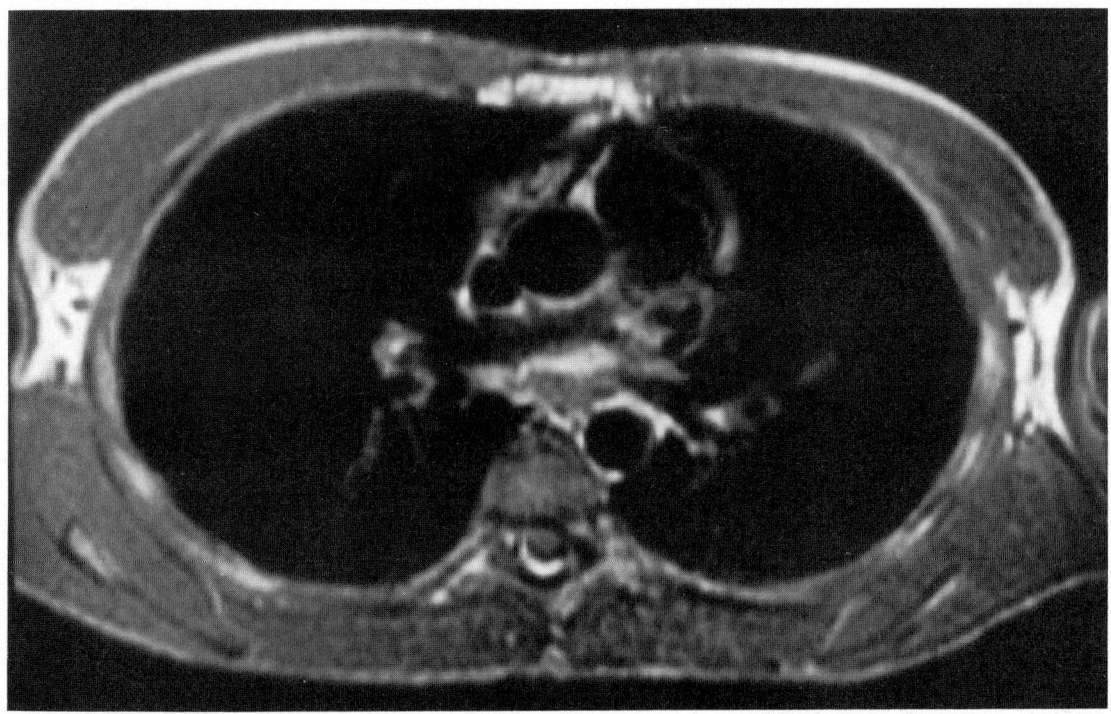

2-12 Chest, axial view (TR 1667; TE 20).

Chest, Axial

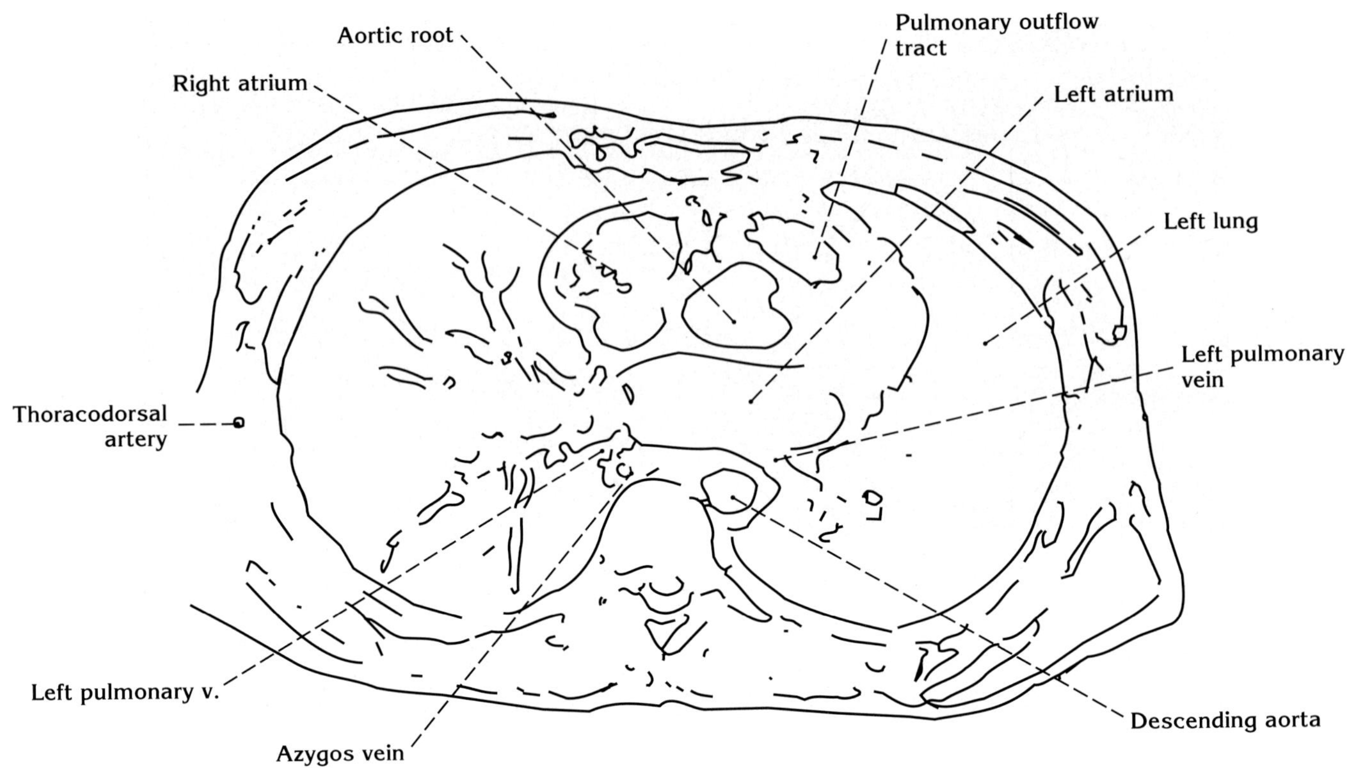
Aortic root
Pulmonary outflow tract
Right atrium
Left atrium
Left lung
Left pulmonary vein
Thoracodorsal artery
Left pulmonary v.
Azygos vein
Descending aorta

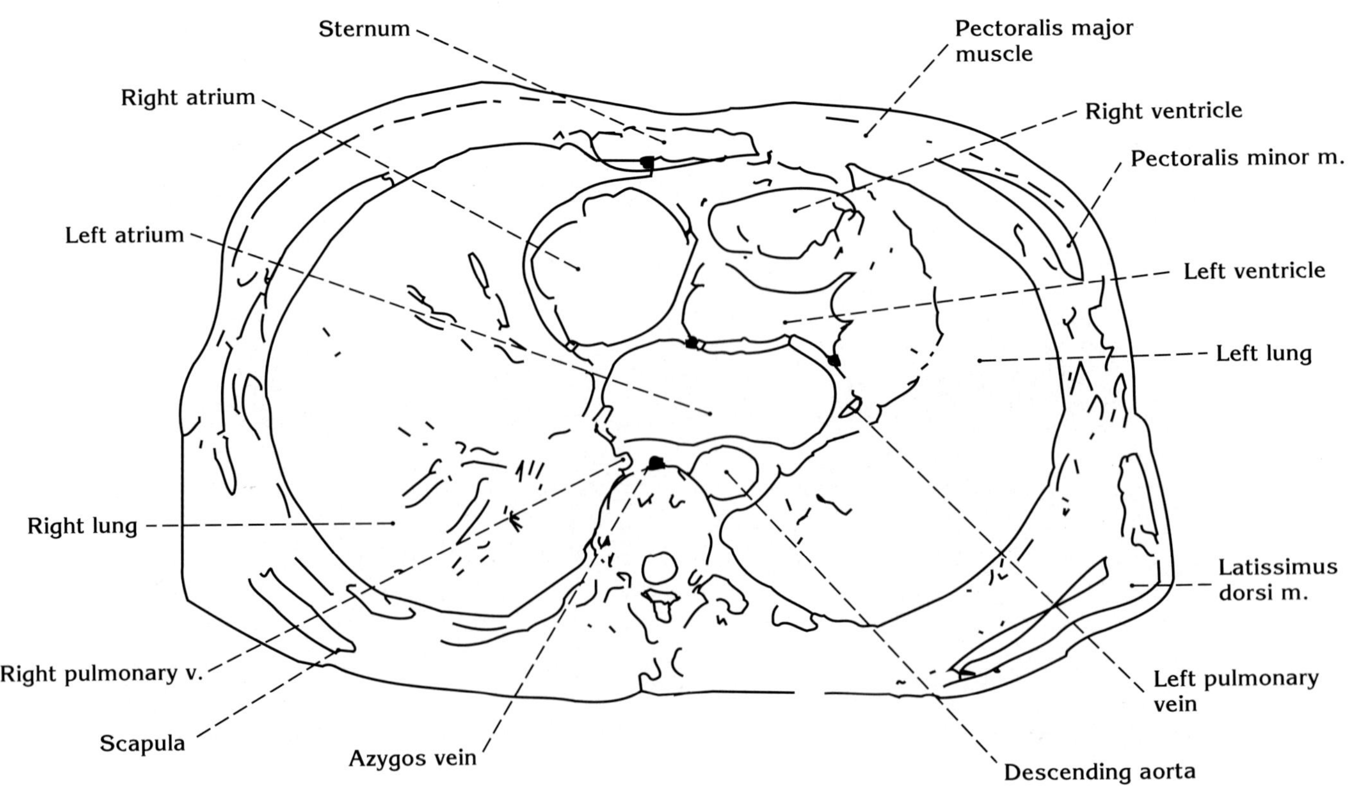
Sternum
Pectoralis major muscle
Right atrium
Right ventricle
Pectoralis minor m.
Left atrium
Left ventricle
Left lung
Right lung
Latissimus dorsi m.
Right pulmonary v.
Scapula
Azygos vein
Left pulmonary vein
Descending aorta

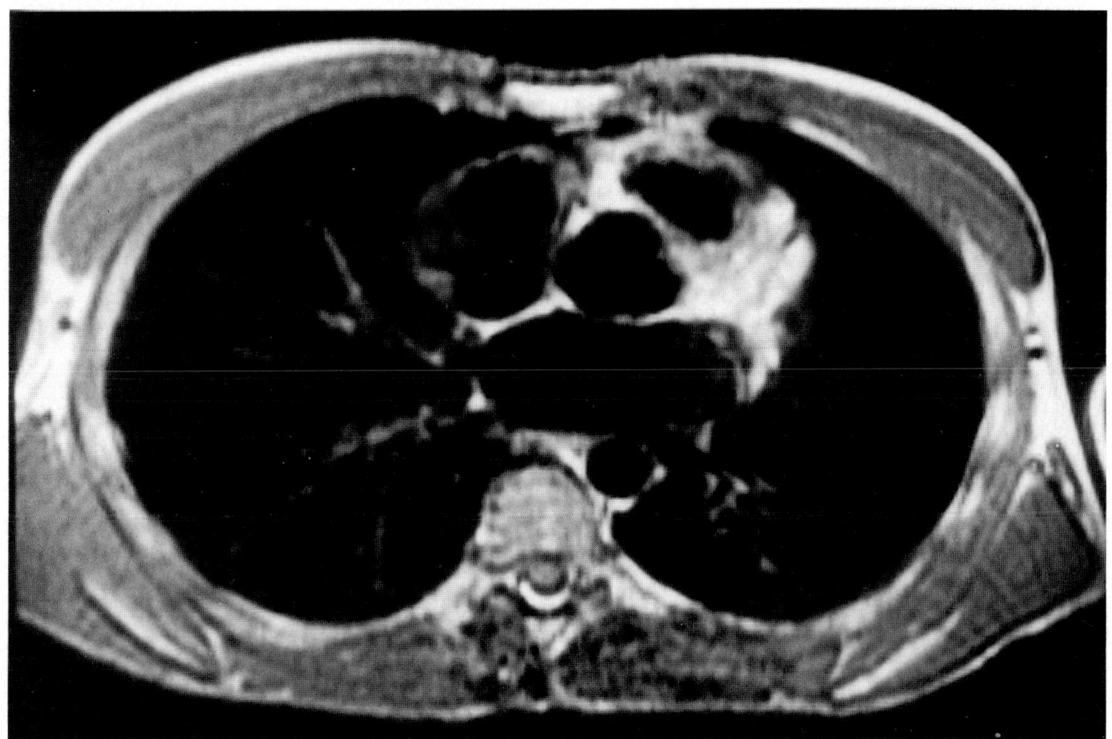

2-13 Chest, axial view (TR 1667; TE 20).

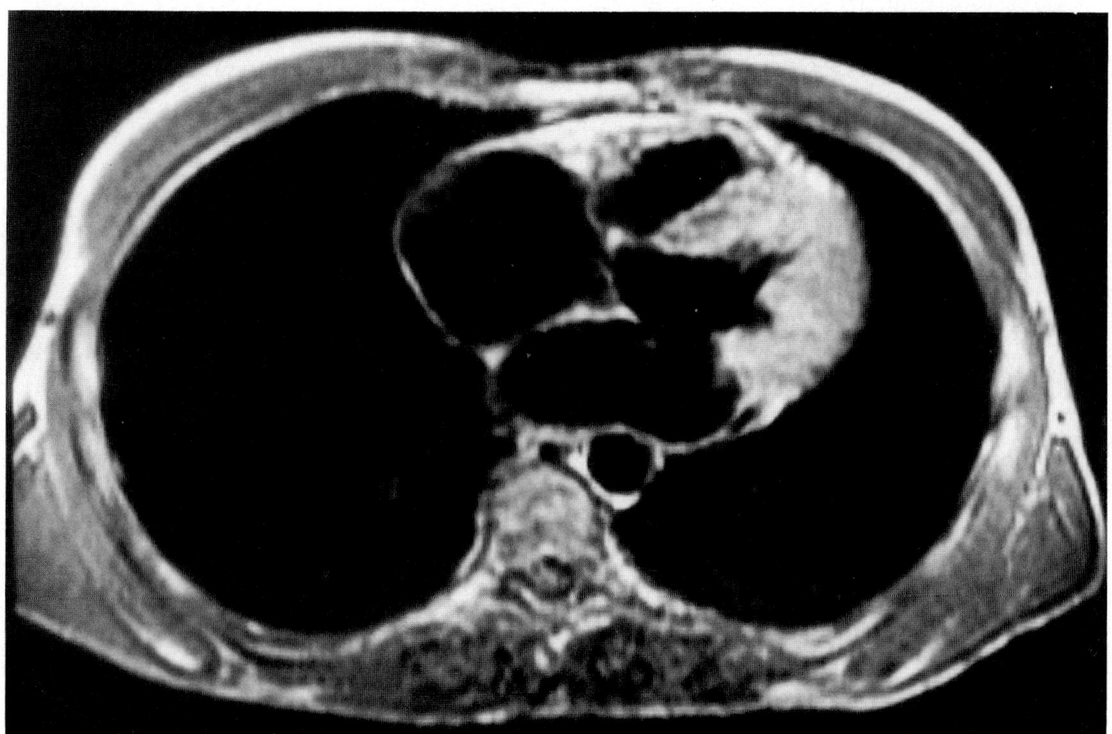

2-14 Chest, axial view (TR 1667; TE 20).

Chest, Axial

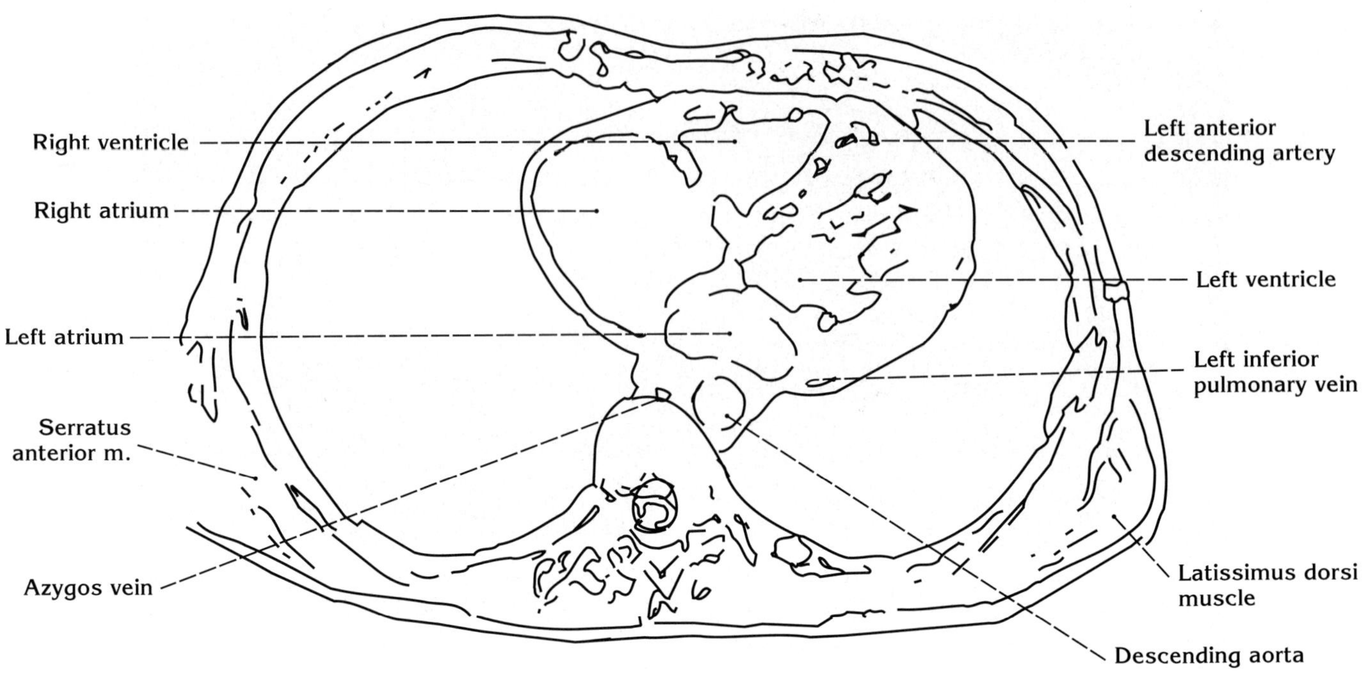
Right ventricle
Right atrium
Left atrium
Serratus anterior m.
Azygos vein
Left anterior descending artery
Left ventricle
Left inferior pulmonary vein
Latissimus dorsi muscle
Descending aorta

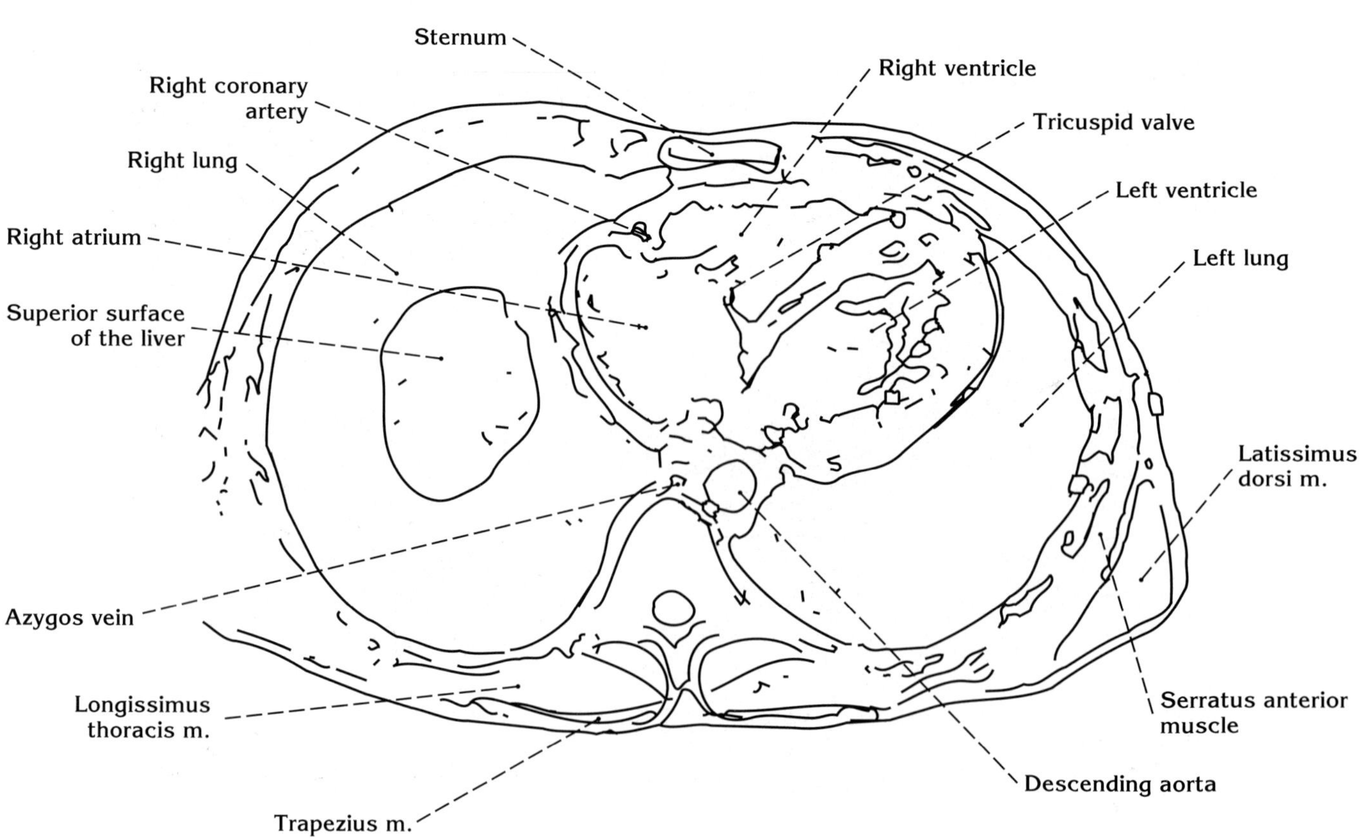
Sternum
Right coronary artery
Right lung
Right atrium
Superior surface of the liver
Azygos vein
Longissimus thoracis m.
Trapezius m.
Right ventricle
Tricuspid valve
Left ventricle
Left lung
Latissimus dorsi m.
Serratus anterior muscle
Descending aorta

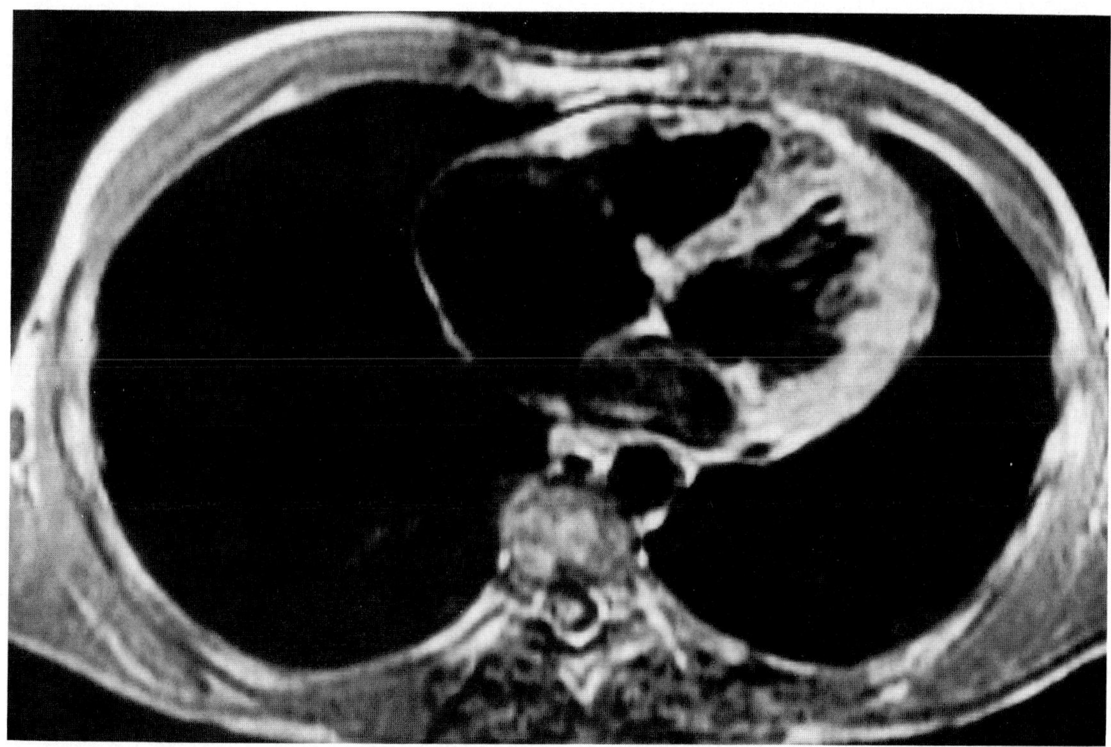

2-15 Chest, axial view (TR 1667; TE 20).

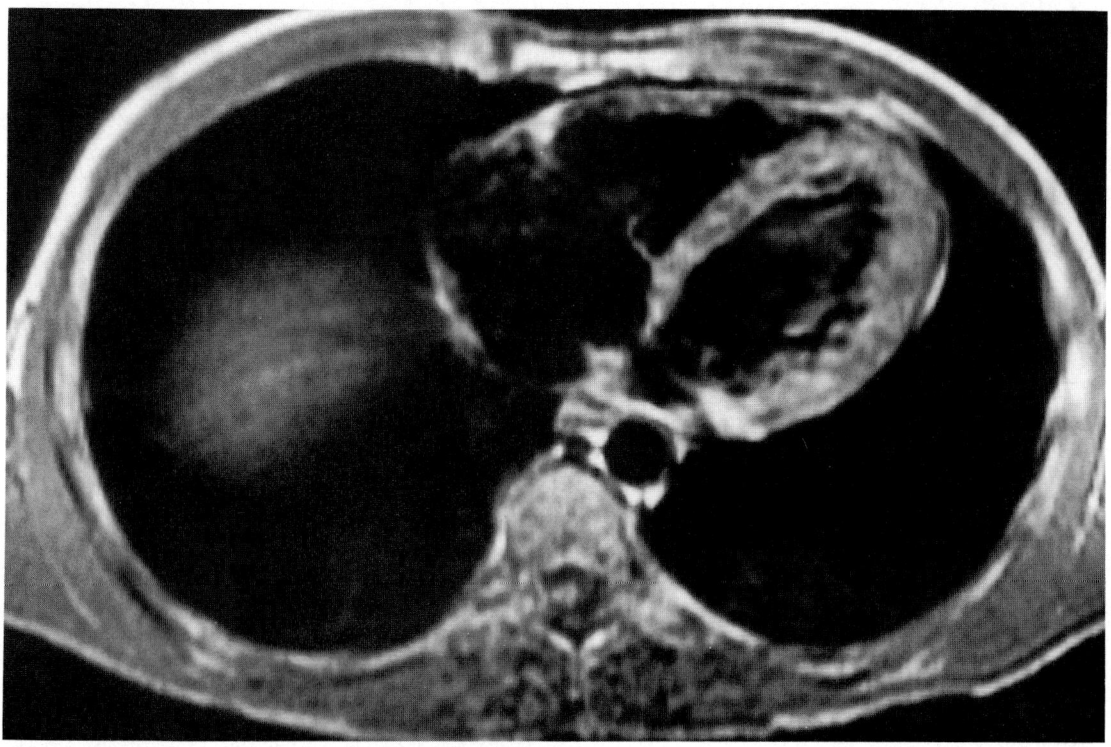

2-16 Chest, axial view (TR 1667; TE 20).

Chest, Axial

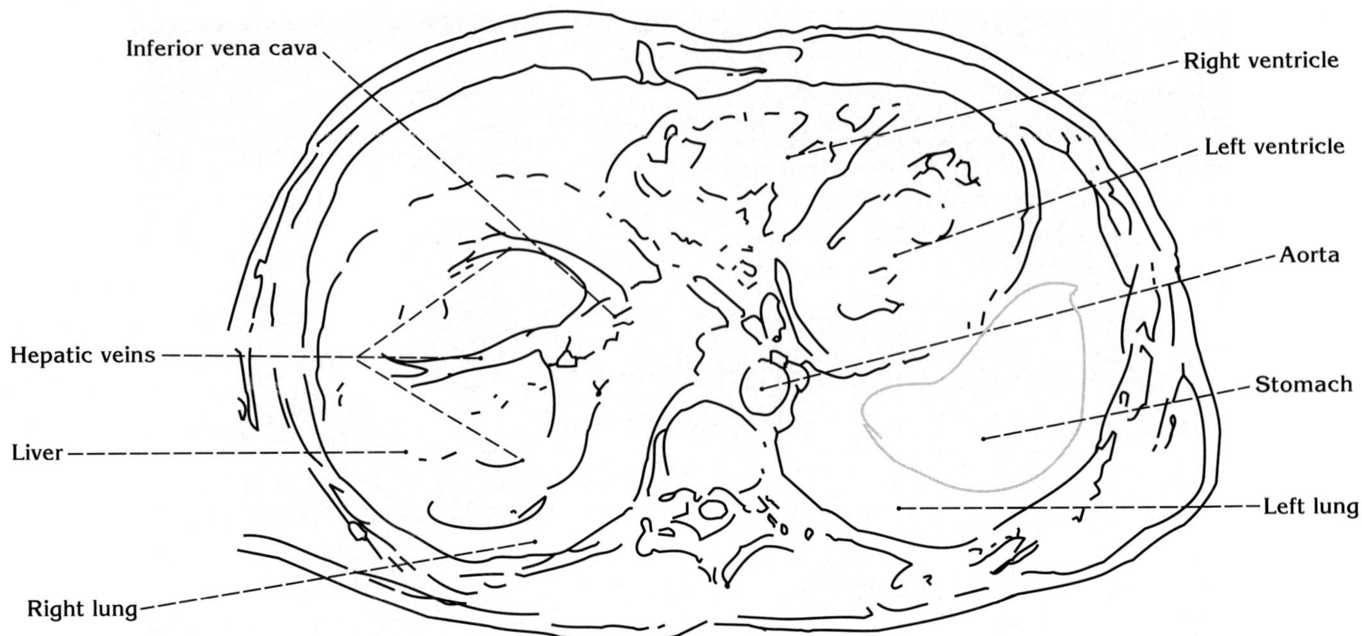
Inferior vena cava
Right ventricle
Left ventricle
Aorta
Hepatic veins
Stomach
Liver
Left lung
Right lung

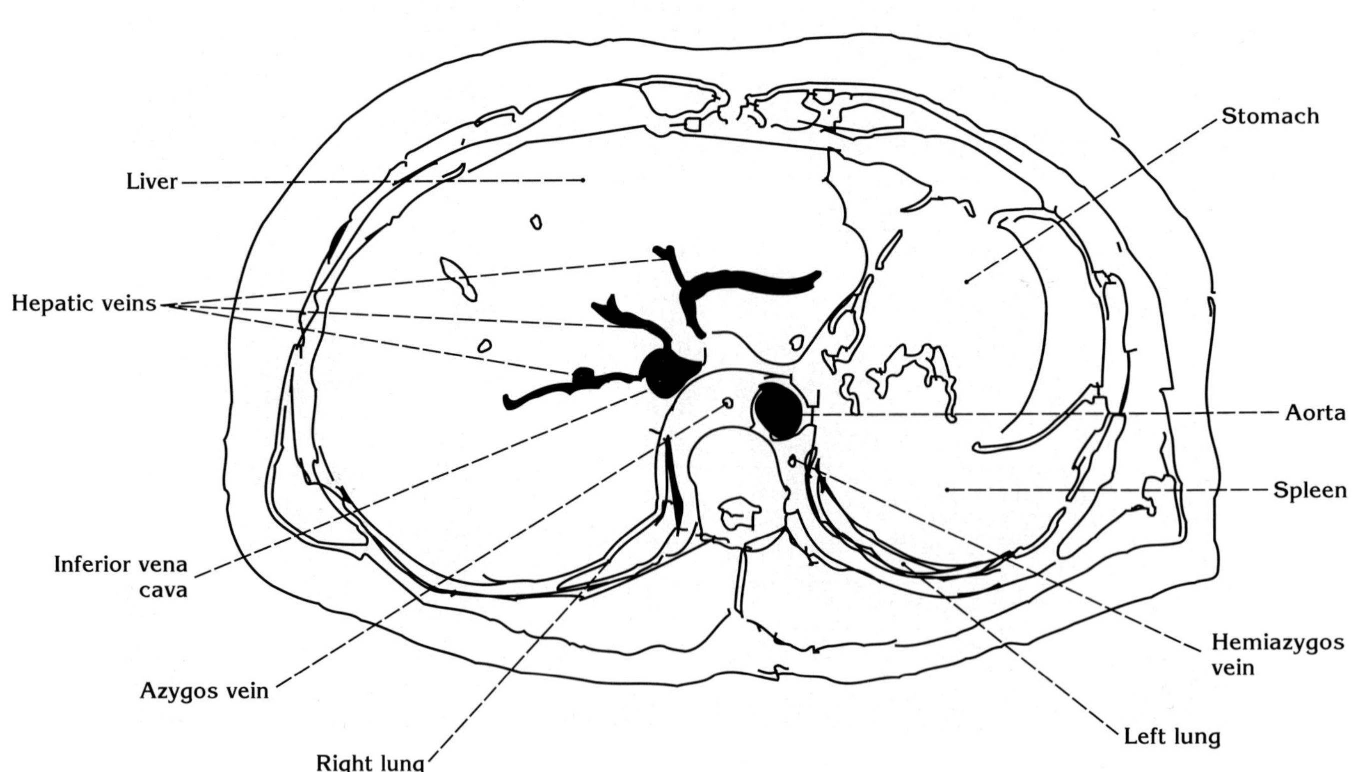
Stomach
Liver
Hepatic veins
Aorta
Spleen
Inferior vena cava
Hemiazygos vein
Azygos vein
Left lung
Right lung

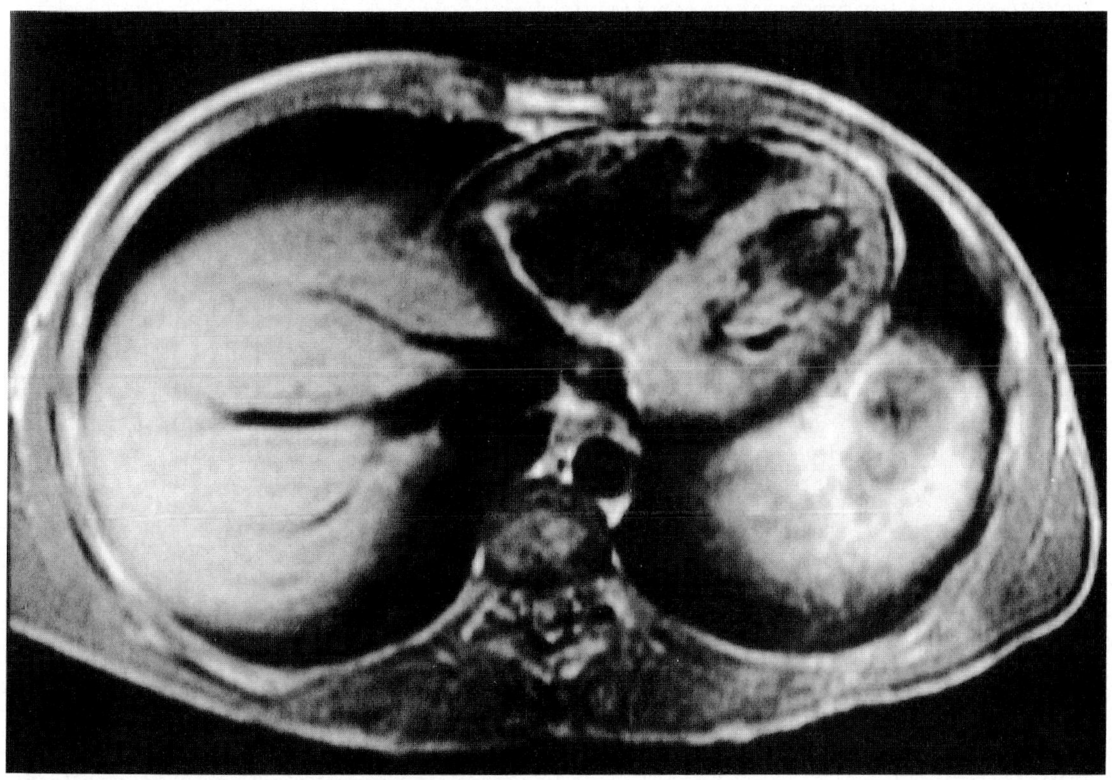

2-17 Chest, axial view (TR 1200; TE 20).

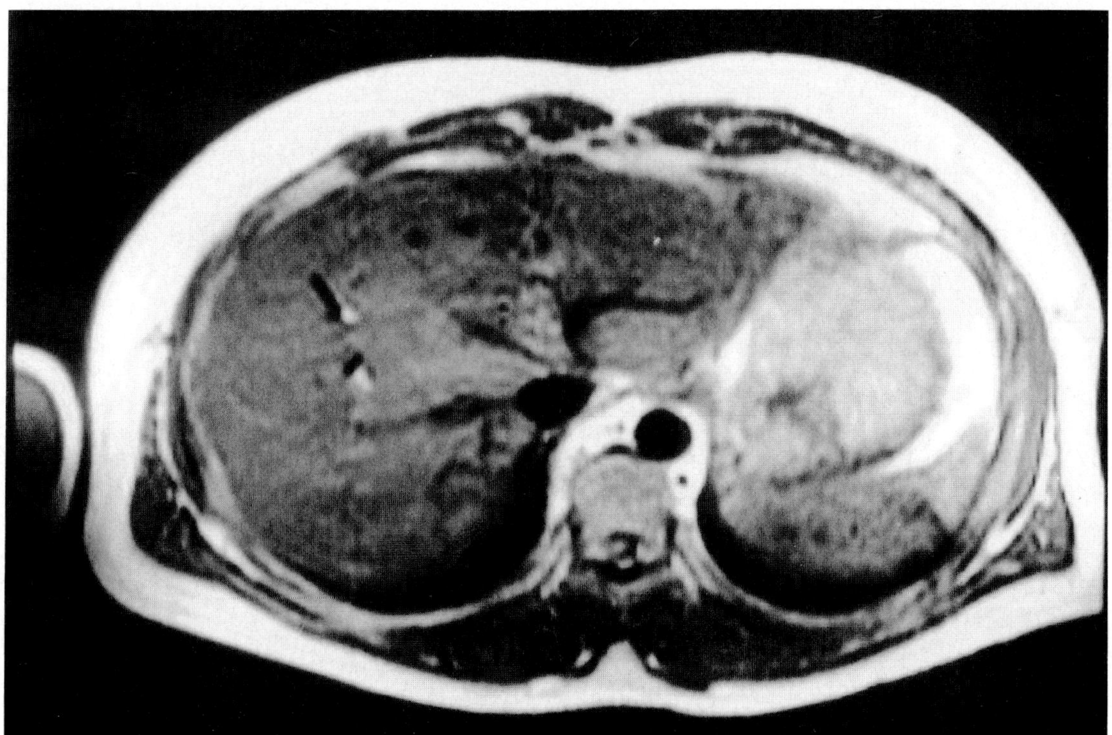

2-18 Chest, axial view (TR 1667; TE 20).

Upper Abdomen, Axial

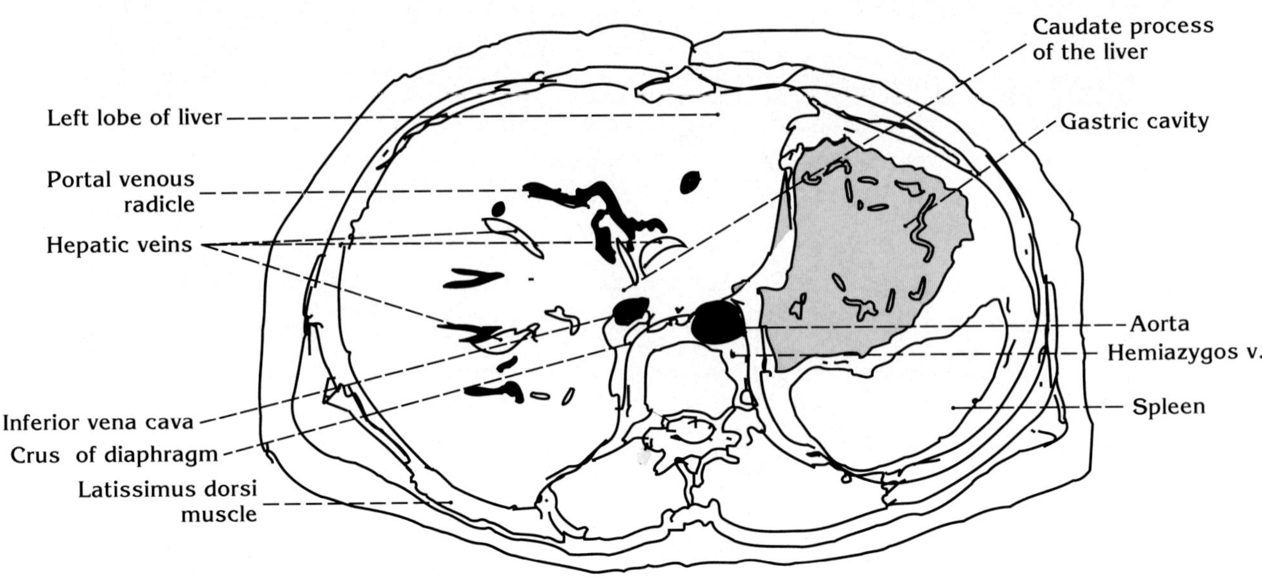

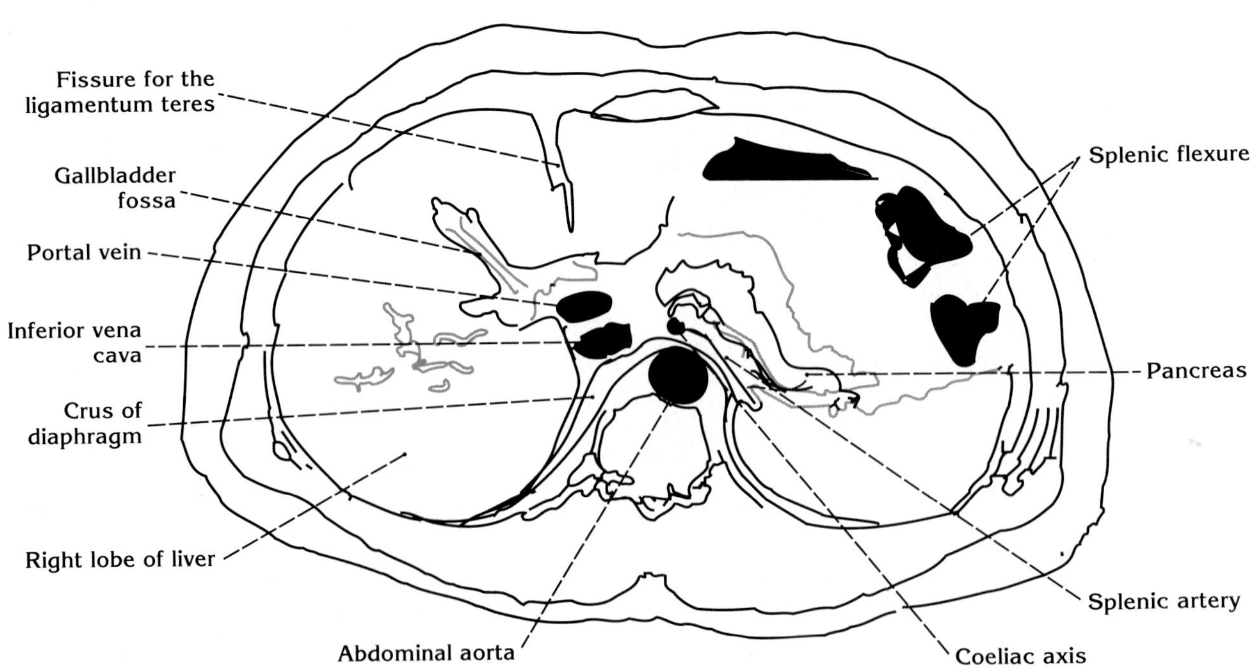

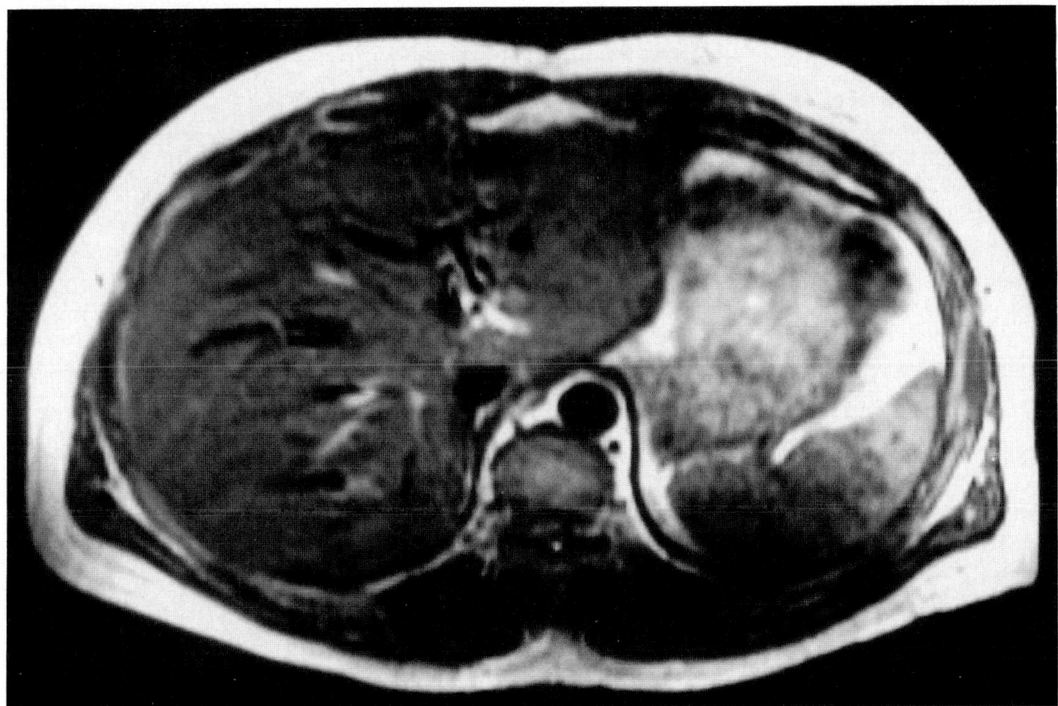

3-1 Upper abdomen, axial view (TR 1667, TE 20).

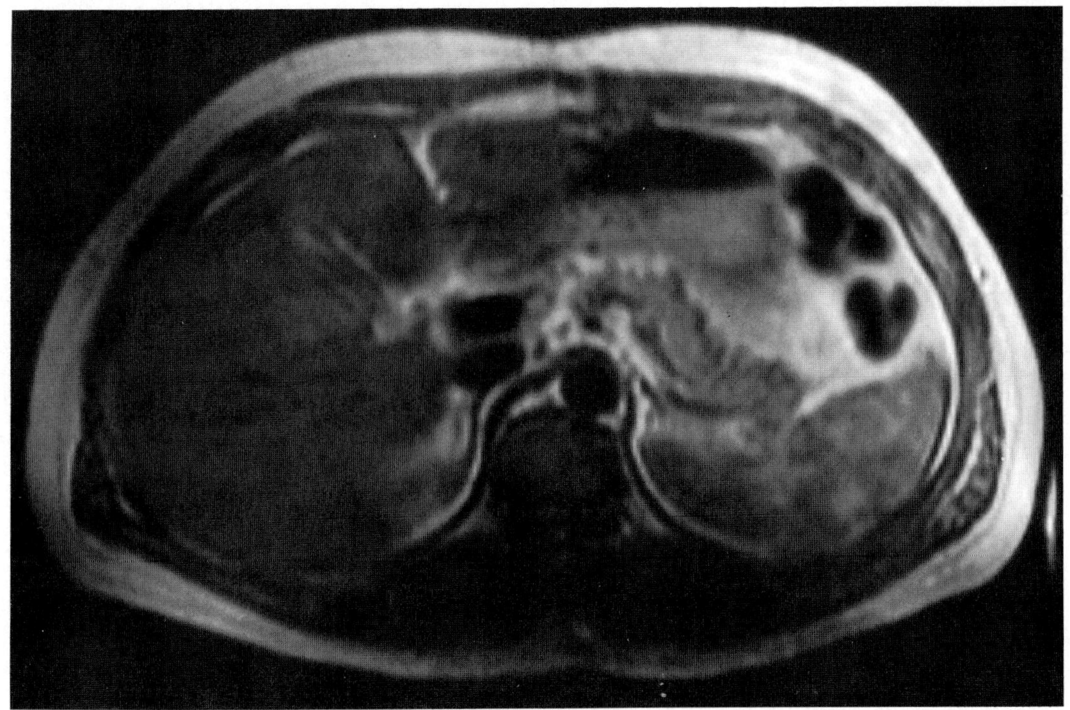

3-2 Upper abdomen, axial view (TR 2000, TE 20).

Upper Abdomen, Axial

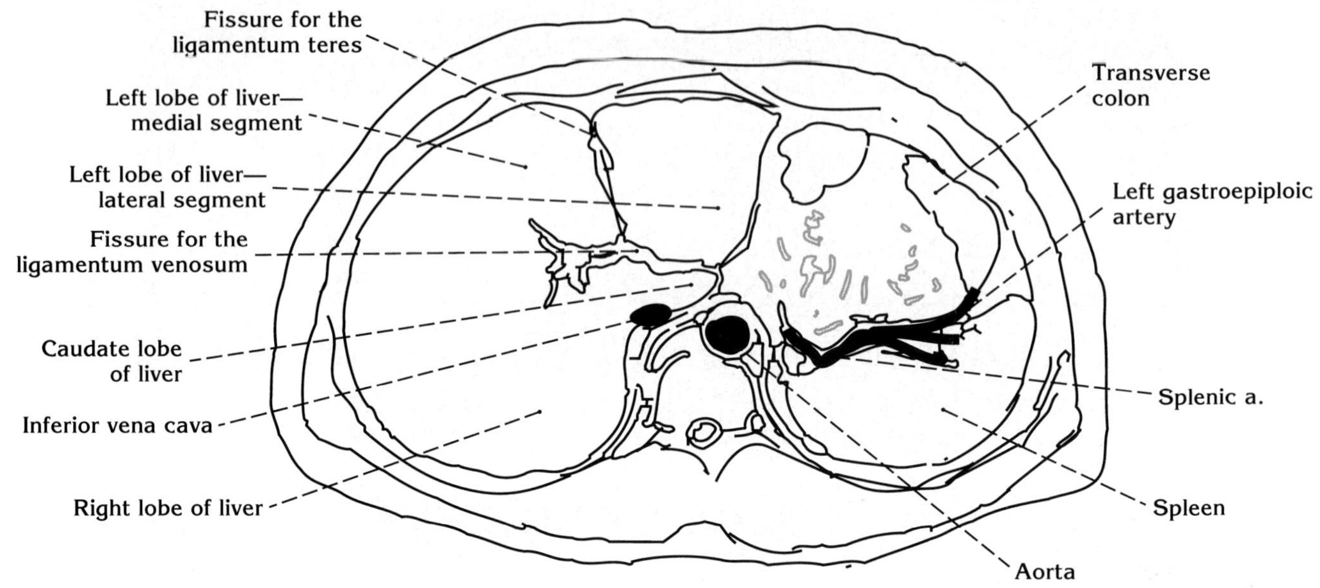

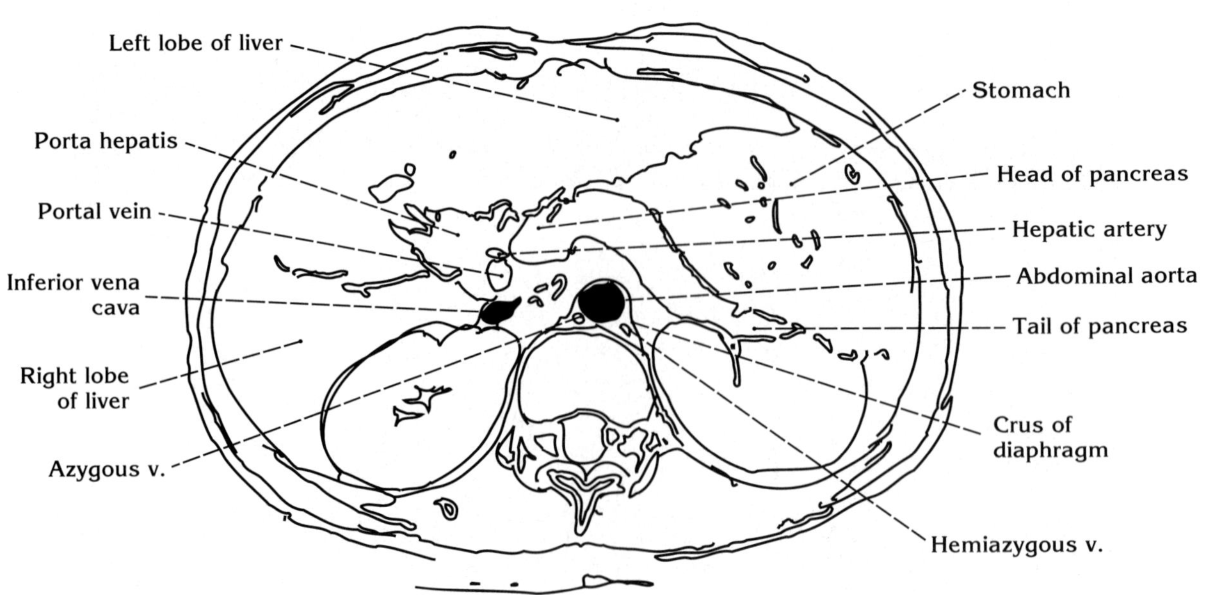

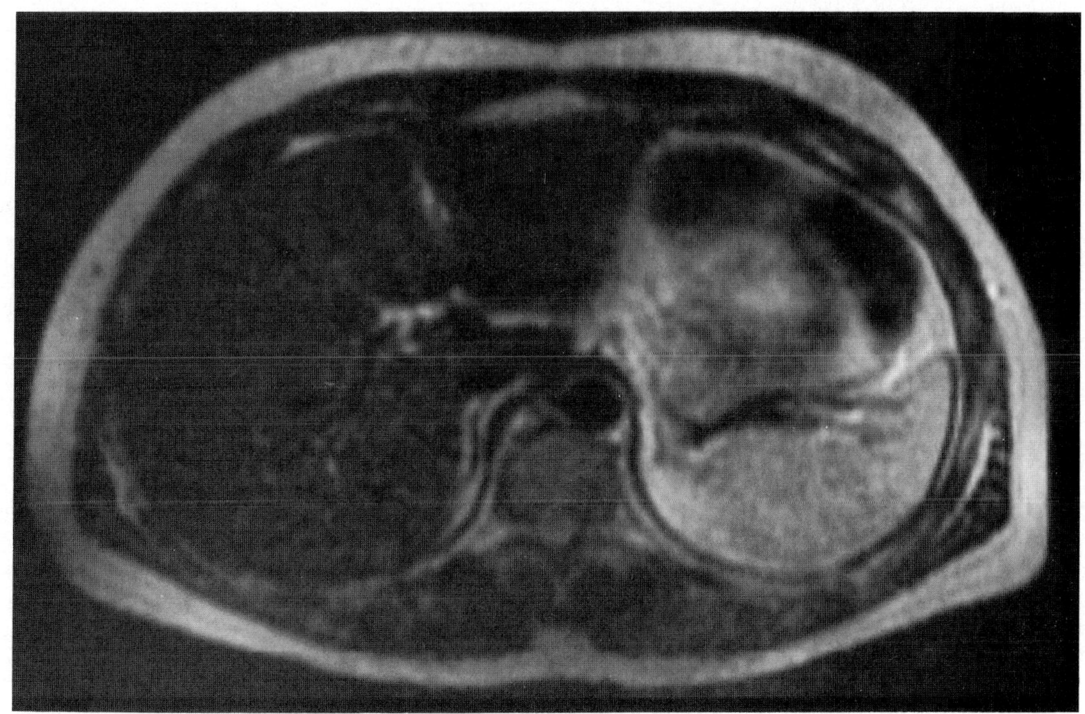

3-3 Upper abdomen, axial view (TR 1661, TE 80).

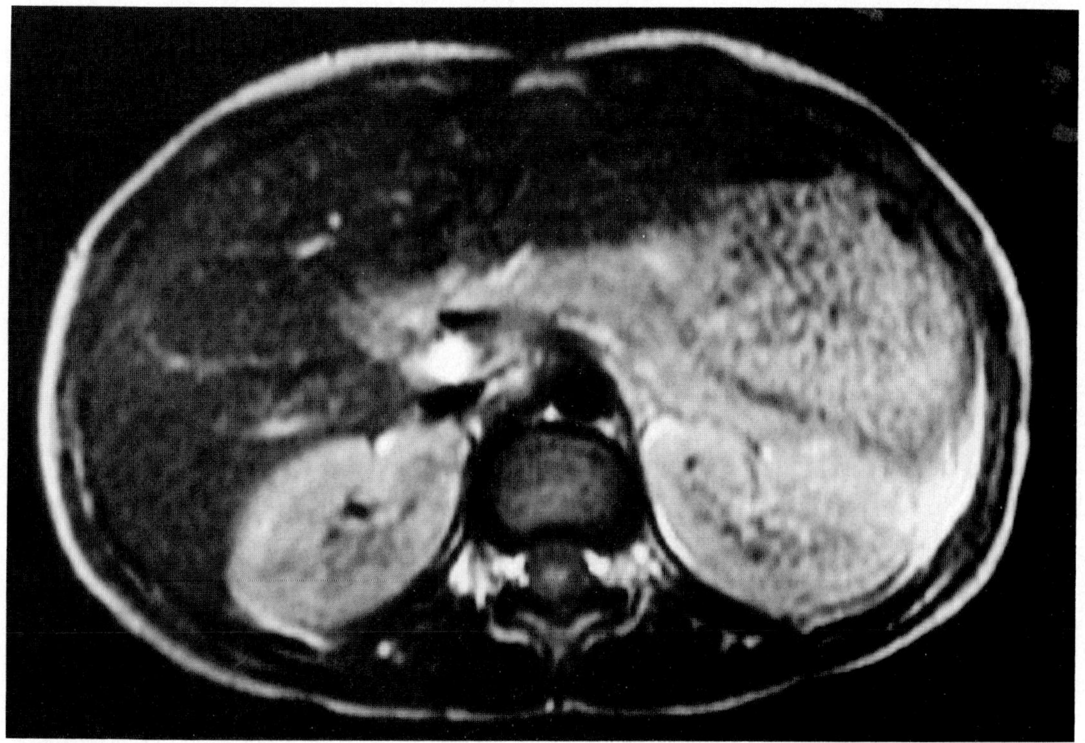

3-4 Upper abdomen, axial view showing the pancreas (TR 2000, TE 30).

Mid Abdomen, Axial

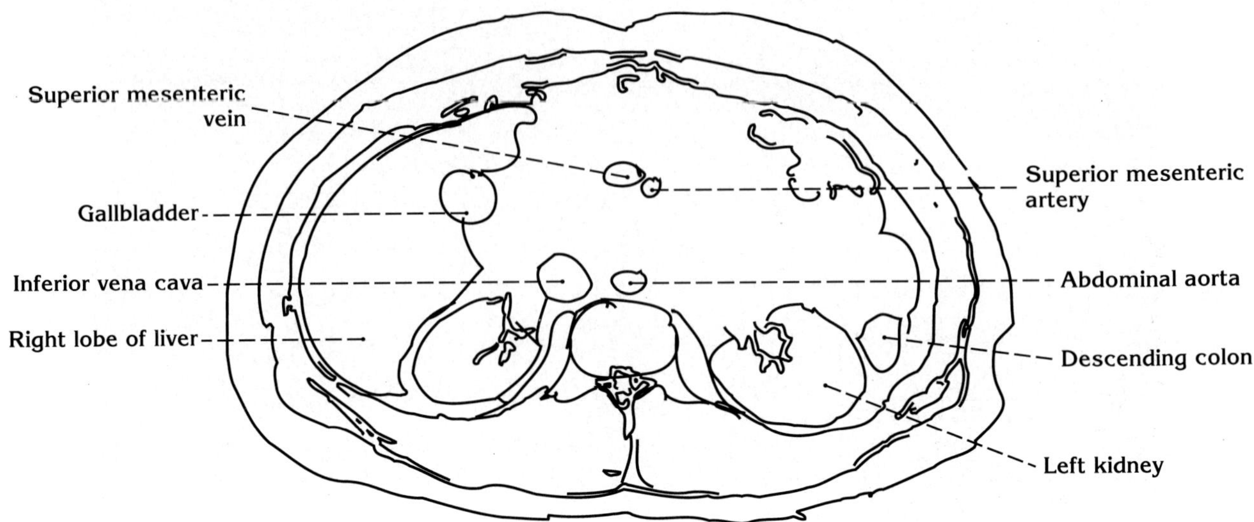

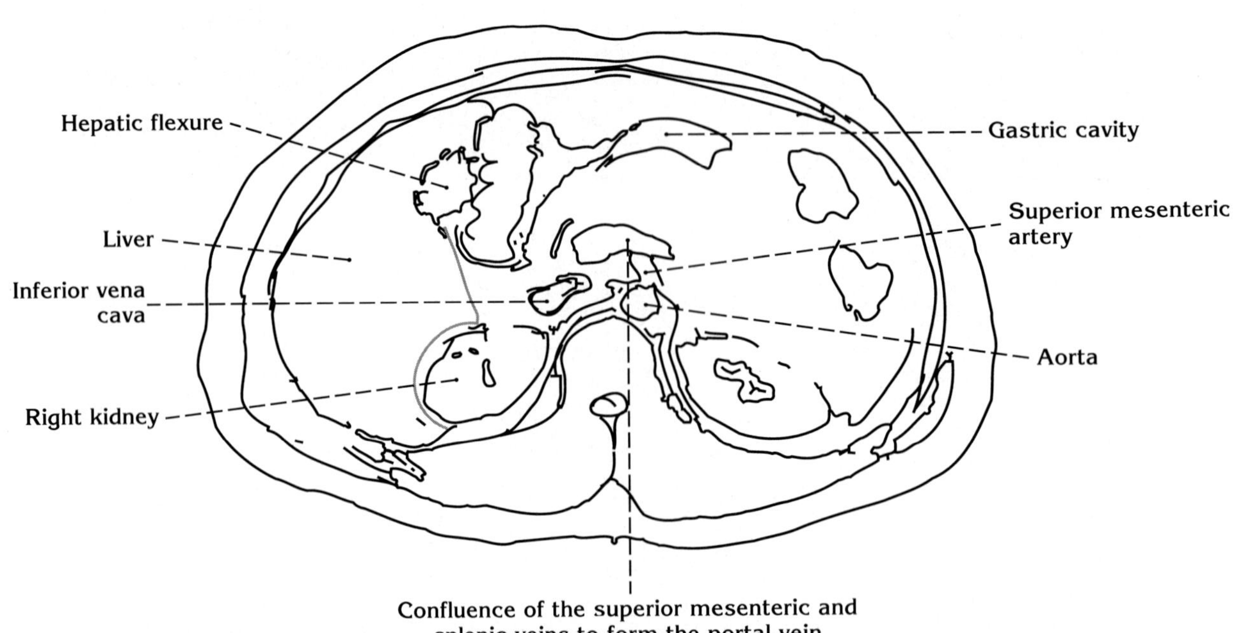

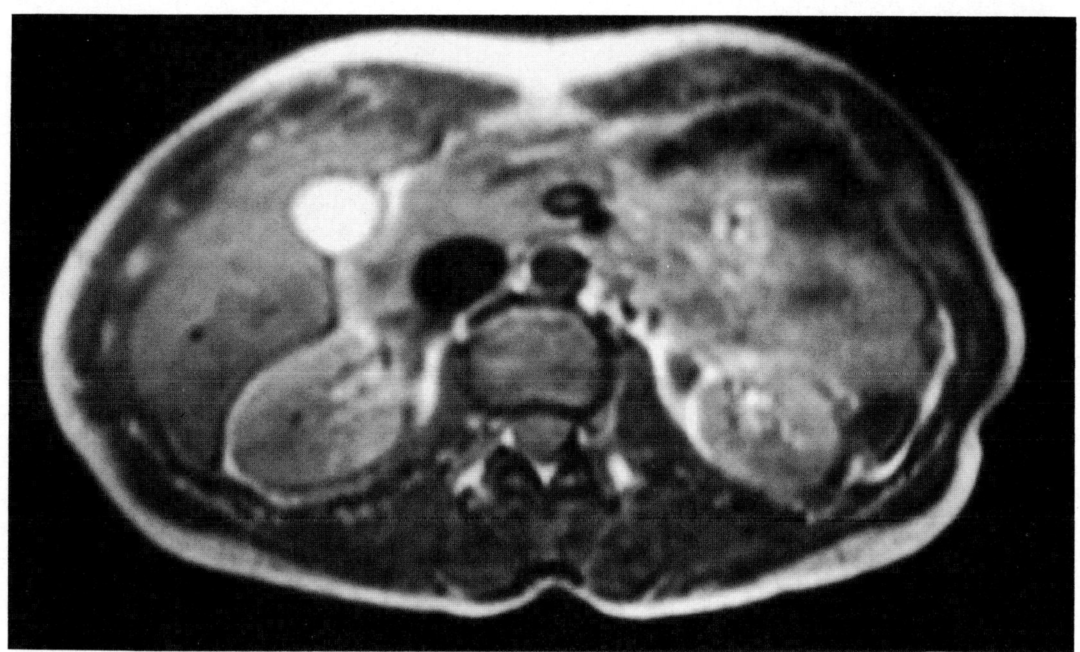

3-5 Mid abdomen, axial view (TR 1878, TE 20).

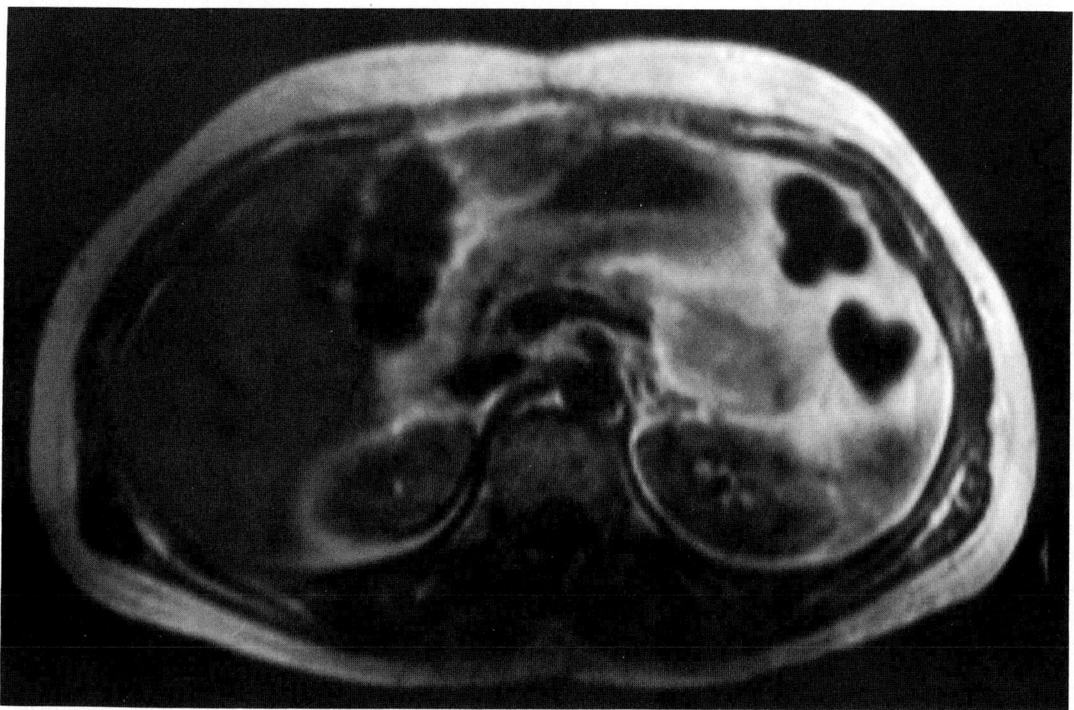

3-6 Mid abdomen, axial view showing the splenomesenteric confluence (TR 2000, TE 80).

Mid Abdomen, Axial

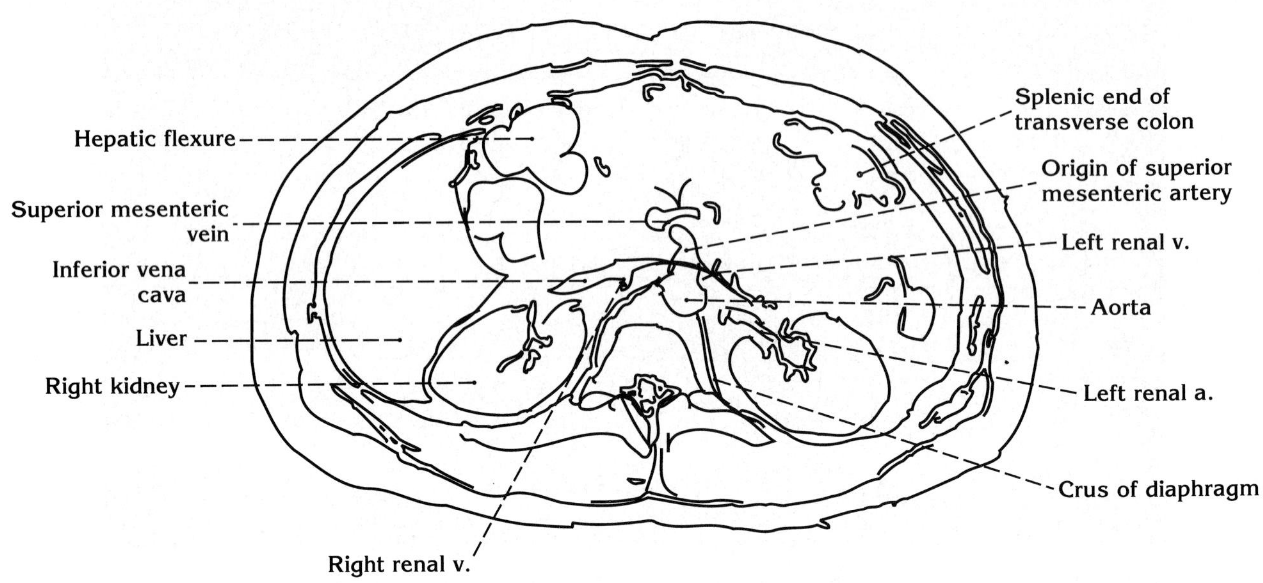

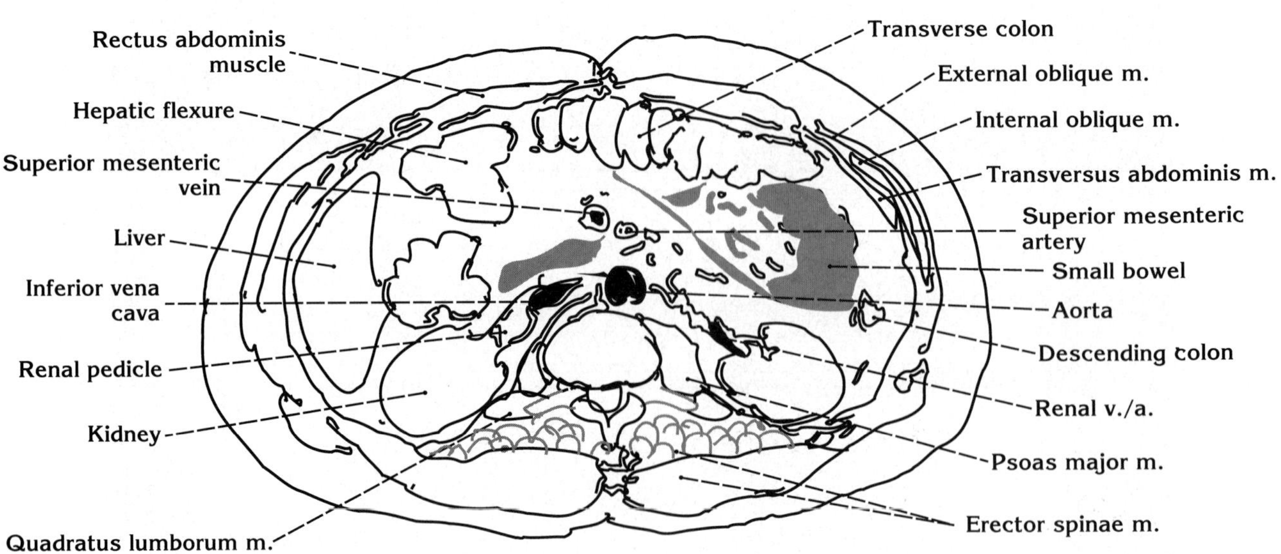

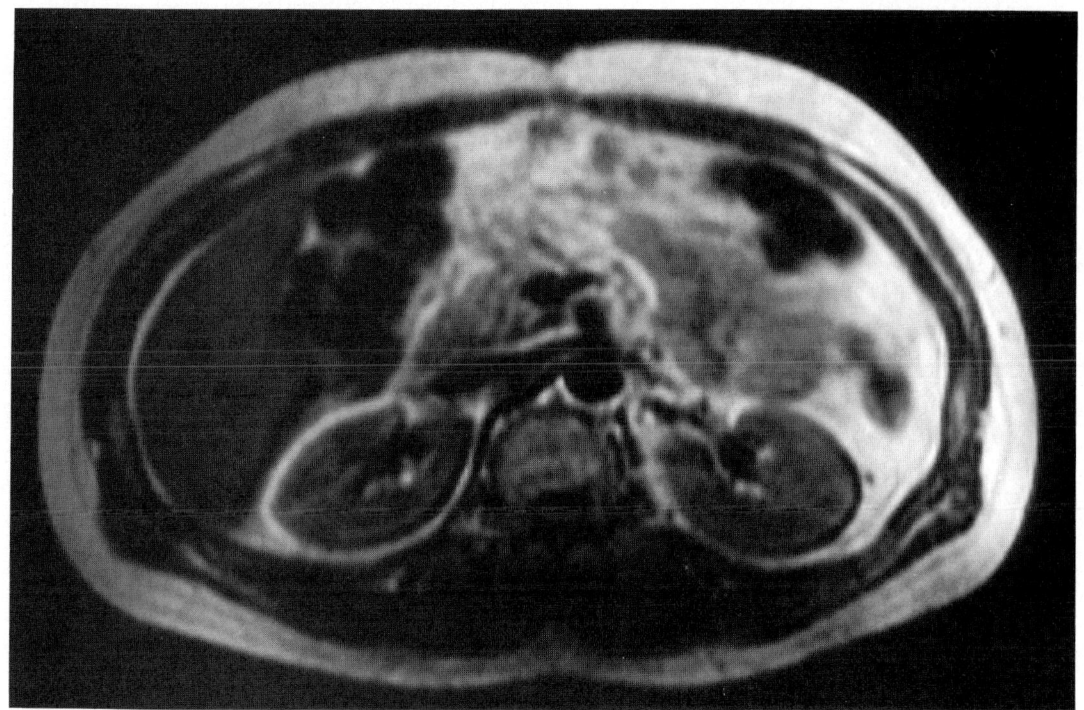

3-7 Mid abdomen, axial view (TR 2000, TE 80).

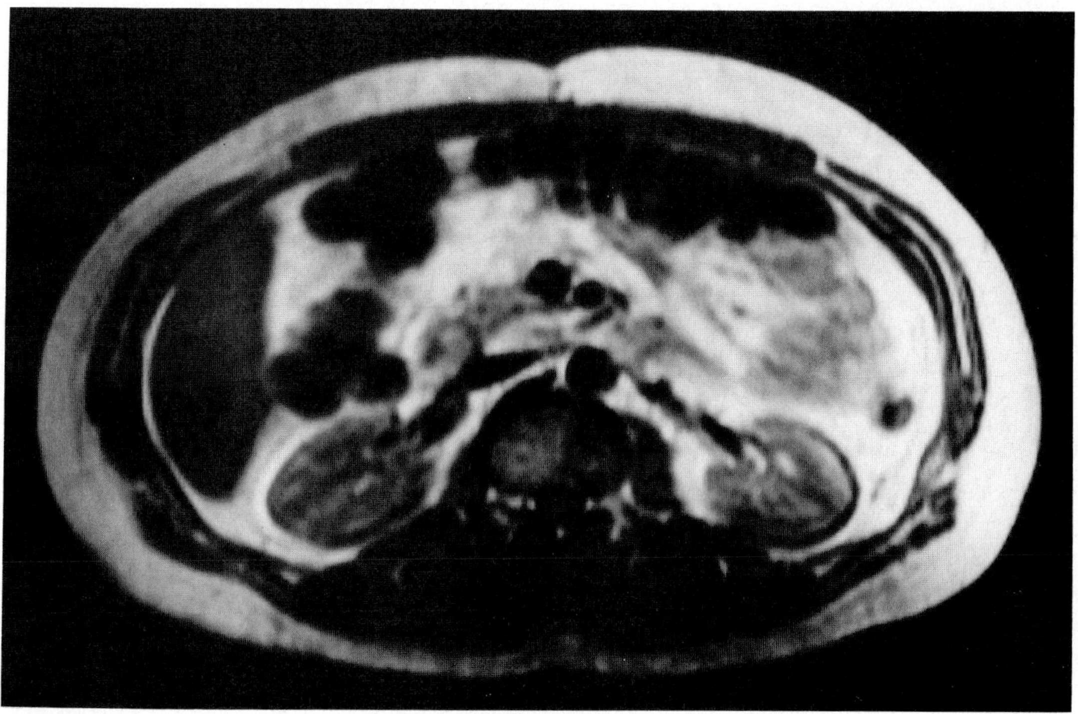

3-8 Mid abdomen, axial view (TR 2000, TE 20).

Mid Abdomen, Axial

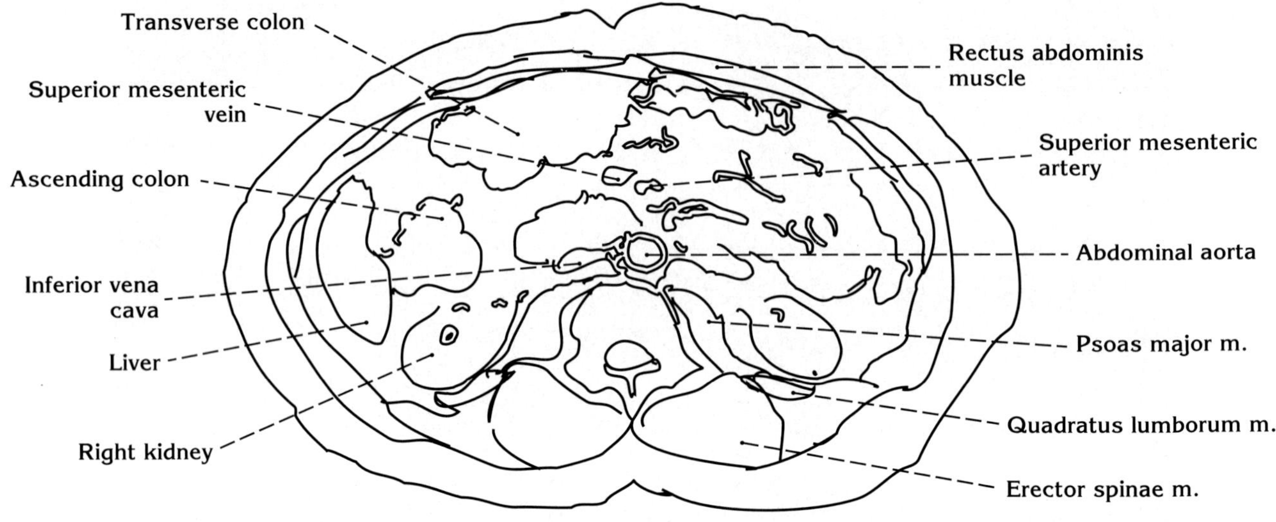

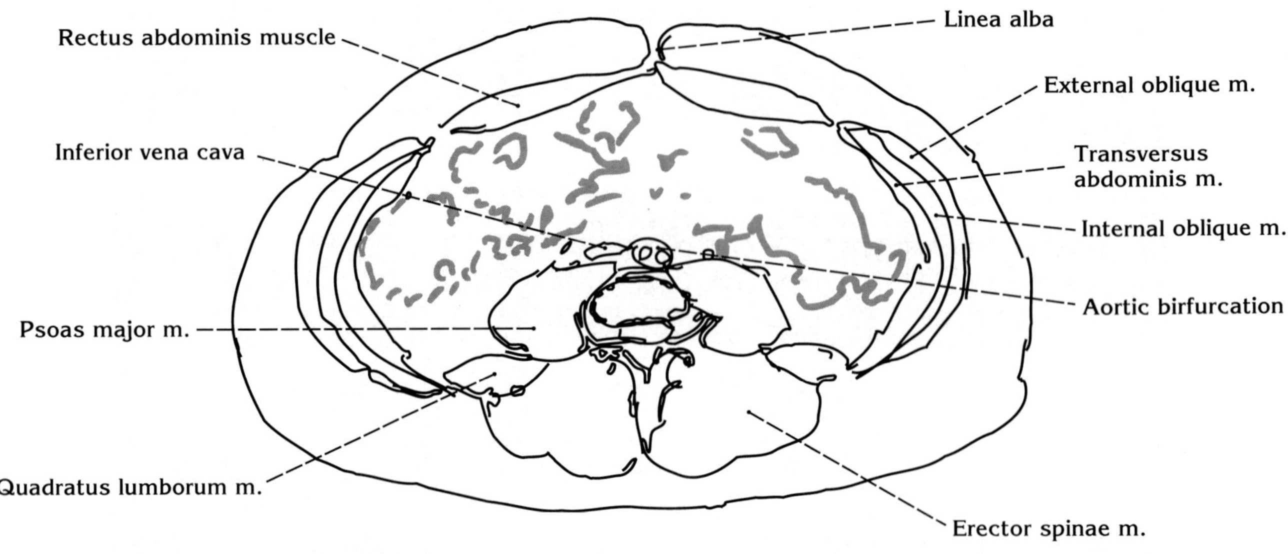

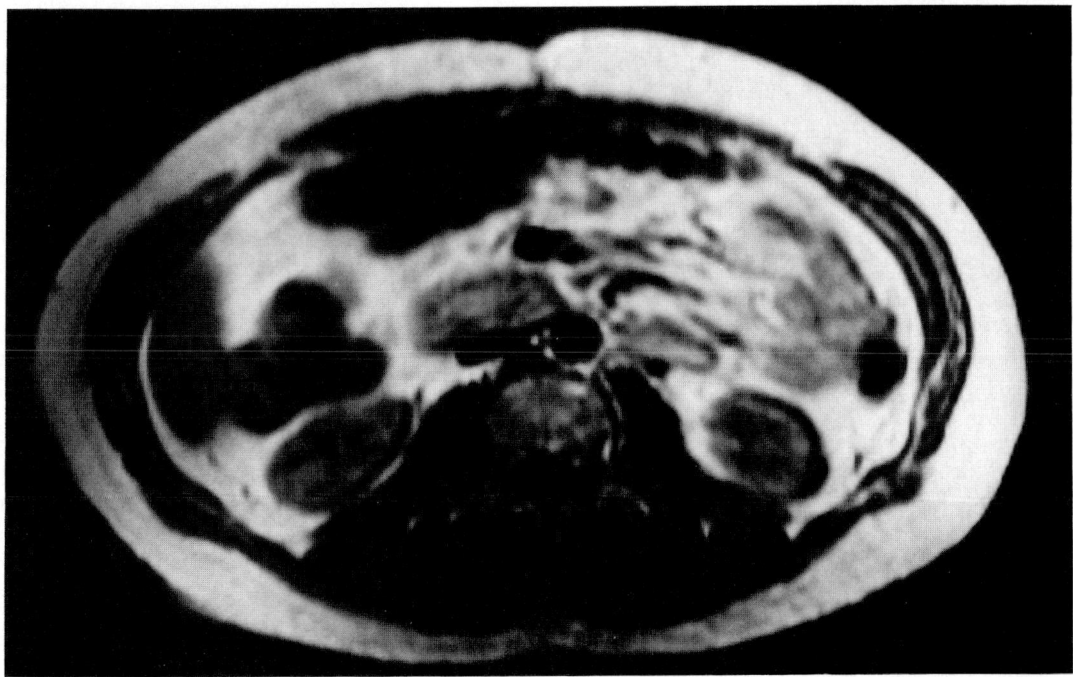

3-9 Mid abdomen, axial view (TR 2000, TE 80).

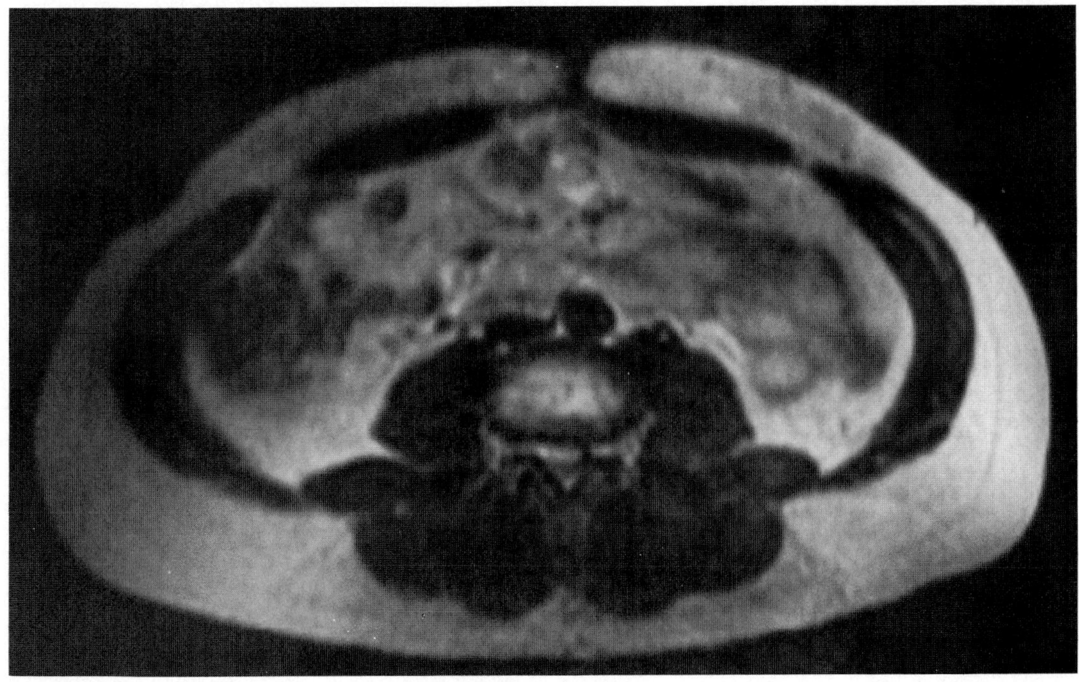

3-10 Mid abdomen, axial view (TR 2000, TE 80).

Abdomen, Coronal

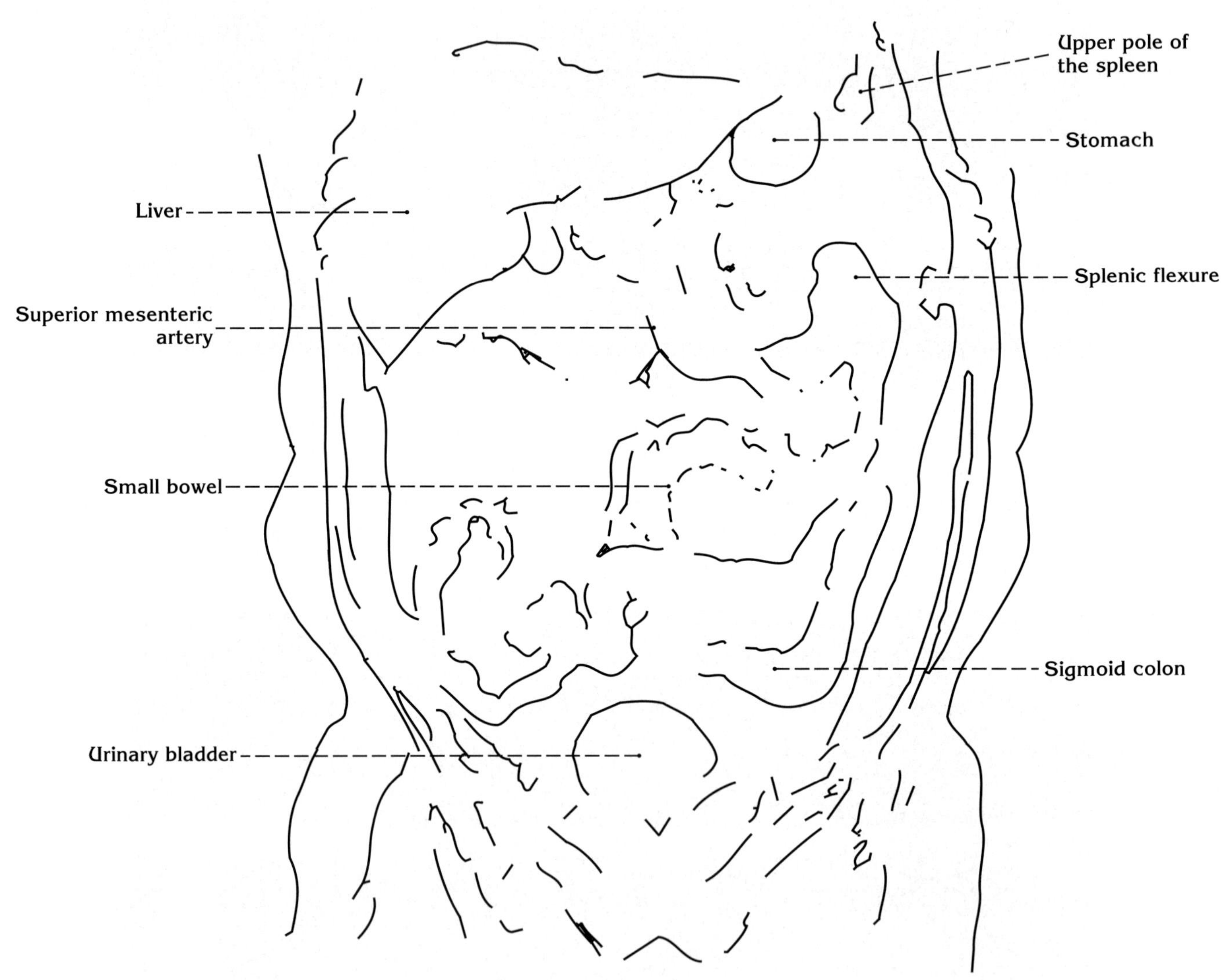

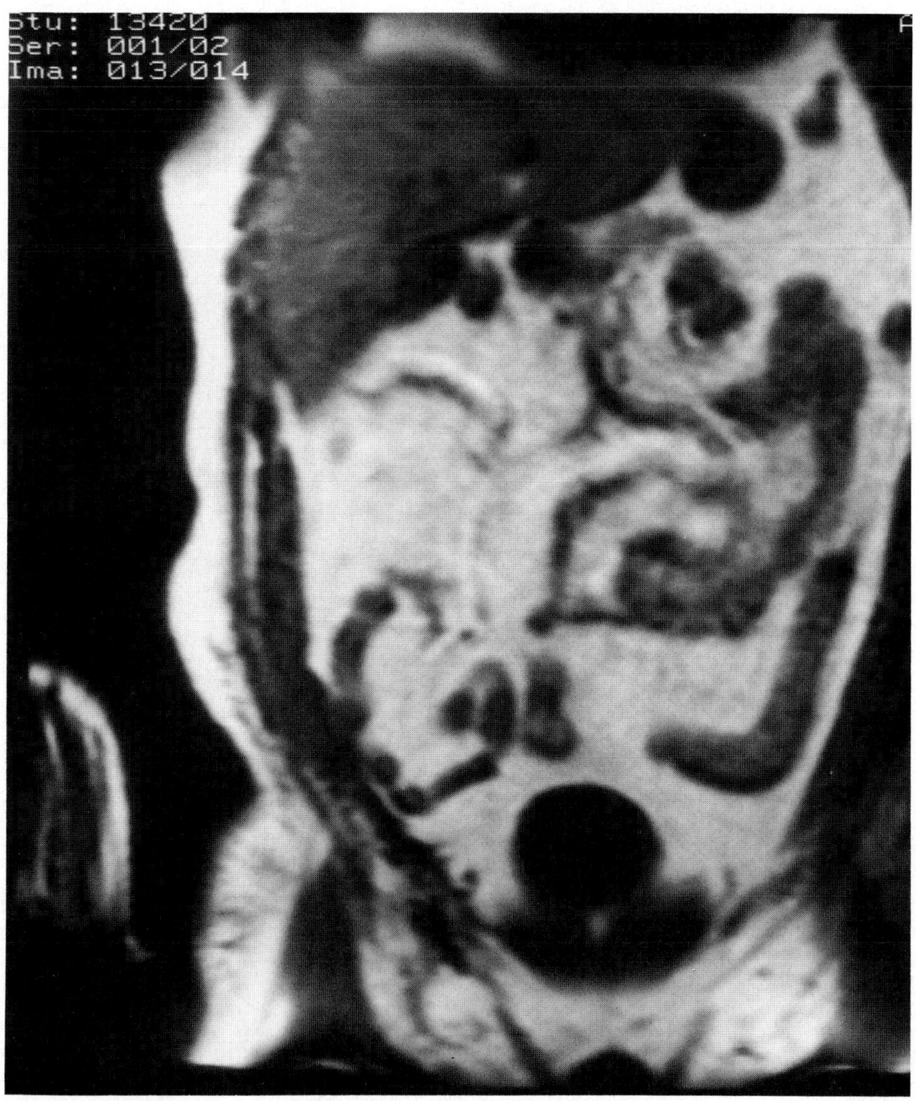

3-11 Abdomen, coronal view (TR 600, TE 20).

Abdomen, Coronal

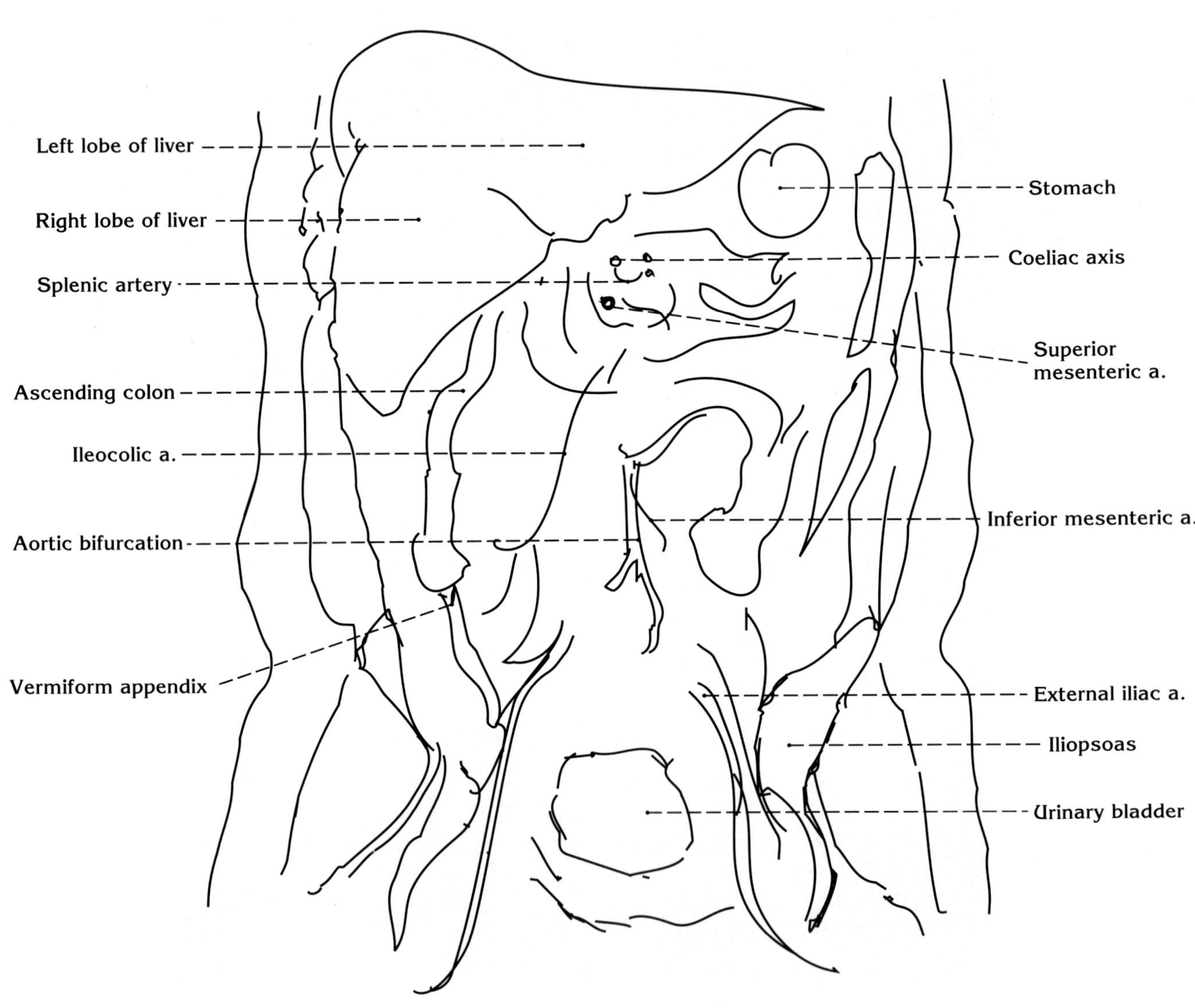

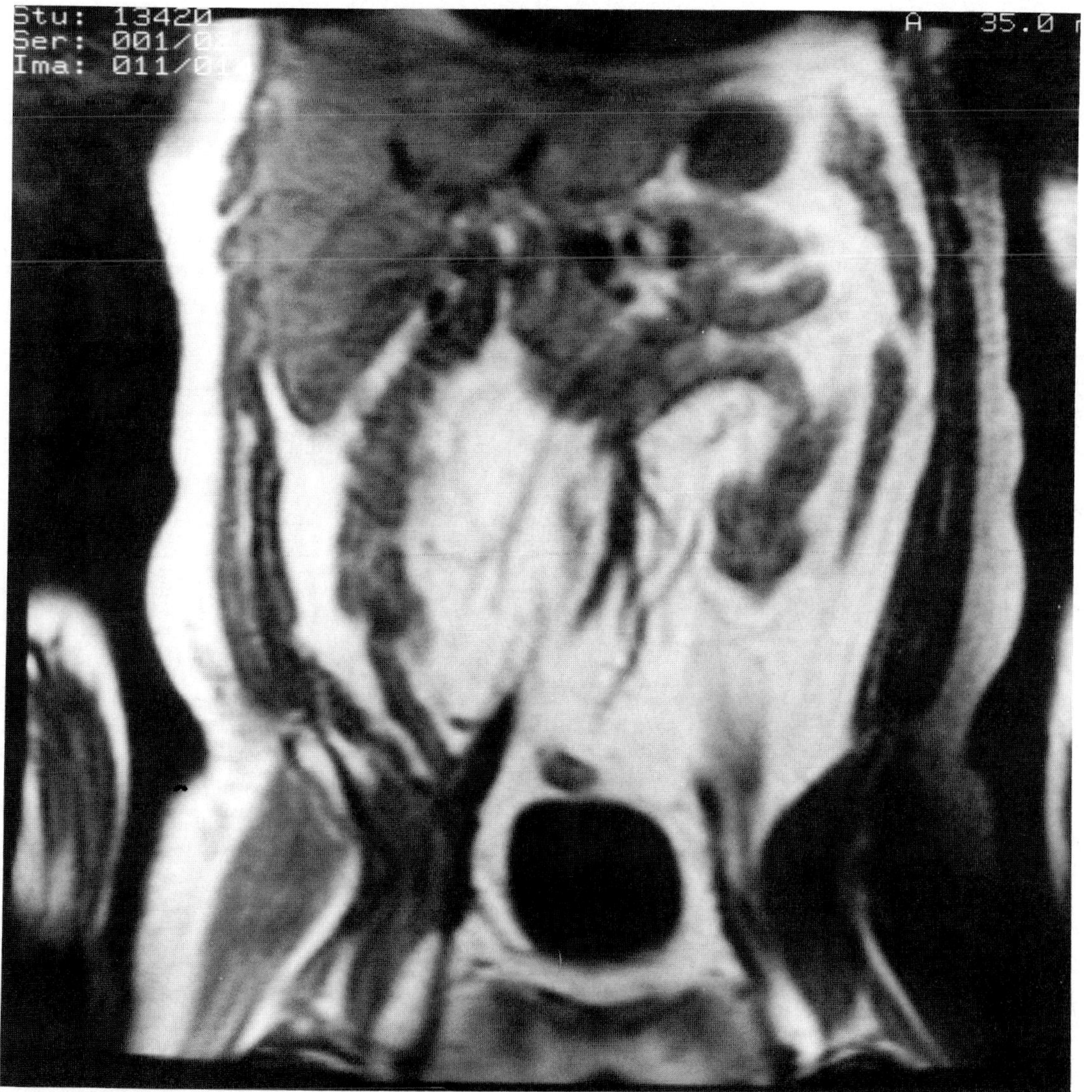

3-12 Abdomen, coronal view showing branches of the abdominal aorta (TR 600, TE 20).

Abdomen, Coronal

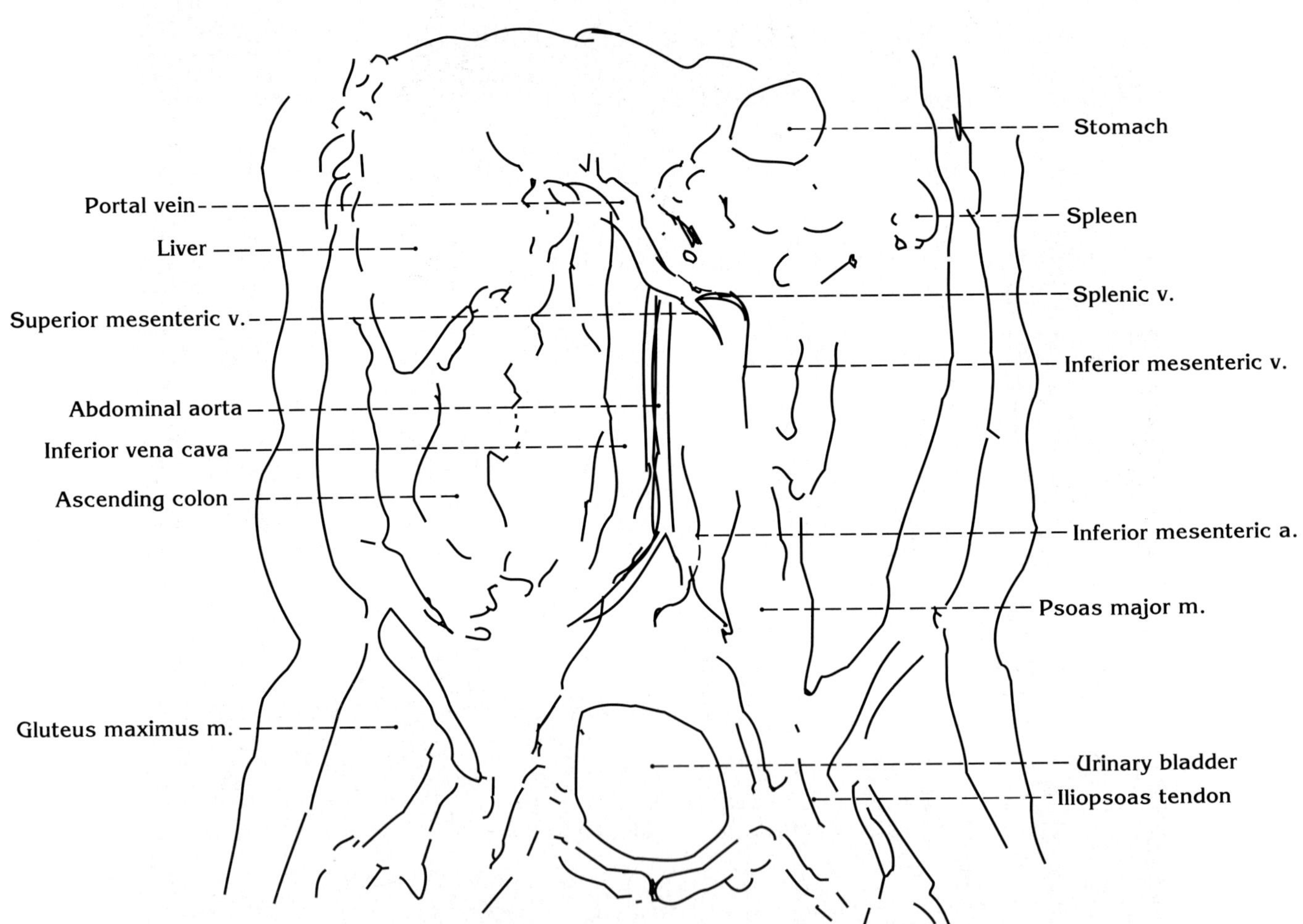

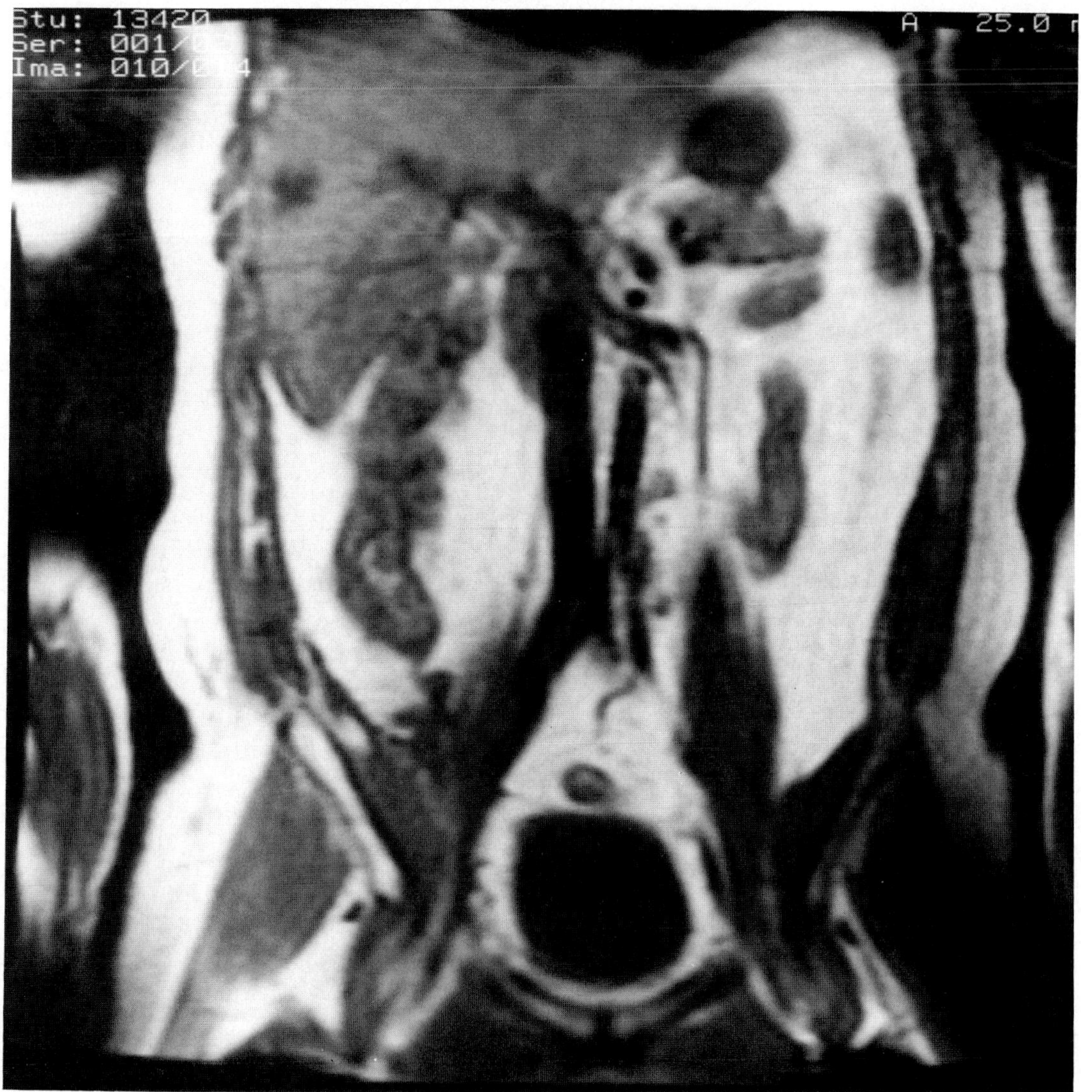

3-13 Abdomen, coronal view (TR 600, TE 20).

Male Abdomen, Coronal

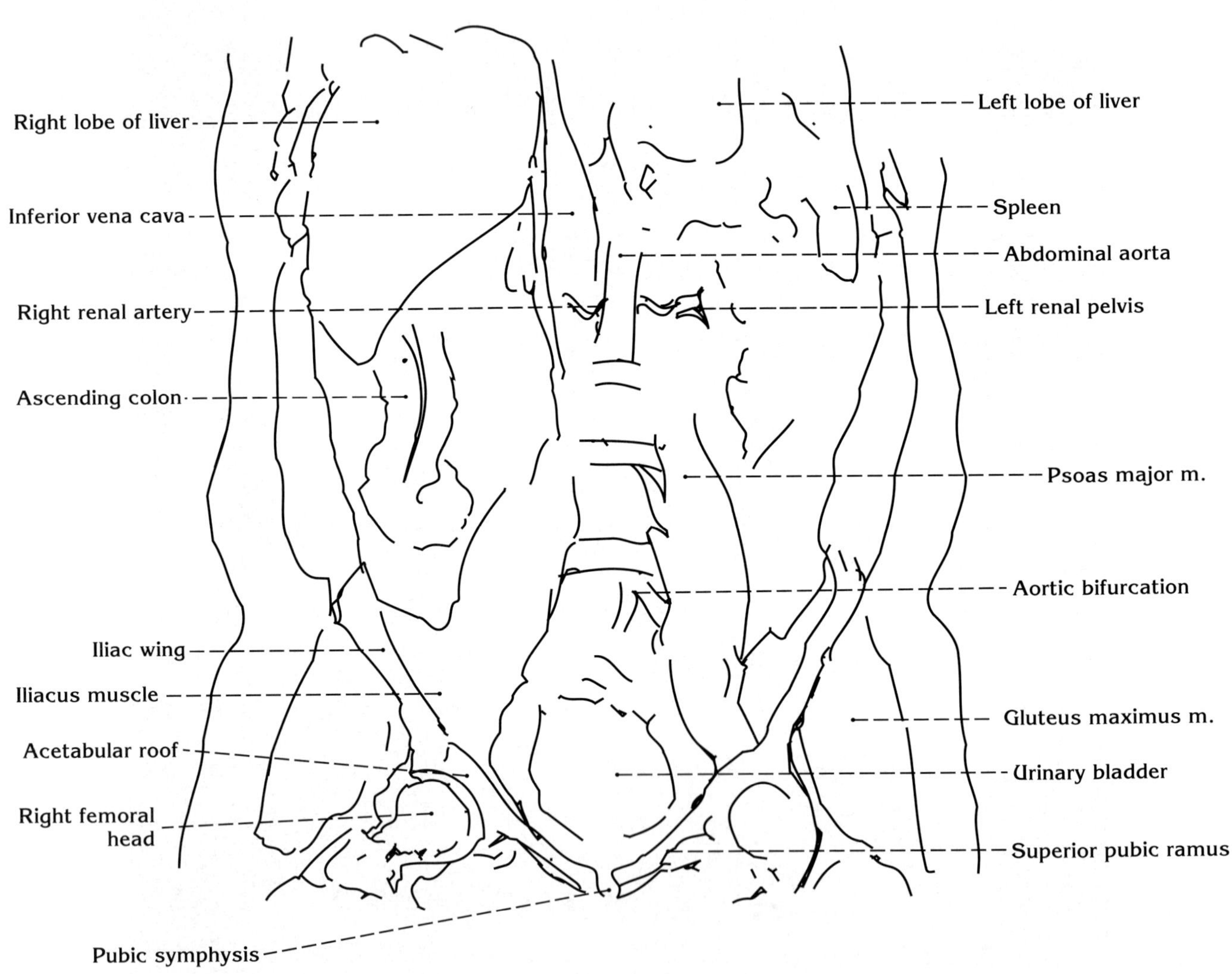

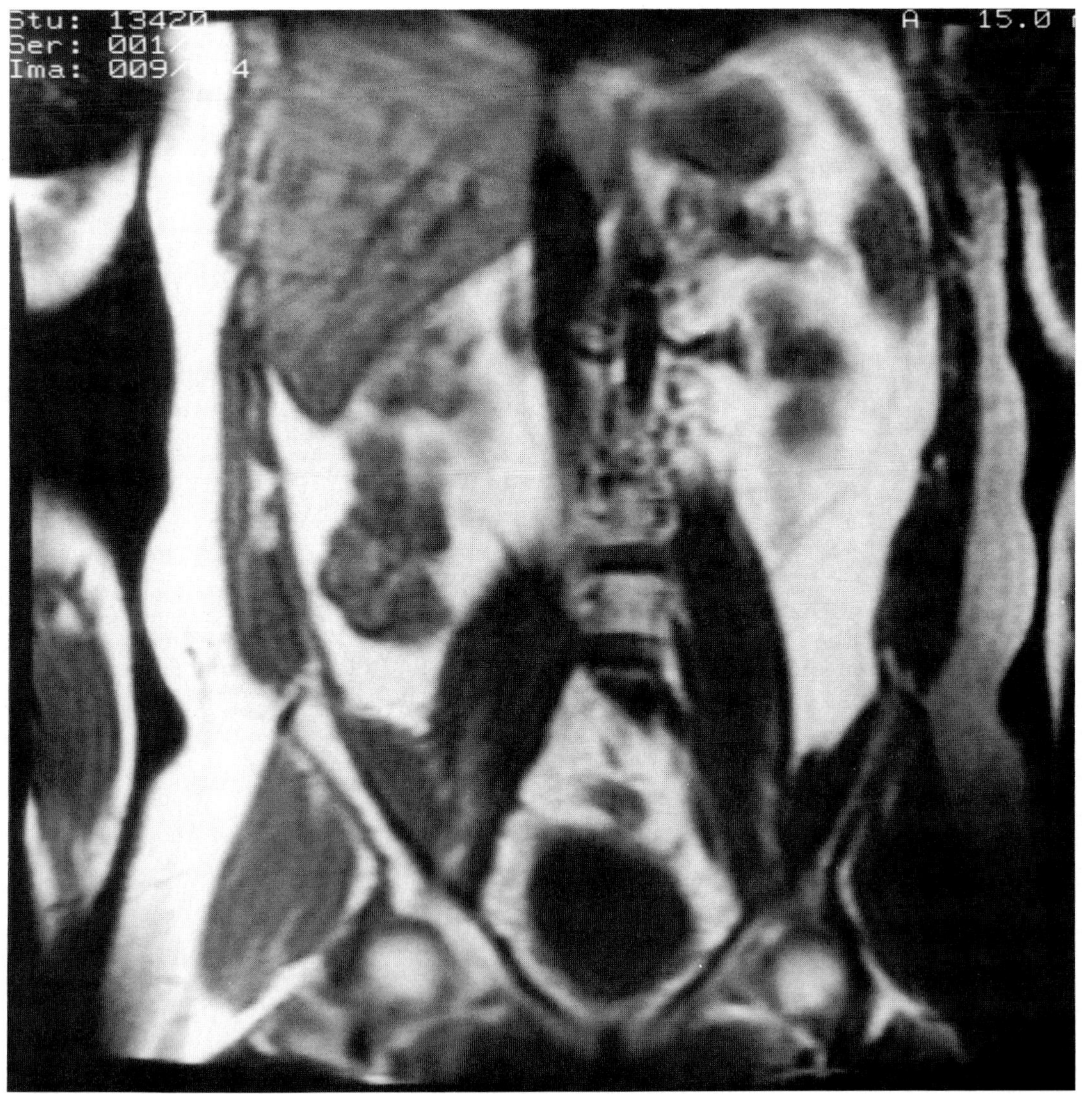

3-14 Male abdomen, coronal view (TR 600, TE 20).

Abdomen, Coronal

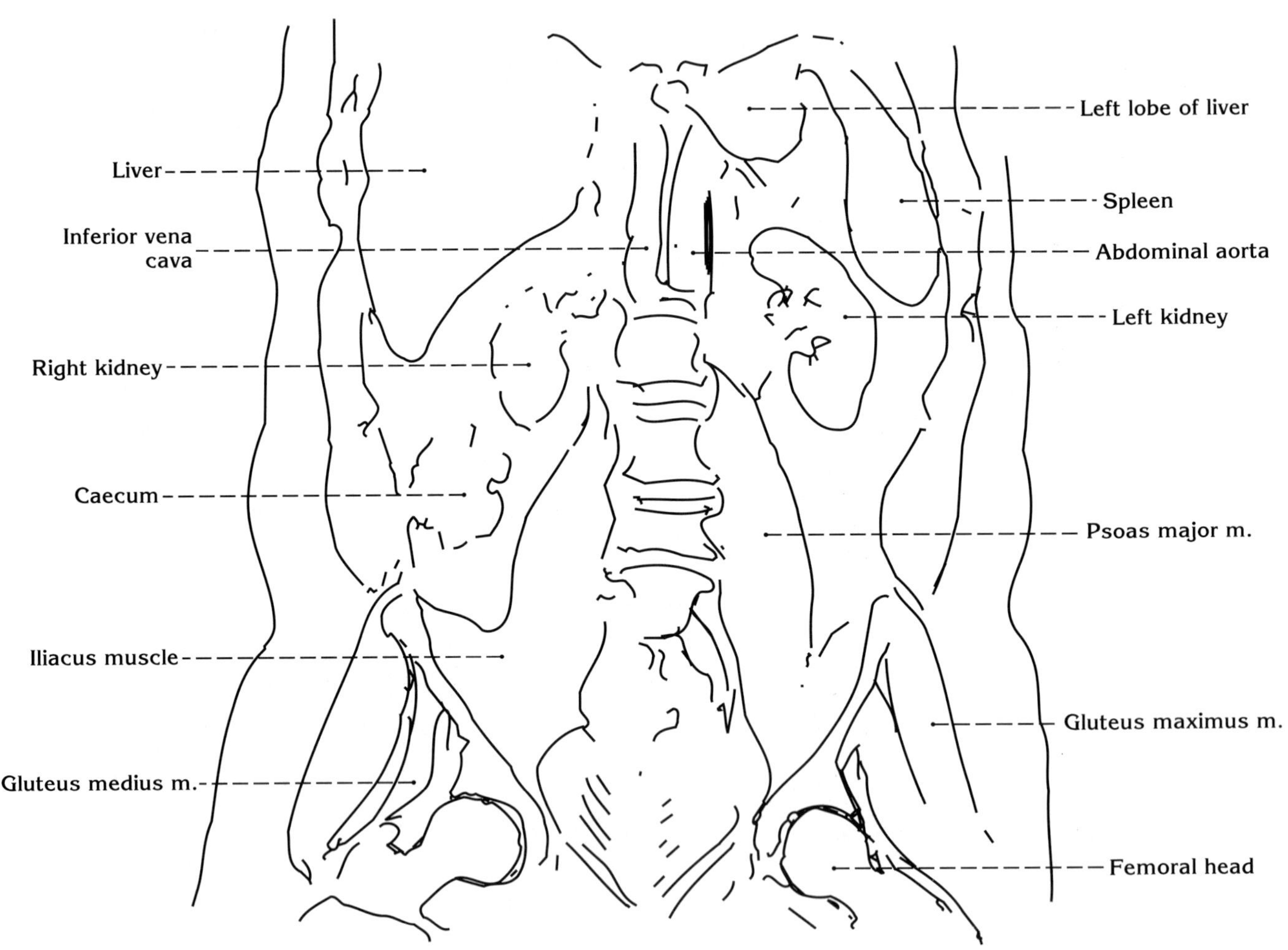

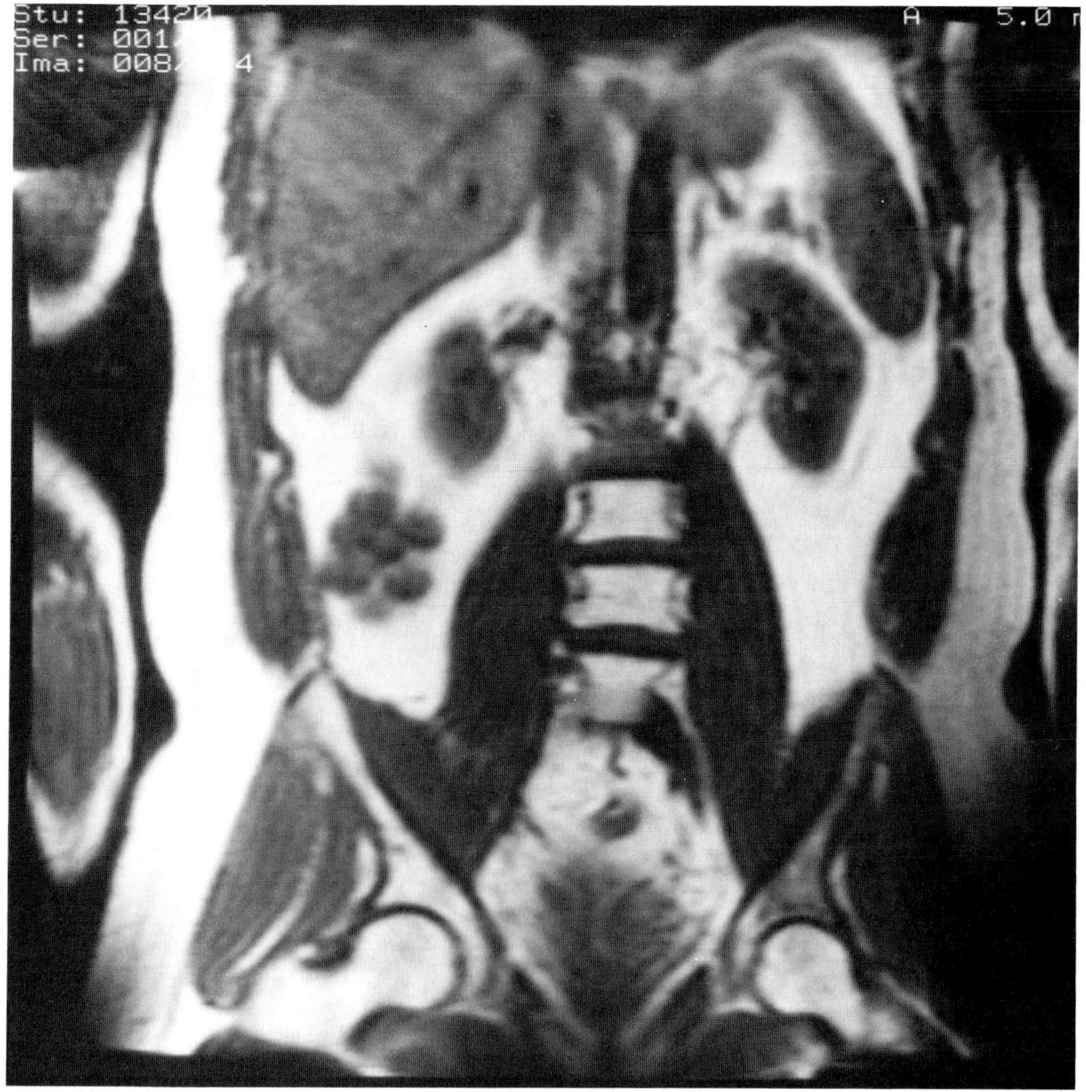

3-15 Abdomen, coronal view (TR 600, TE 20).

Abdomen, Coronal

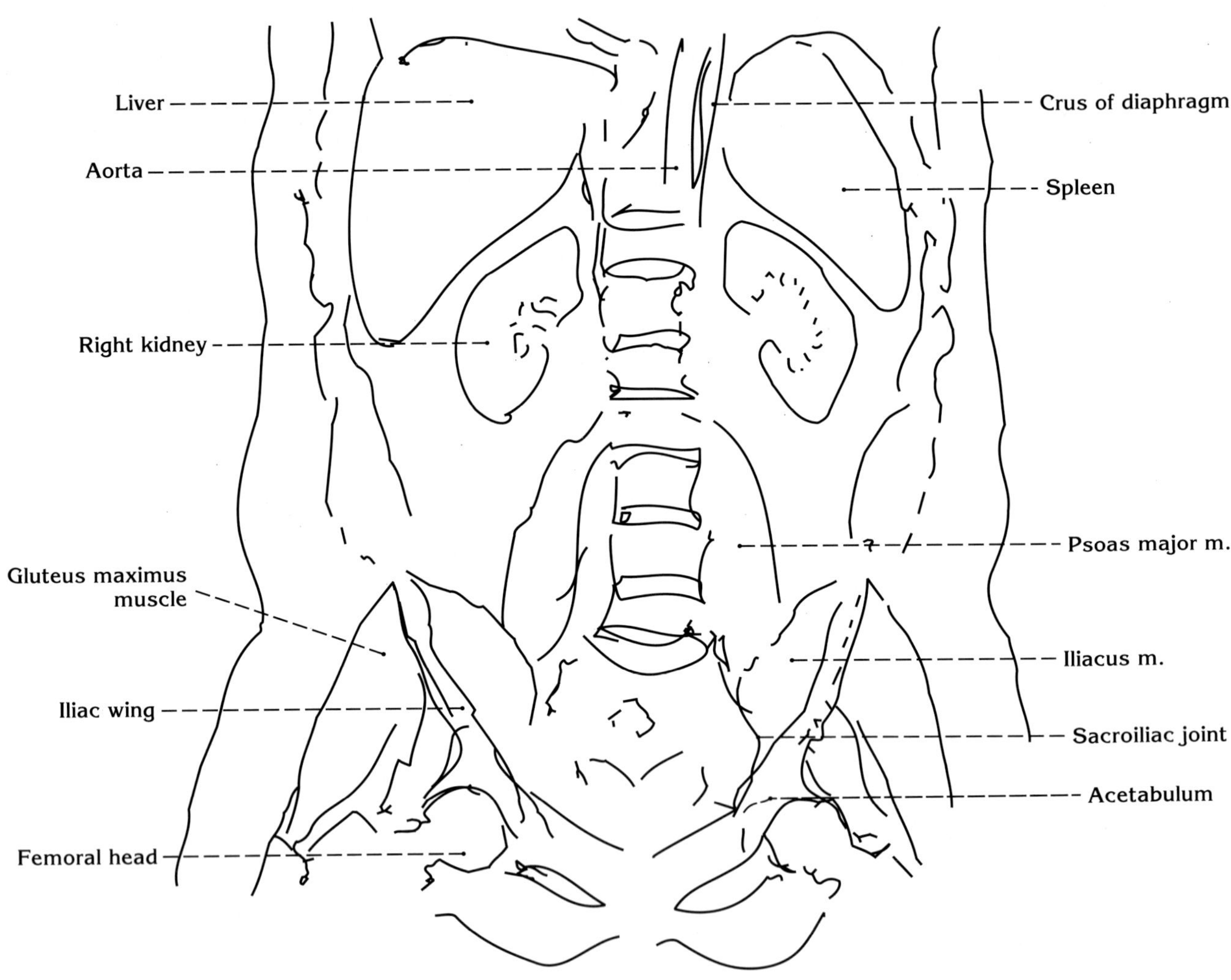

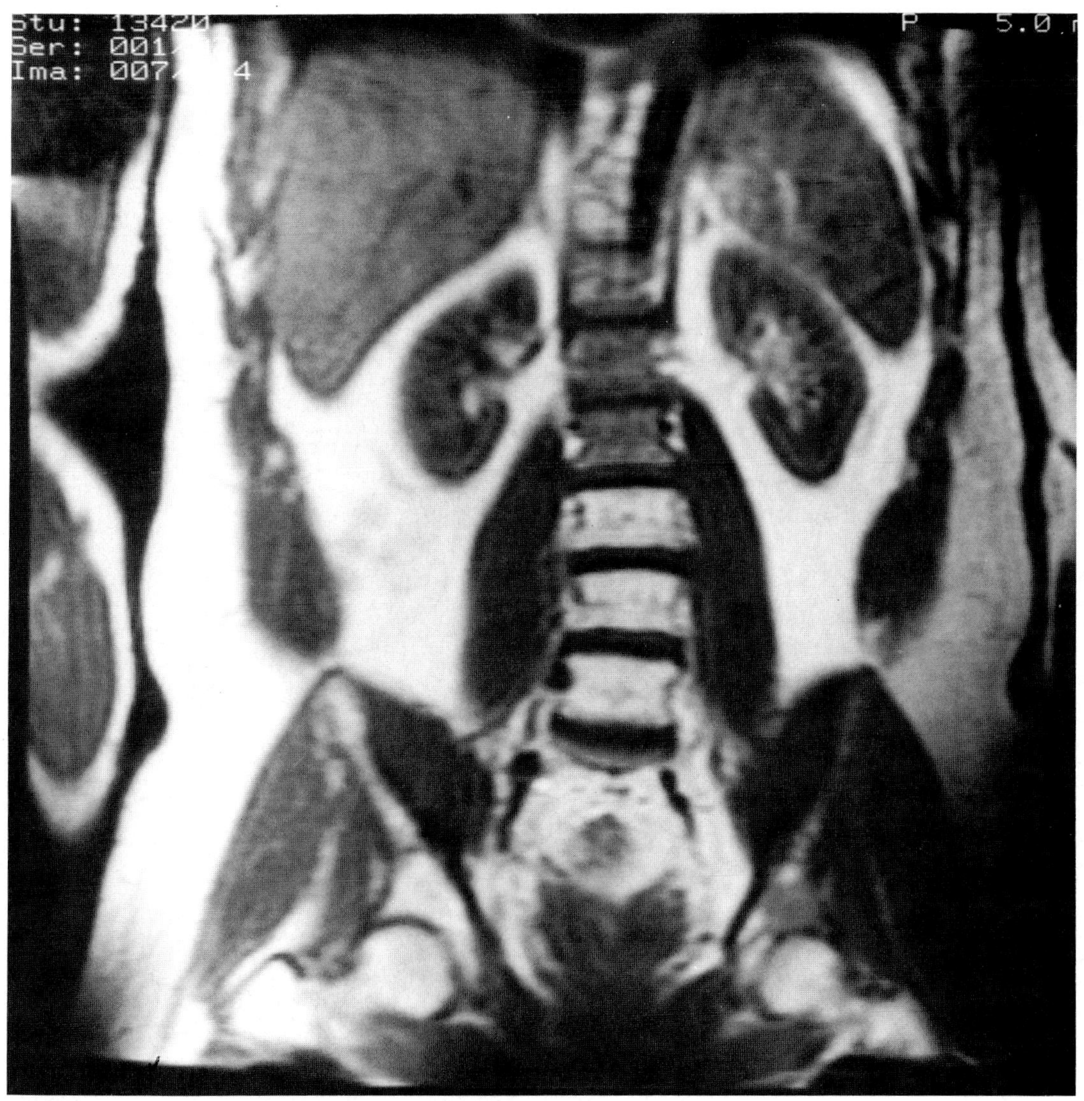

3-16 Abdomen, coronal view (TR 600, TE 20).

Abdominal Vessels, Axial

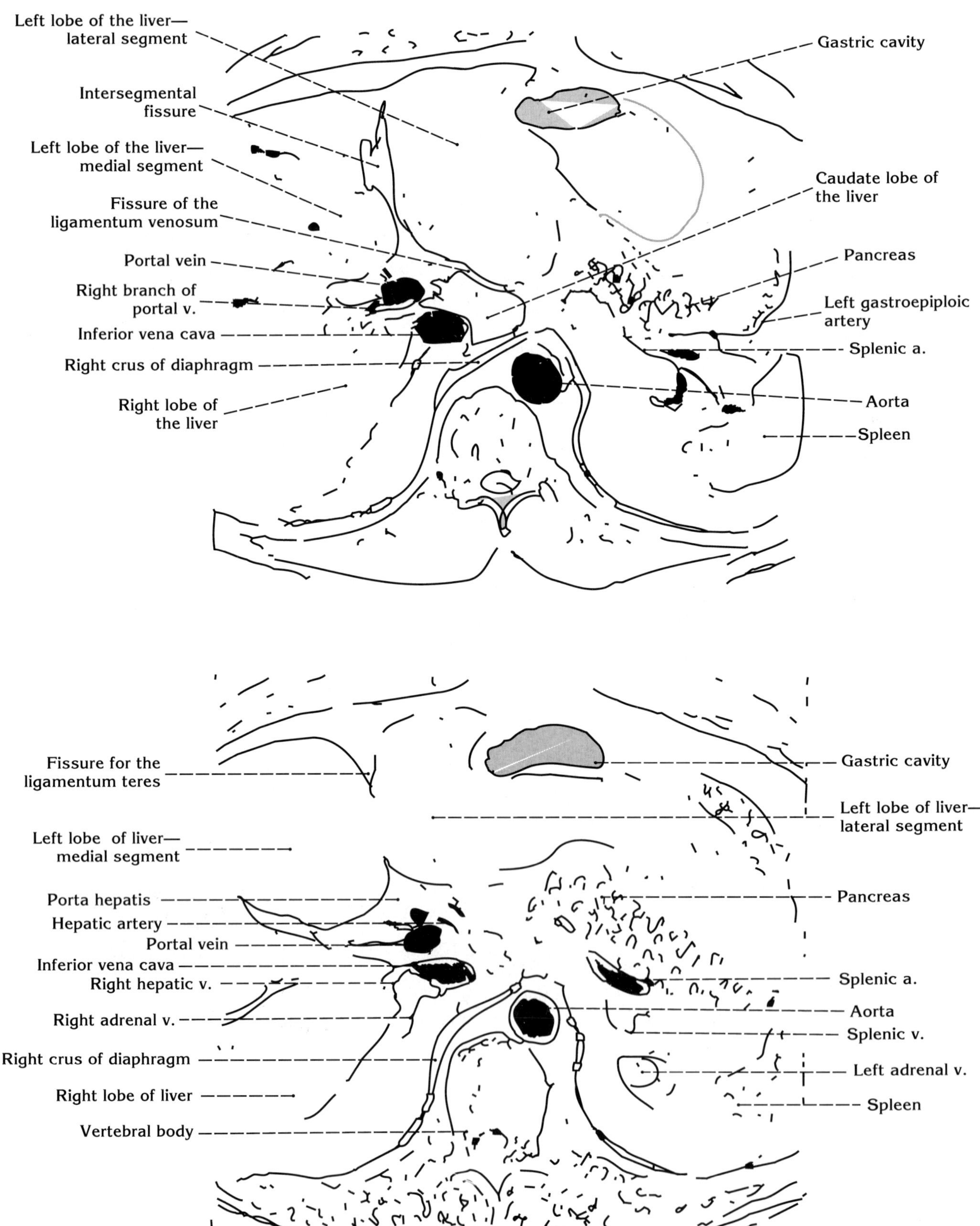

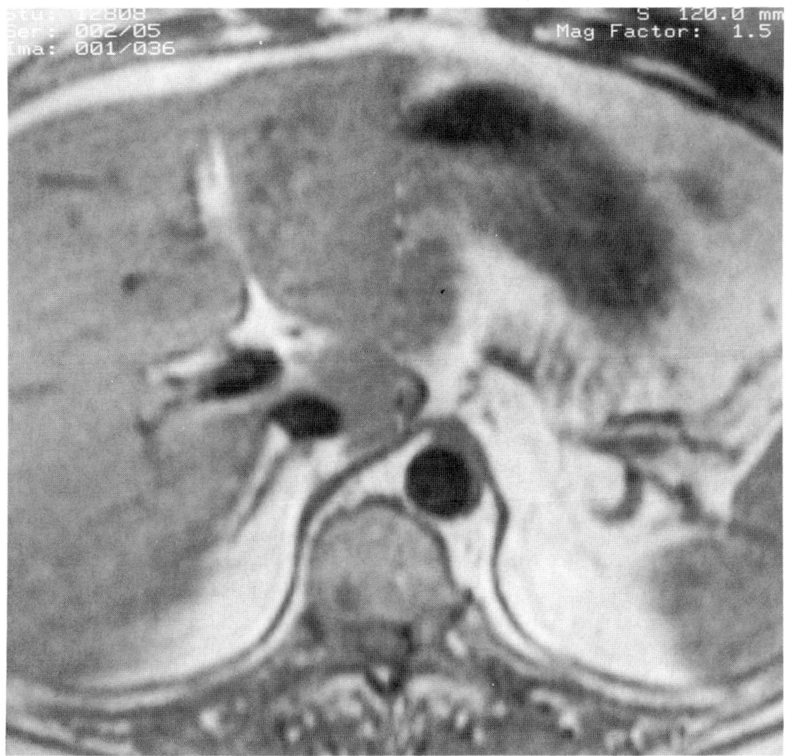

3-17 Abdomen, axial view showing the abdominal vessels (TR 2000, TE 20).

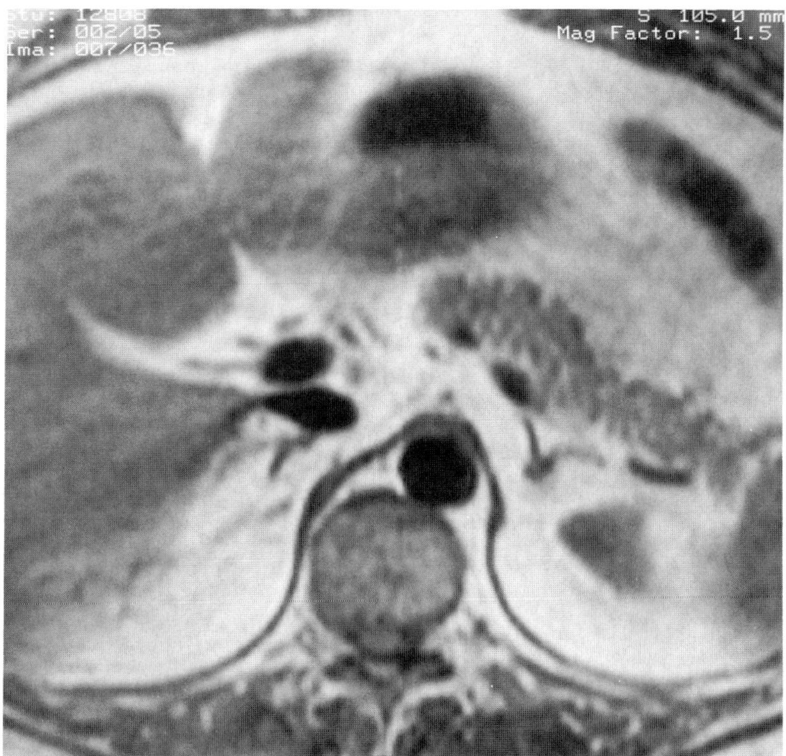

3-18 Abdomen, axial view showing the abdominal vessels (TR 2000, TE 20).
(This patient had a right adrenal mass, which may account for the unusual adrenal vein.)

Abdominal Vessels, Axial

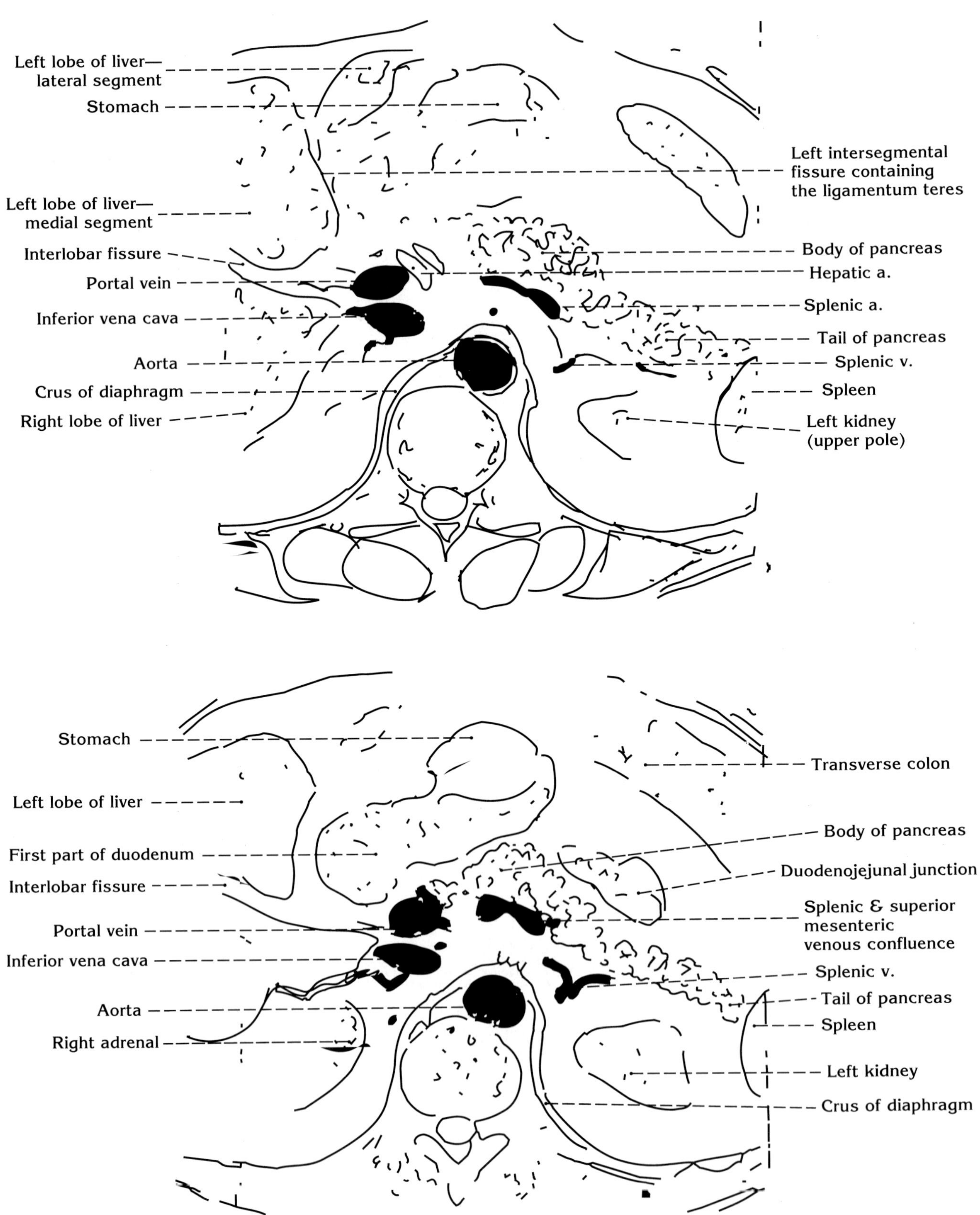

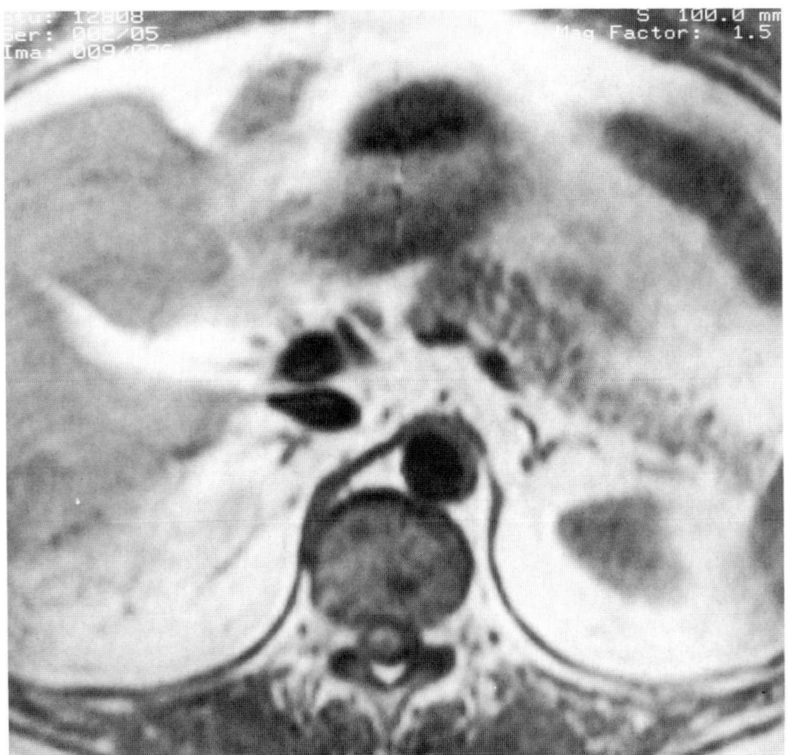

3-19 Abdomen, axial view showing the abdominal vessels (TR 2000, TE 20).

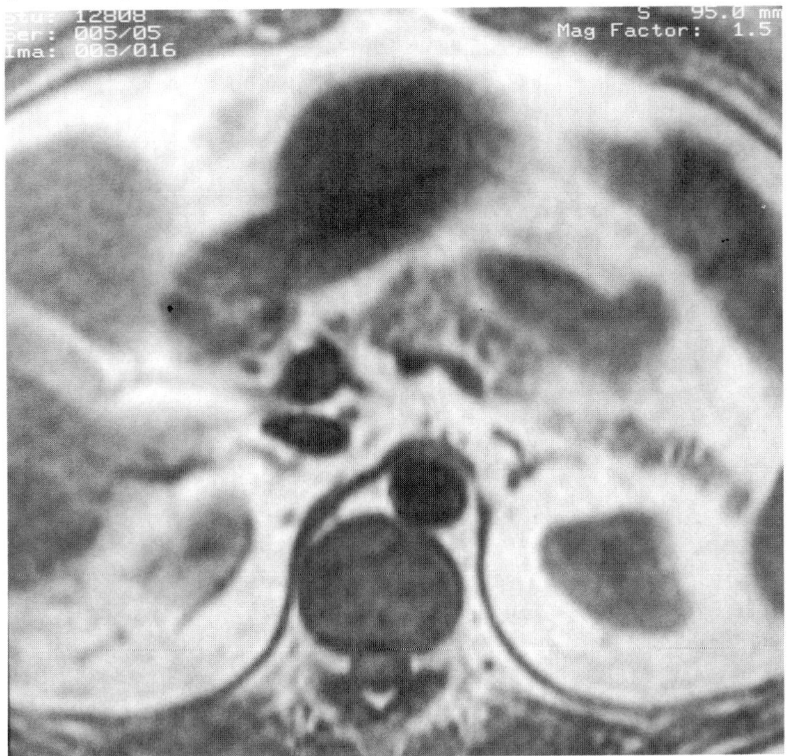

3-20 Abdomen, axial view showing the abdominal vessels (TR 2000, TE 20).

Abdominal Vessels, Axial

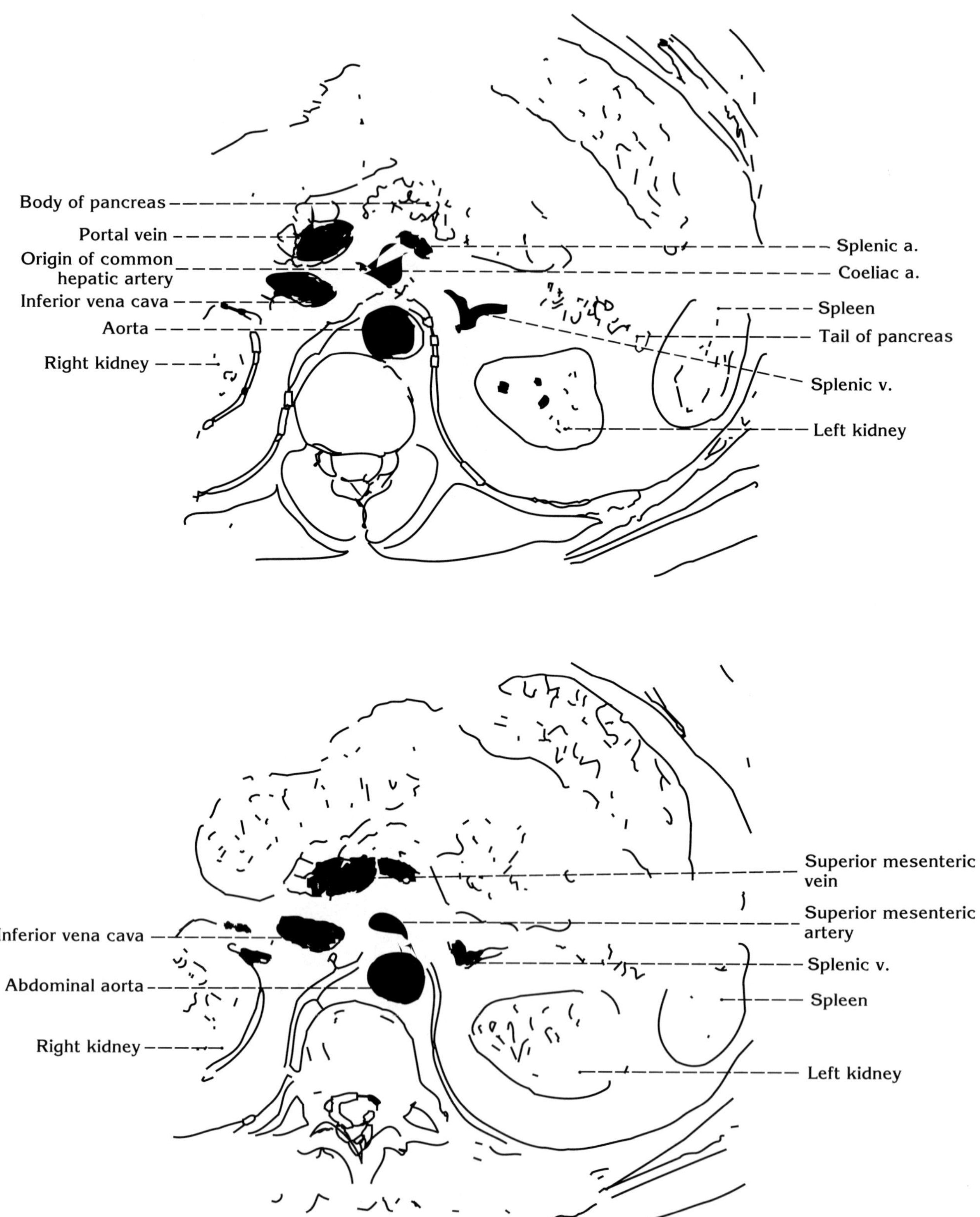

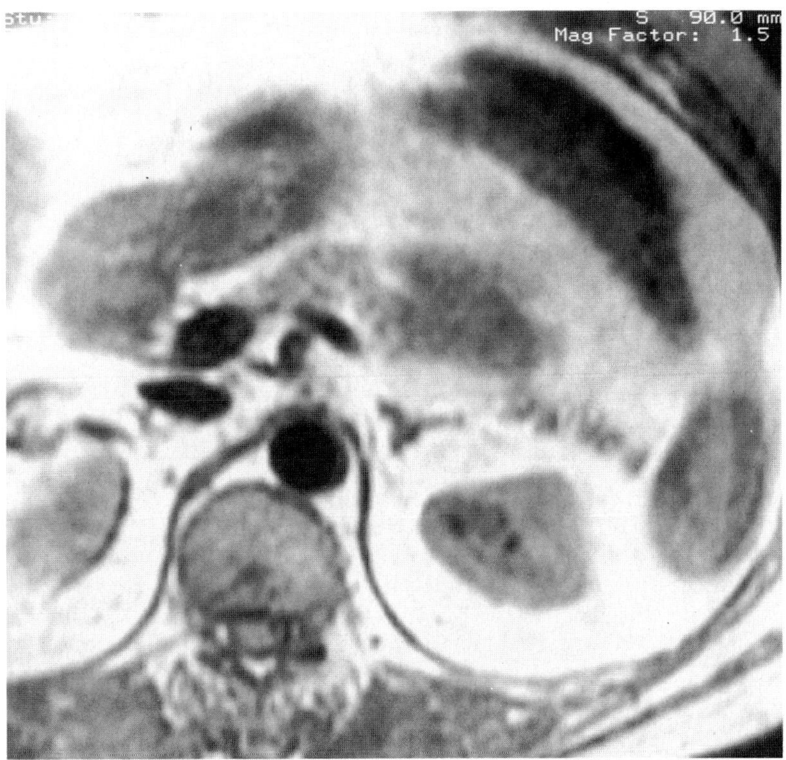

3-21 Abdomen, axial view showing the abdominal vessels (TR 2000, TE 20).

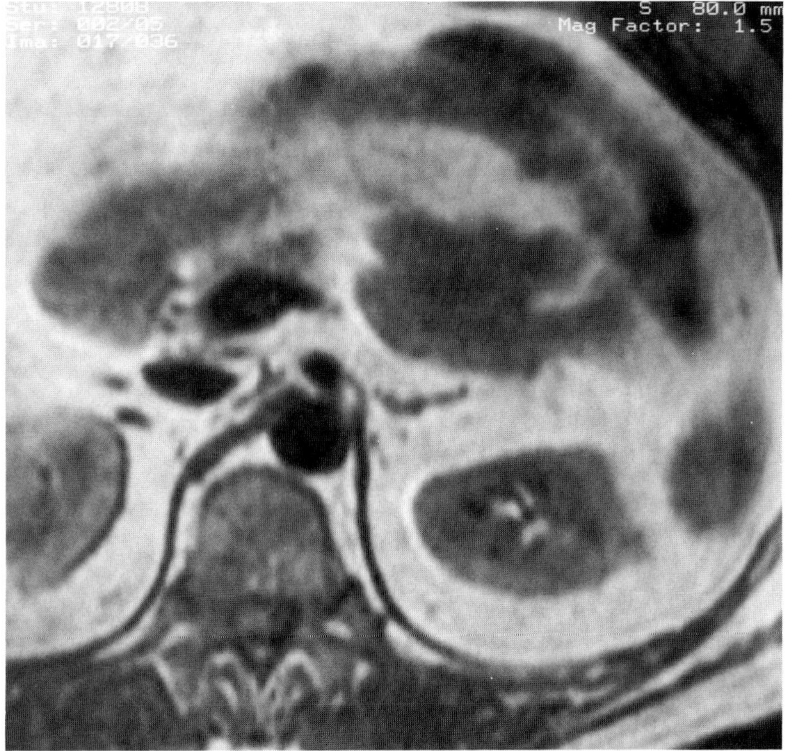

3-22 Abdomen, axial view showing the abdominal vessels (TR 2000, TE 20).

Abdominal Vessels, Axial

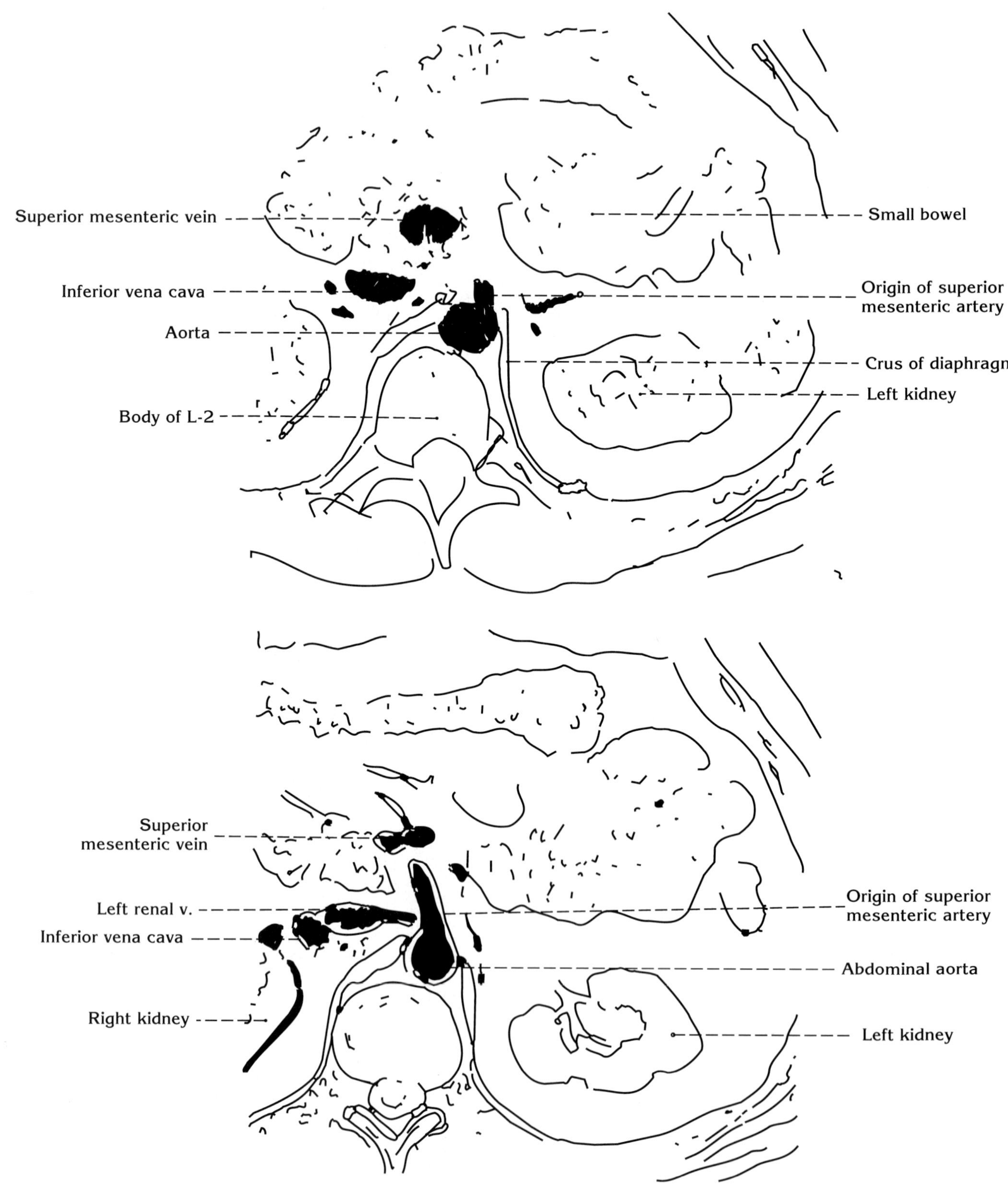

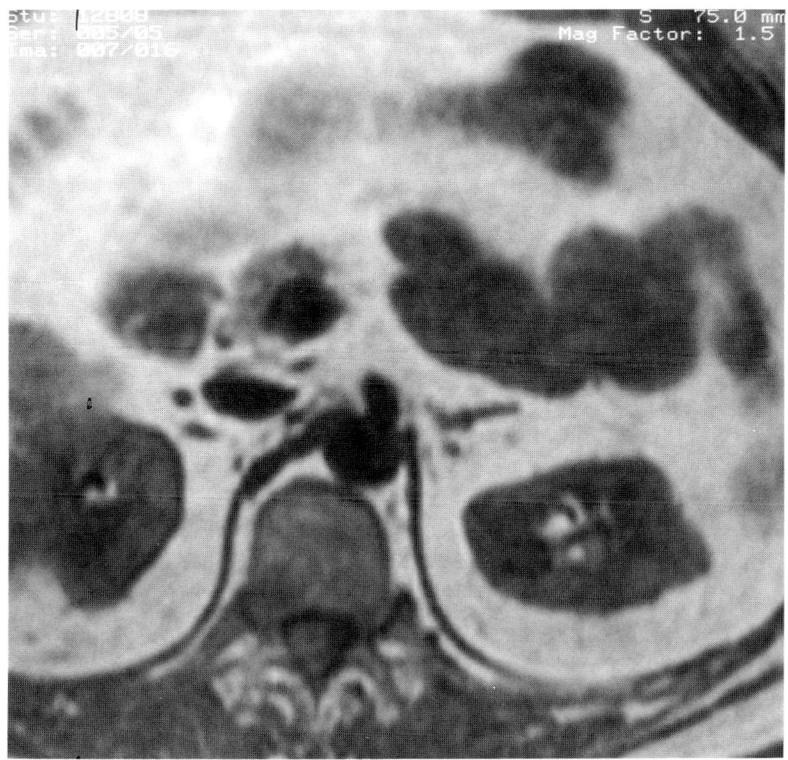

3-23 Abdomen, axial view showing the abdominal vessels (TR 2000, TE 20).

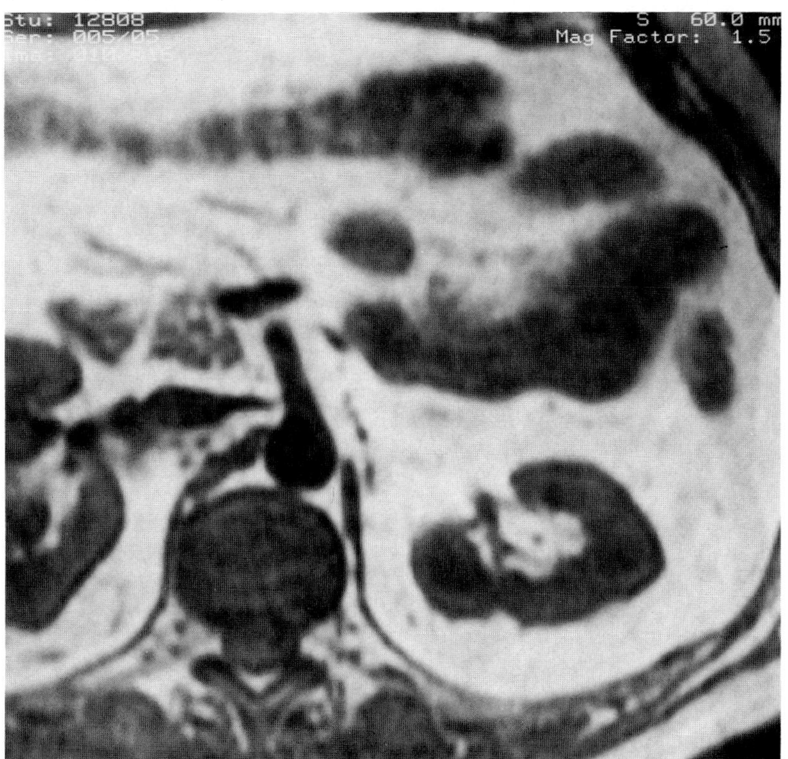

3-24 Abdomen, axial view showing the abdominal vessels (TR 2000, TE 20).

Abdominal Vessels, Axial

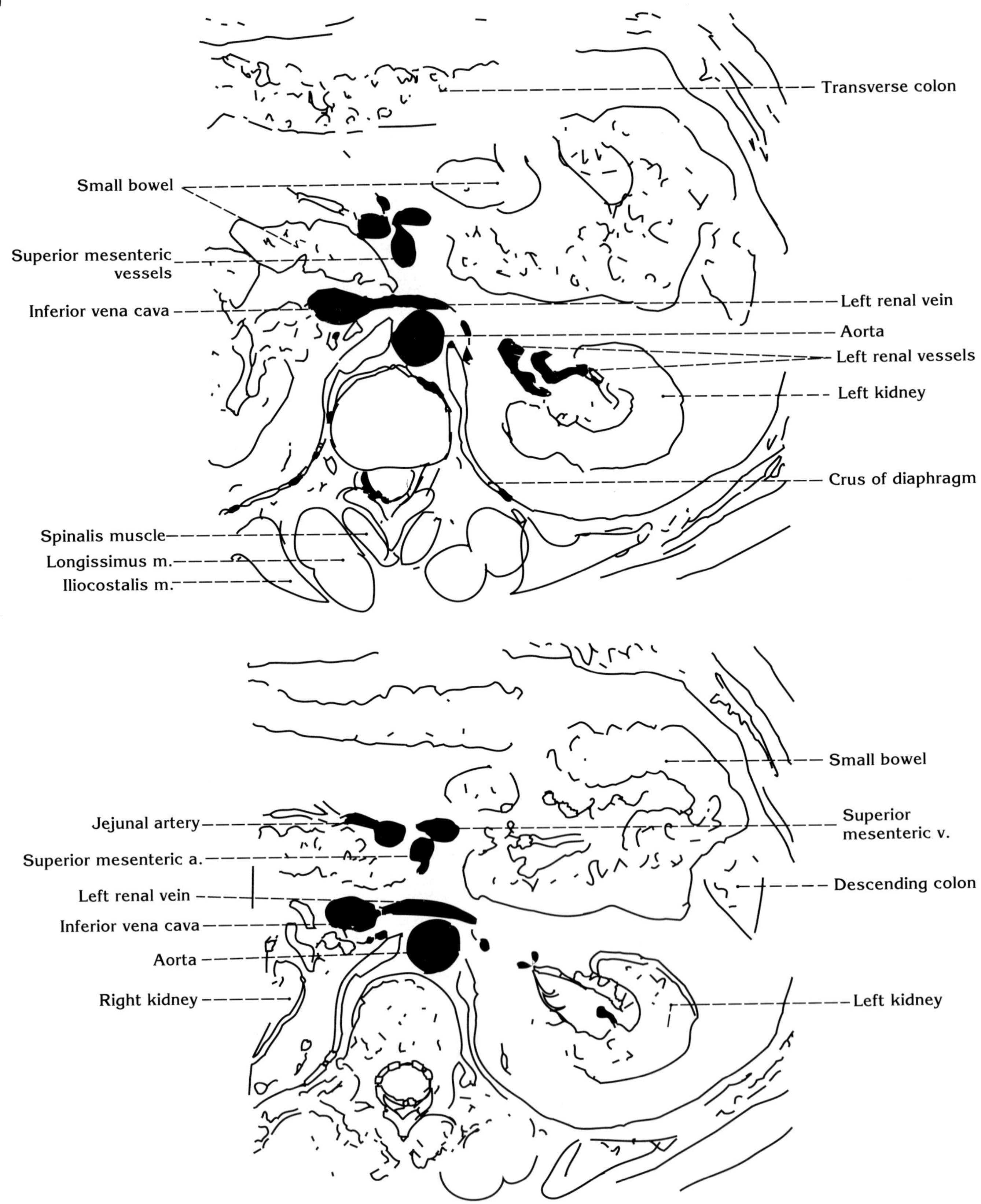

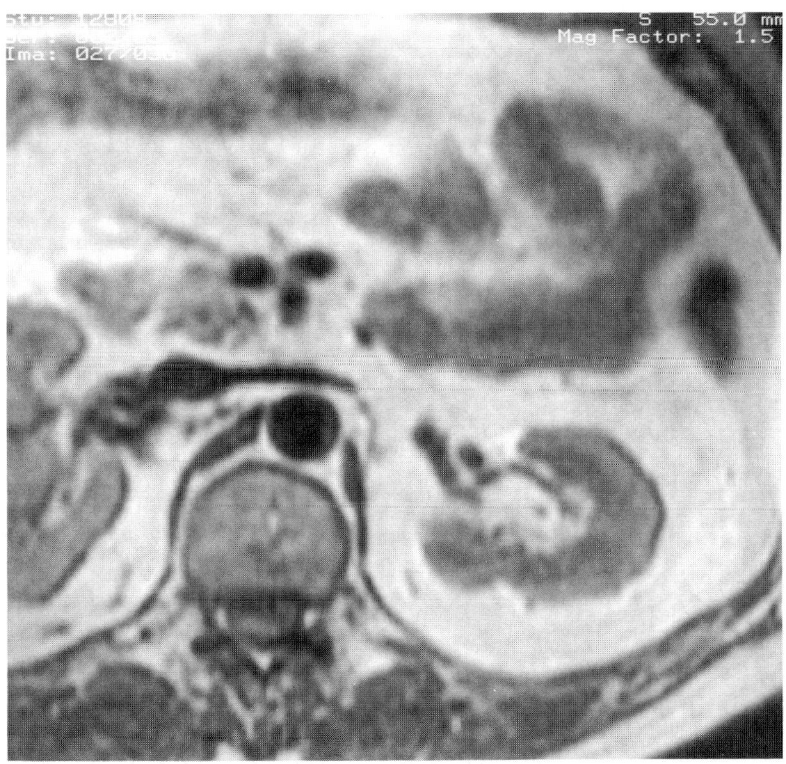

3-25 Abdomen, axial view showing the abdominal vessels (TR 2000, TE 20).

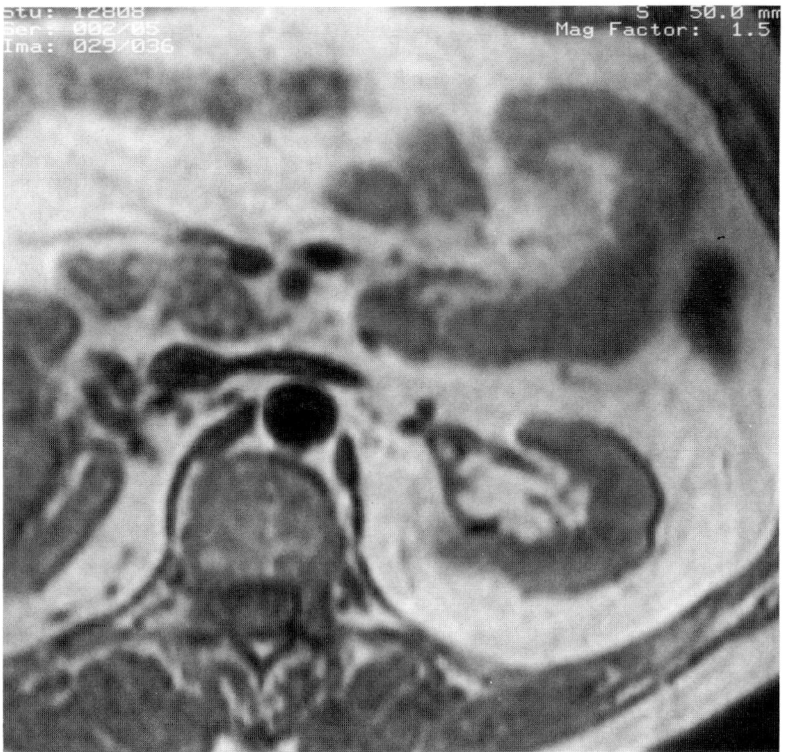

3-26 Abdomen, axial view showing the abdominal vessels (TR 2000, TE 20).

Abdominal Vessels, Axial

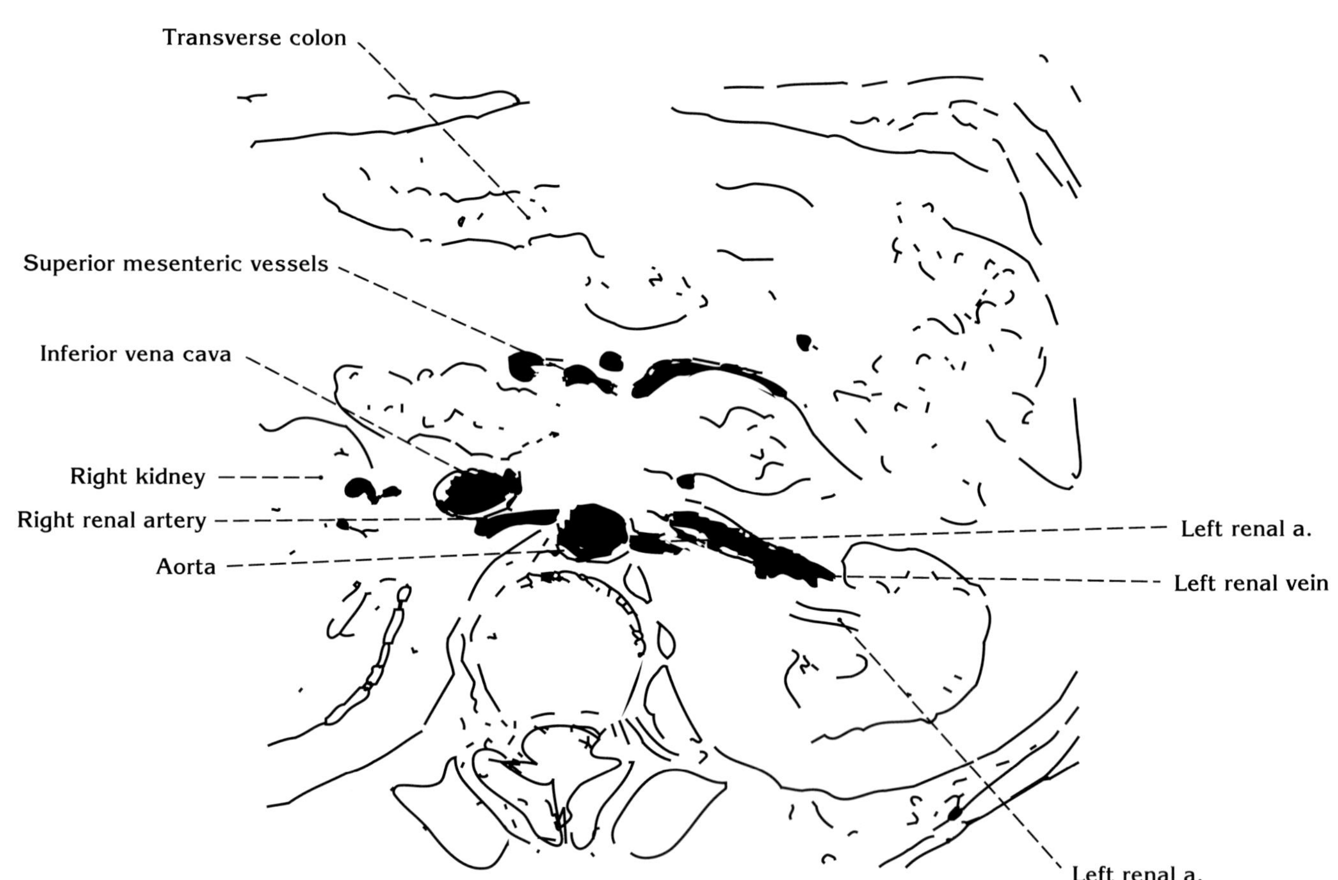

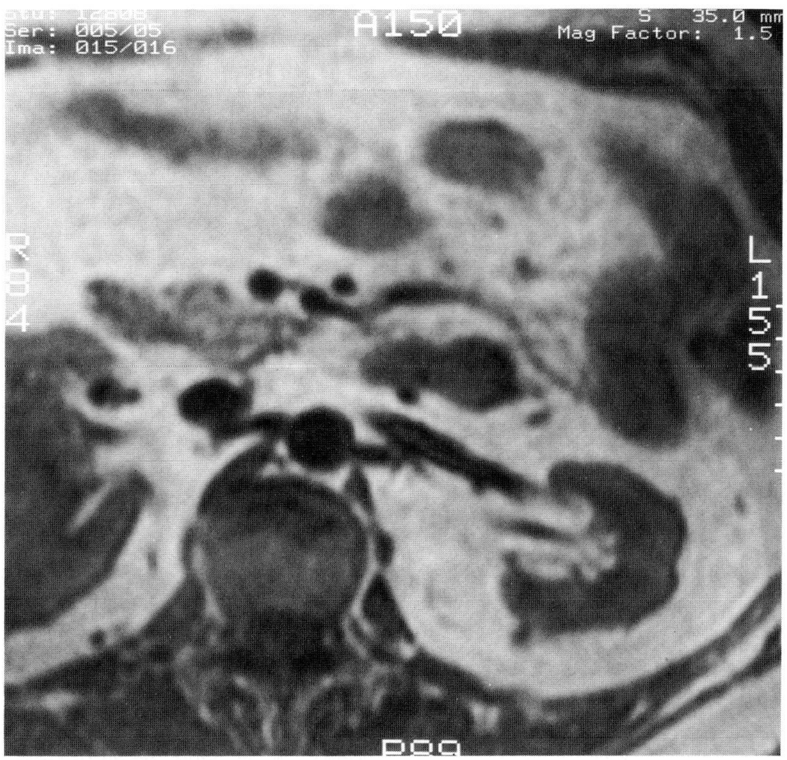

3-27 Abdomen, axial view showing the abdominal vessels (TR 2000, TE 20).

Female Pelvis, Sagittal

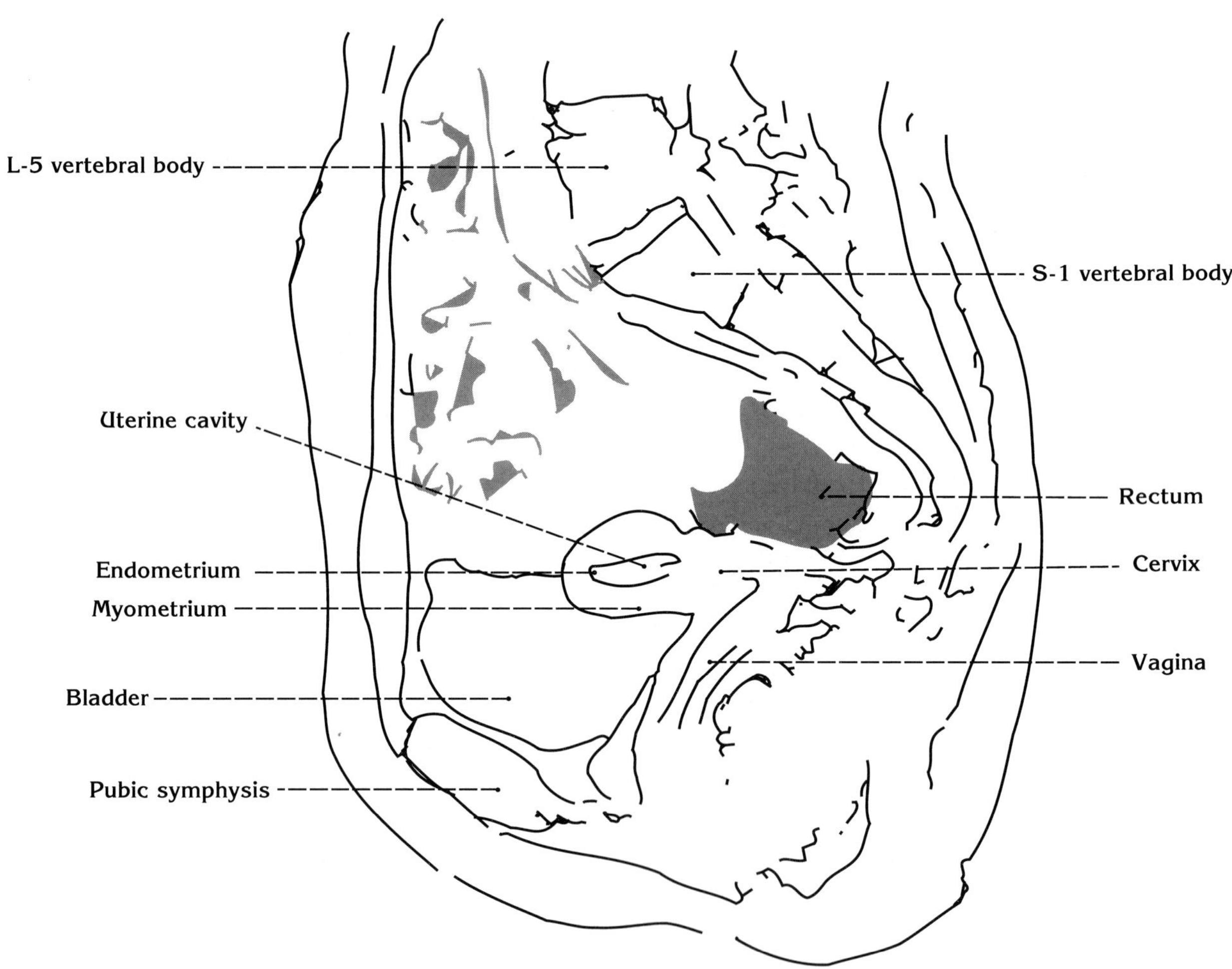

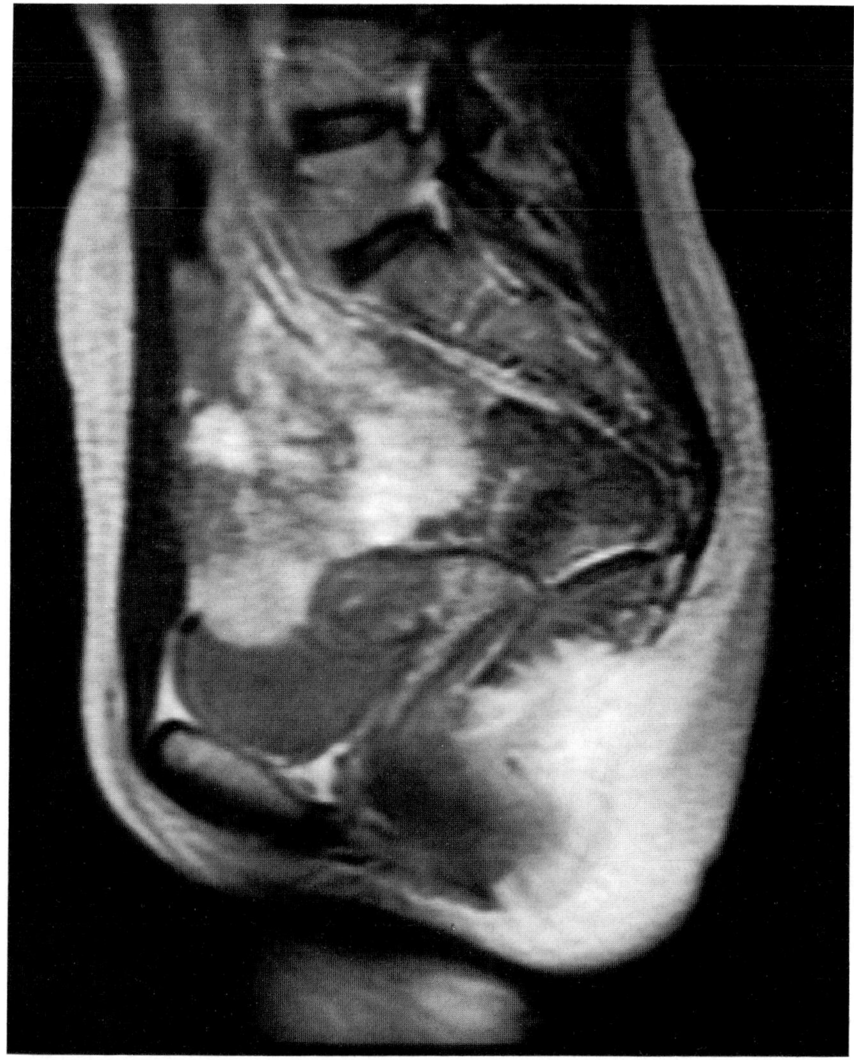

3-28 Female pelvis, sagittal view (TR 2000, TE 30).

Male Pelvis, Sagittal

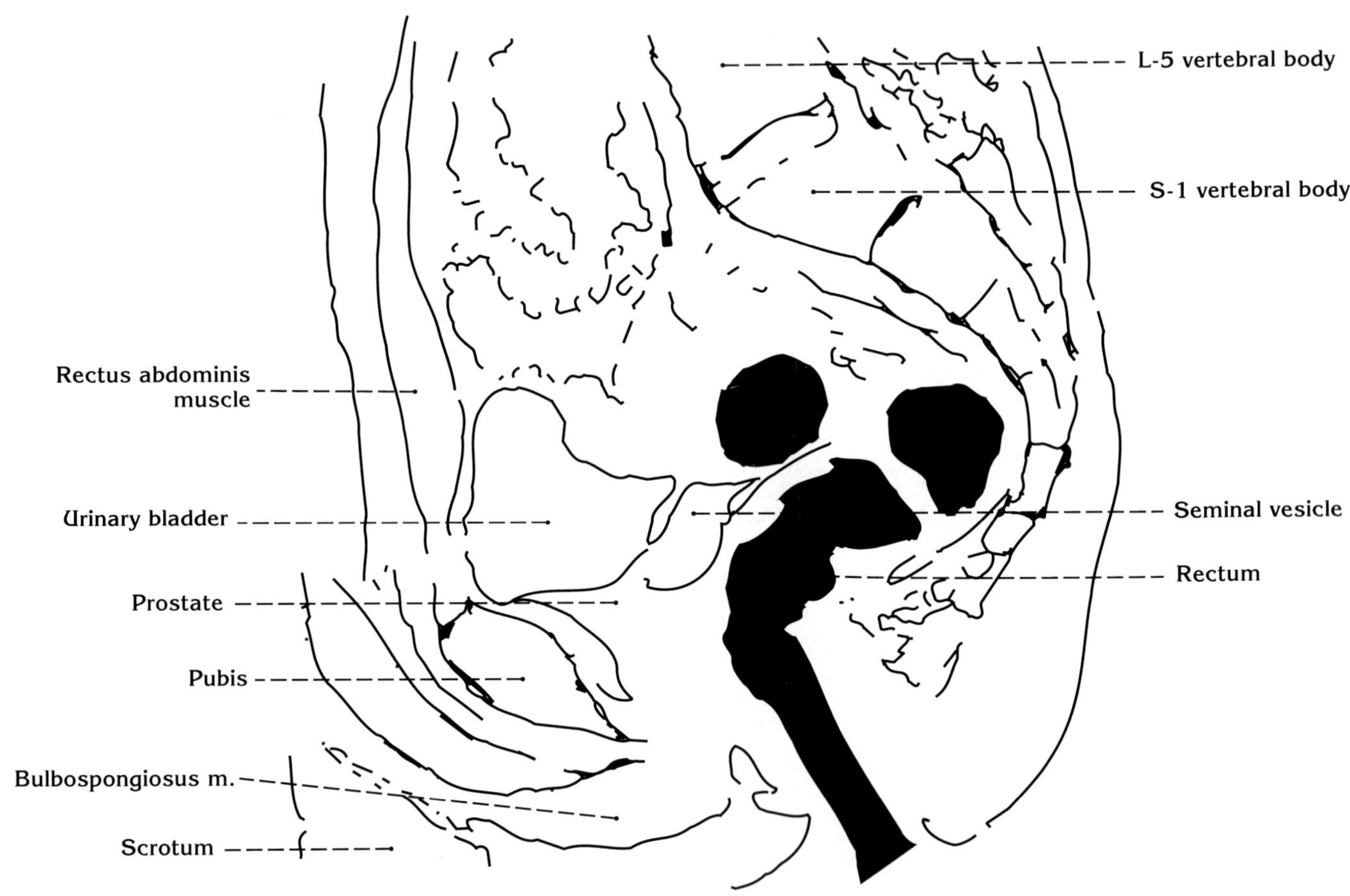

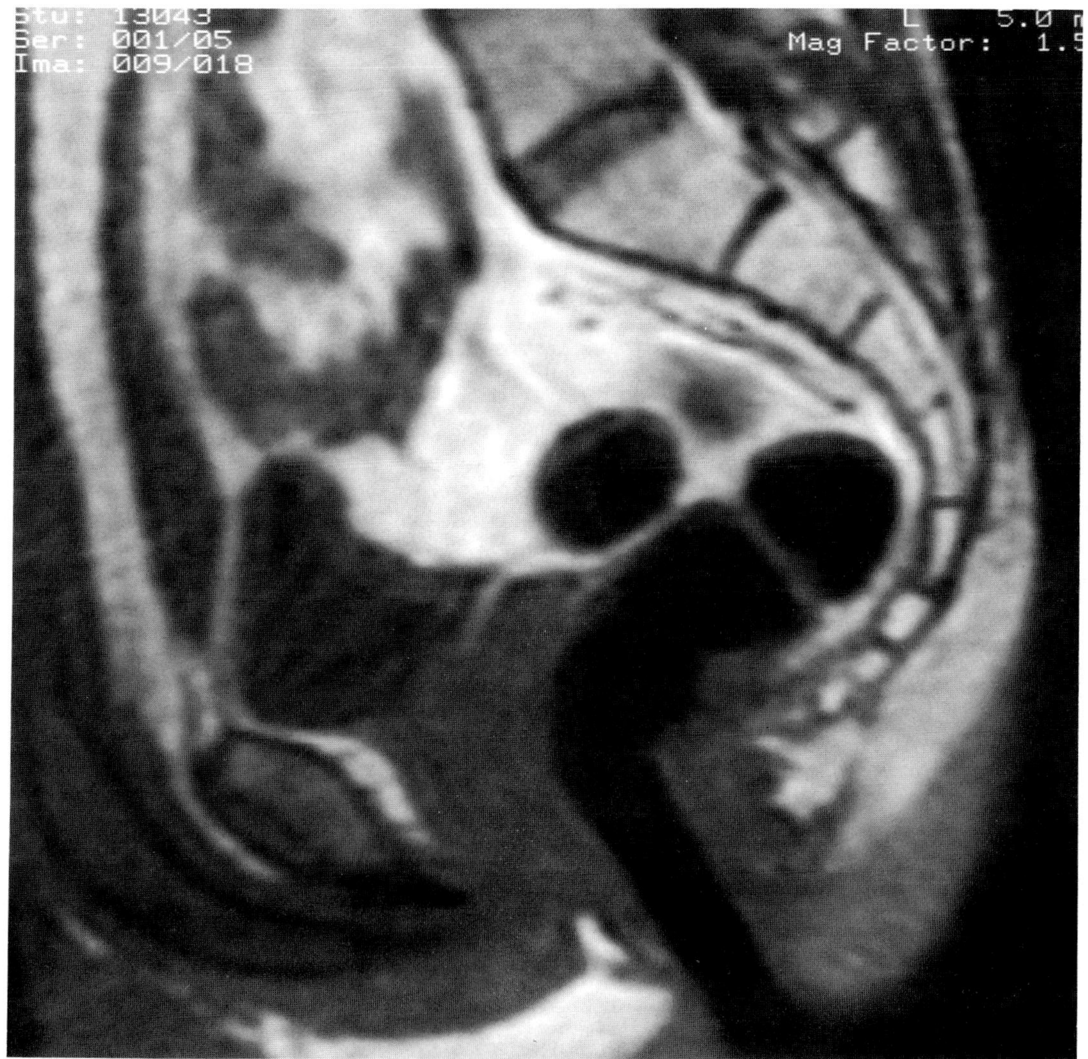

3-29 Male pelvis, sagittal view (TR 2000, TE 20).

Female Pelvis, Coronal

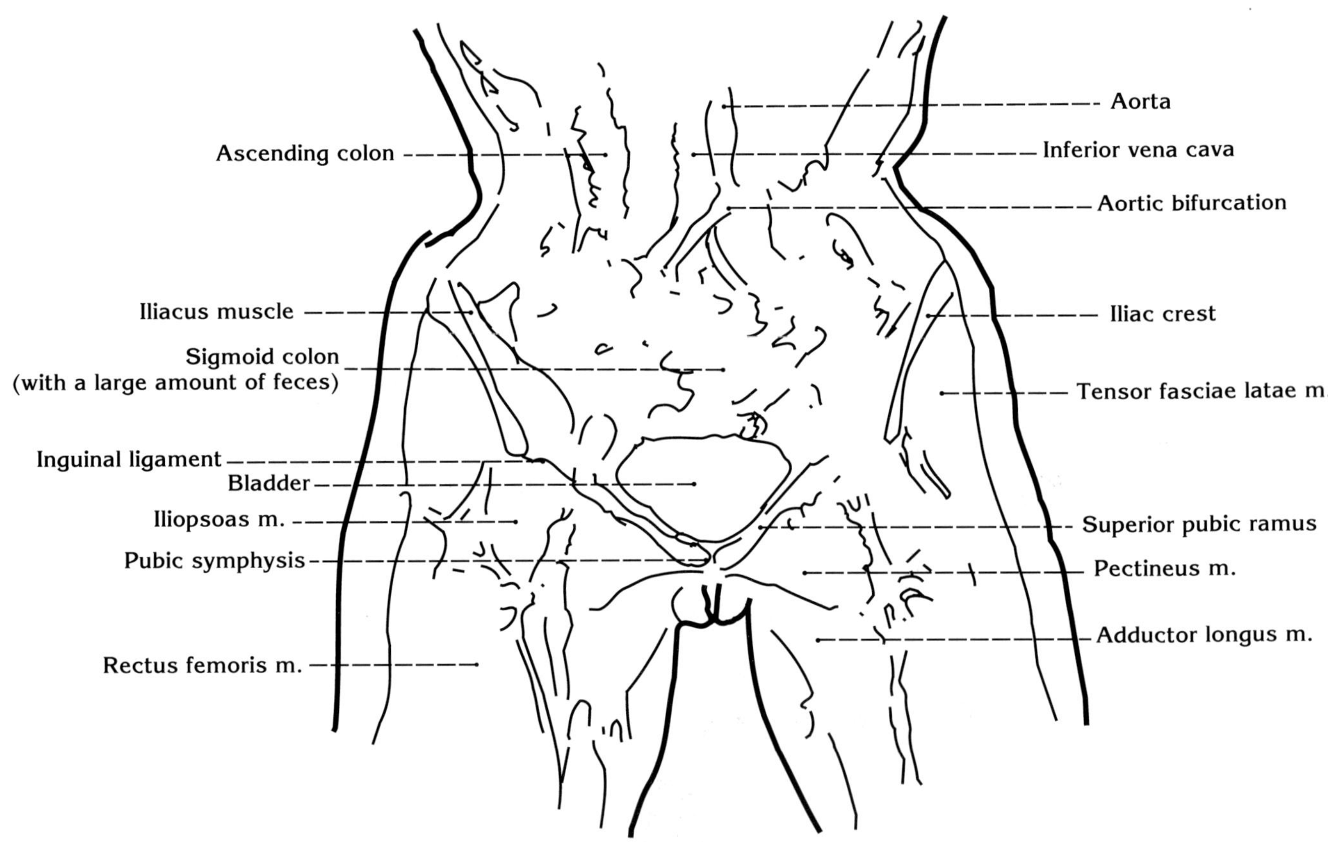

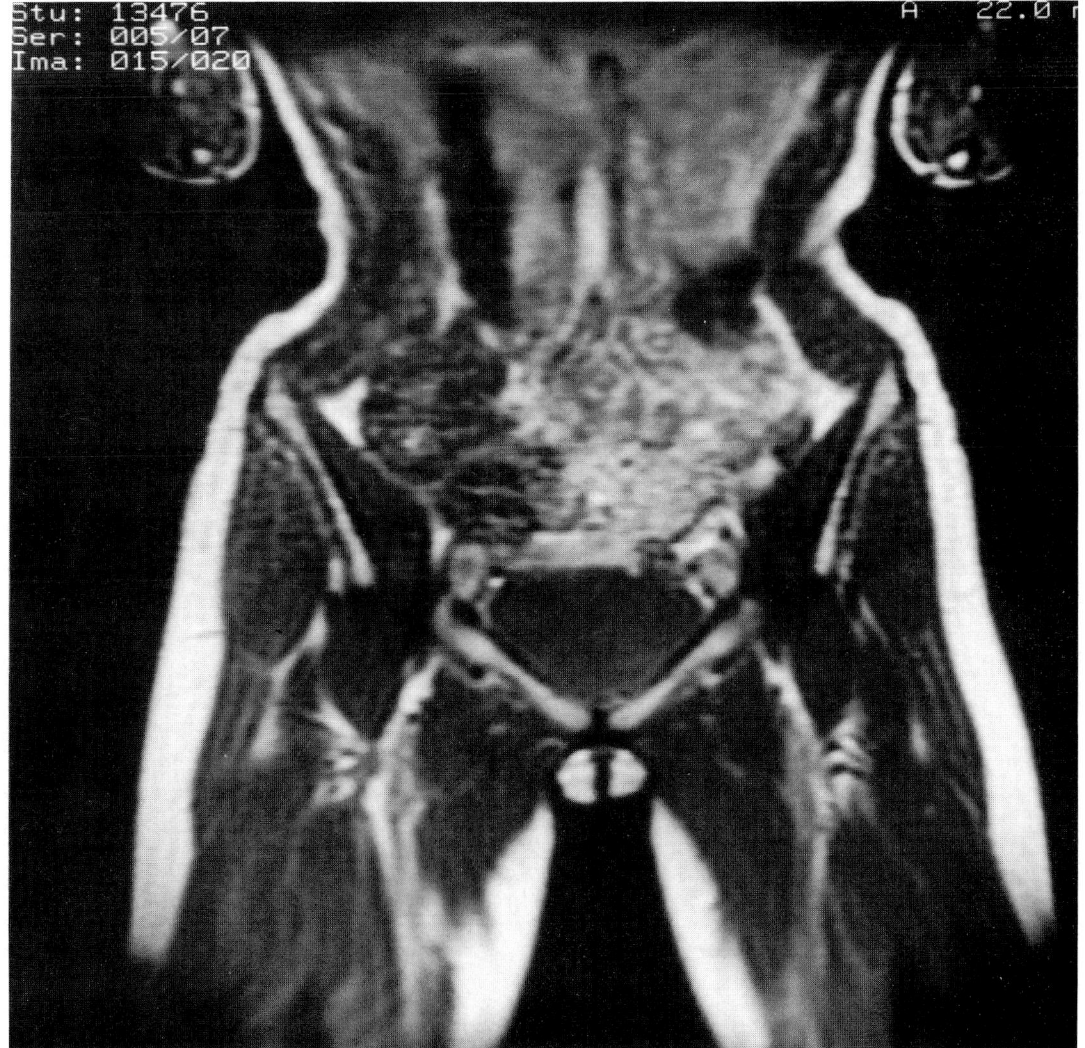

3-30 Female pelvis, coronal view (TR 800, TE 30).

Female Pelvis, Coronal

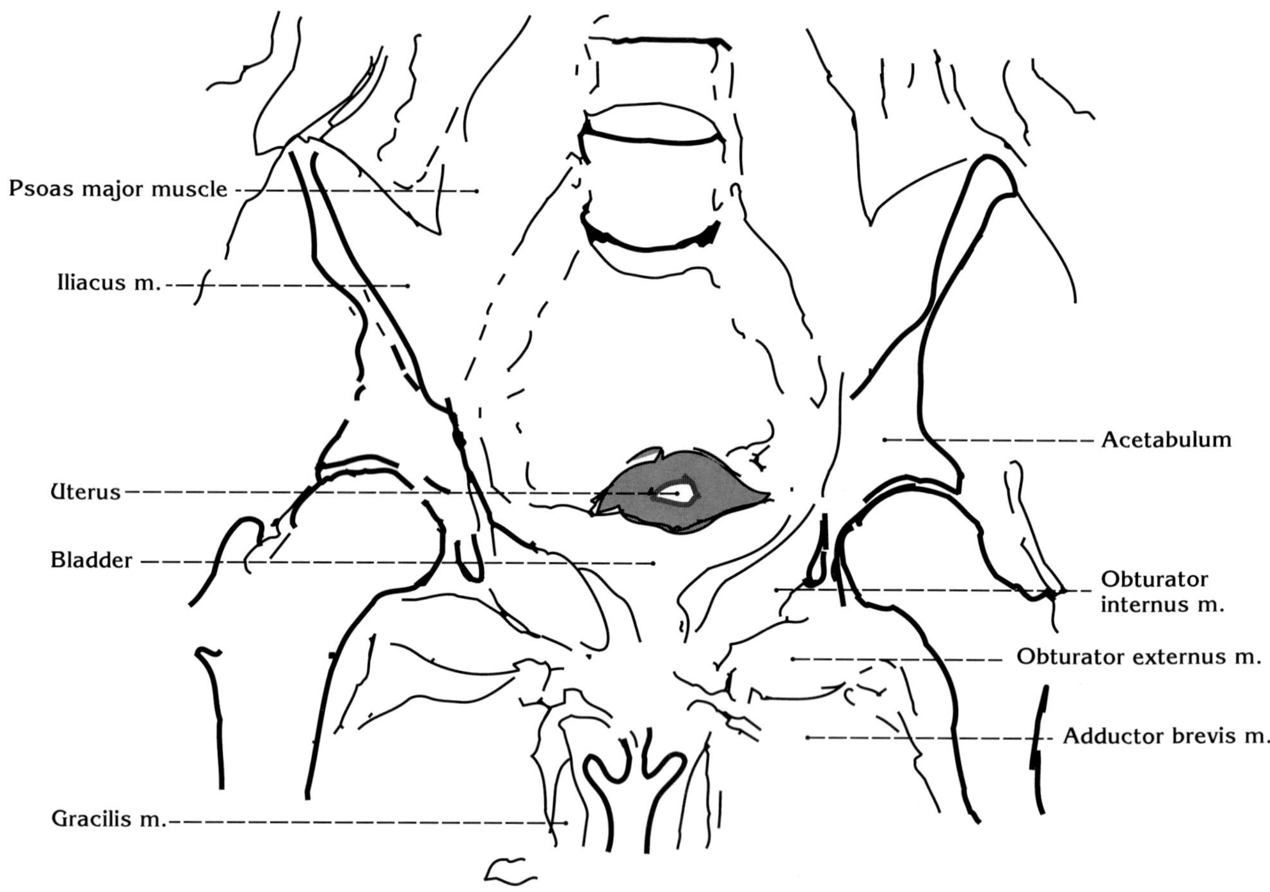

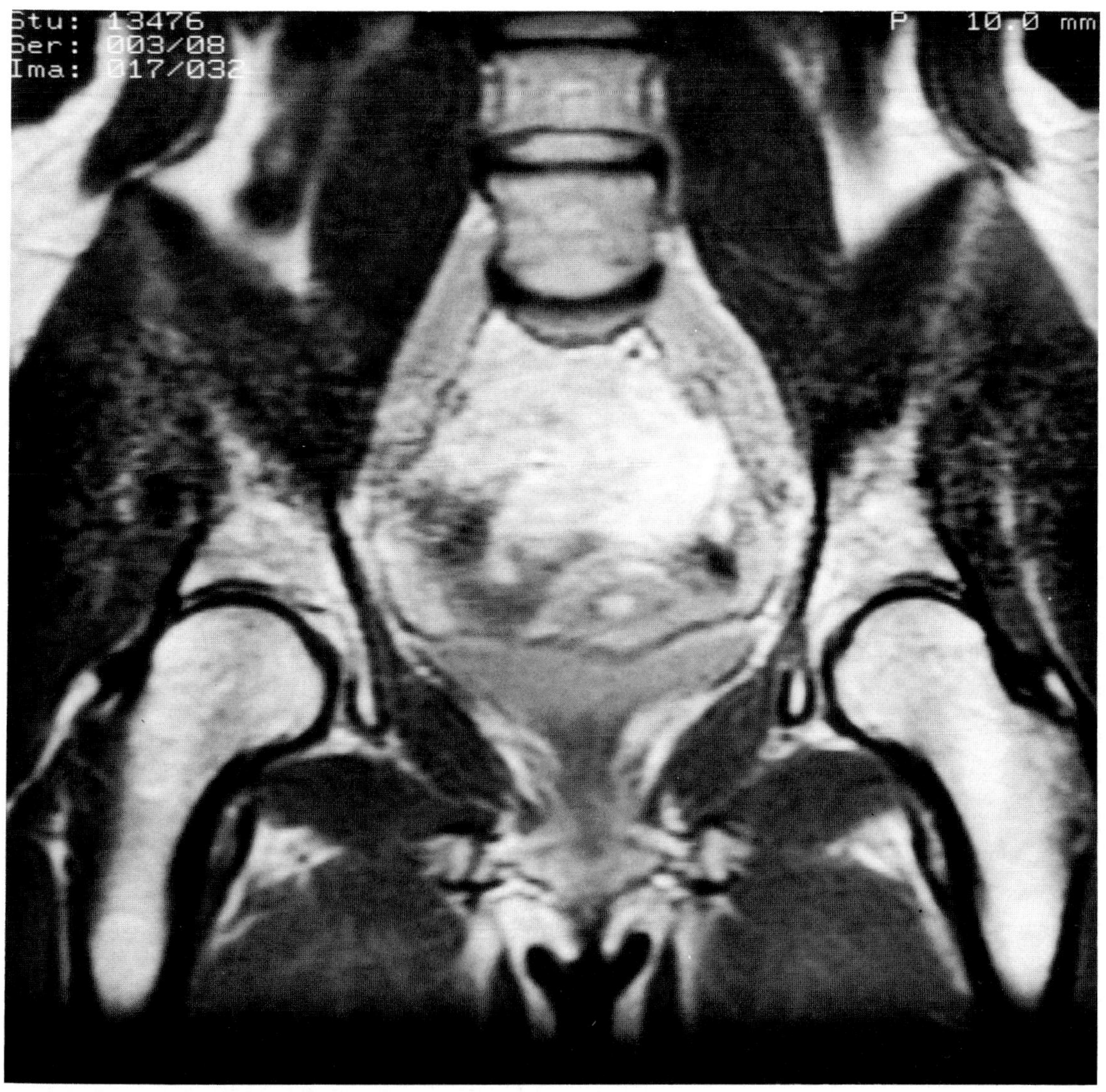

3-31 Female pelvis, coronal view (TR 2000, TE 30).

Male Pelvis, Coronal

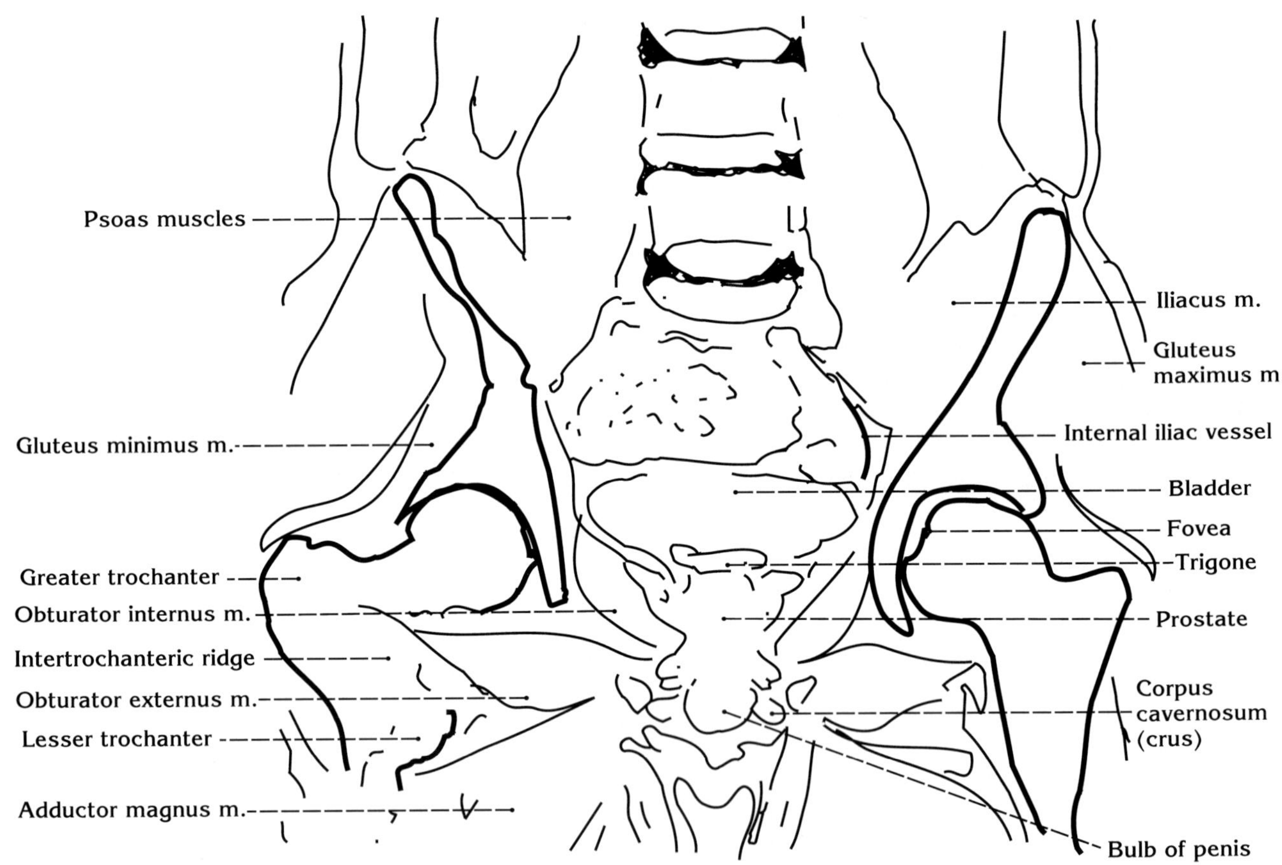

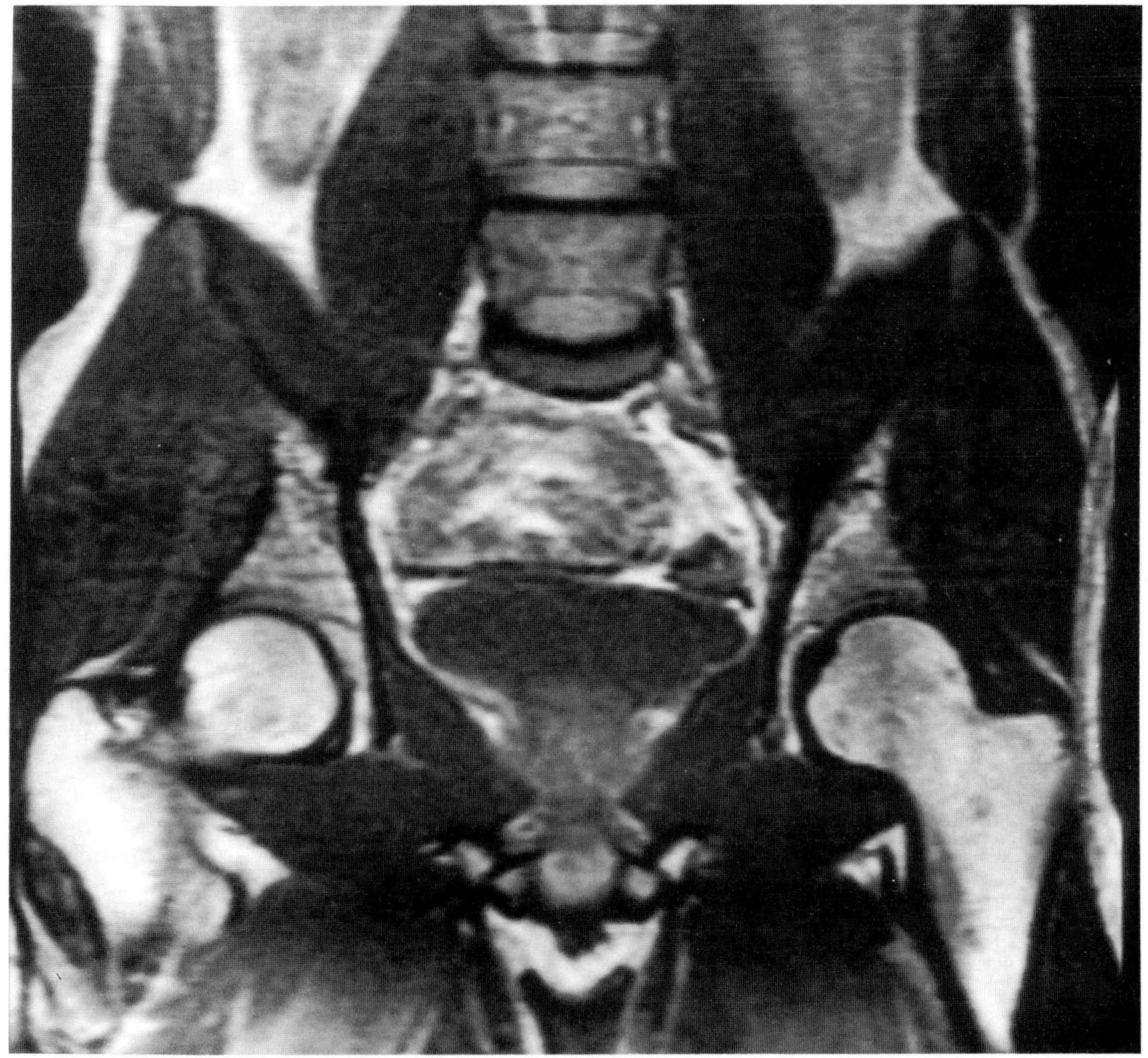

3-32 Male pelvis, coronal view (TR 2000, TE 30).

Female Pelvis, Coronal

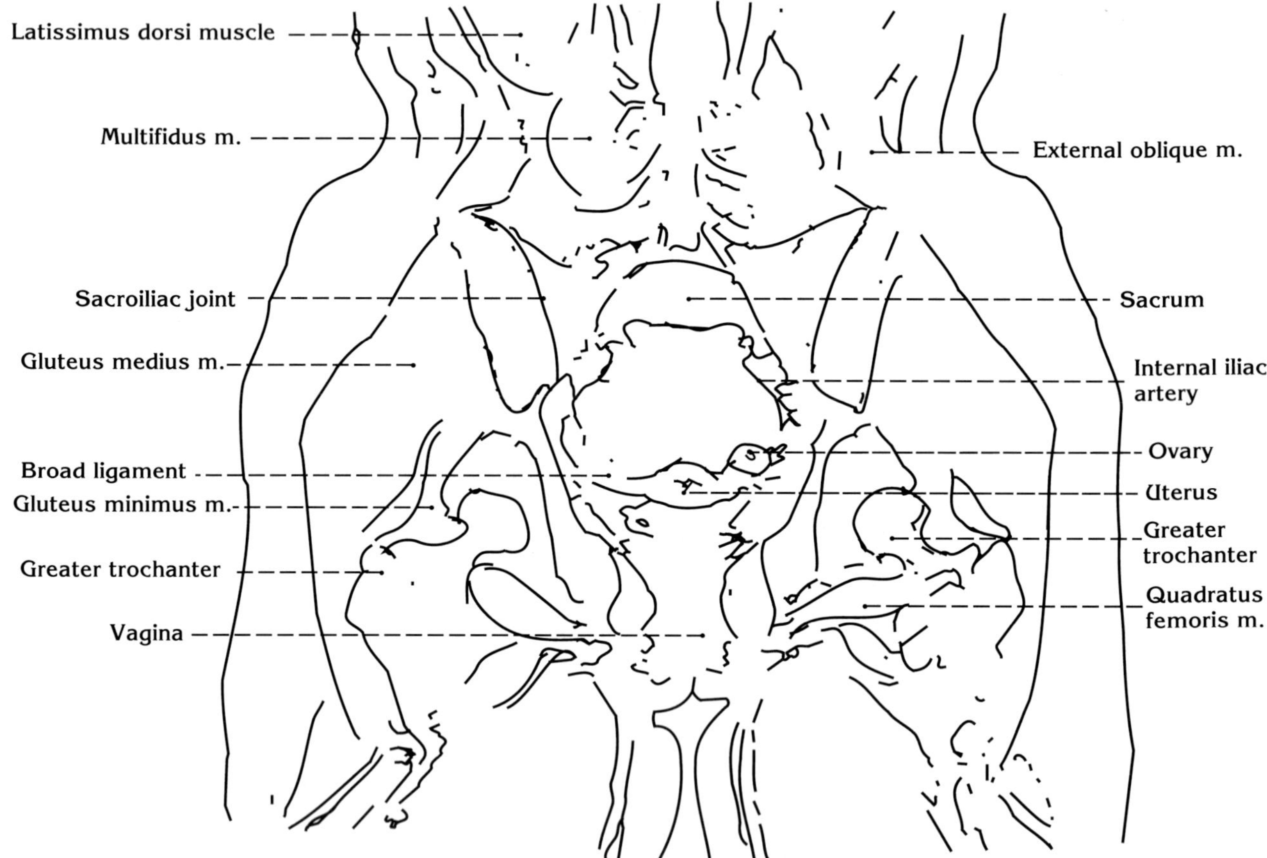

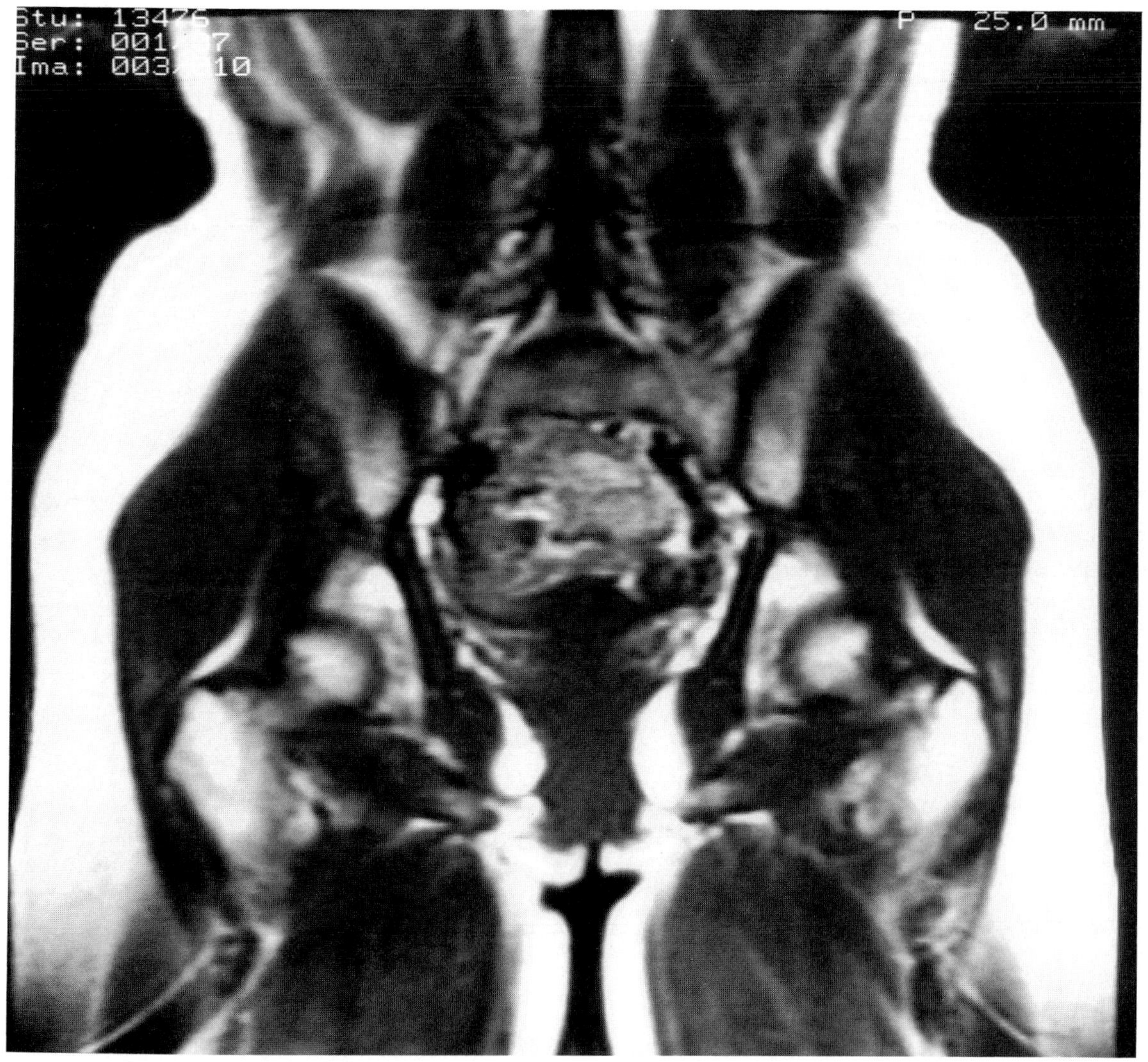

3-33 Female pelvis and upper thigh, coronal view (TR 400, TE 20).

Female Pelvis, Coronal

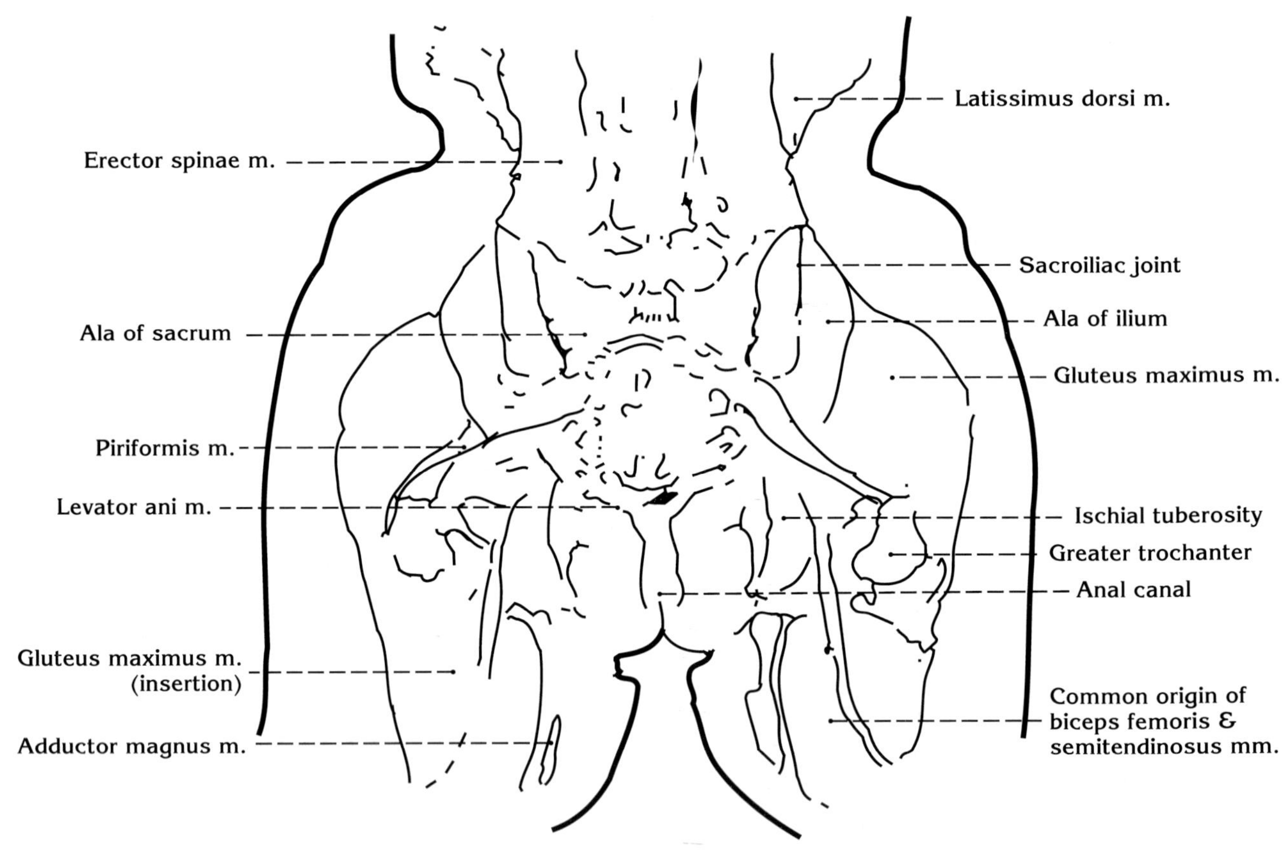

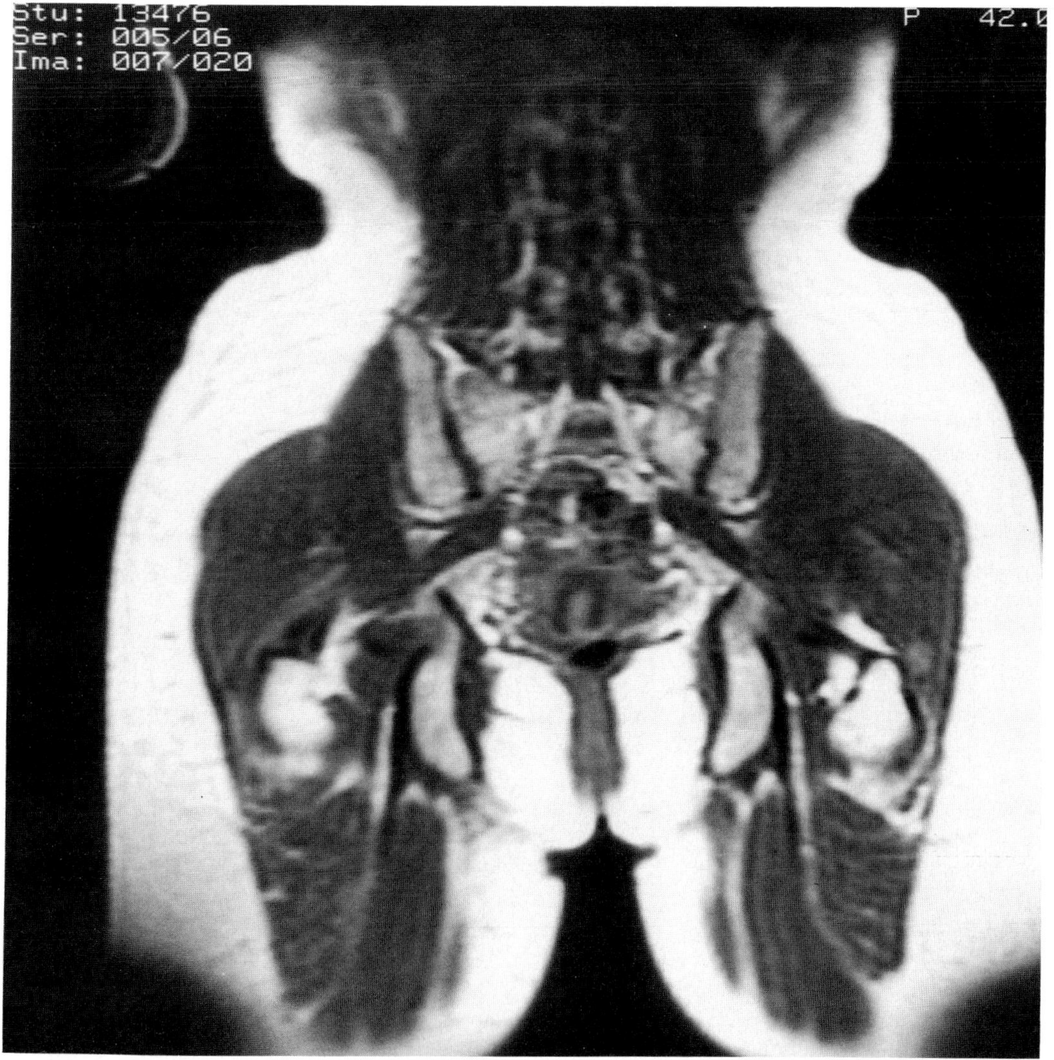

3-34 Female pelvis and upper thigh, coronal view (TR 800, TE 30).

Male Pelvis, Coronal

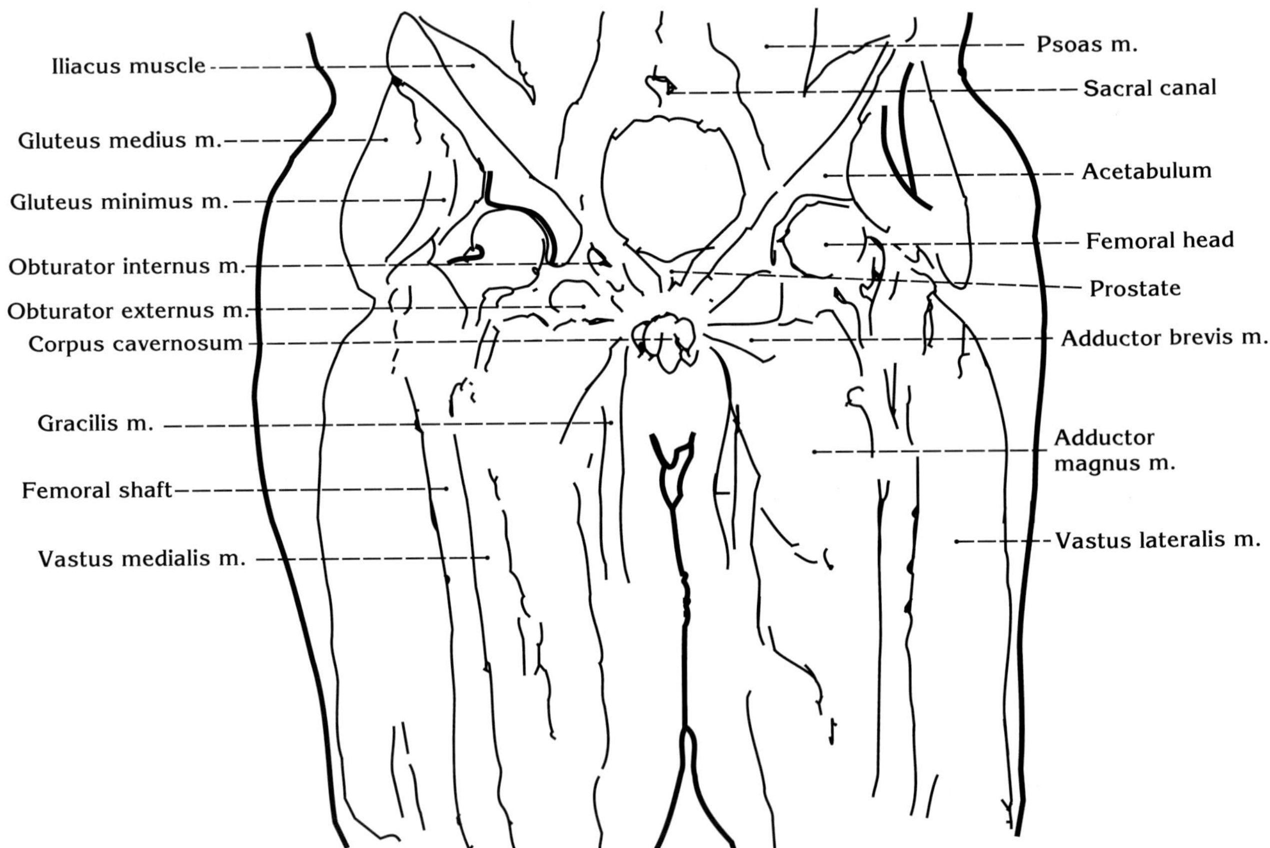

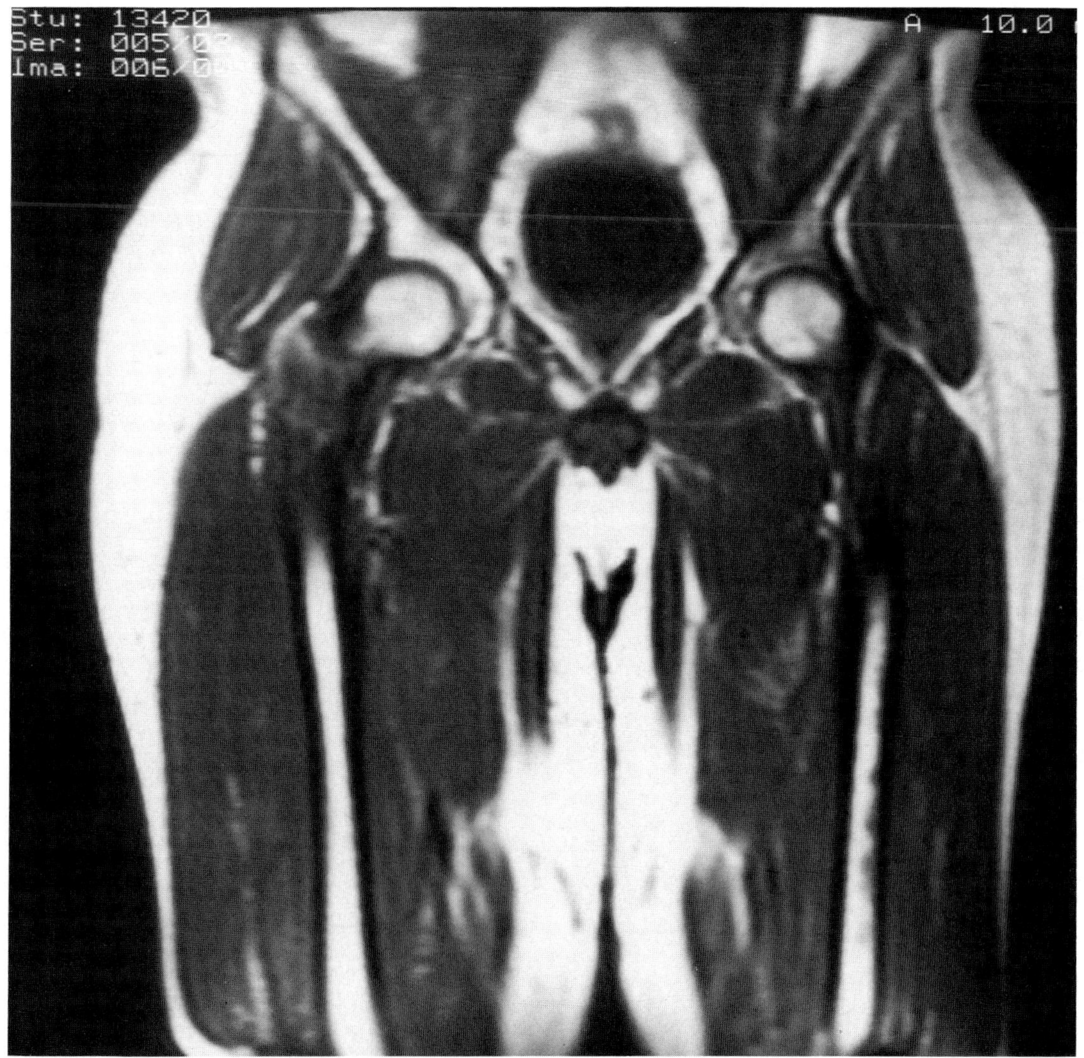

3-35 Male pelvis and upper thigh, coronal view (TR 400, TE 20).

Male Pelvis, Coronal

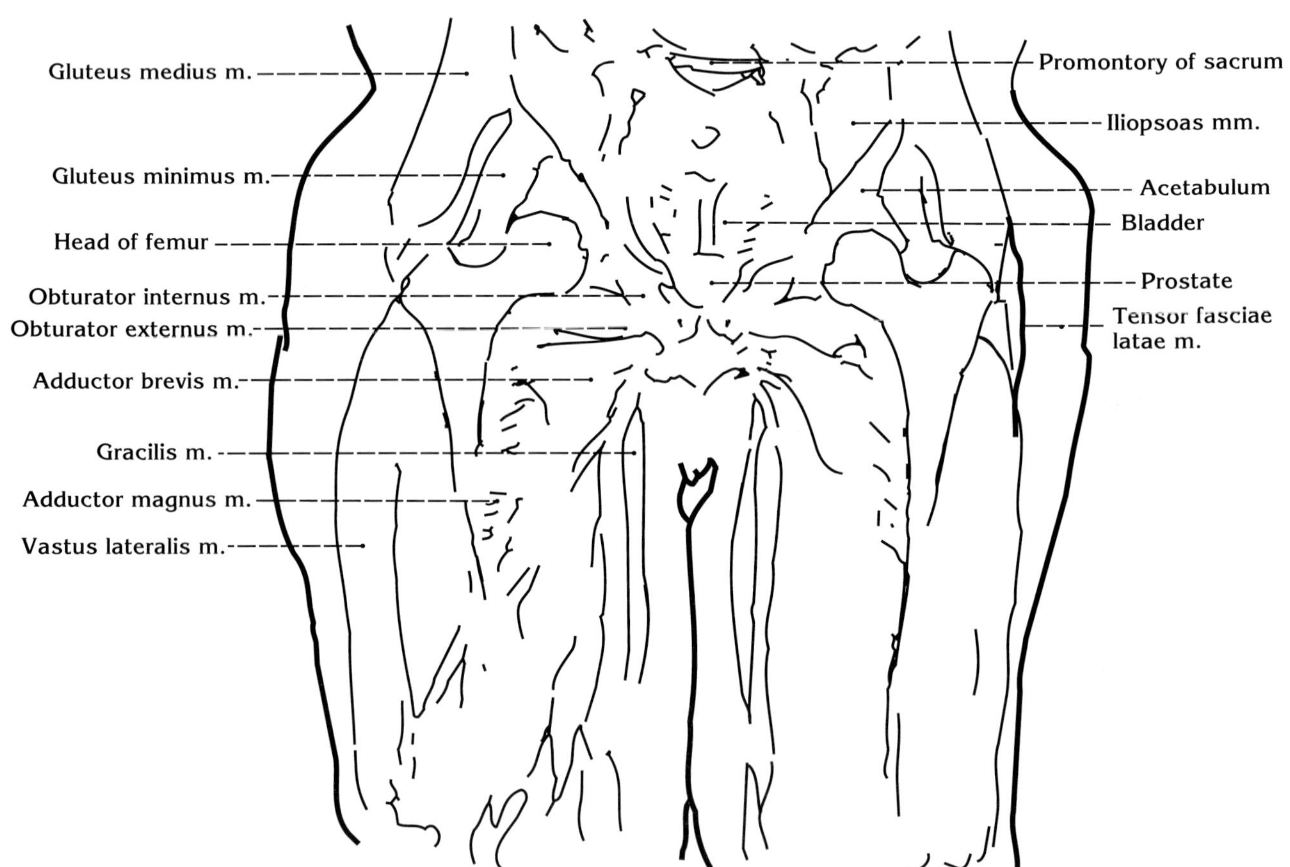

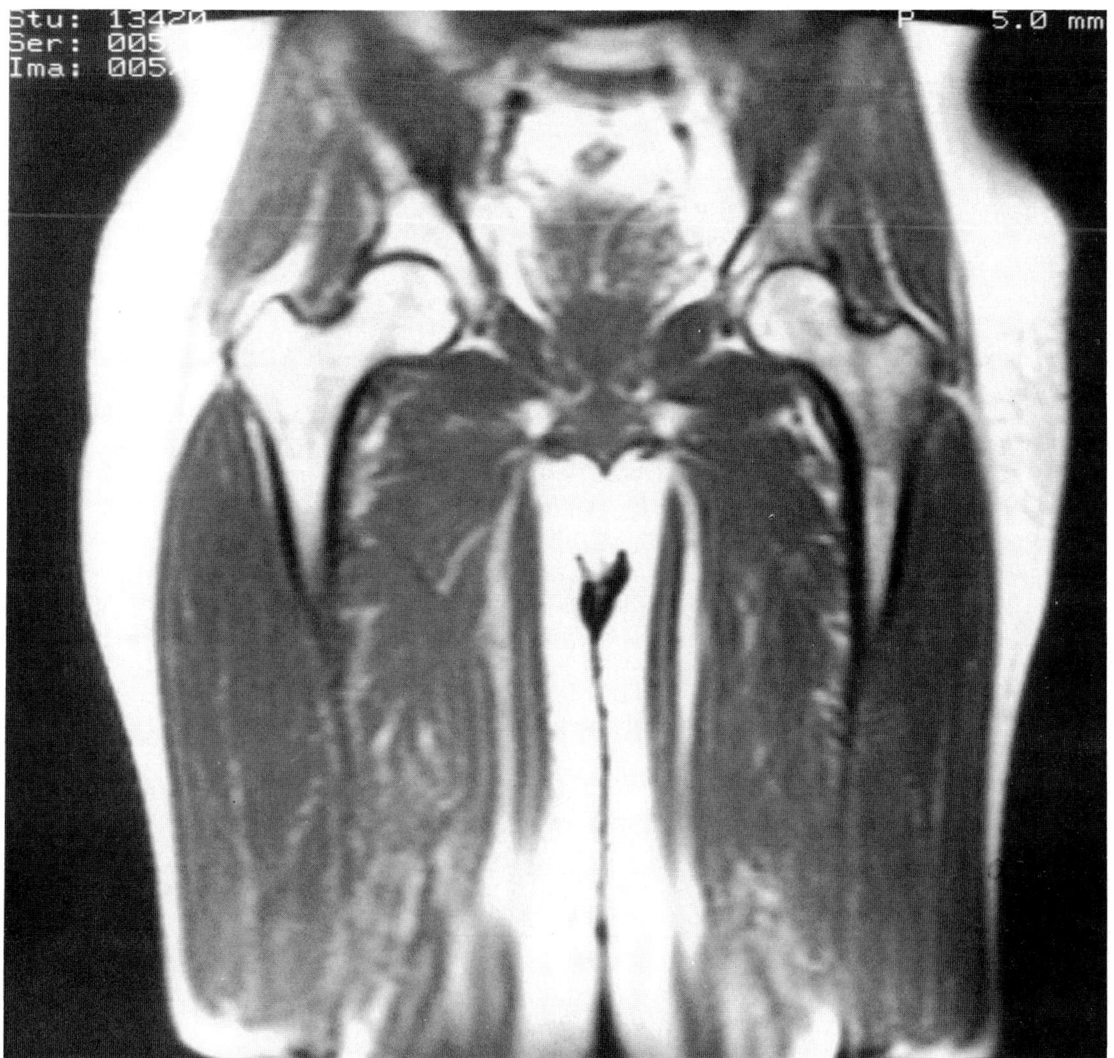

3-36 Male pelvis and upper thigh, coronal view (TR 400, TE 20).

Pelvis, Coronal

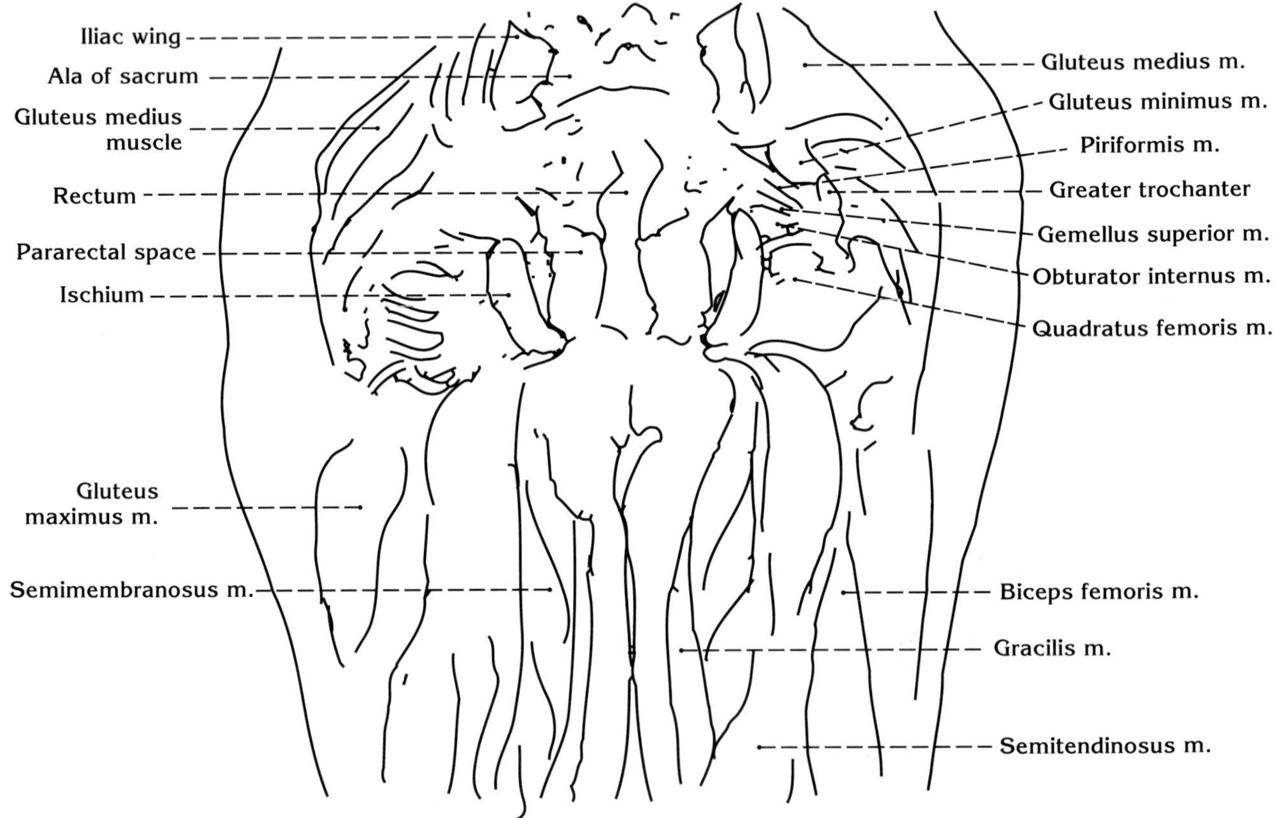

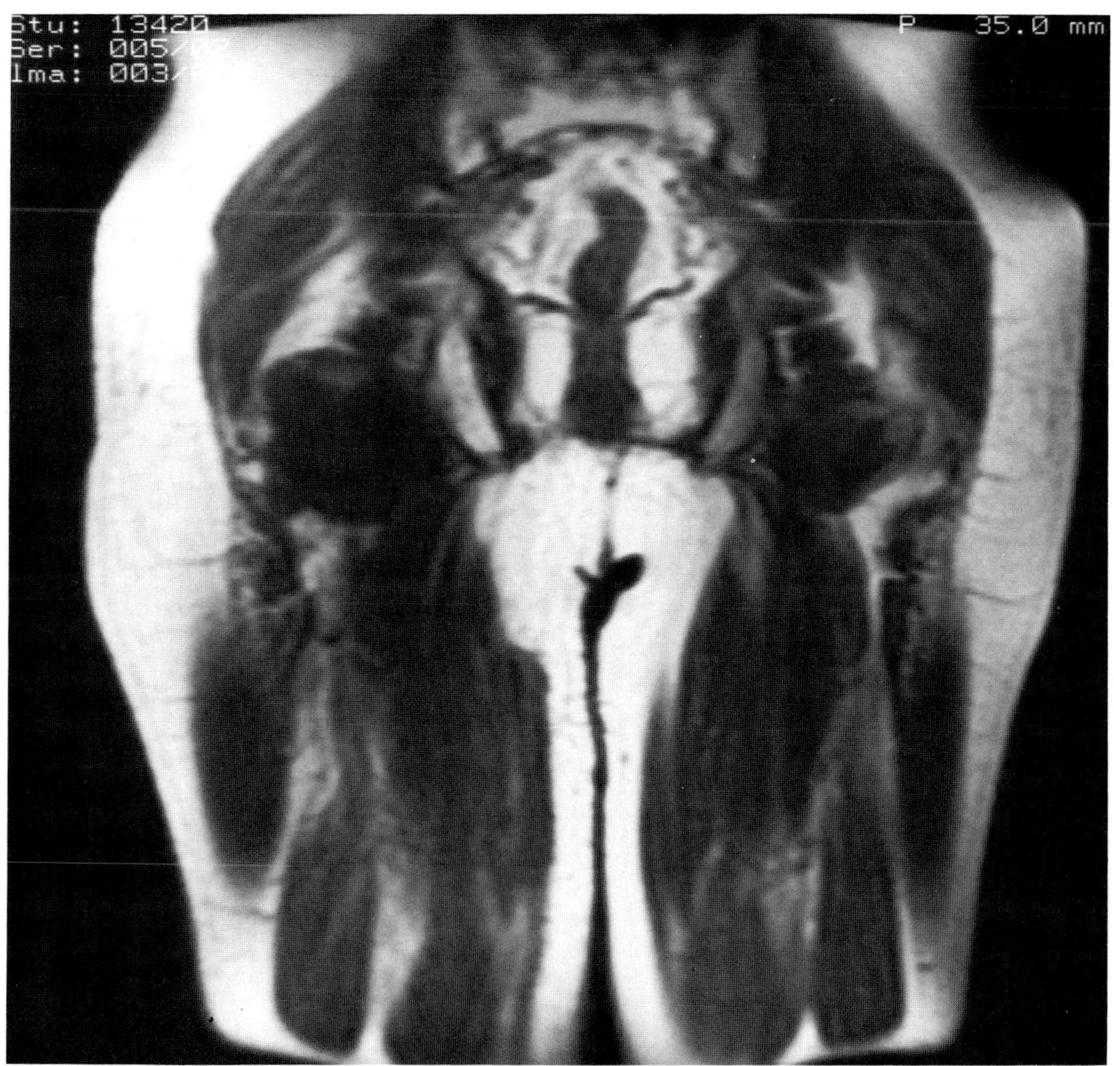

3-37 Pelvis and upper thigh, coronal view (TR 400, TE 20).

Pelvis, Coronal

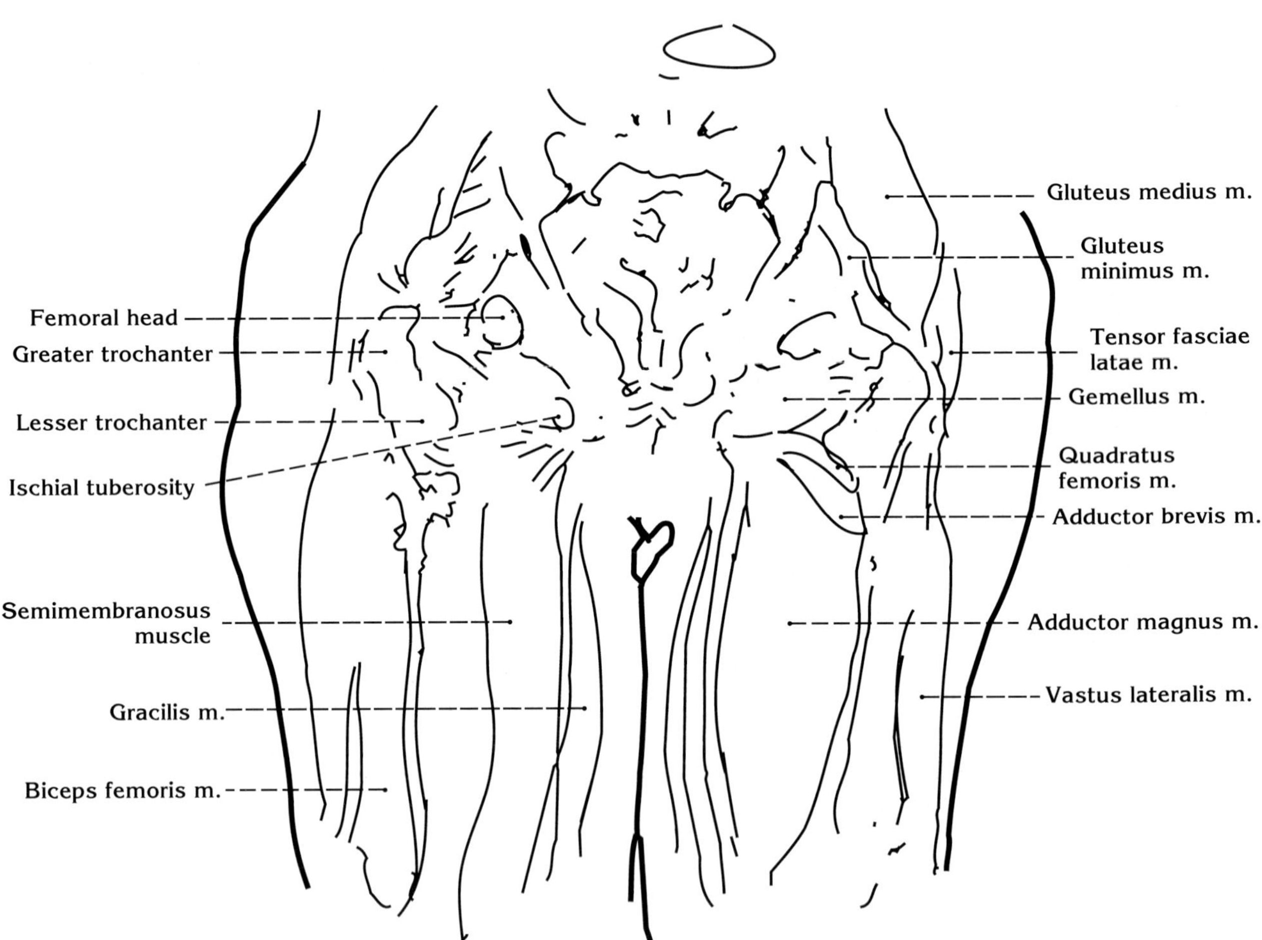

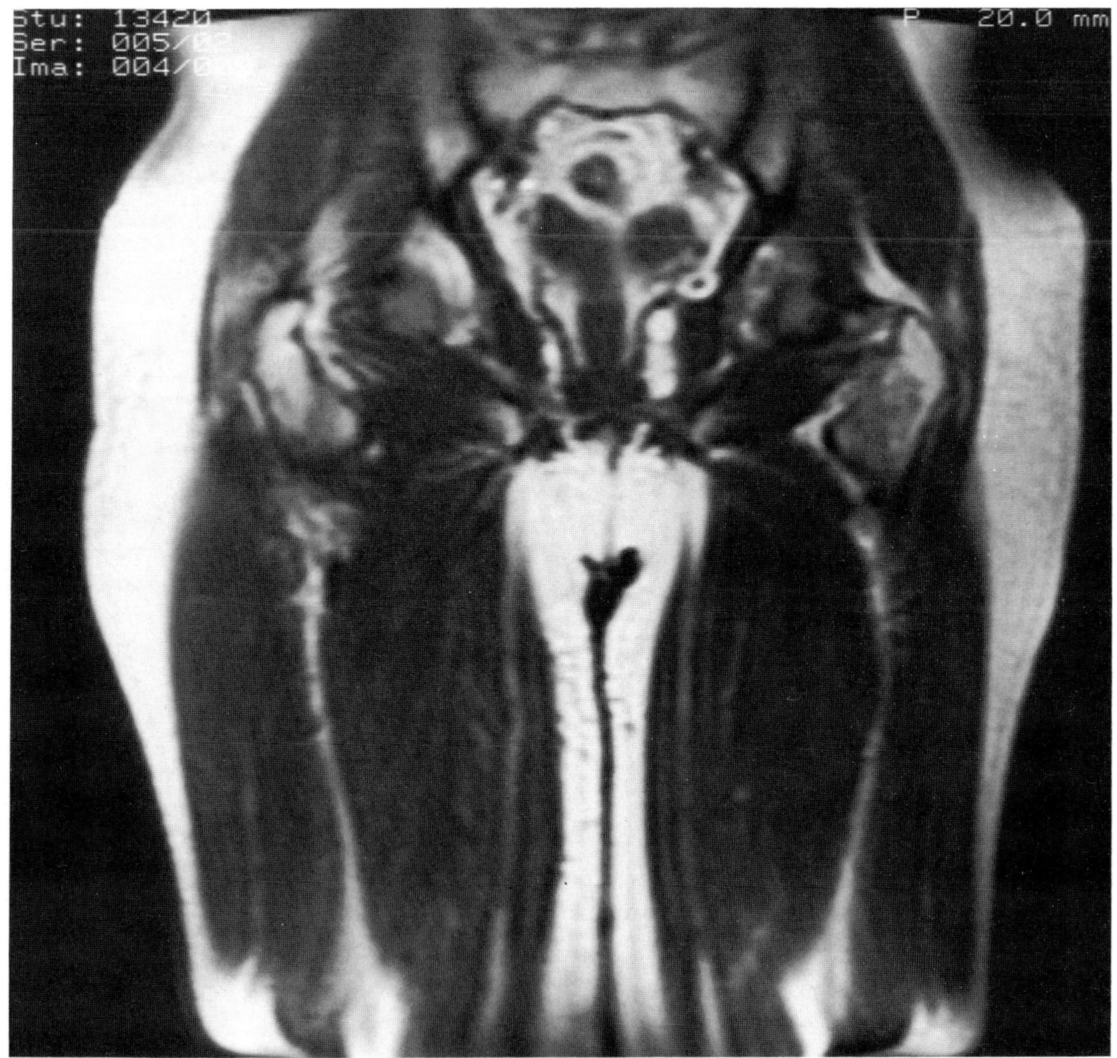

3-38 Pelvis and upper thigh, coronal view (TR 400, TE 20).

Pelvis, Coronal

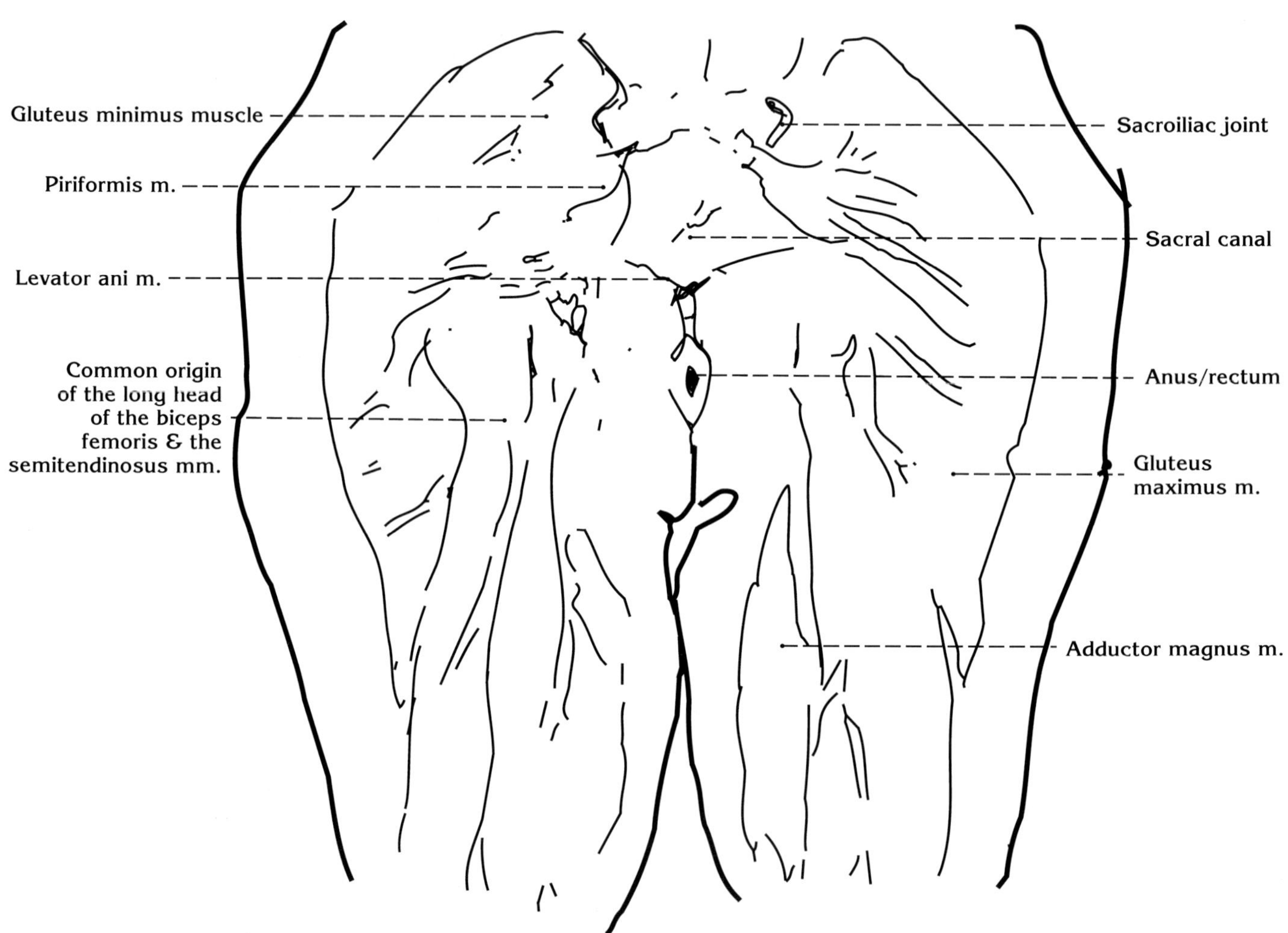

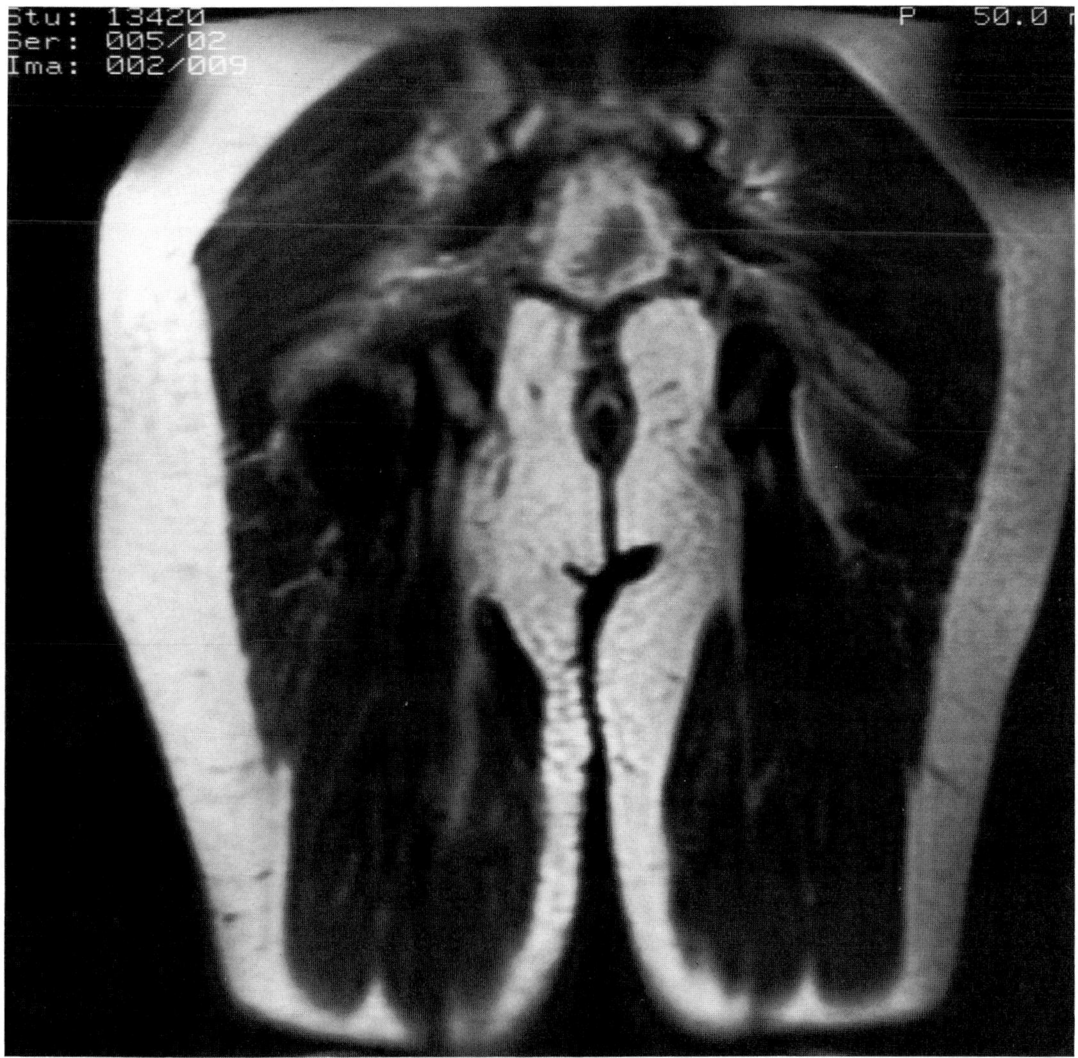

3-39 Pelvis and upper thigh, coronal view (TR 400, TE 20).

Pelvis, Coronal

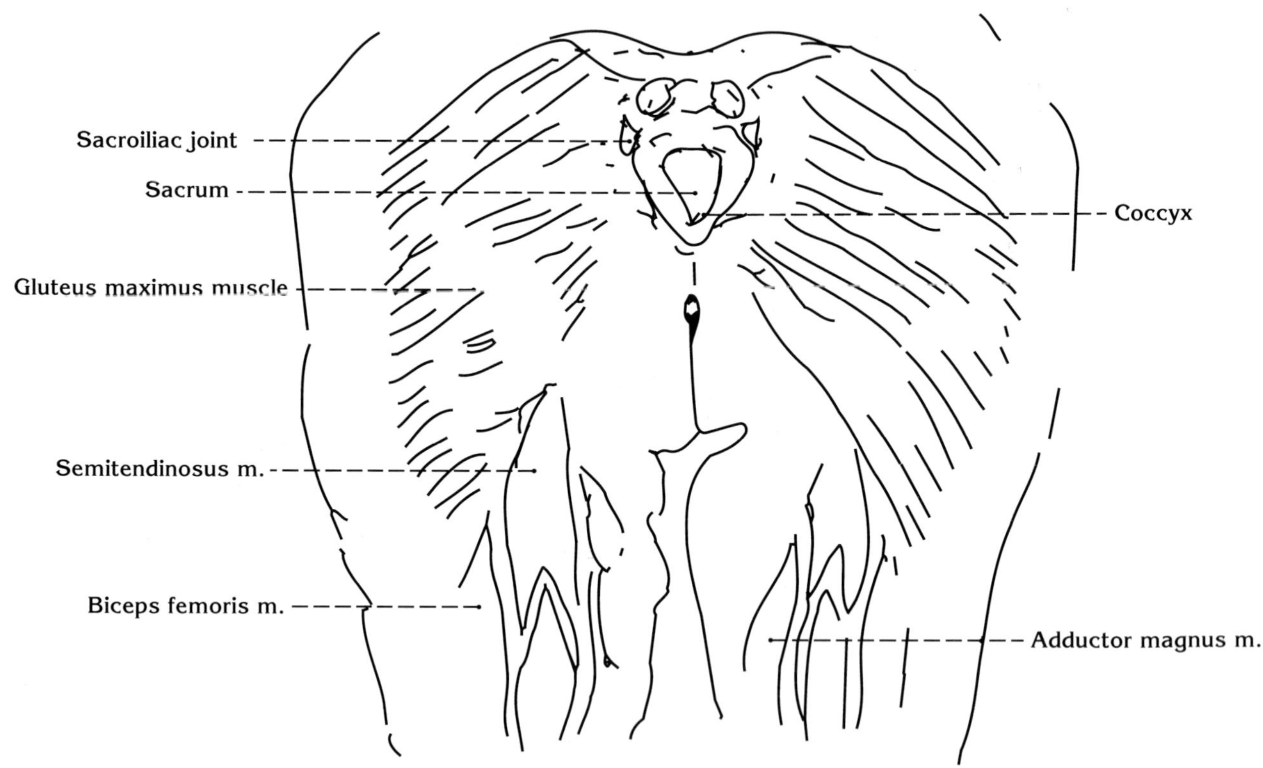

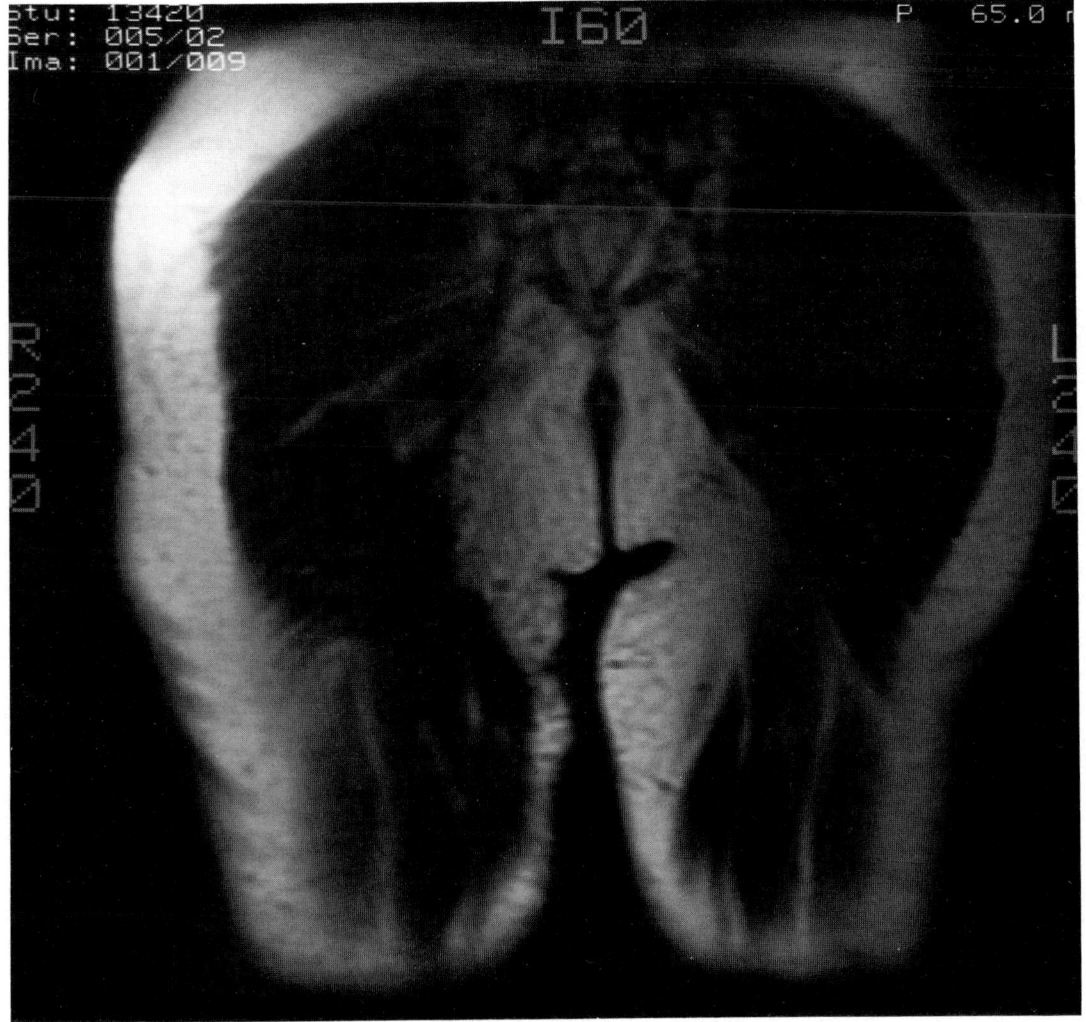

3-40 Pelvis and upper thigh, coronal view (TR 400, TE 20).

Upper Pelvis, Axial

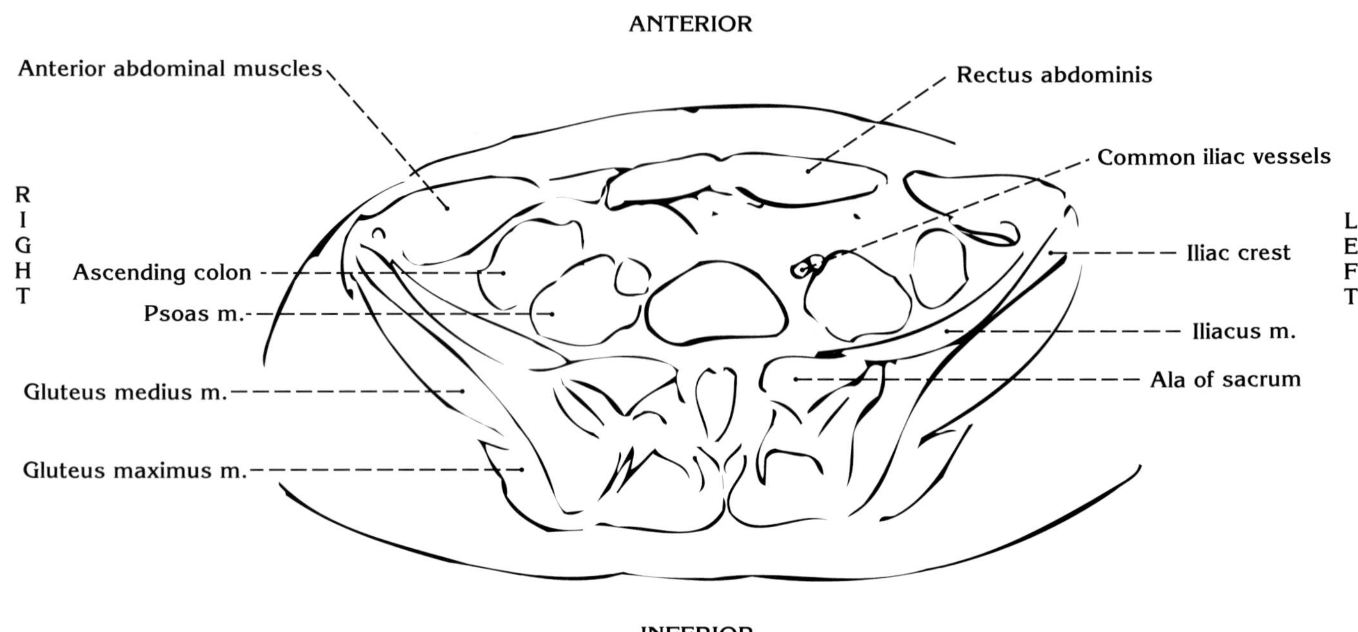

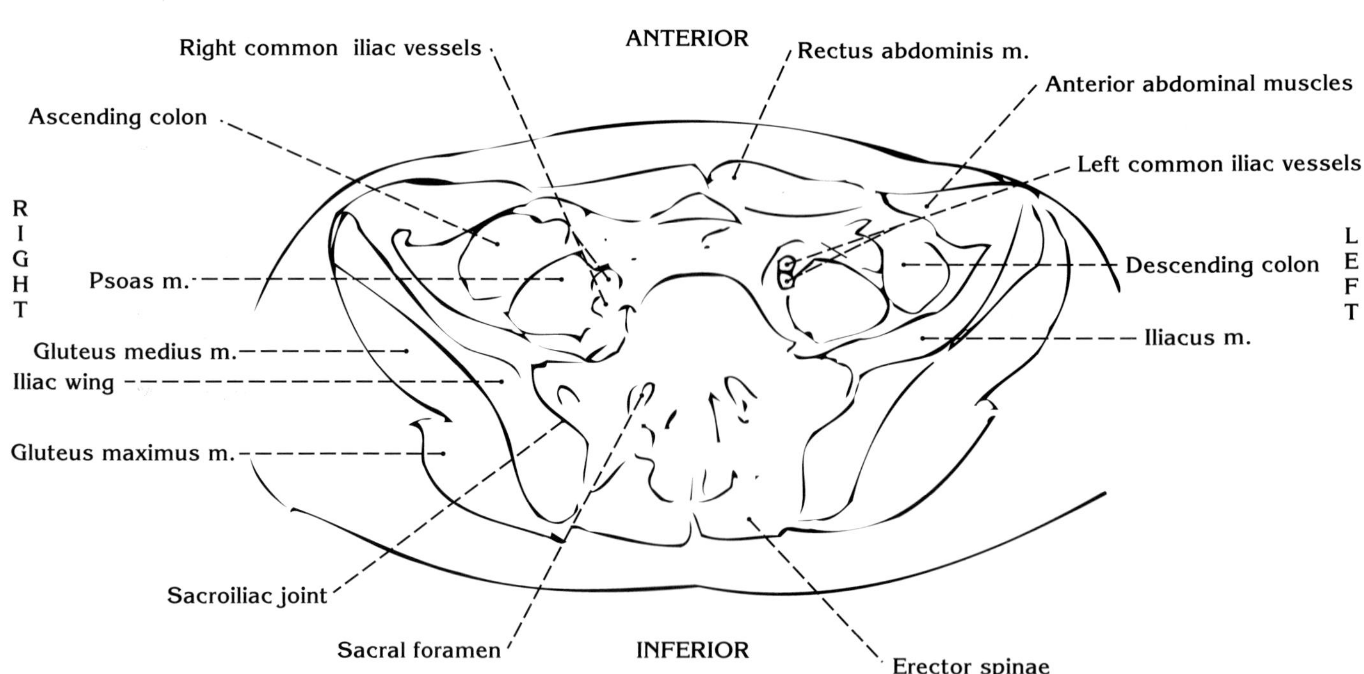

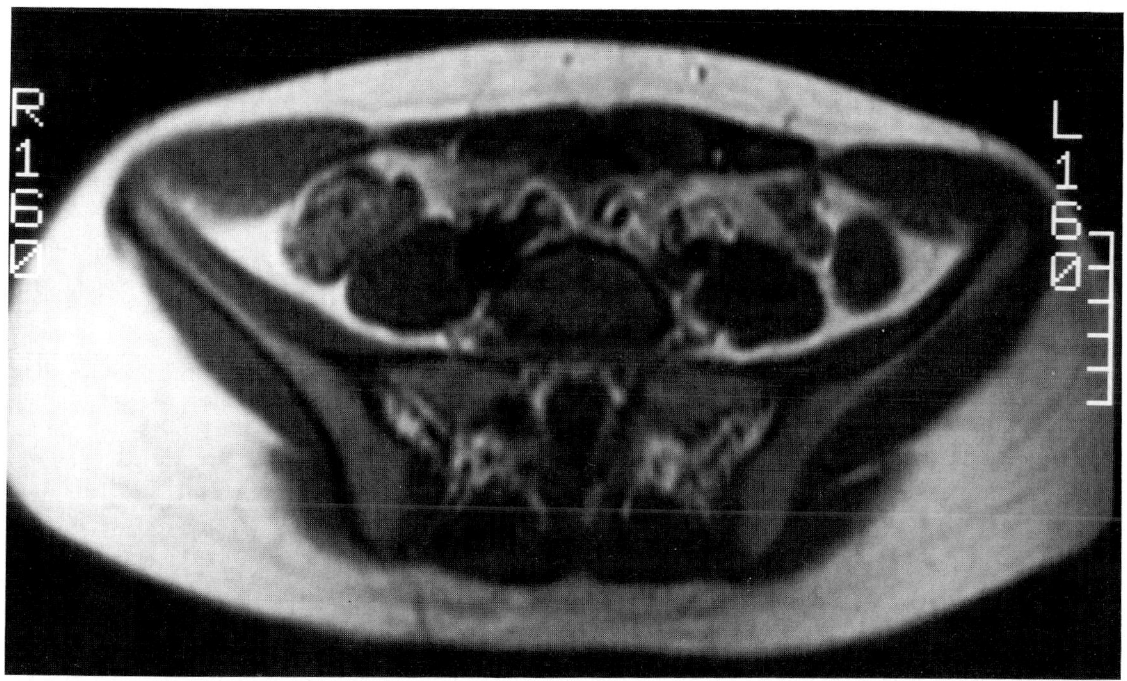

3-41 Upper pelvis, axial view (TR 800, TE 20).

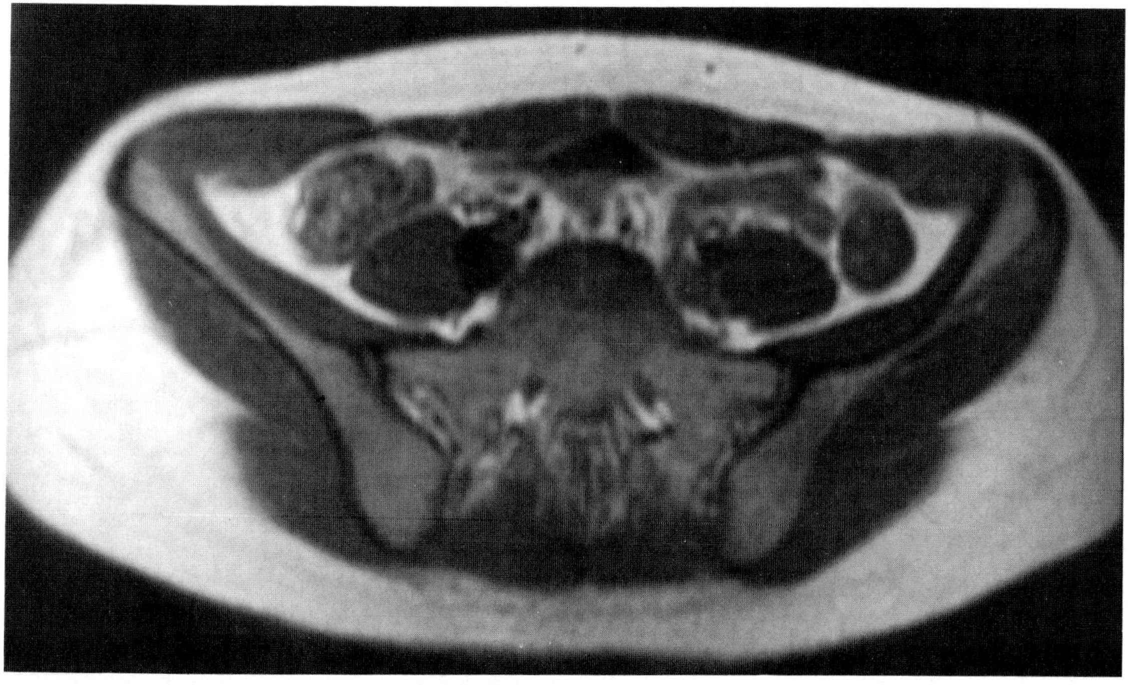

3-42 Upper pelvis, axial view (TR 800, TE 20).

Upper Pelvis, Axial

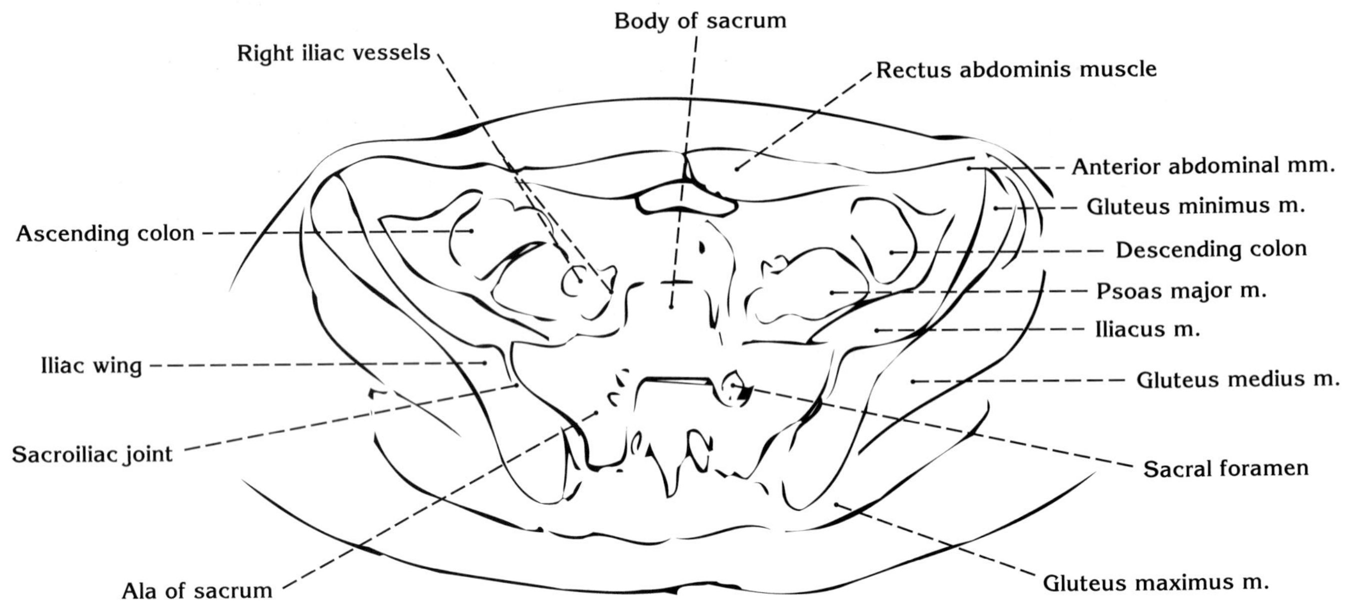

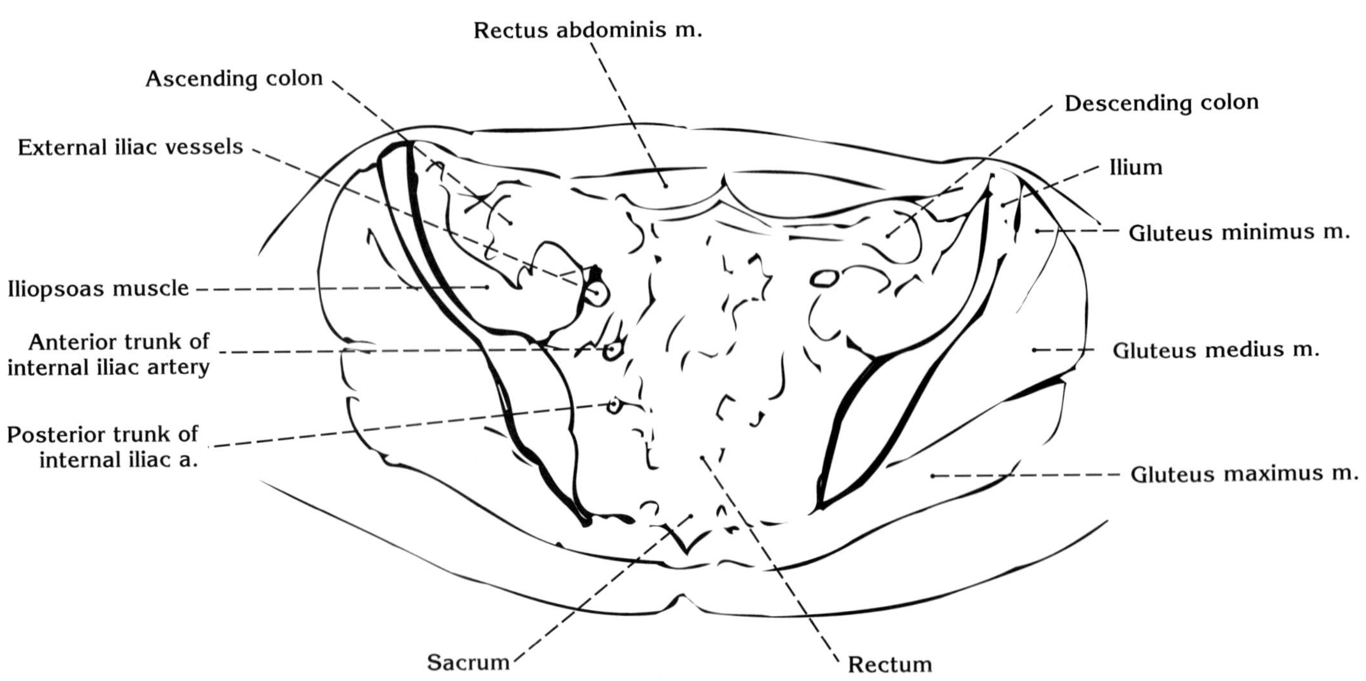

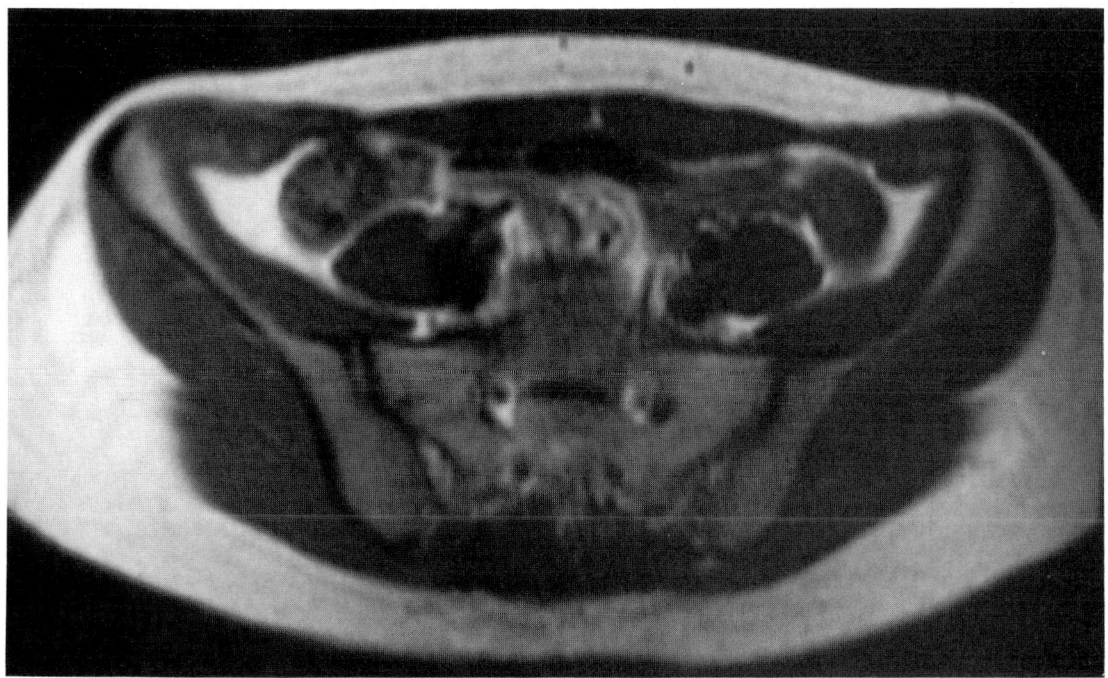

3-43 Upper pelvis, axial view (TR 800, TE 20).

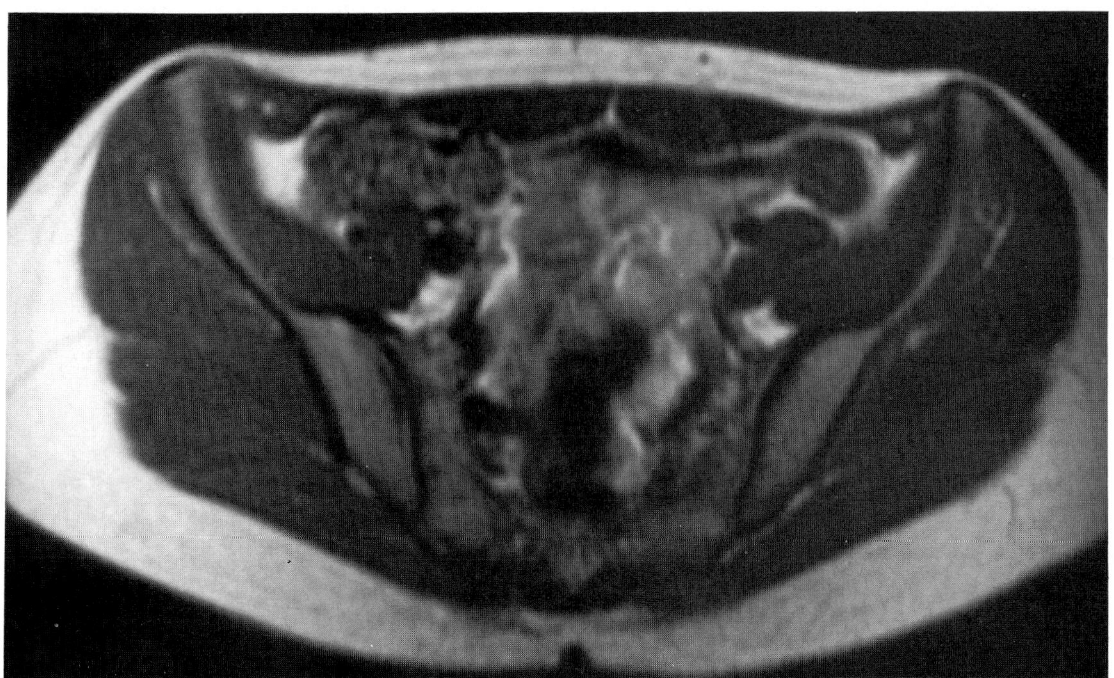

3-44 Upper pelvis, axial view (TR 800, TE 20).

Upper Pelvis, Axial

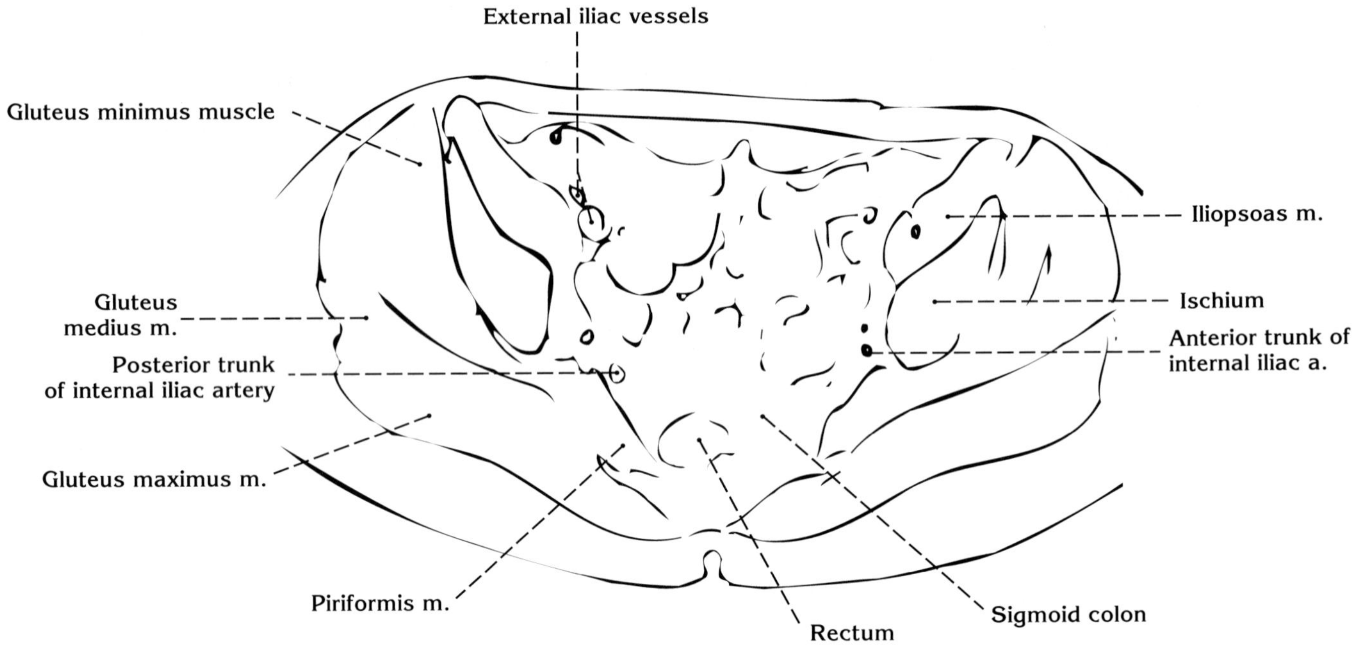

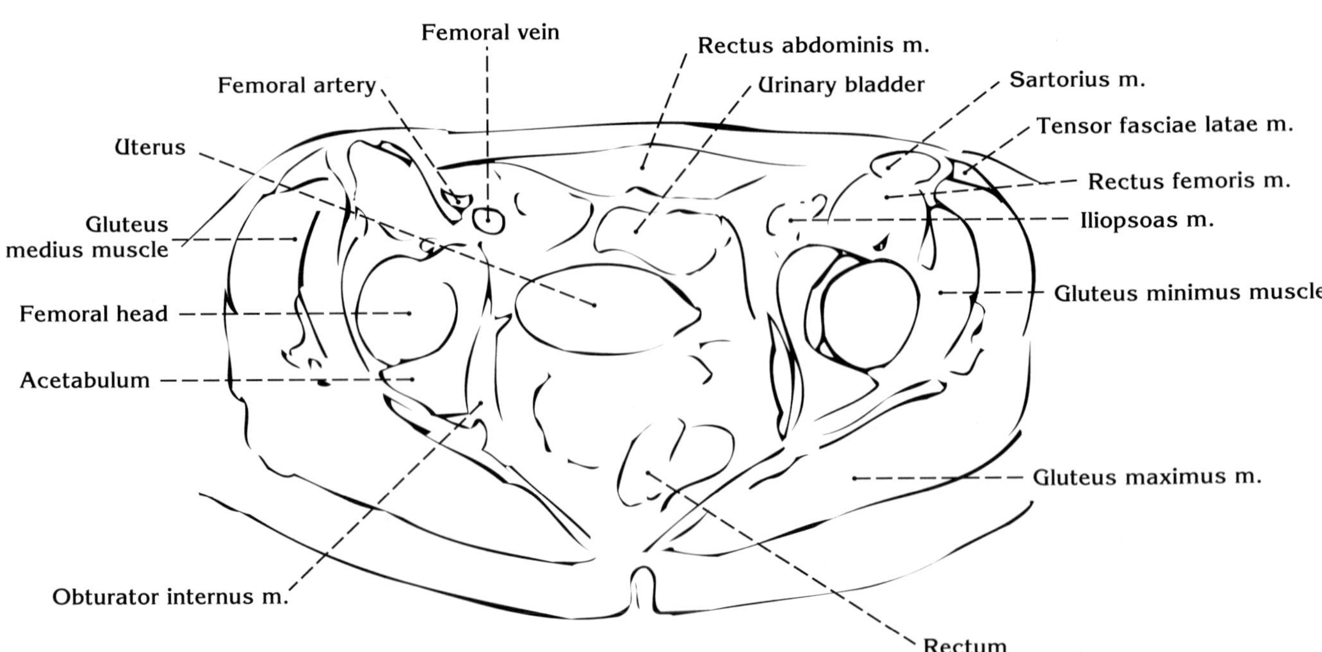

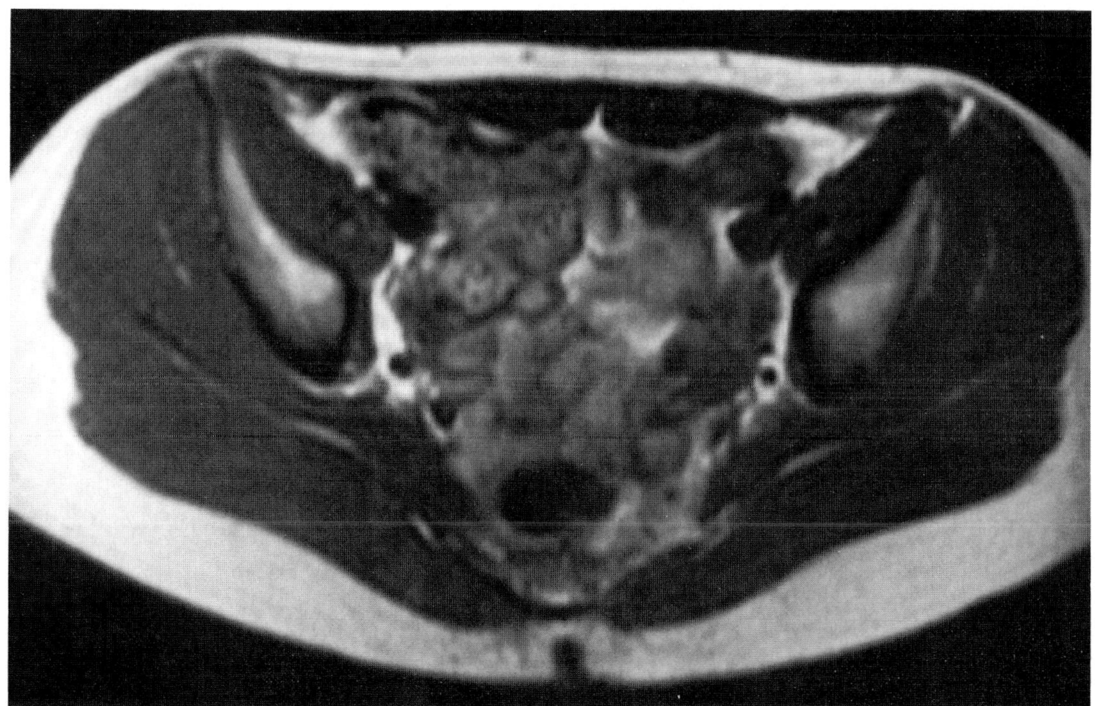

3-45 Upper pelvis, axial view (TR 800, TE 20).

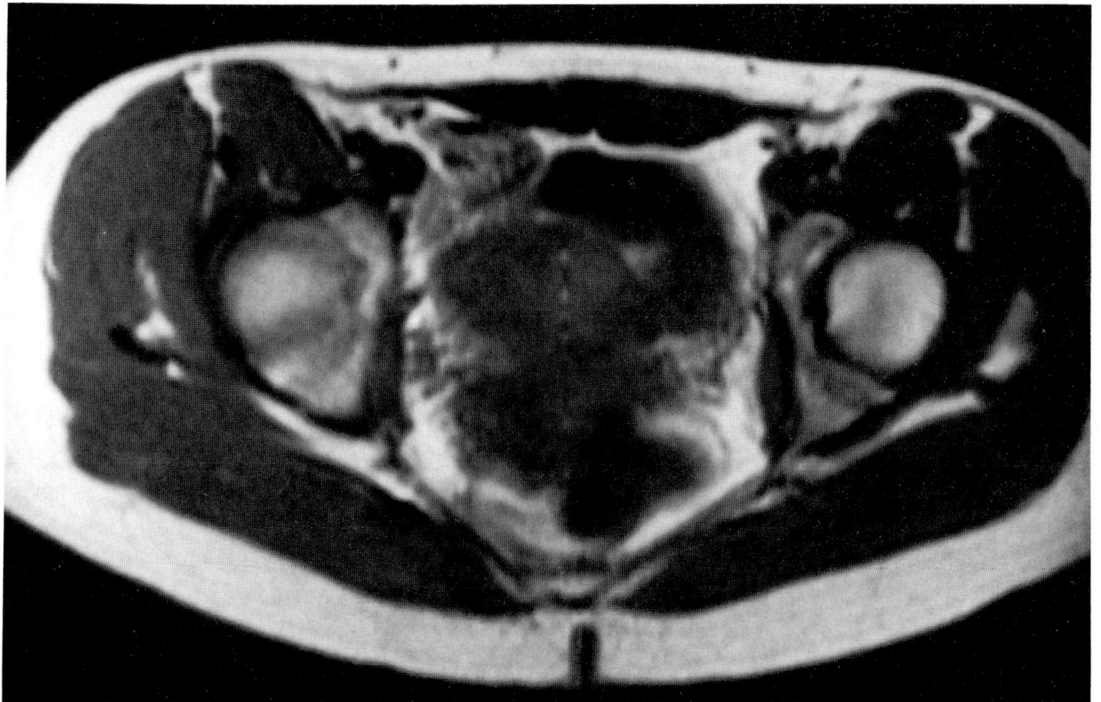

3-46 Upper pelvis, axial view (TR 800, TE 20).

Female Pelvis, Axial

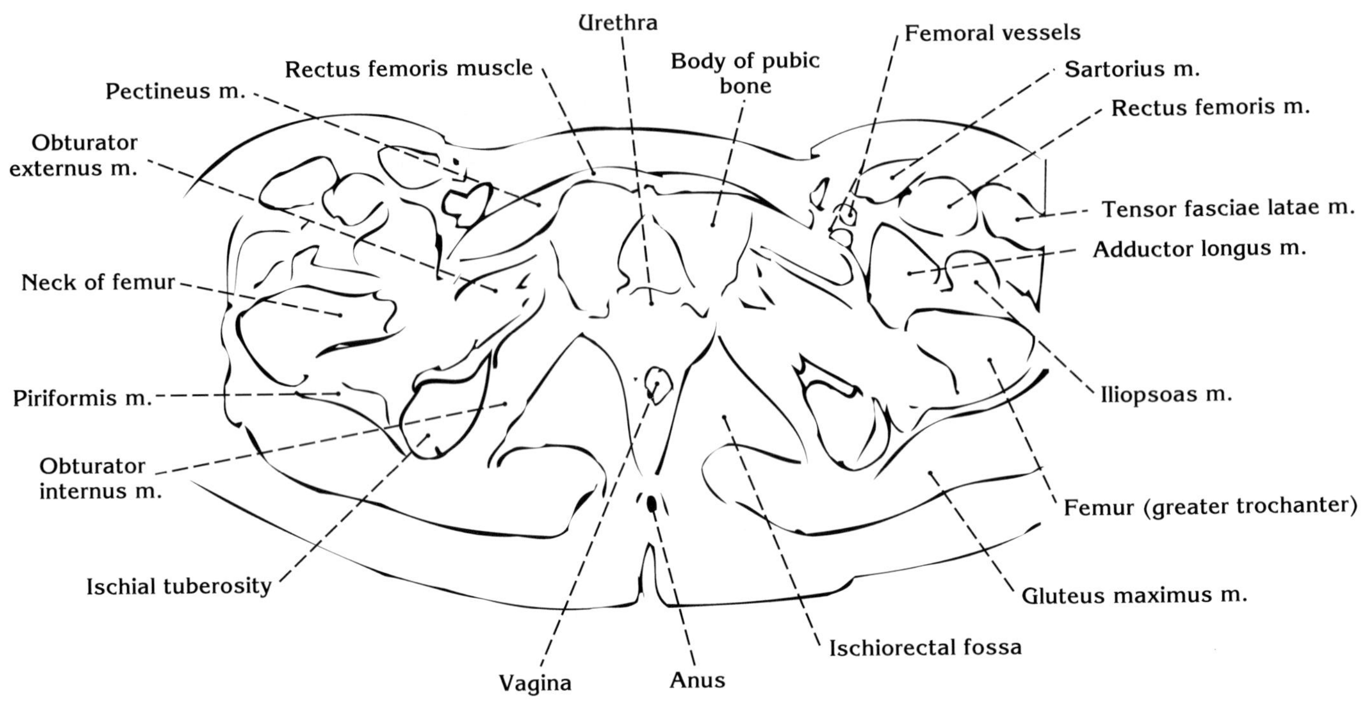

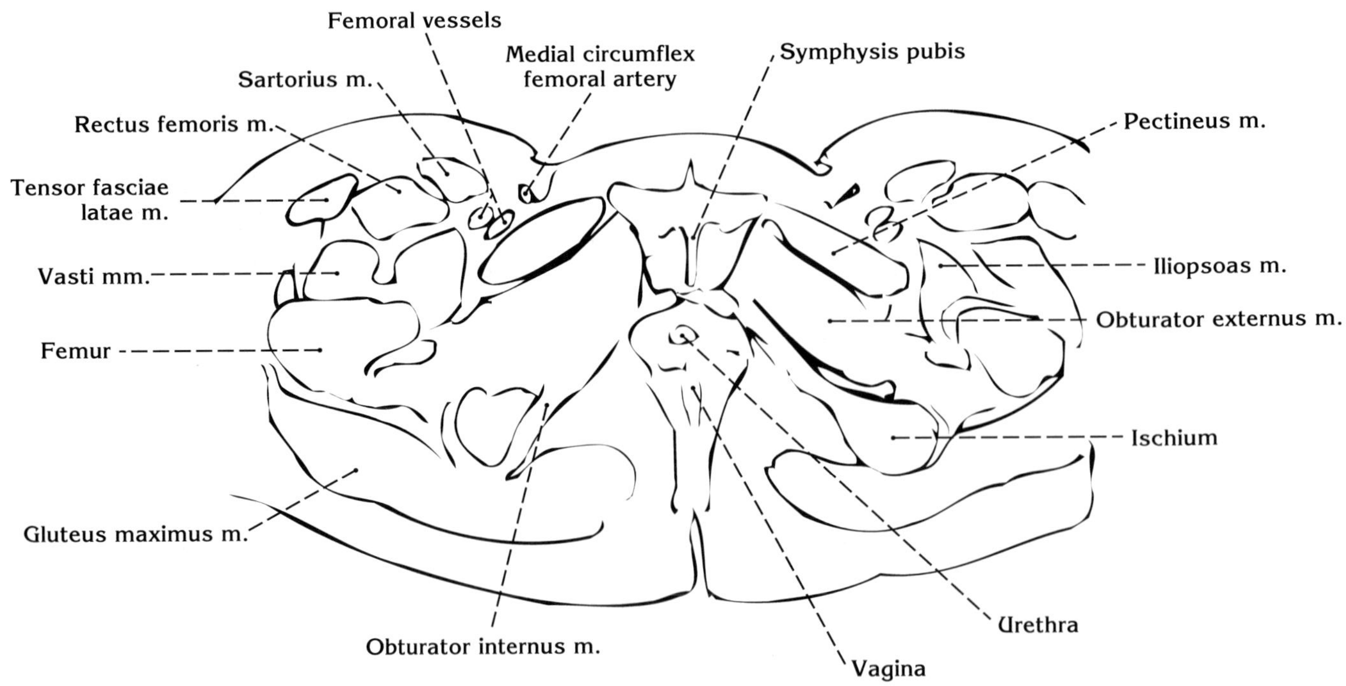

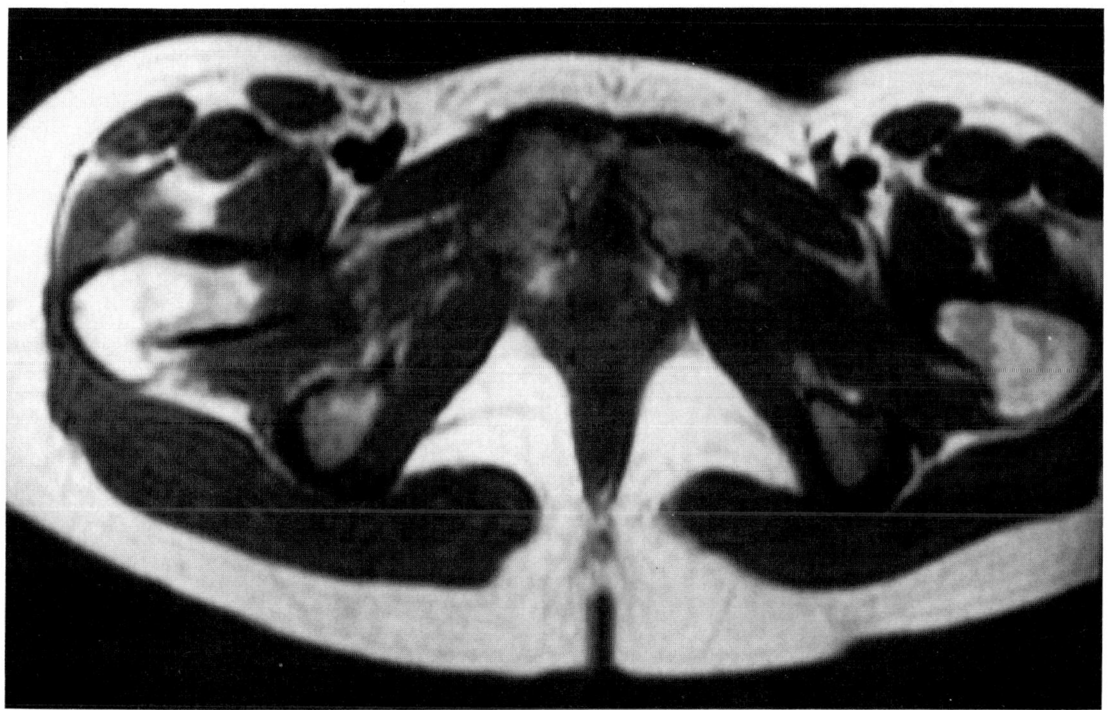

3-47 Female pelvis, axial view (TR 800, TE 20).

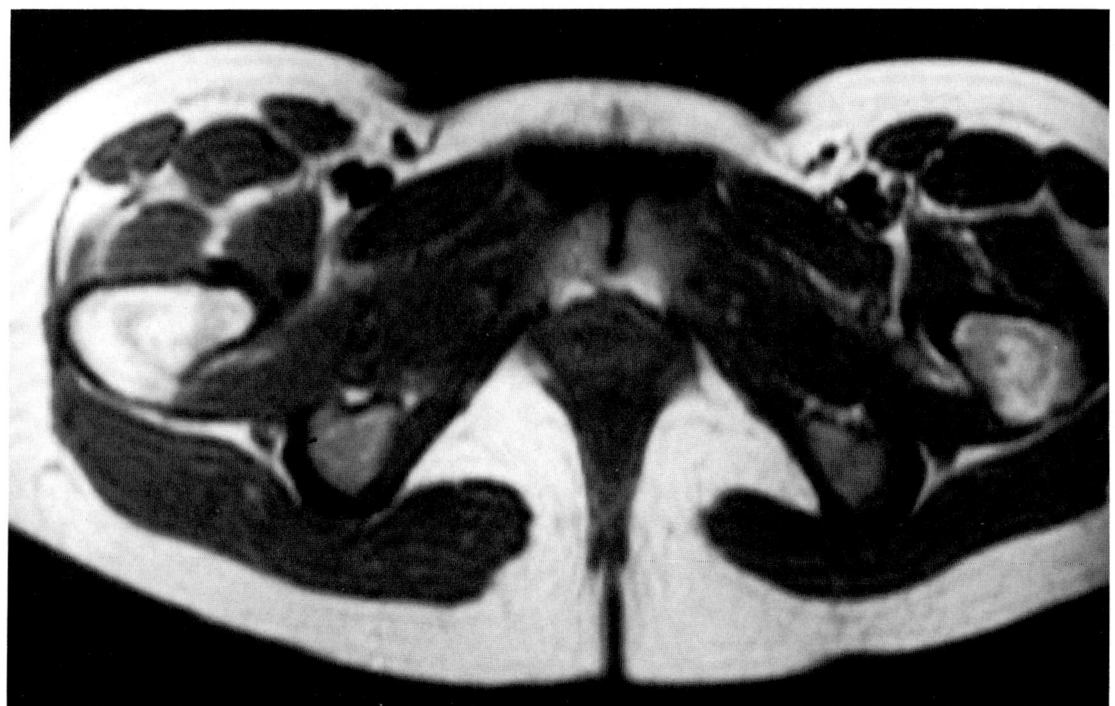

3-48 Female pelvis, axial view (TR 800, TE 20).

Female and Male Pelvis, Axial

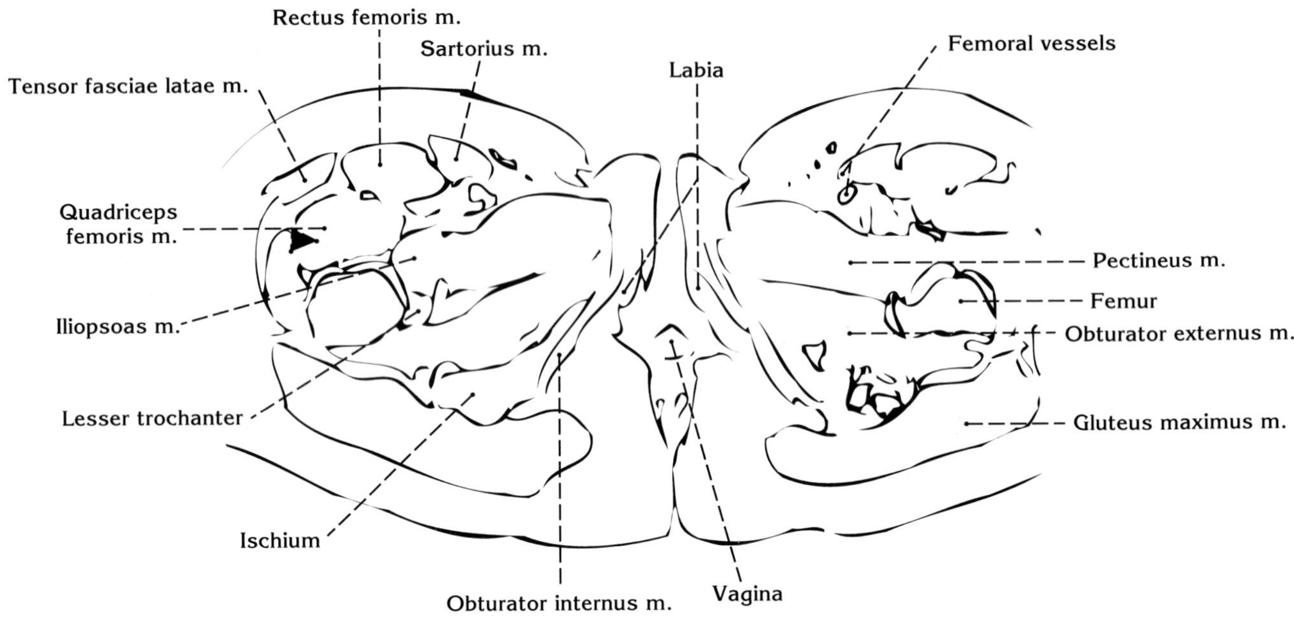

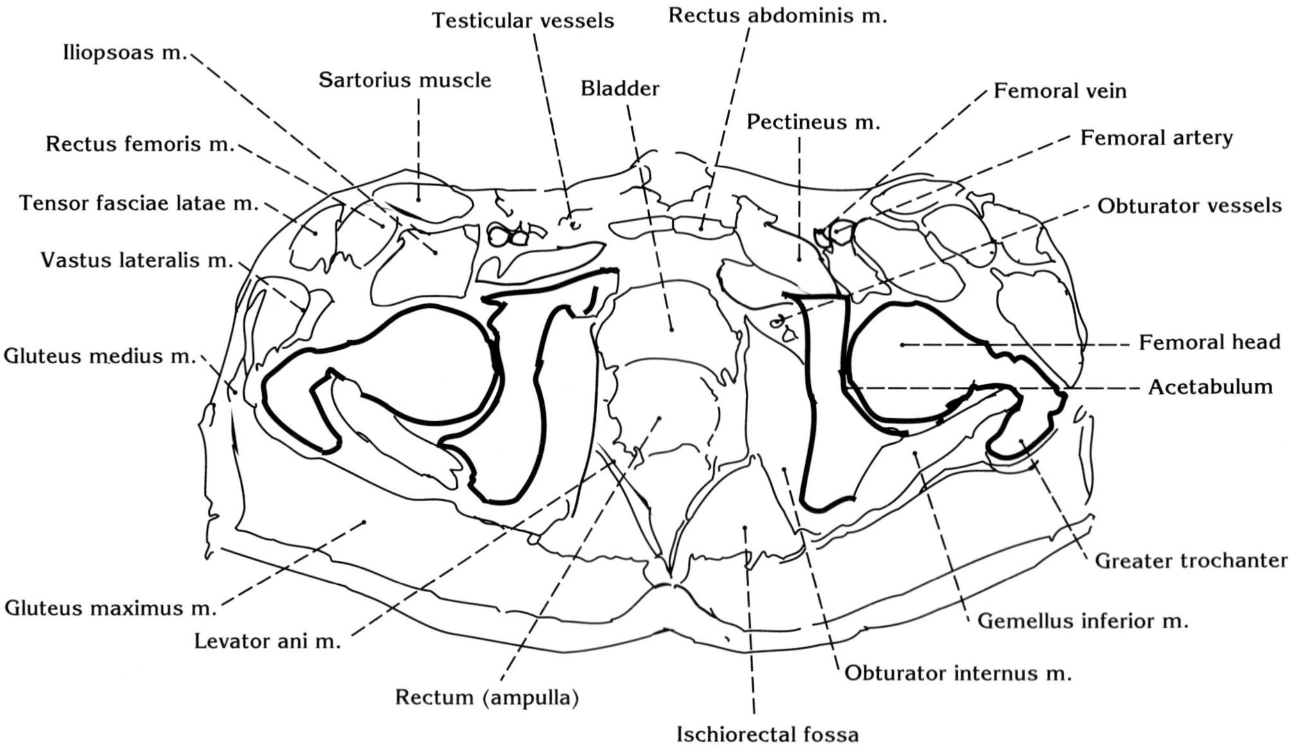

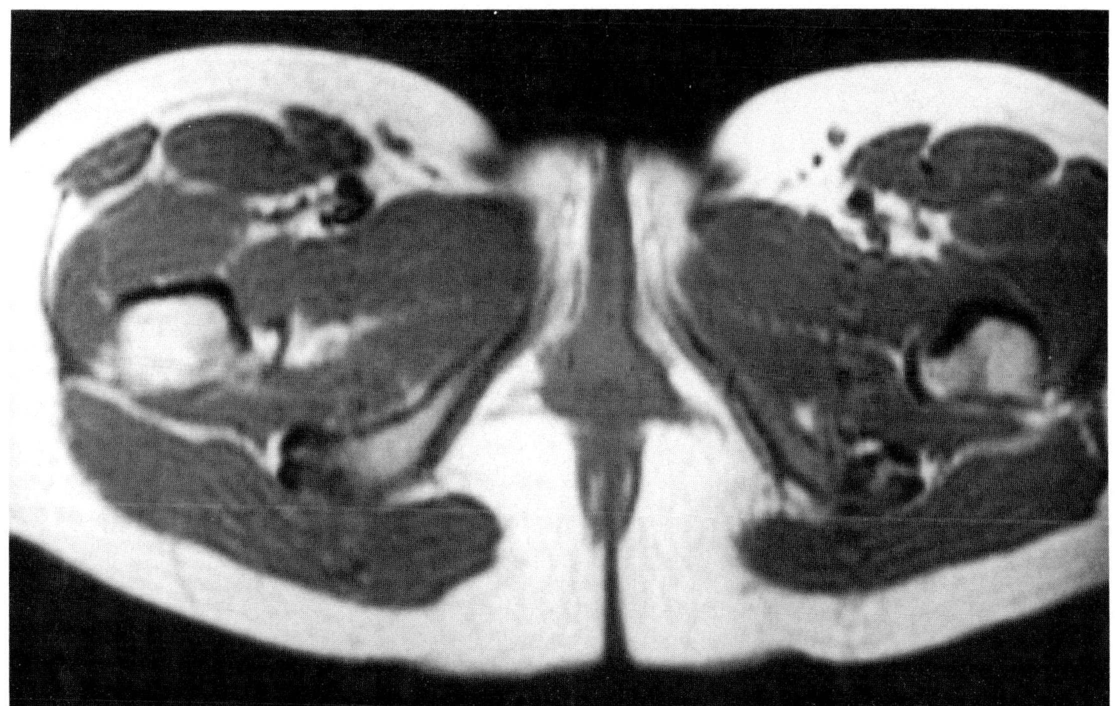

3-49 Female pelvis, axial view (TR 800, TE 20).

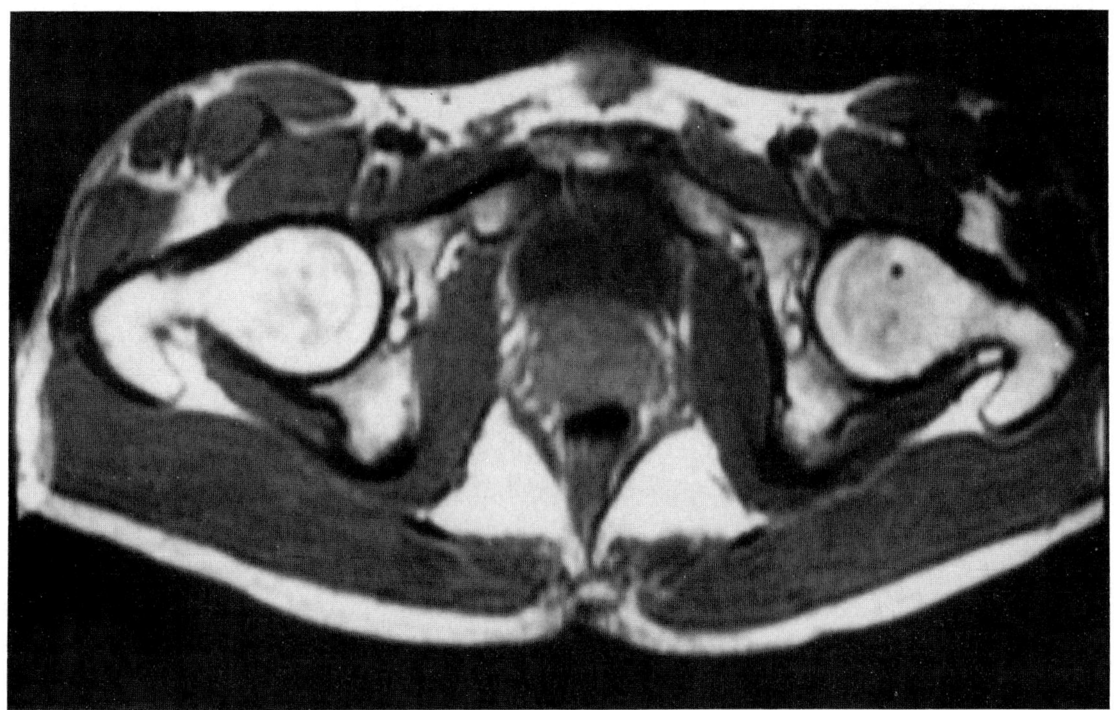

3-50 Male pelvis, axial view (TR 2000, TE 20).

Male Pelvis, Axial

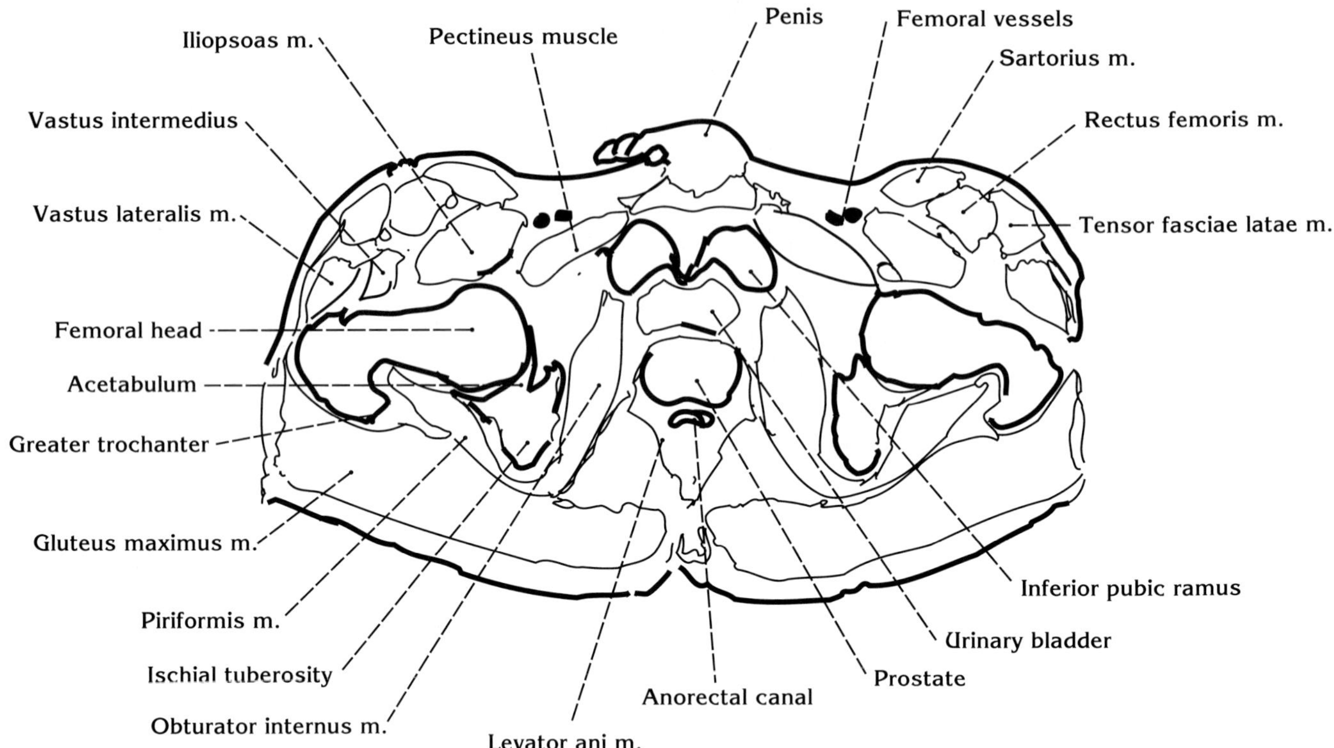

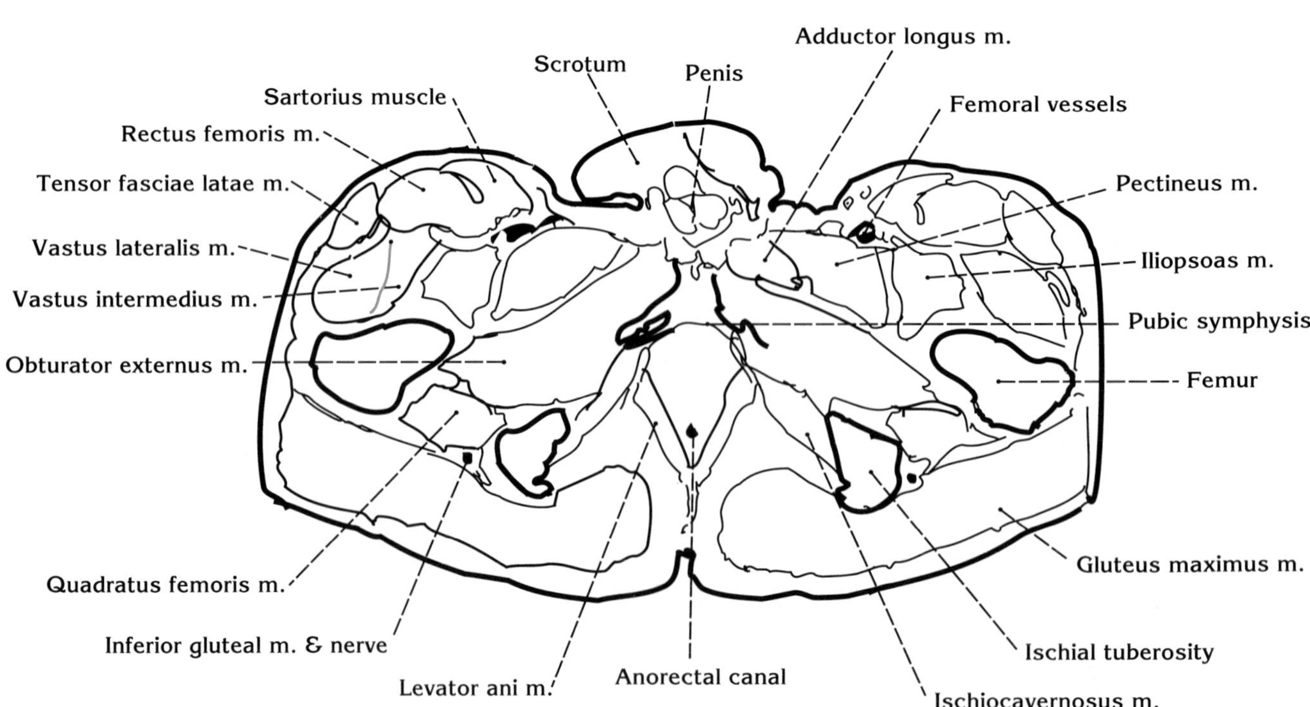

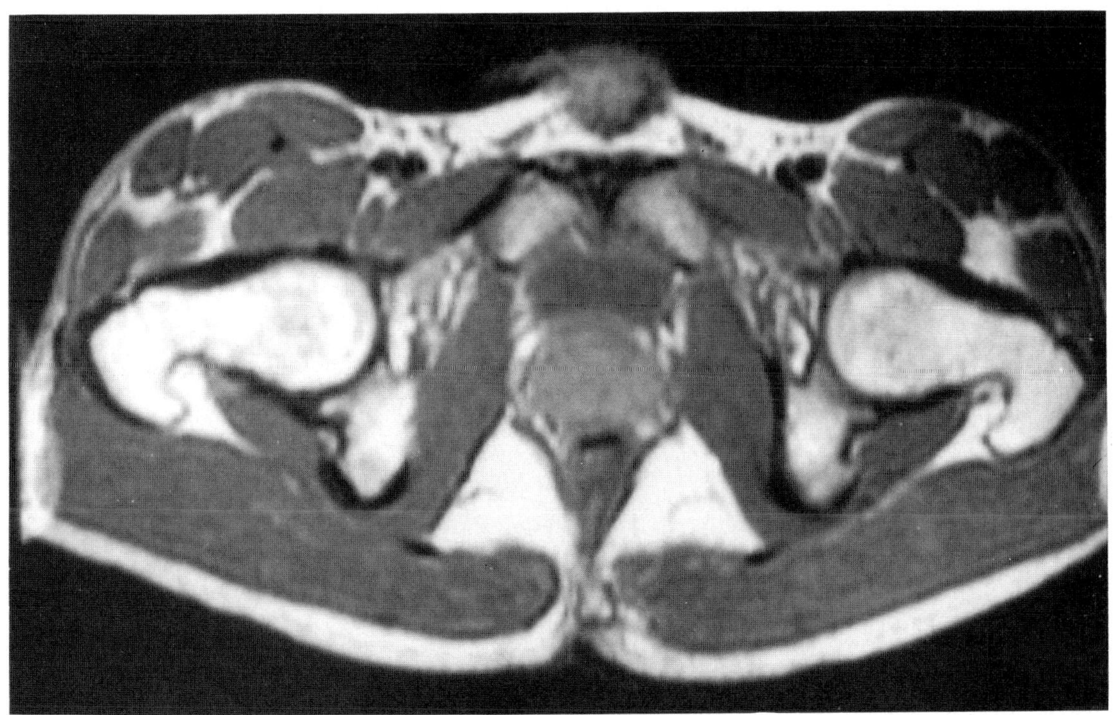

3-51 Male pelvis, axial view (TR 2000, TE 20).

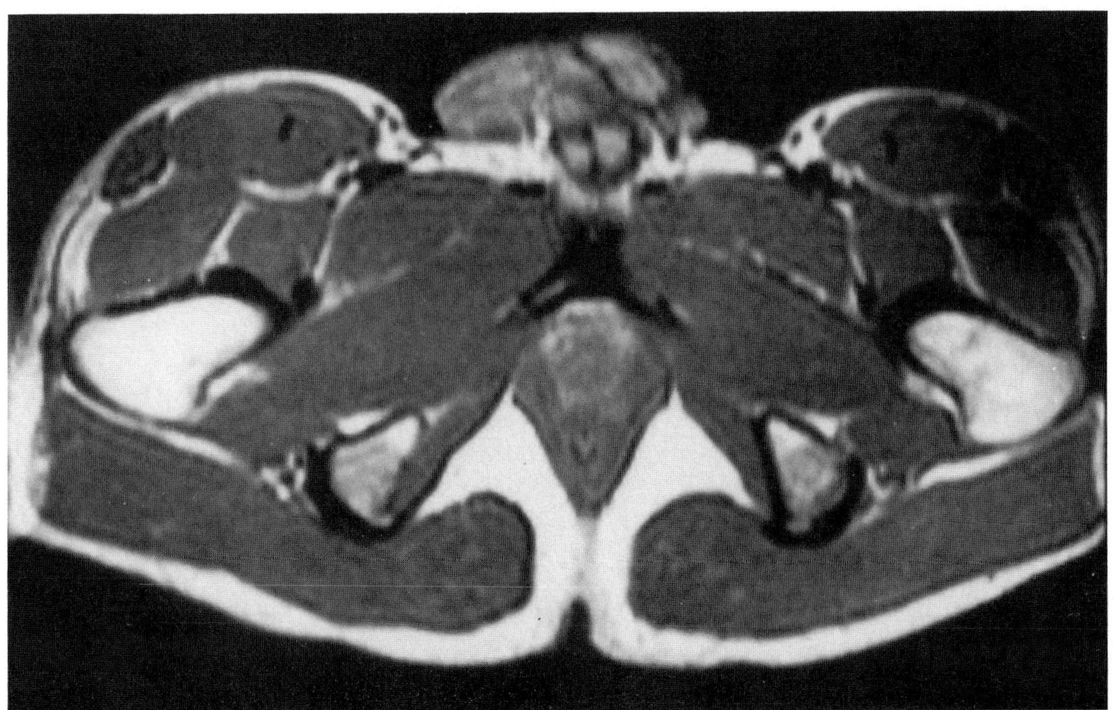

3-52 Male pelvis, axial view (TR 2000, TE 20).

Shoulder, Coronal and Axial

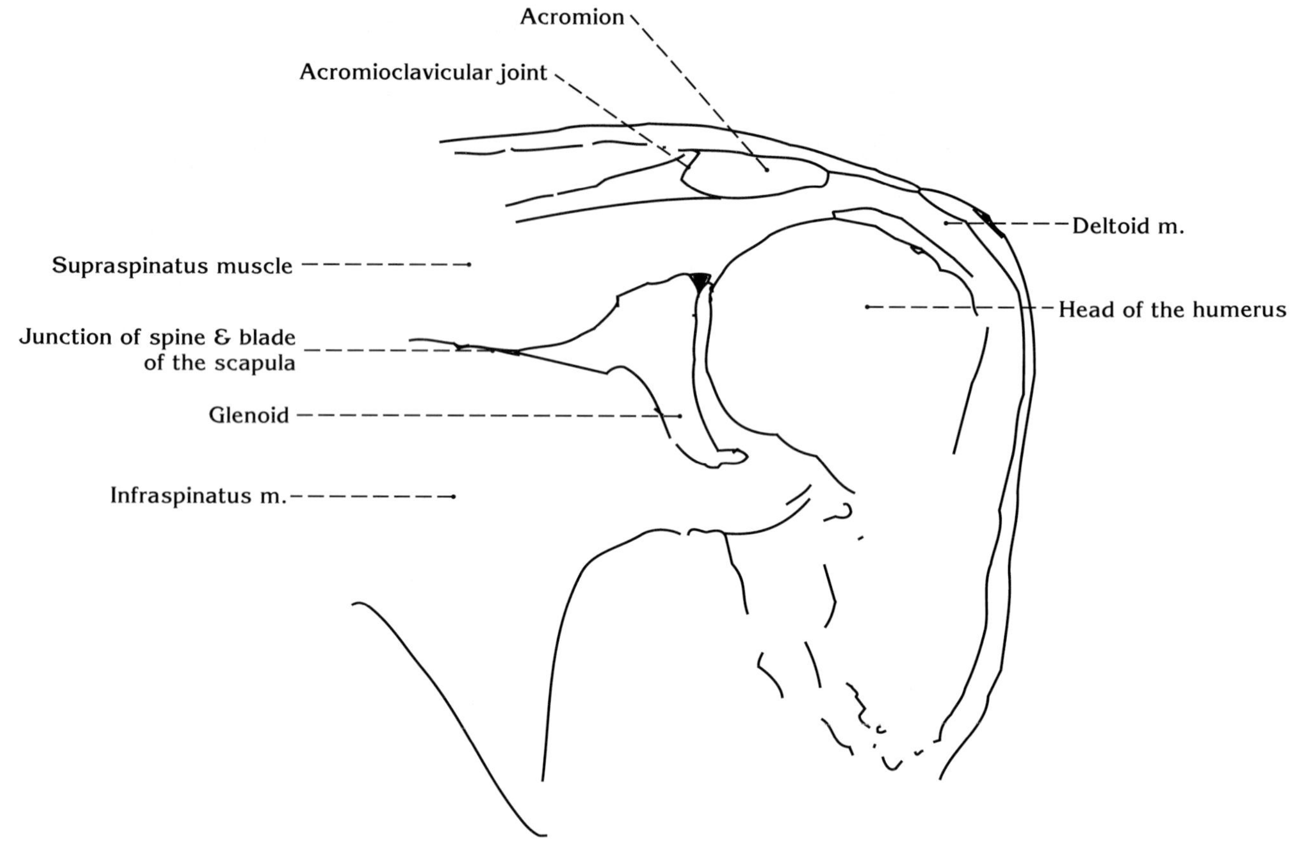

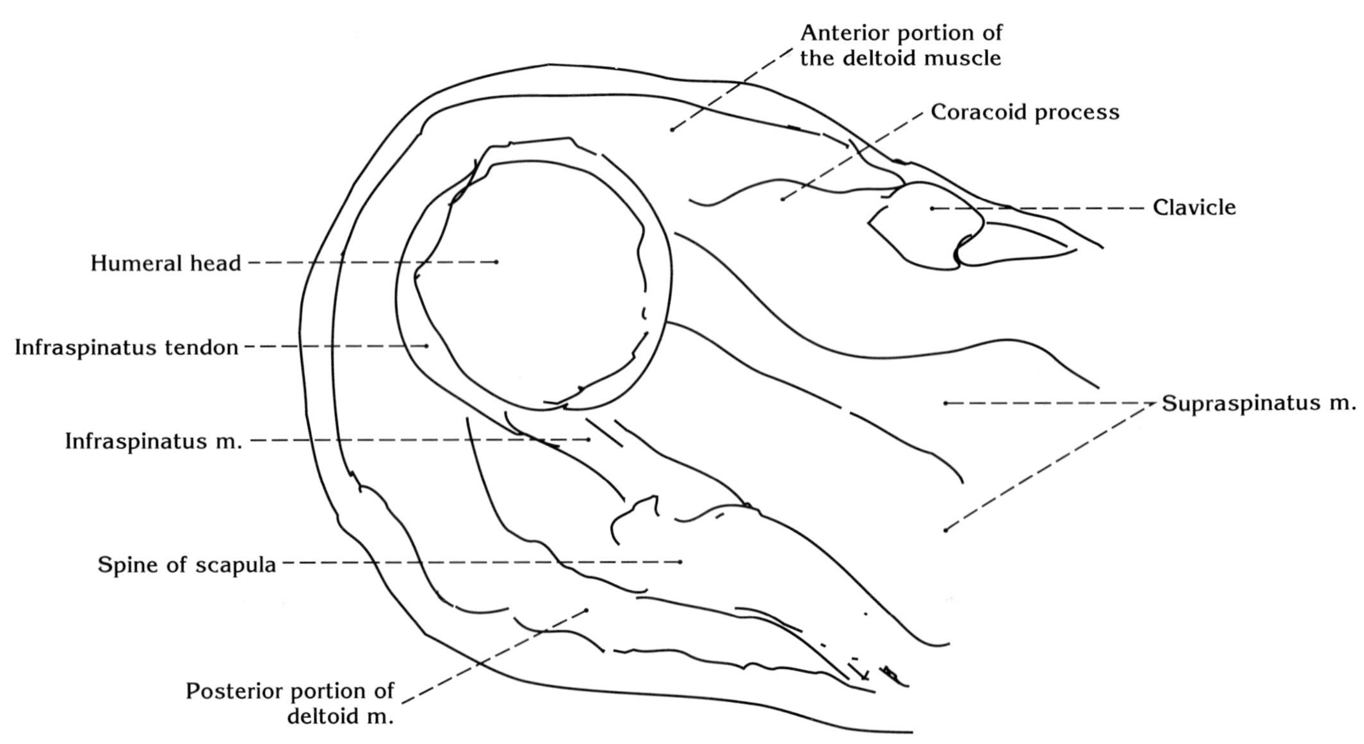

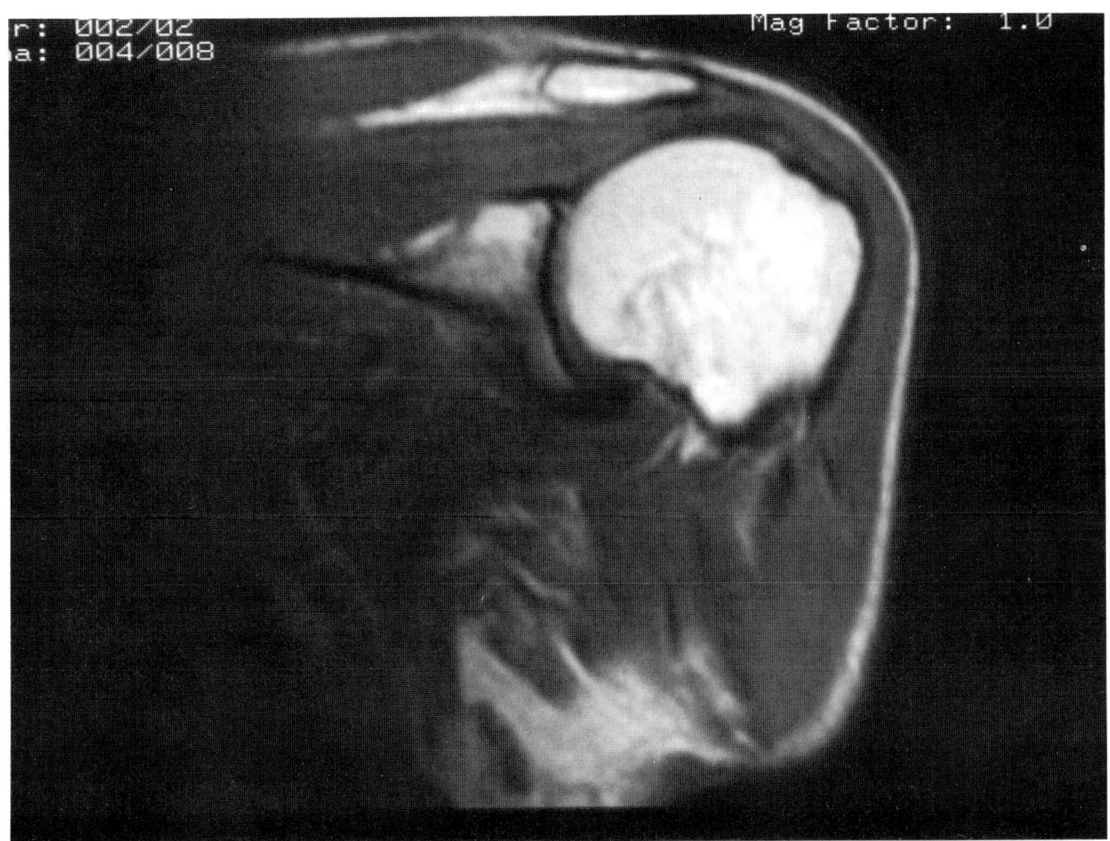

4-1 The shoulder, coronal view (TR 2000; TE 20). *Note:* This is a modified coronal section taken parallel to the body of the scapula.

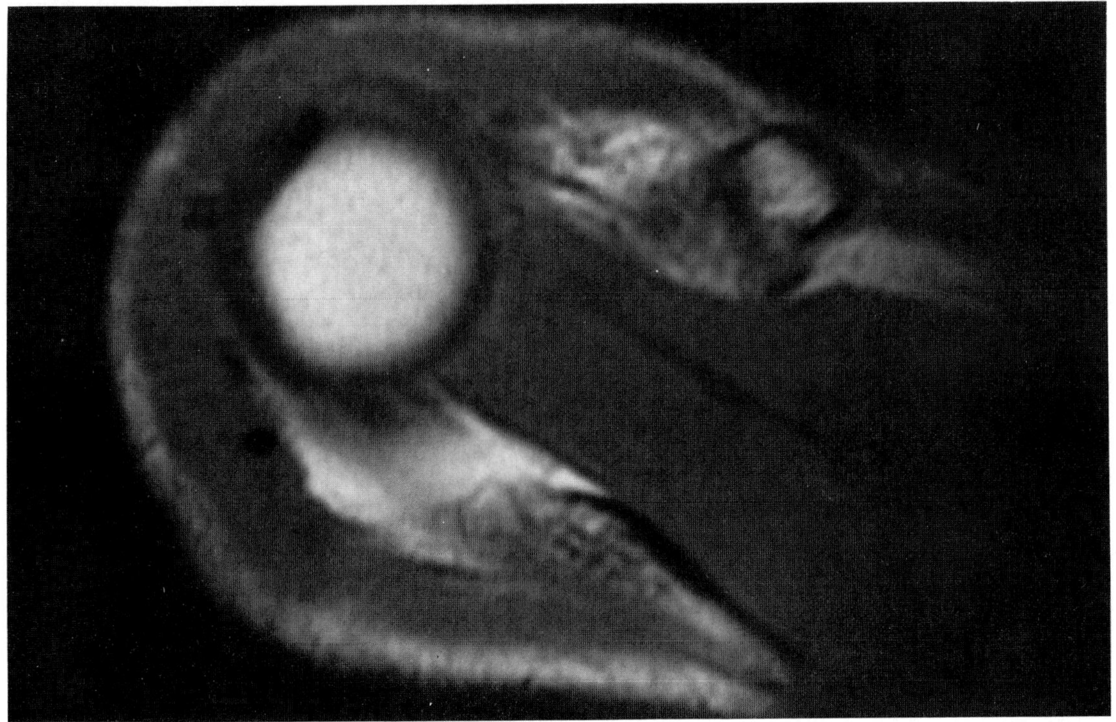

4-2 The shoulder, axial view (TR 2000; TE 20).

Shoulder, Axial

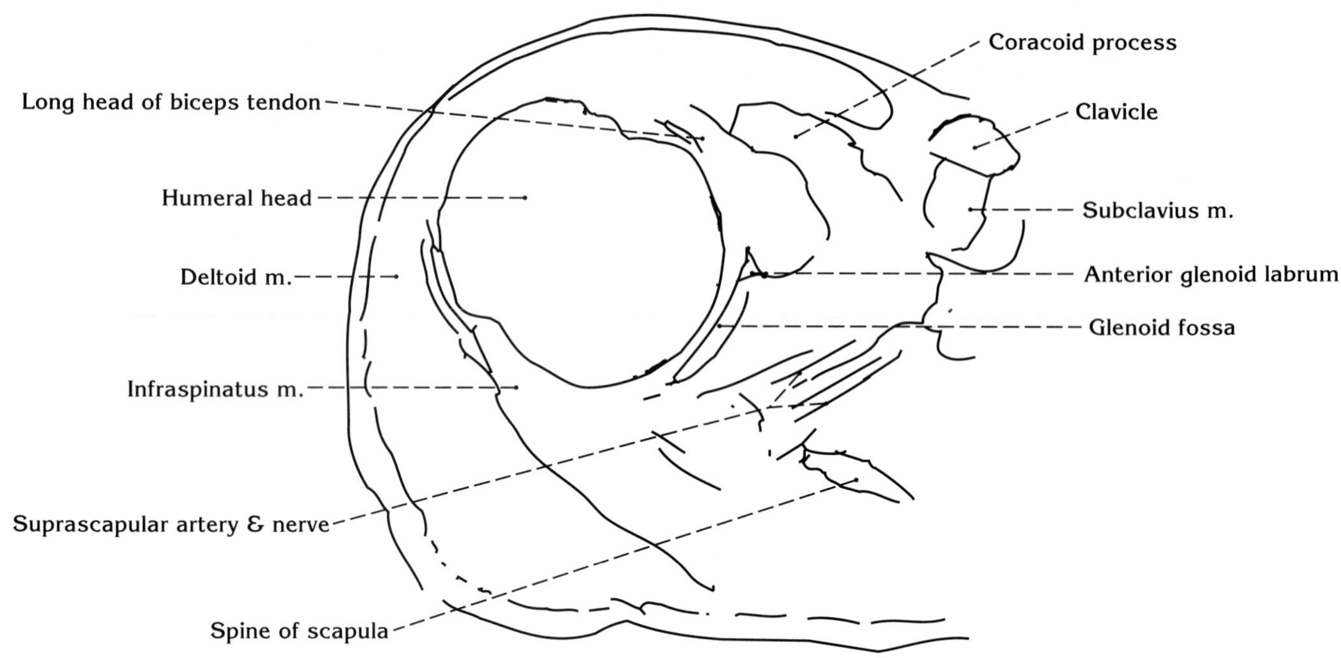

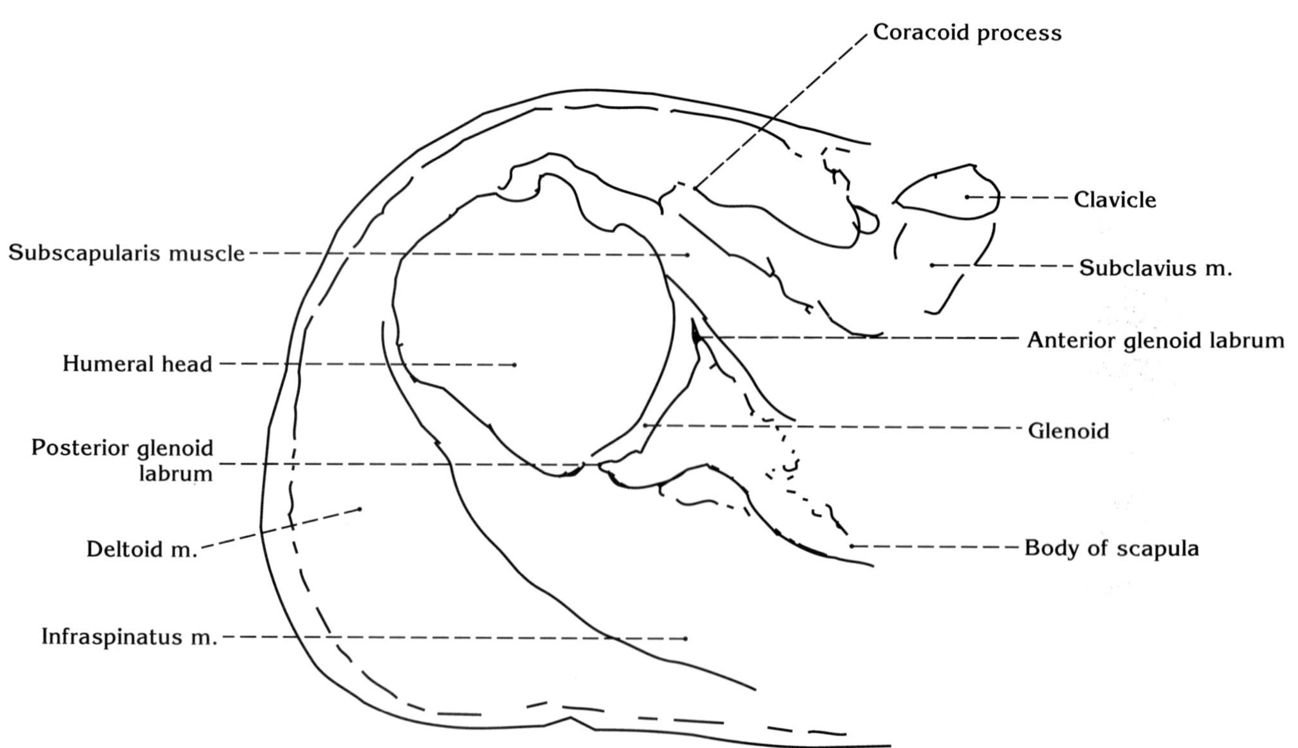

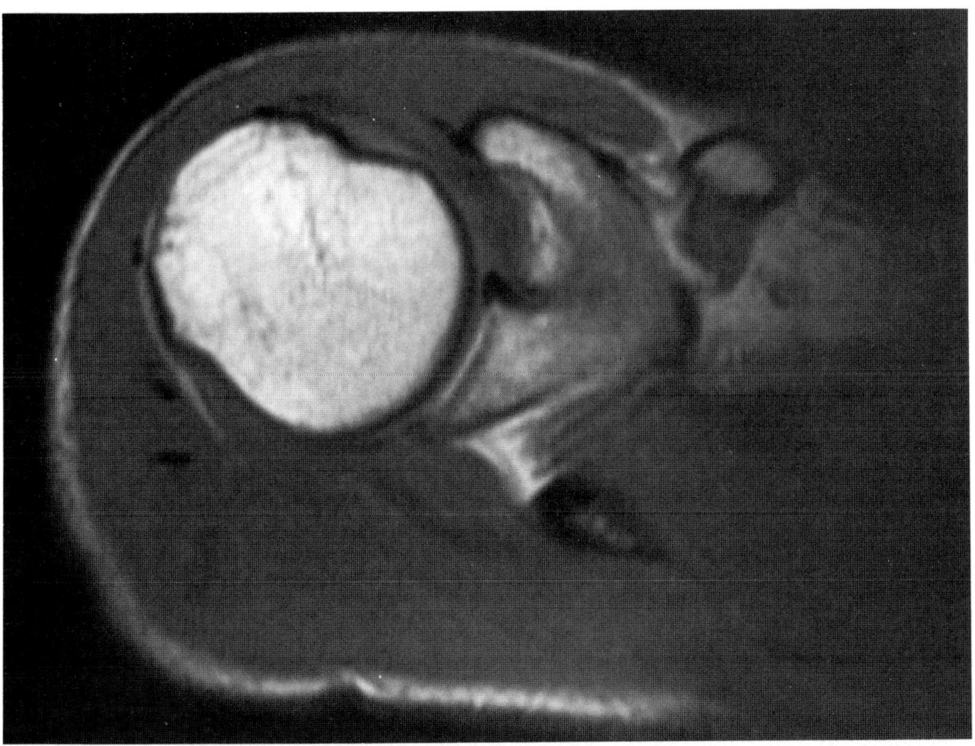

4-3 The shoulder, axial view (TR 2000; TE 20).

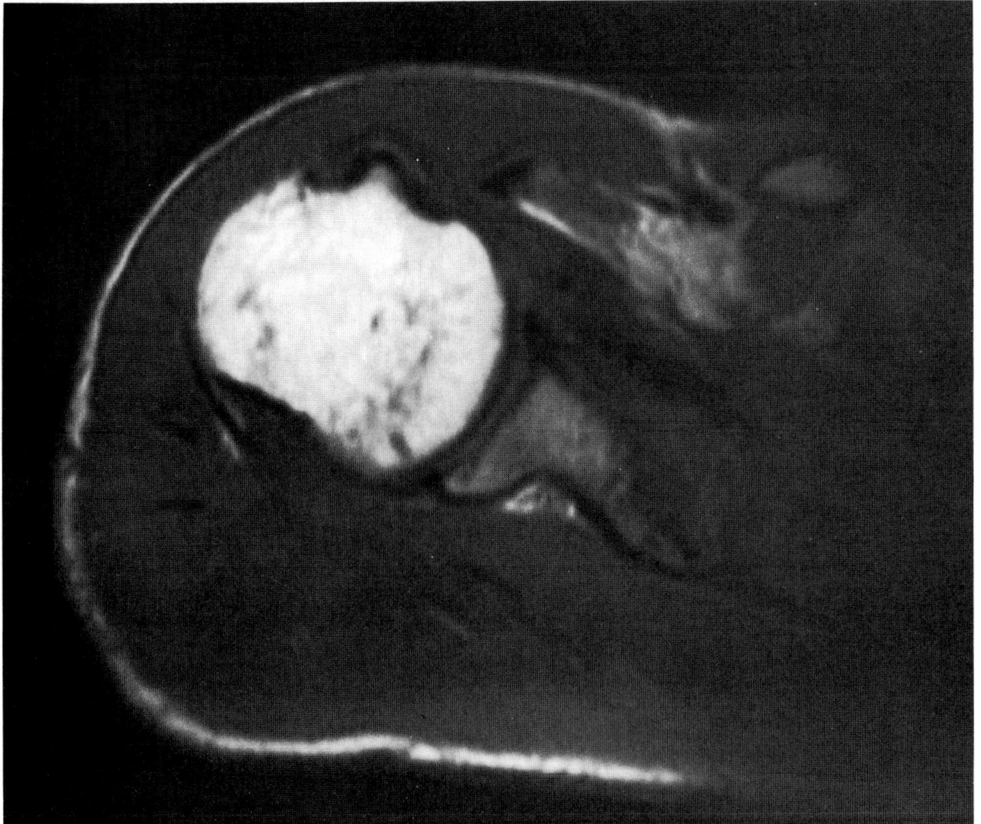

4-4 The shoulder, axial view (TR 2000; TE 20).

Shoulder, Sagittal

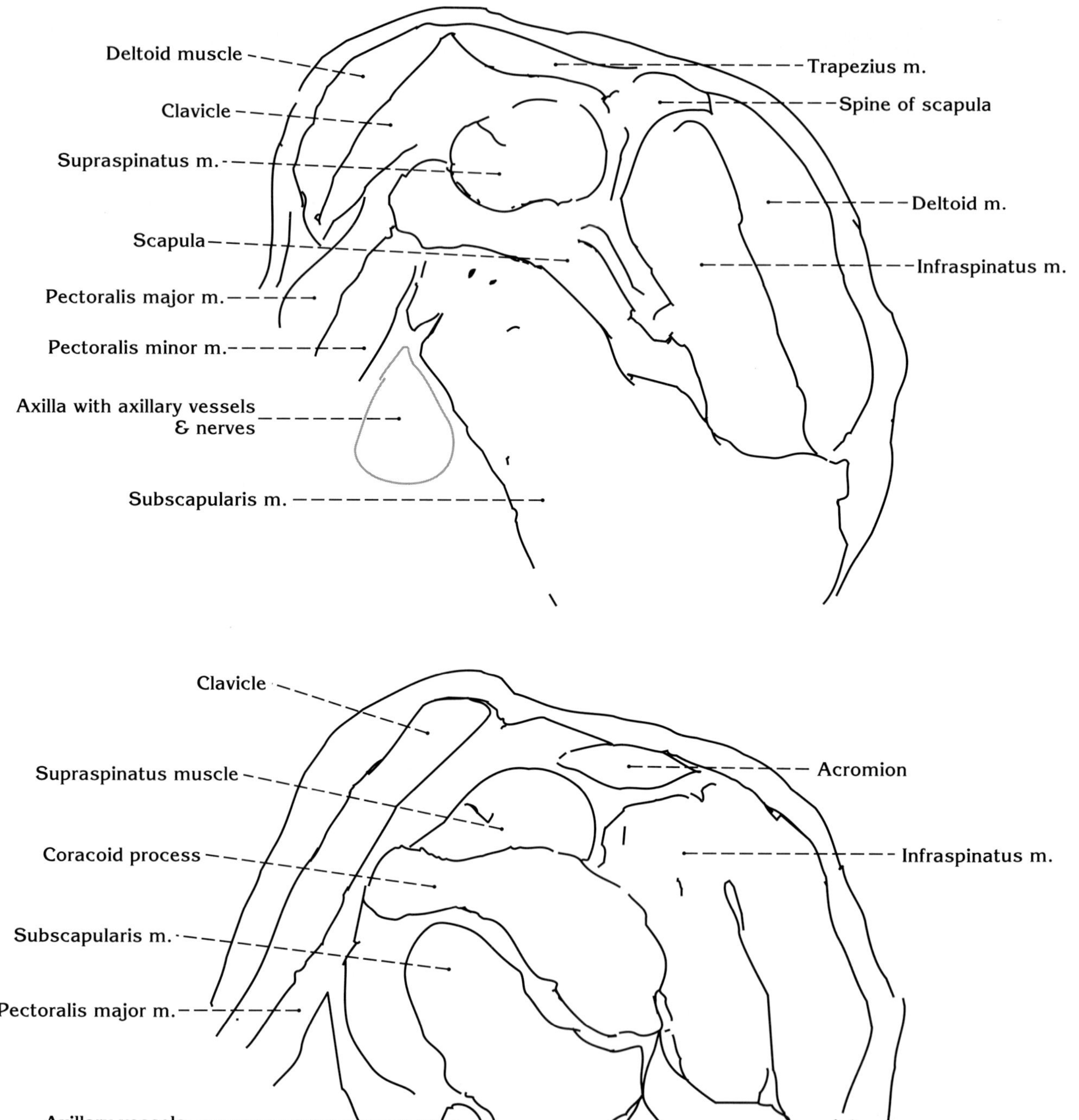

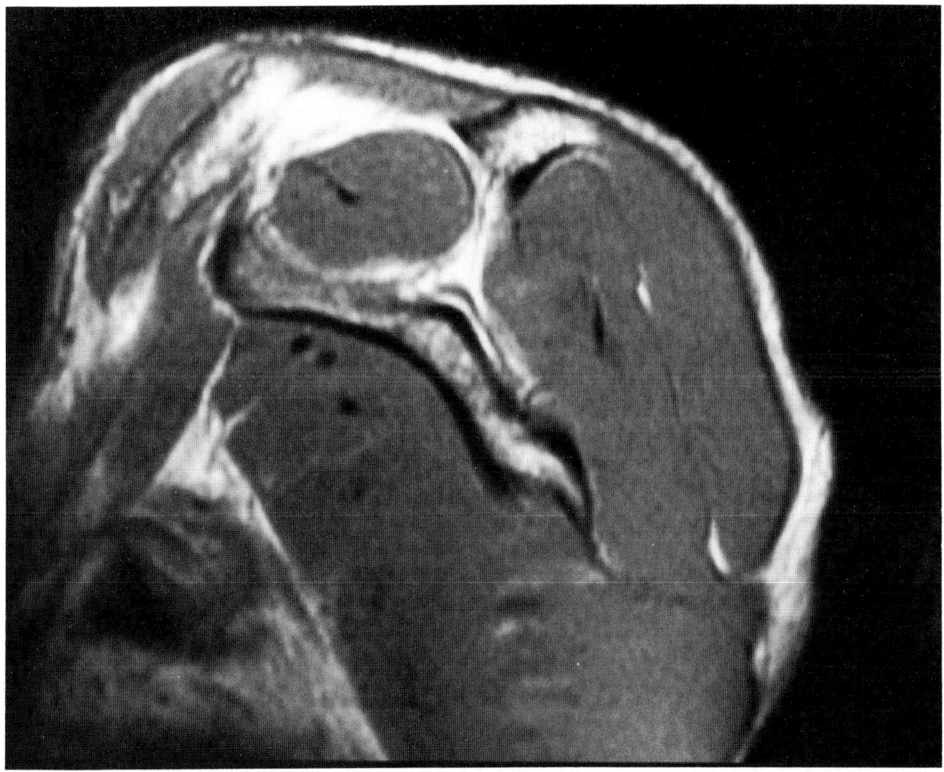

4-5 The shoulder, sagittal/glenoid view (TR 2000; TE 20). *Note:* This section is obtained parallel to the glenoid fossa.

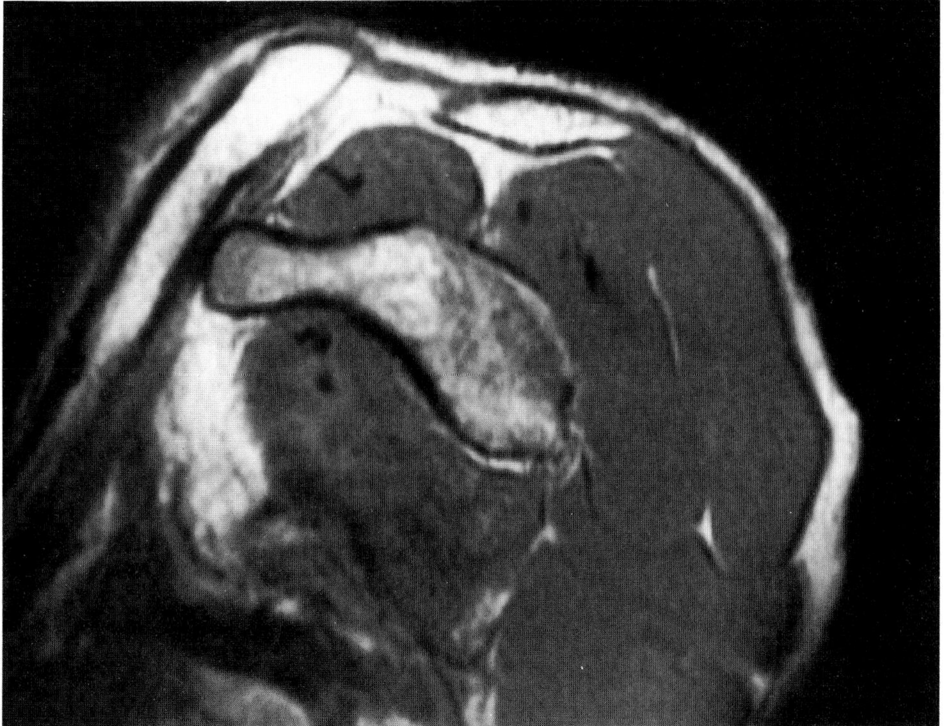

4-6 The shoulder, sagittal/glenoid view (TR 2000; TE 20). *Note:* This section is obtained parallel to the glenoid fossa.

Shoulder, Sagittal

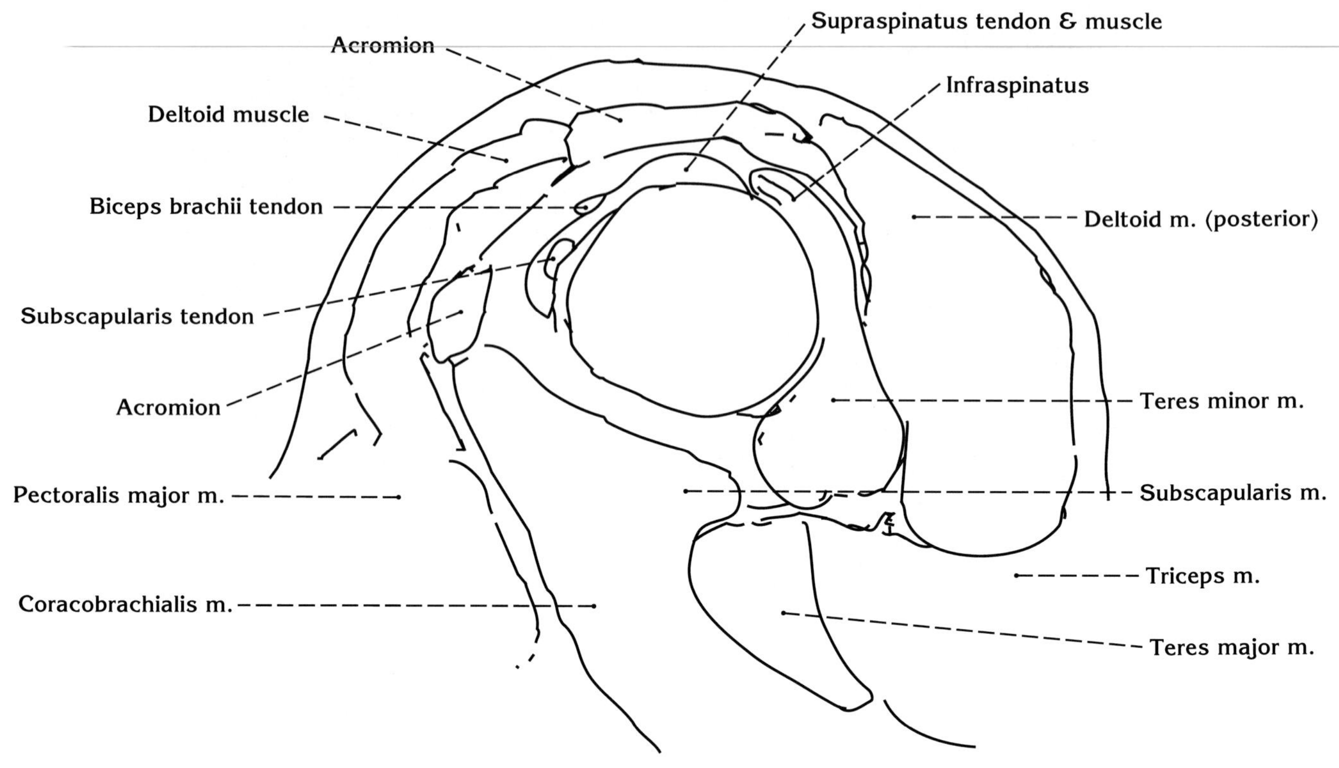

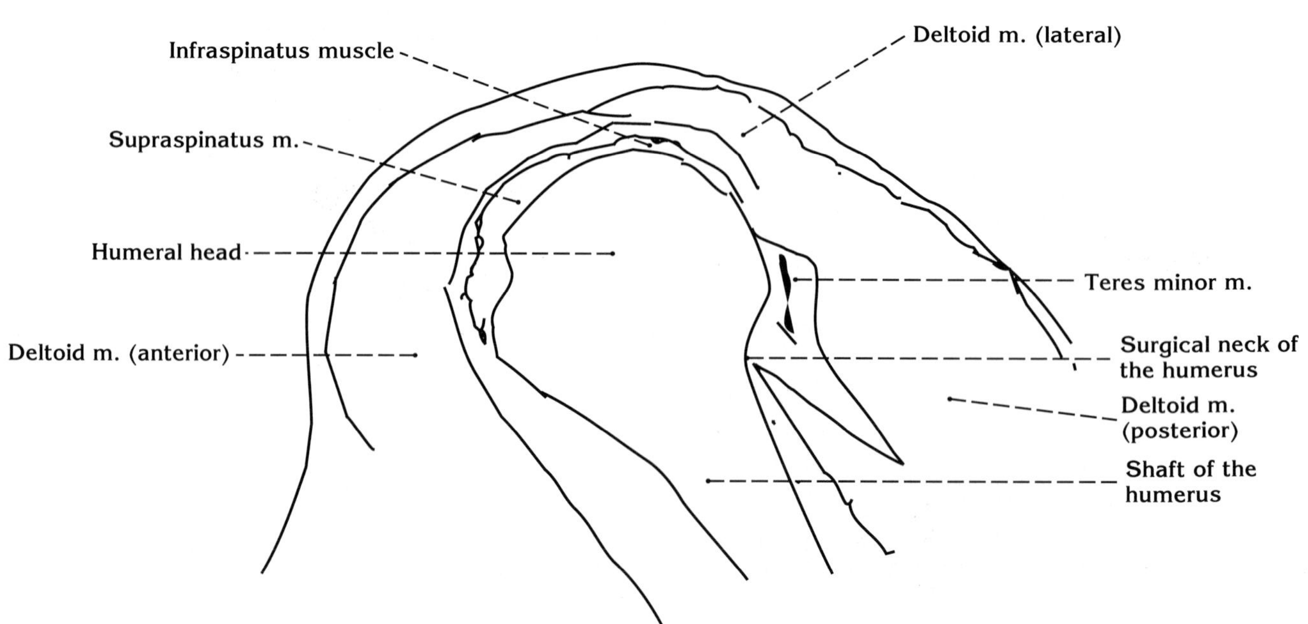

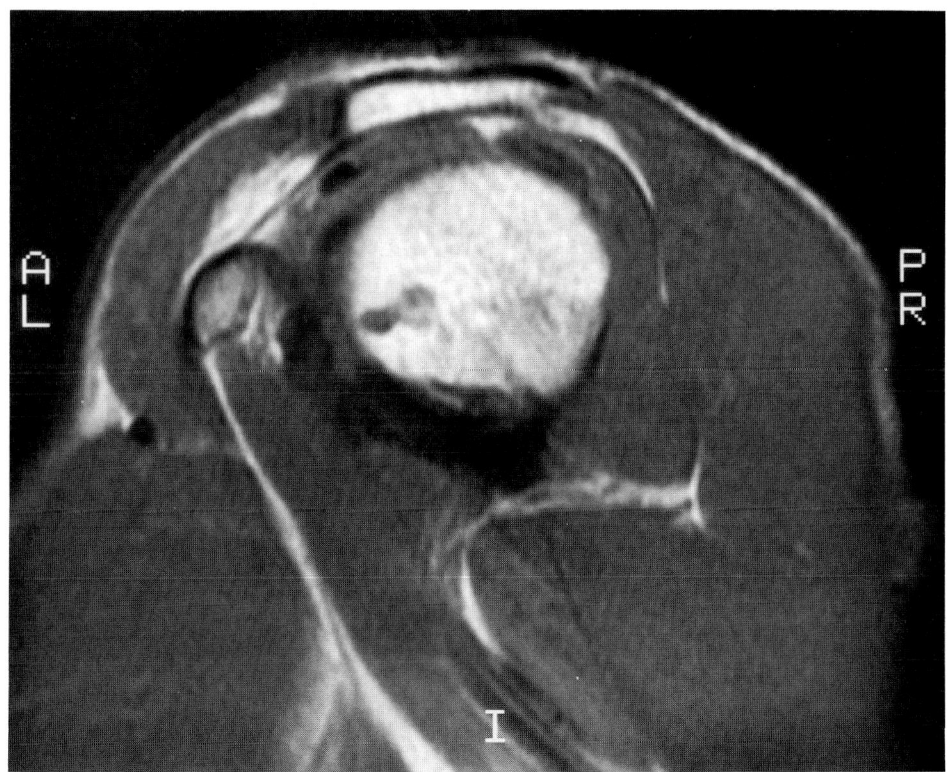

4-7 The shoulder, sagittal/glenoid view (TR 2000; TE 20). *Note:* This section is obtained parallel to the glenoid.

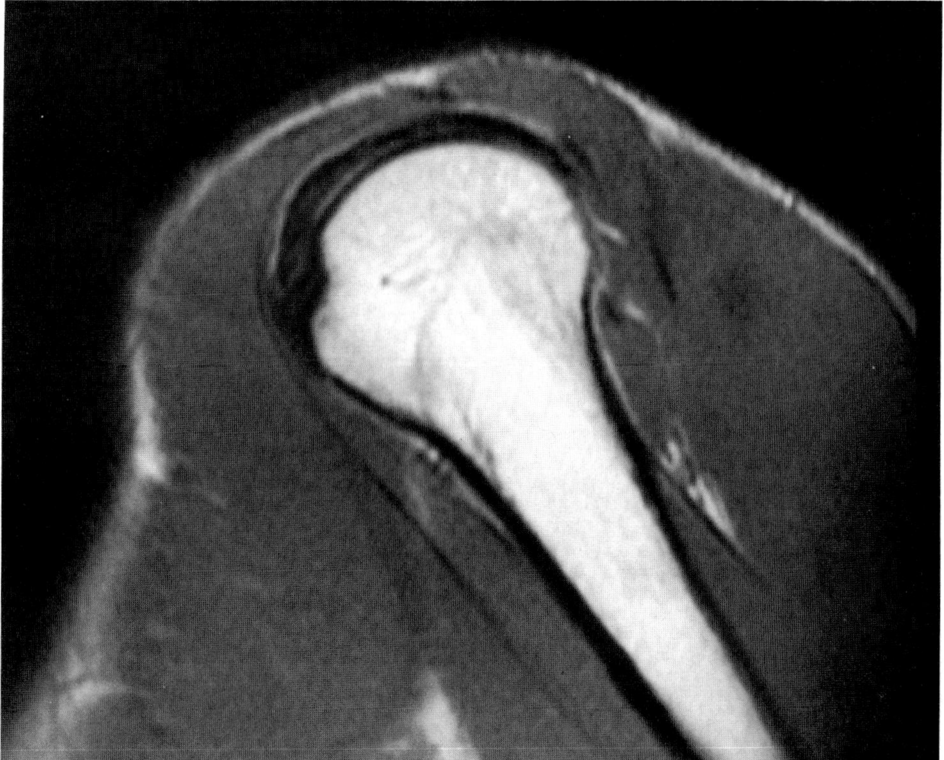

4-8 The shoulder, sagittal/glenoid view (TR 2000; TE 20).

Elbow, Sagittal

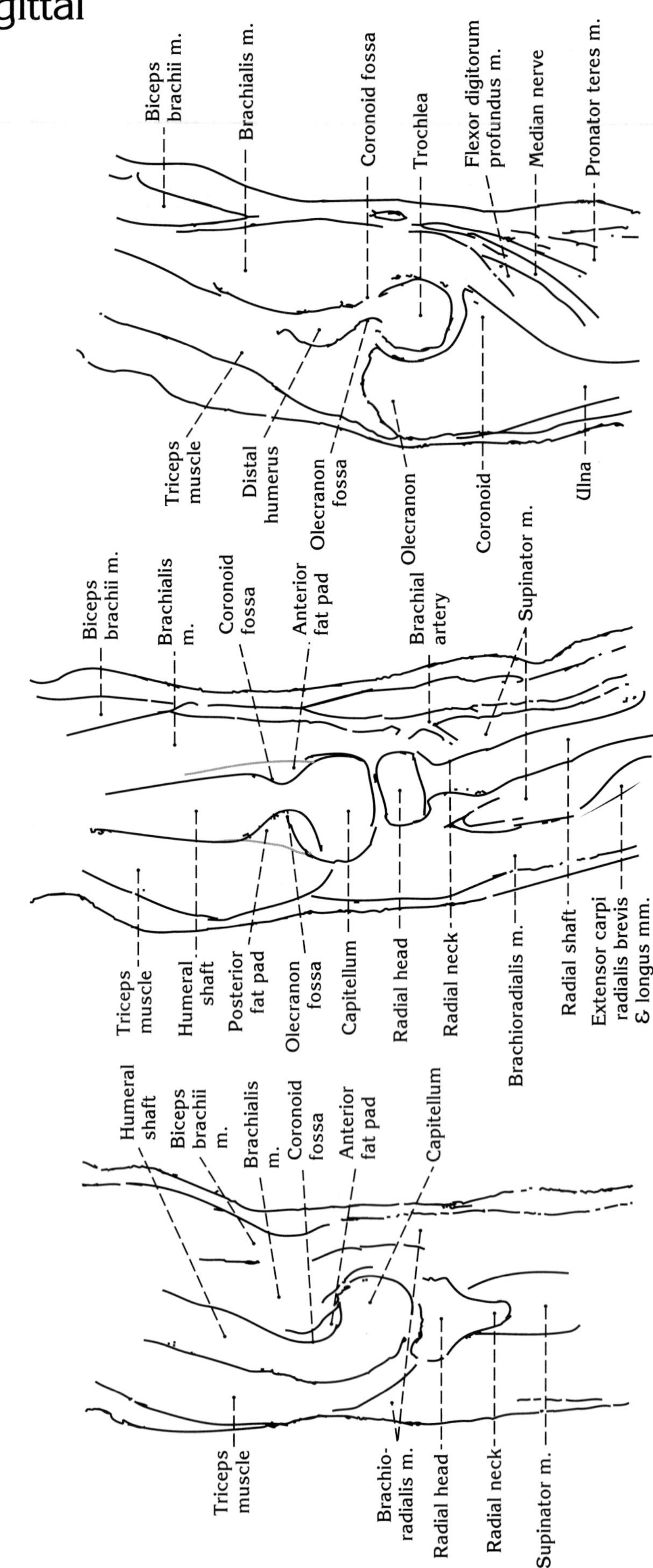

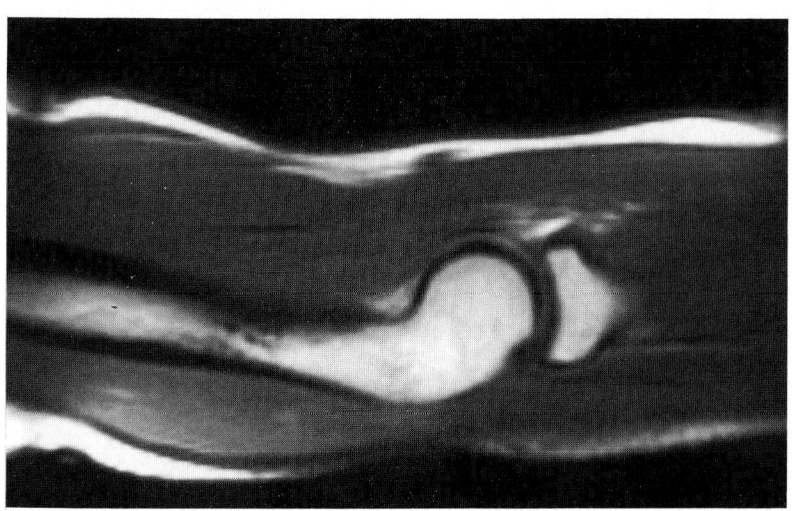

4-9 Elbow, sagittal view (TR 800; TE 30).

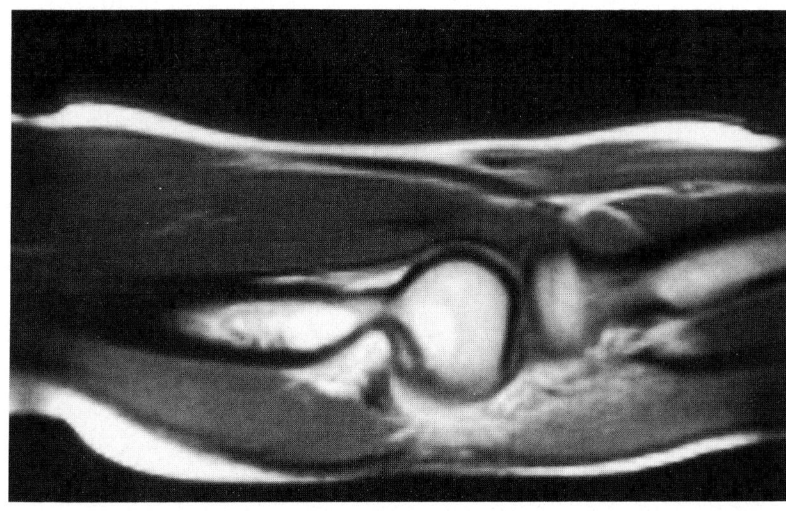

4-10 Elbow, sagittal view (TR 800; TE 30).

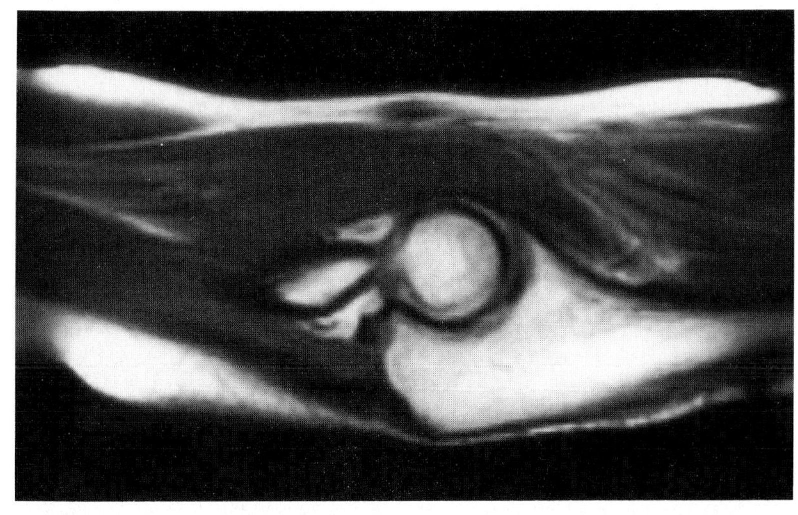

4-11 Elbow, sagittal view (TR 800; TE 30).

Elbow, Axial

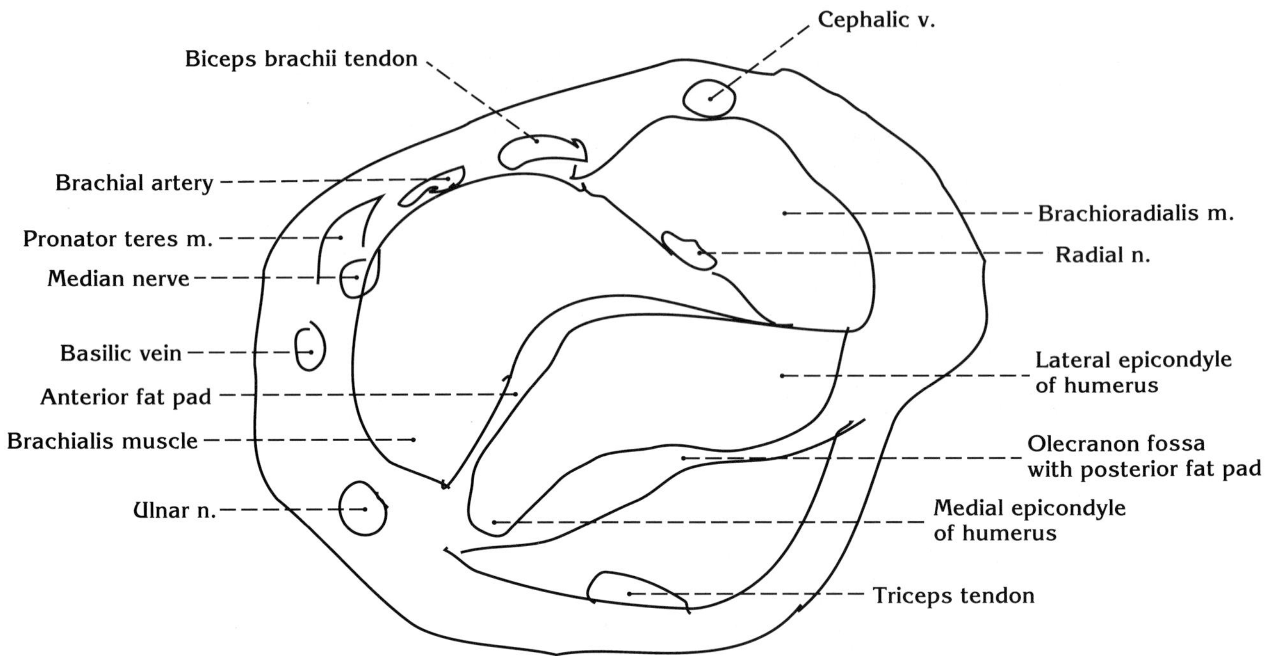
Cephalic v.
Biceps brachii tendon
Brachial artery
Pronator teres m.
Median nerve
Basilic vein
Anterior fat pad
Brachialis muscle
Ulnar n.
Brachioradialis m.
Radial n.
Lateral epicondyle of humerus
Olecranon fossa with posterior fat pad
Medial epicondyle of humerus
Triceps tendon

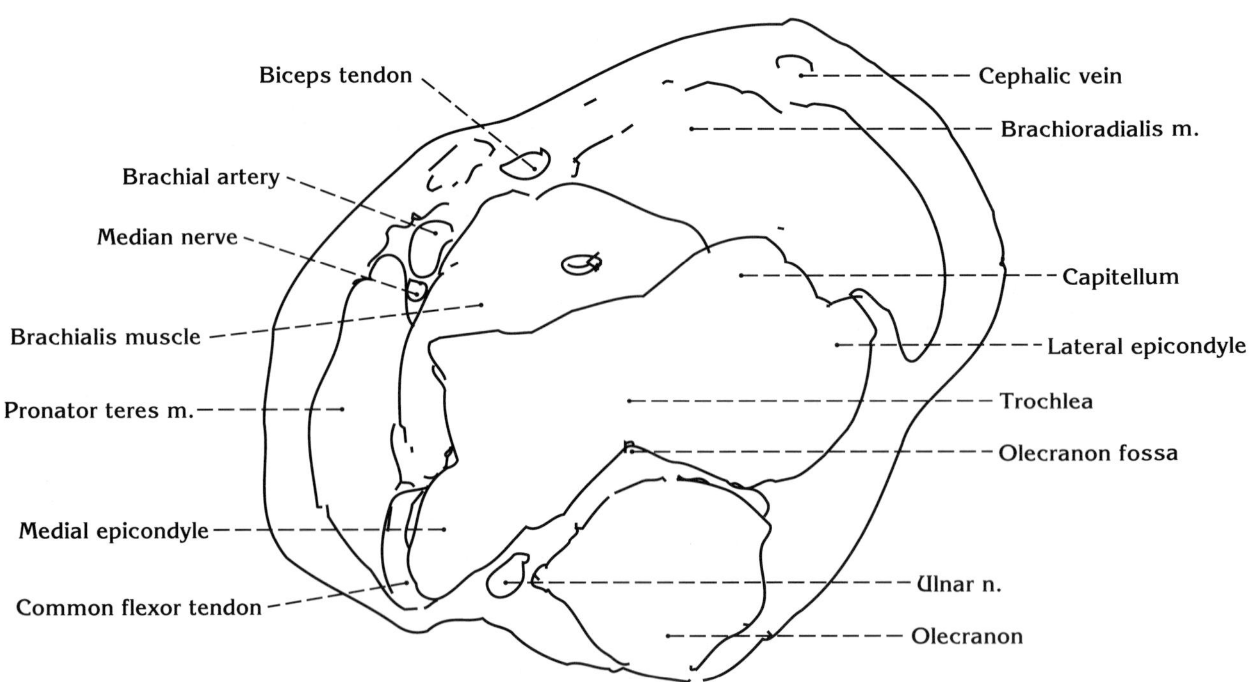
Biceps tendon
Brachial artery
Median nerve
Brachialis muscle
Pronator teres m.
Medial epicondyle
Common flexor tendon
Cephalic vein
Brachioradialis m.
Capitellum
Lateral epicondyle
Trochlea
Olecranon fossa
Ulnar n.
Olecranon

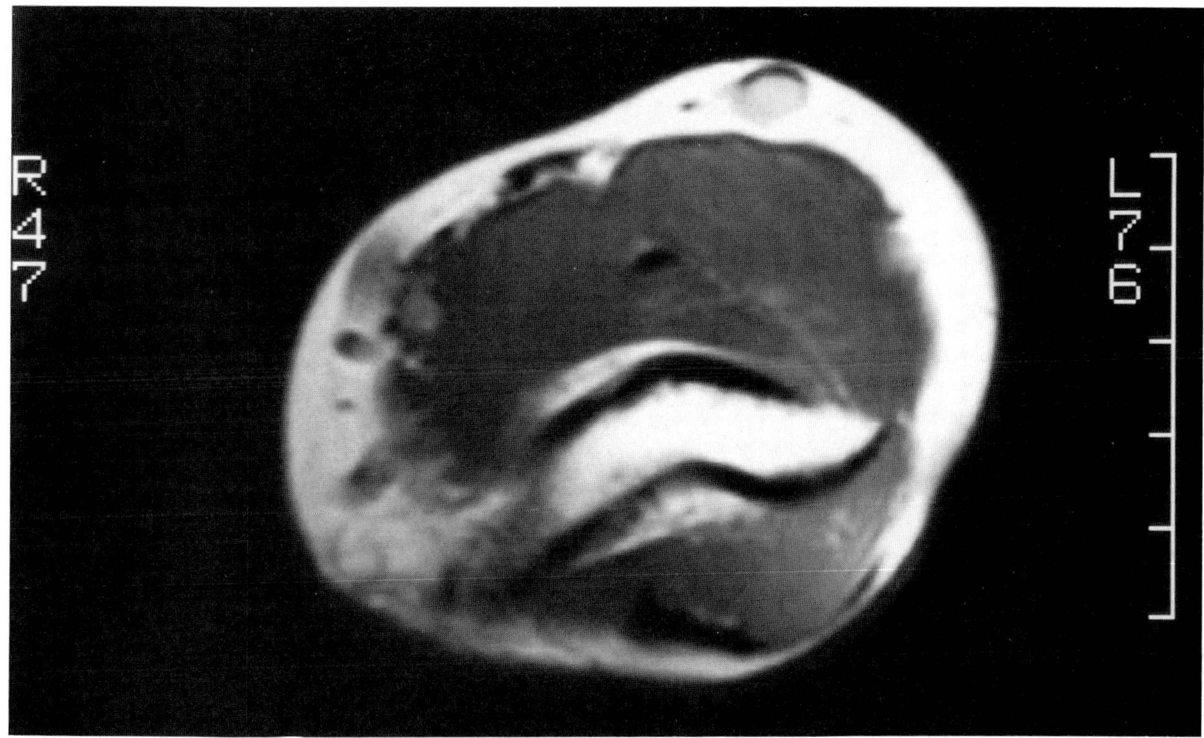

4-12 Elbow, axial view (TR 800; TE 30).

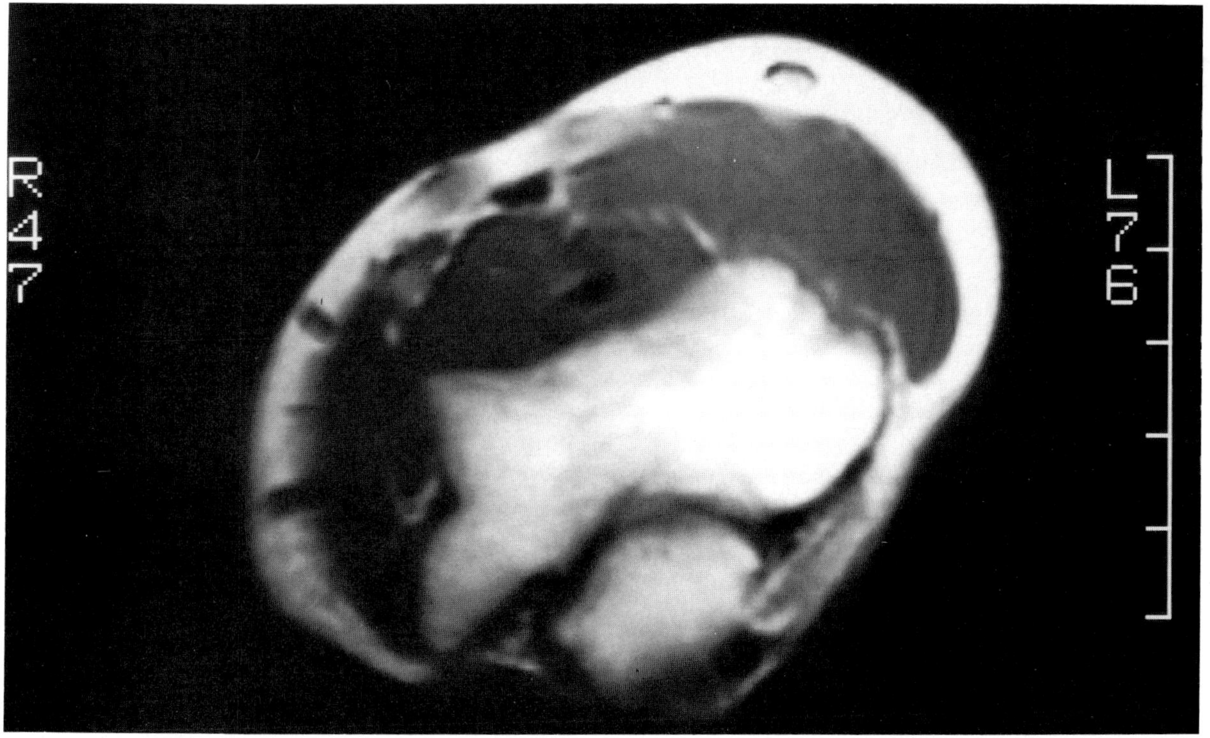

4-13 Elbow, axial view (TR 800; TE 30).

Elbow, Axial

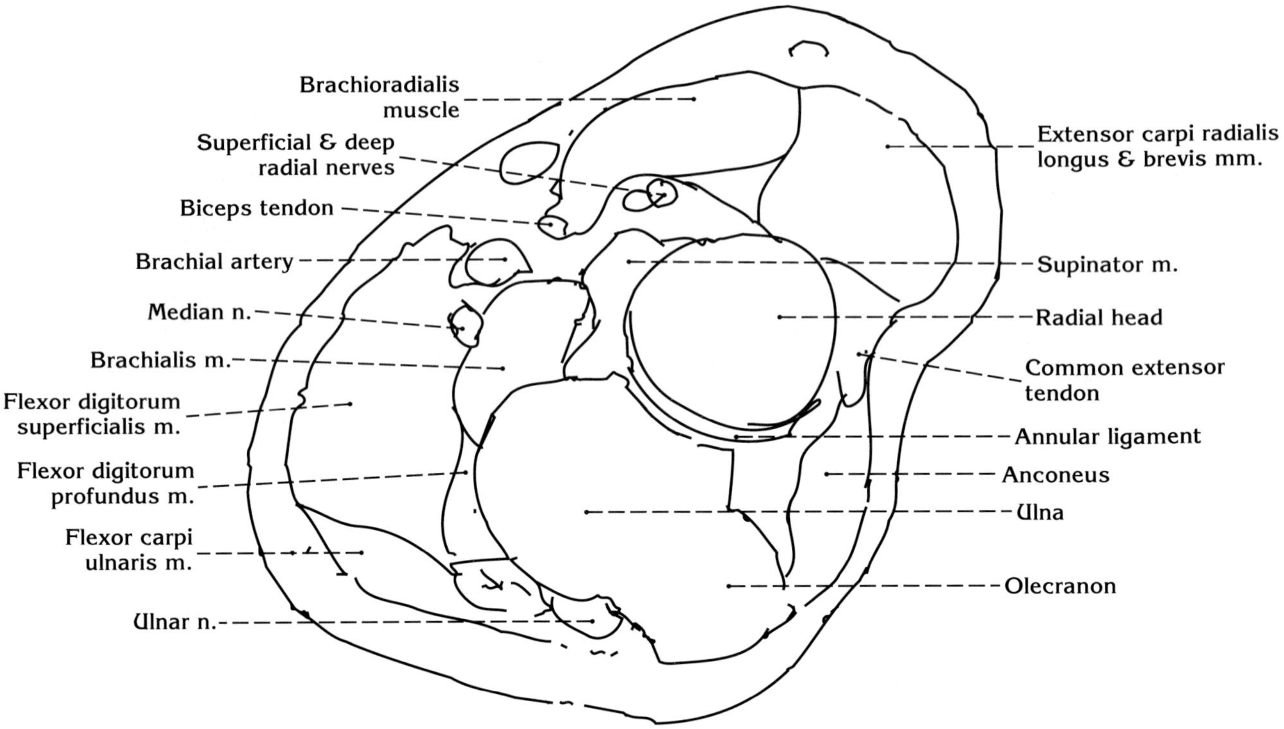

Brachioradialis muscle
Superficial & deep radial nerves
Biceps tendon
Brachial artery
Median n.
Brachialis m.
Flexor digitorum superficialis m.
Flexor digitorum profundus m.
Flexor carpi ulnaris m.
Ulnar n.
Extensor carpi radialis longus & brevis mm.
Supinator m.
Radial head
Common extensor tendon
Annular ligament
Anconeus
Ulna
Olecranon

Extensor carpi radialis longus & brevis muscles
Brachioradialis m.
Pronator teres m.
Biceps tendon
Flexor digitorum superficialis m.
Brachialis m.
Flexor carpi ulnaris m.
Flexor digitorum profundus m.
Extensor digitorum m.
Supinator m.
Radius
Extensor carpi ulnaris m.
Anconeus
Ulna

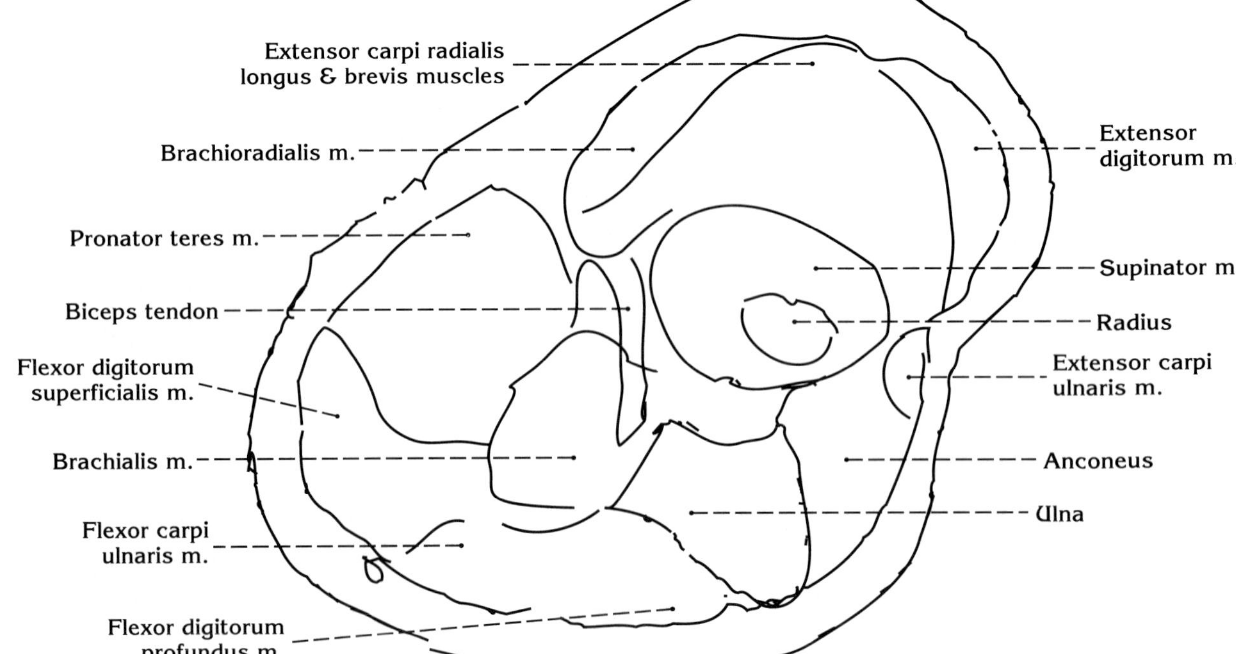

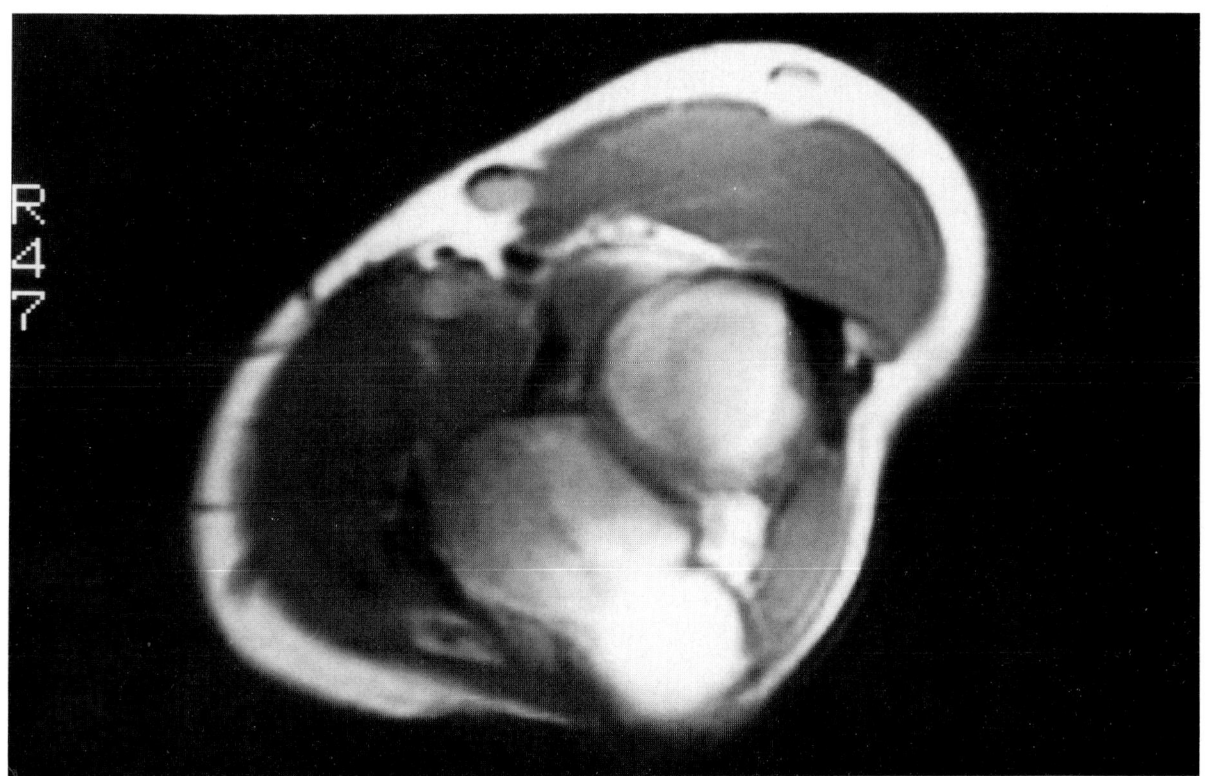

4-14 Elbow, axial view (TR 800; TE 30).

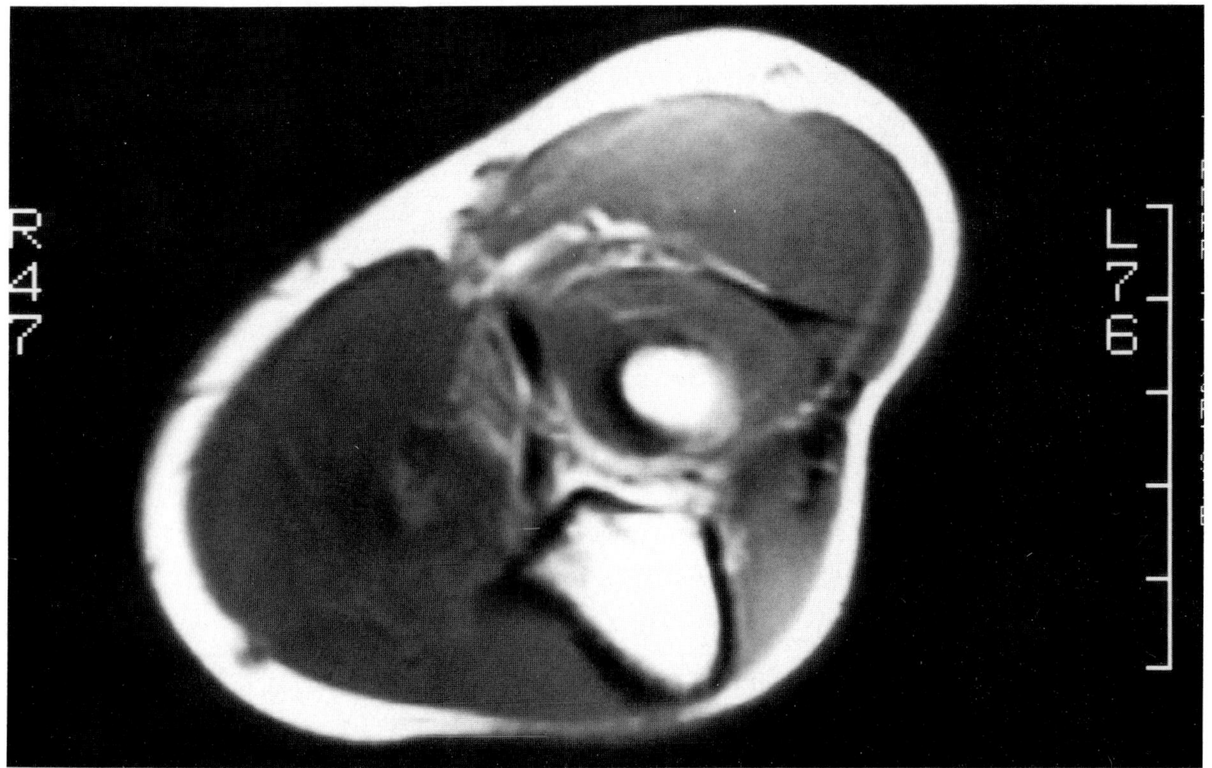

4-15 Elbow, axial view (TR 800; TE 30).

Elbow, Coronal

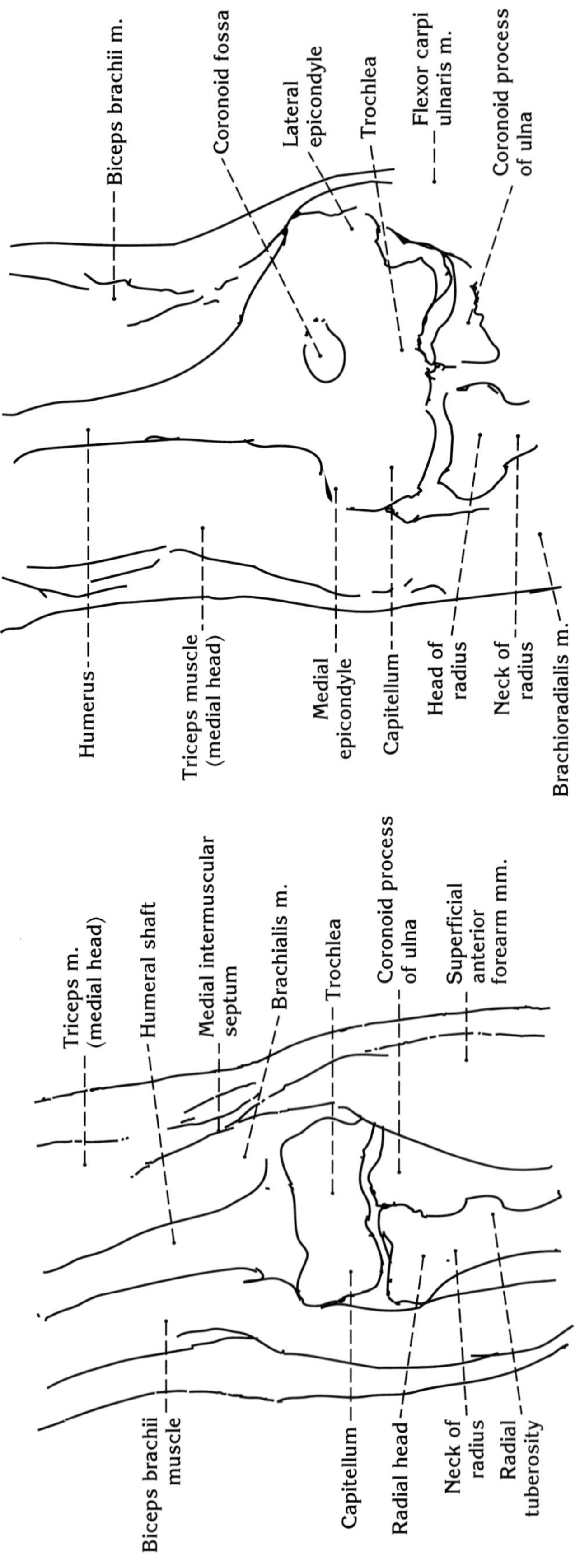

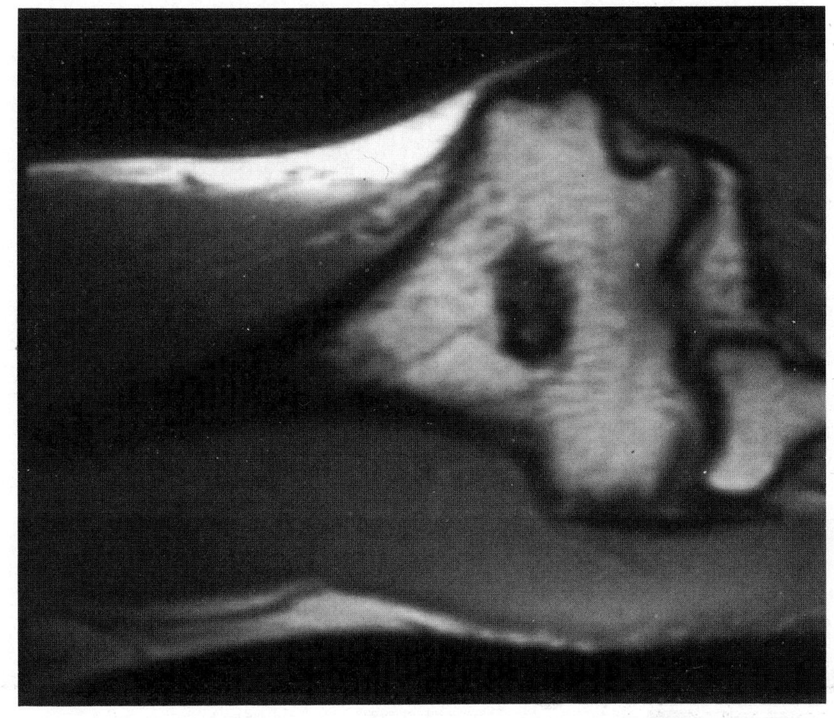

4-17 Elbow, coronal view (TR 2000; TE 20).

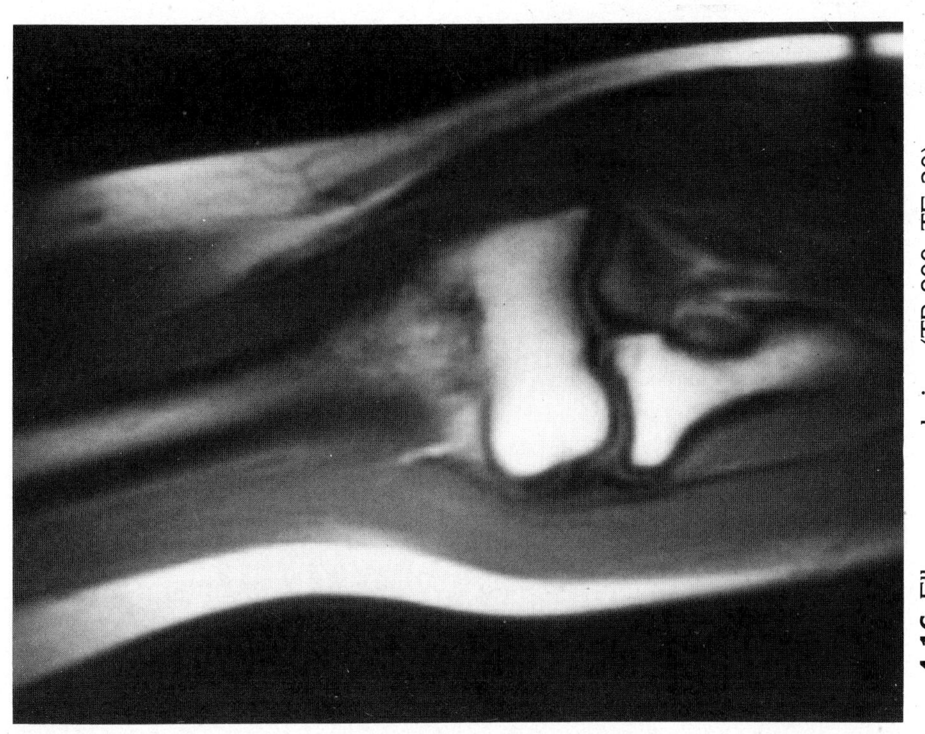

4-16 Elbow, coronal view (TR 800; TE 30).

Elbow, Coronal

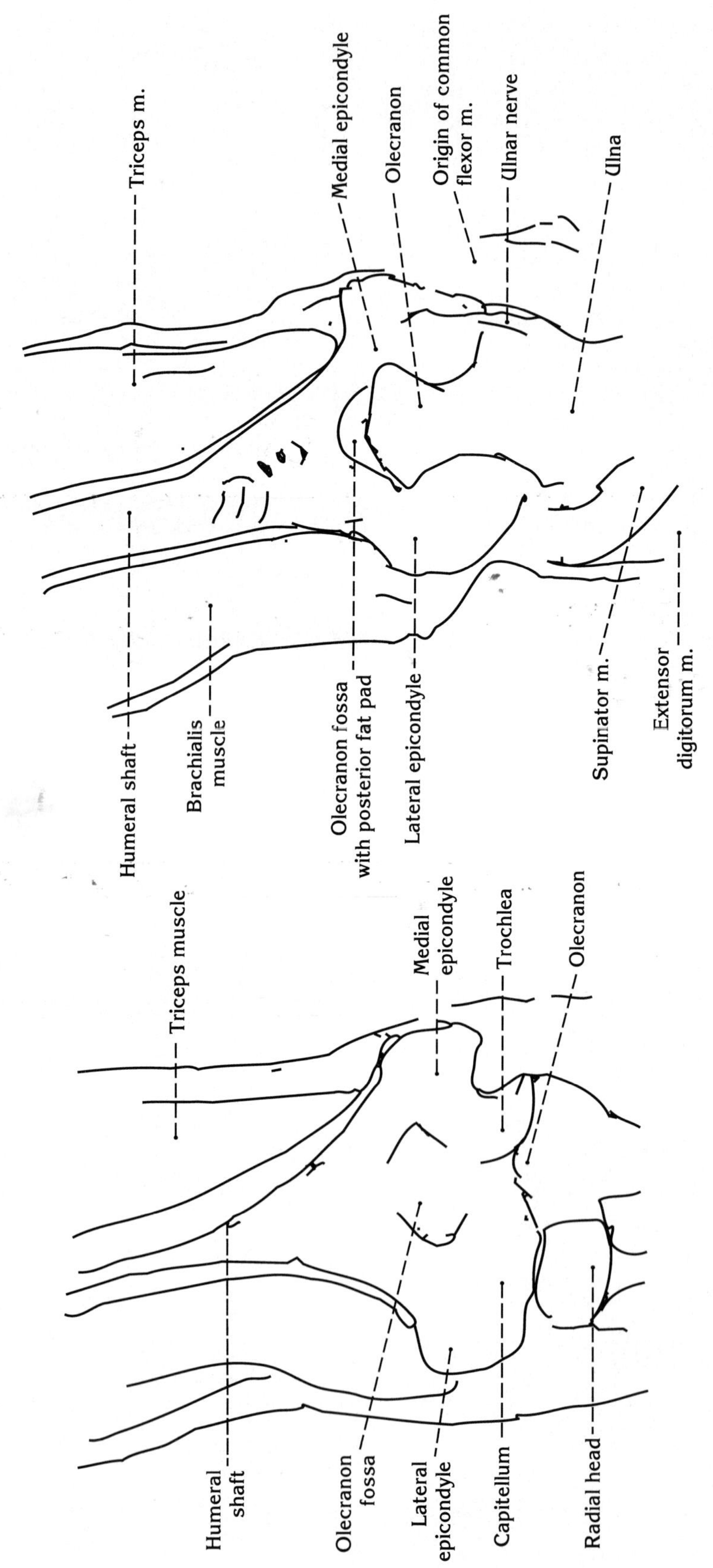

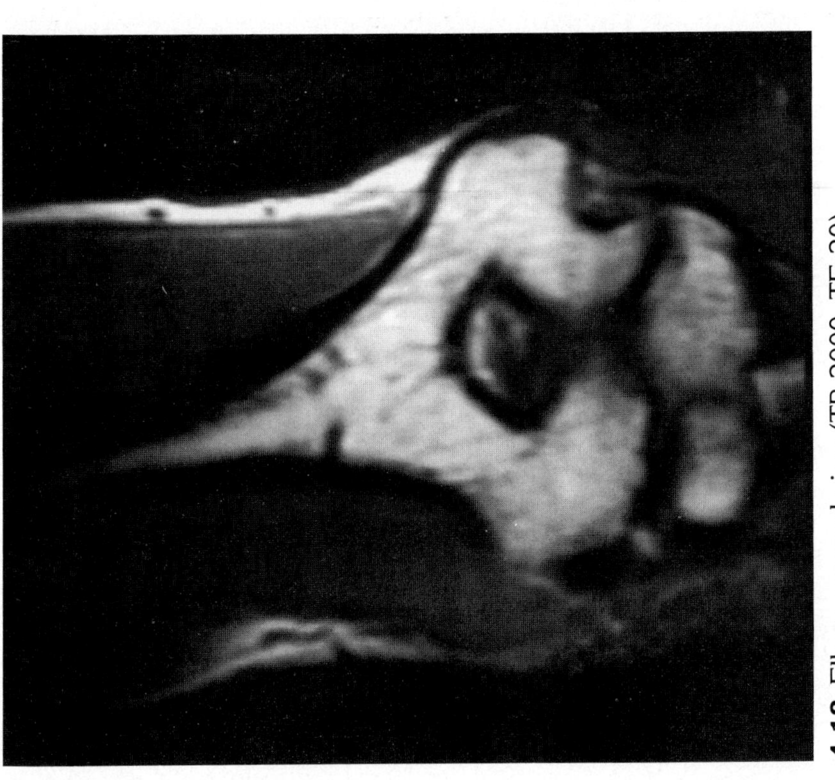

4-18 Elbow, coronal view (TR 2000; TE 20).

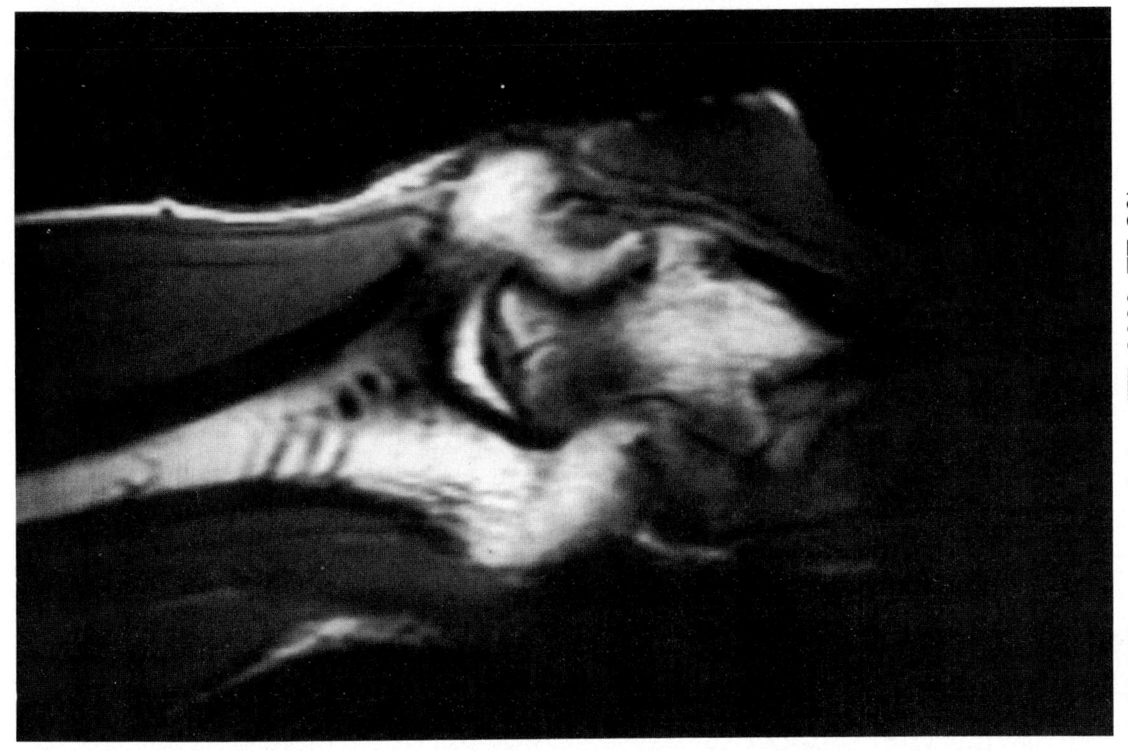

4-19 Elbow, coronal view (TR 2000; TE 20).

Wrist, Sagittal

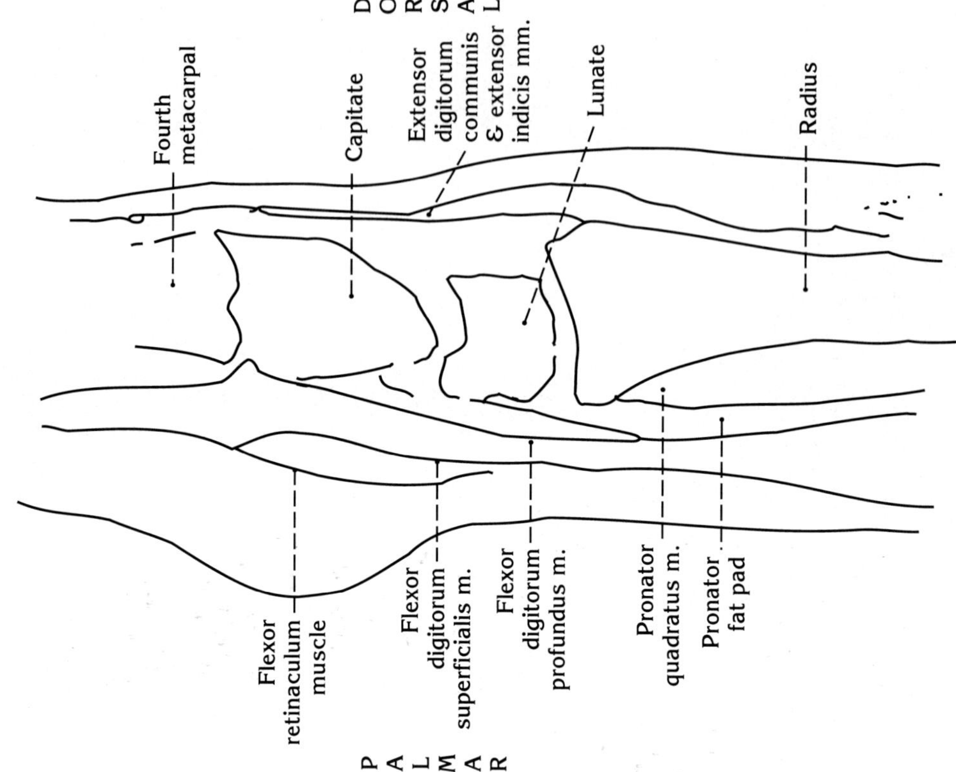

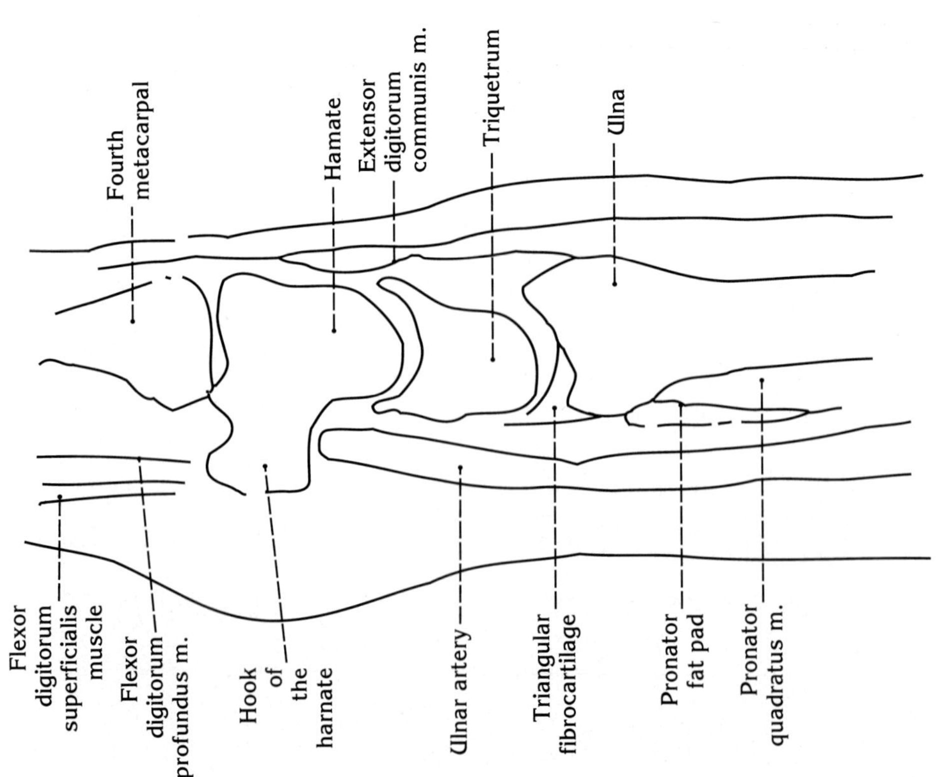

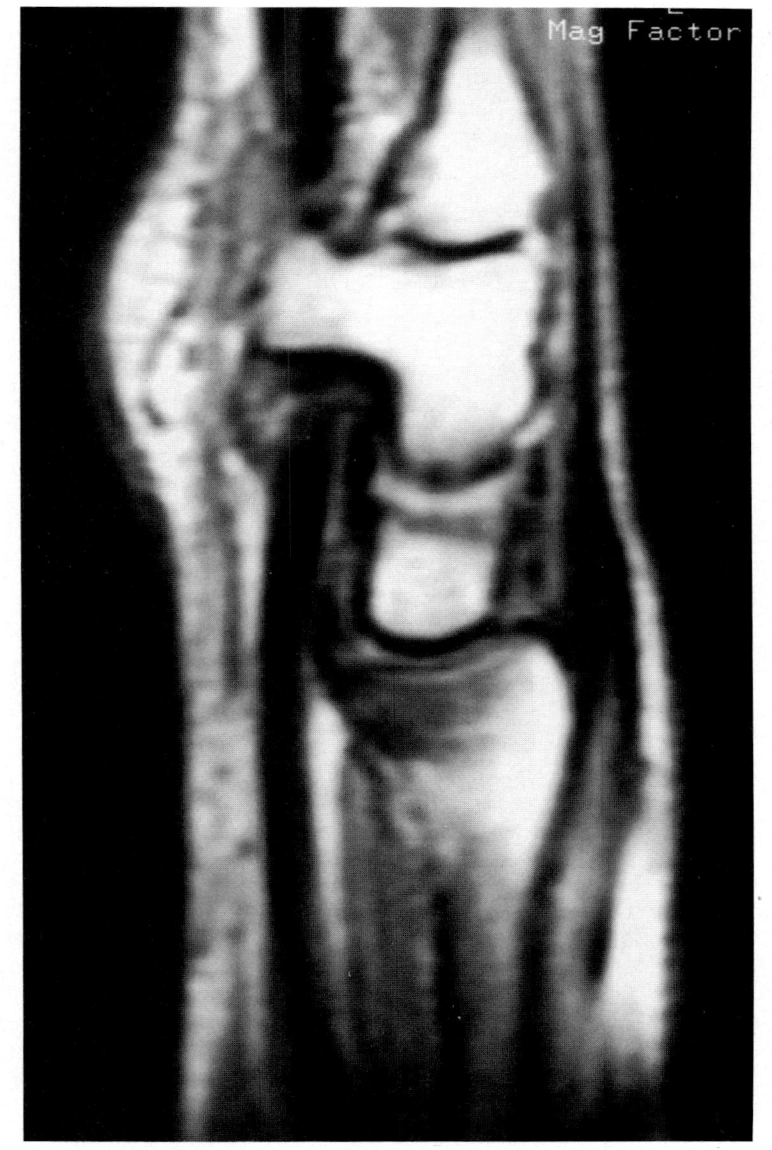

4-20 Wrist, sagittal view (TR 2000; TE 20).

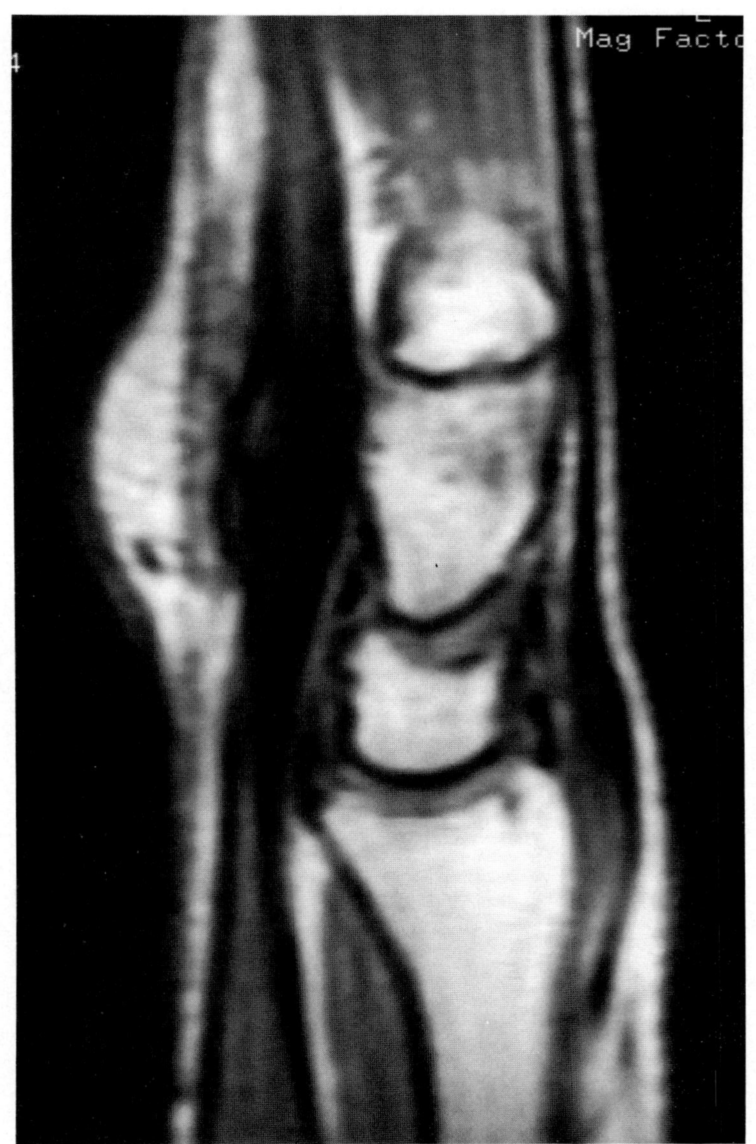

4-21 Wrist, sagittal view (TR 2000; TE 20).

Wrist, Sagittal

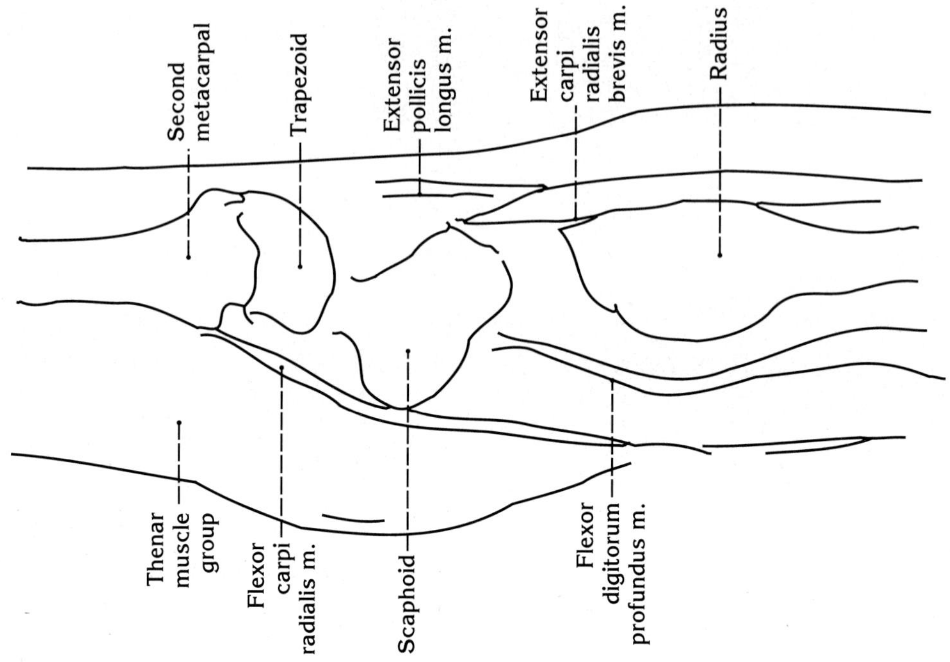

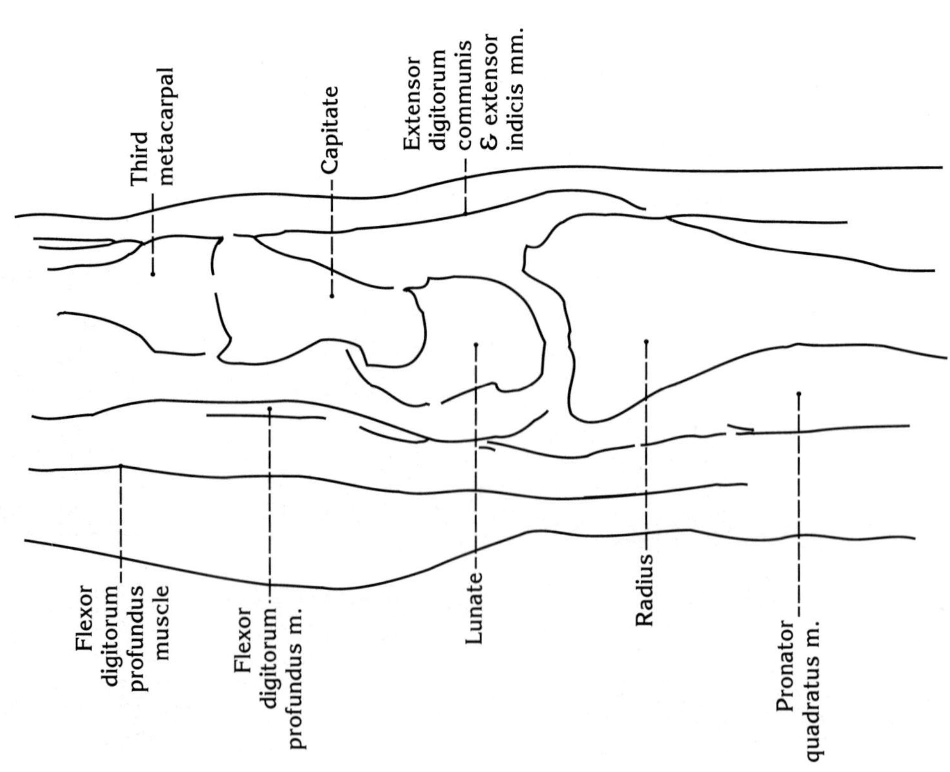

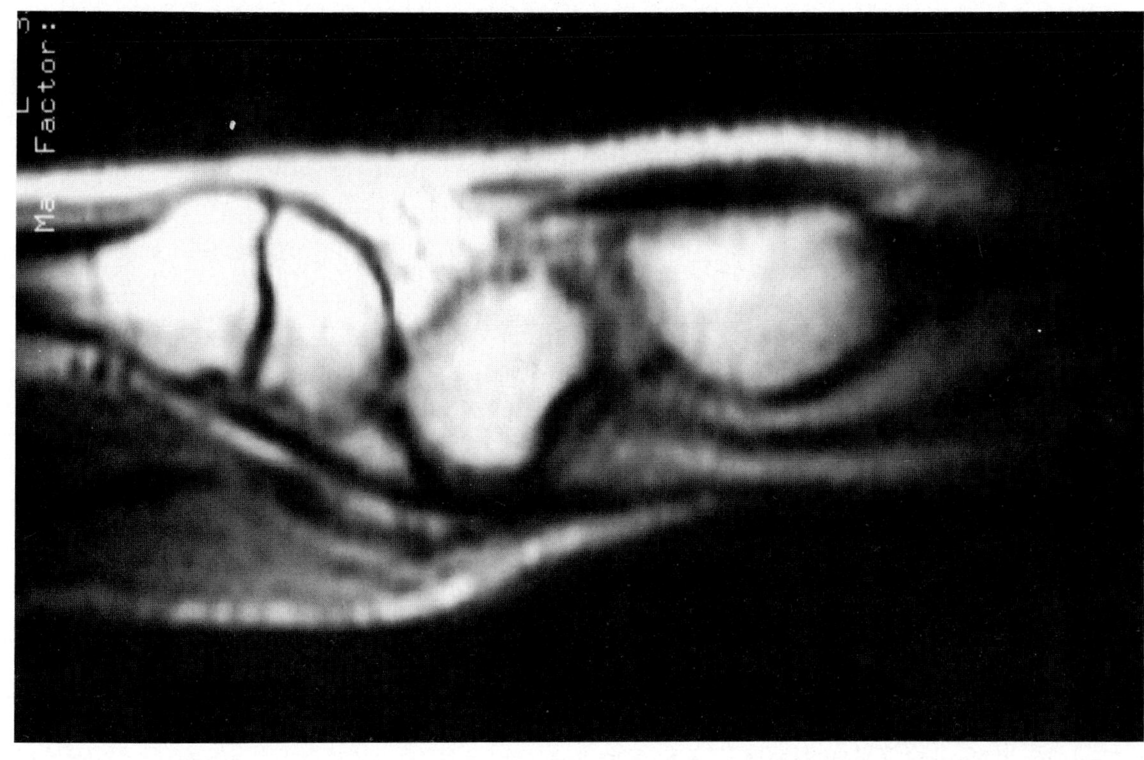

4-23 Wrist, sagittal view (TR 2000; TE 20).

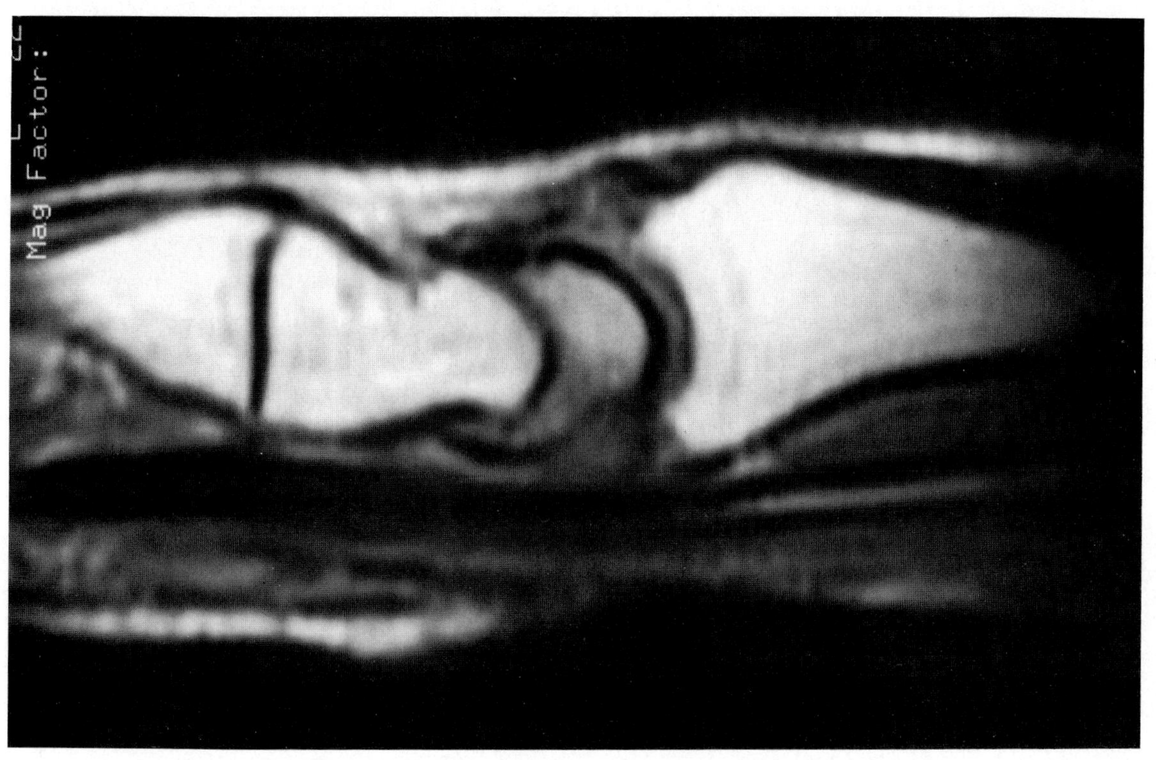

4-22 Wrist, sagittal view (TR 2000; TE 20).

Wrist, Coronal

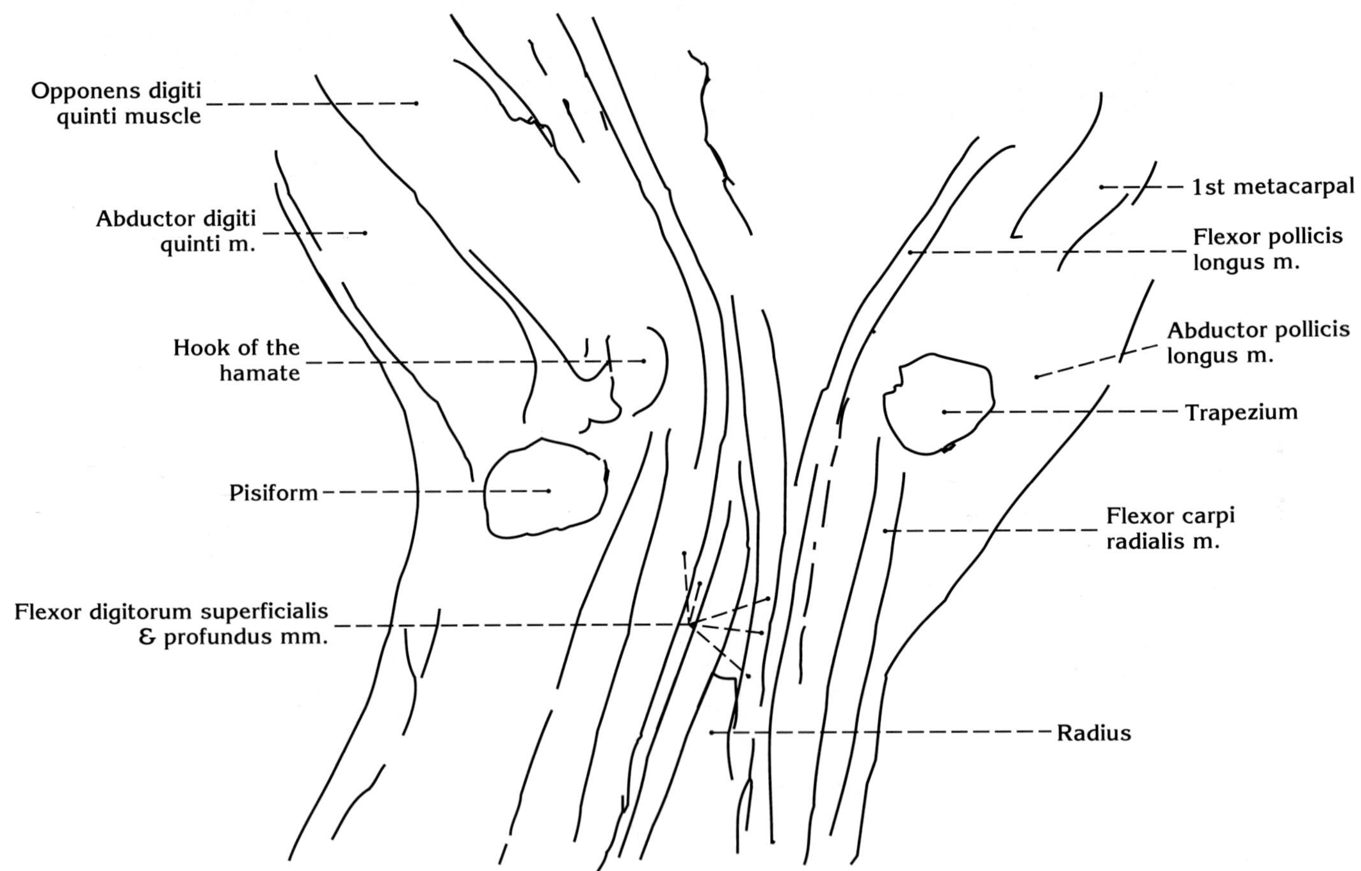

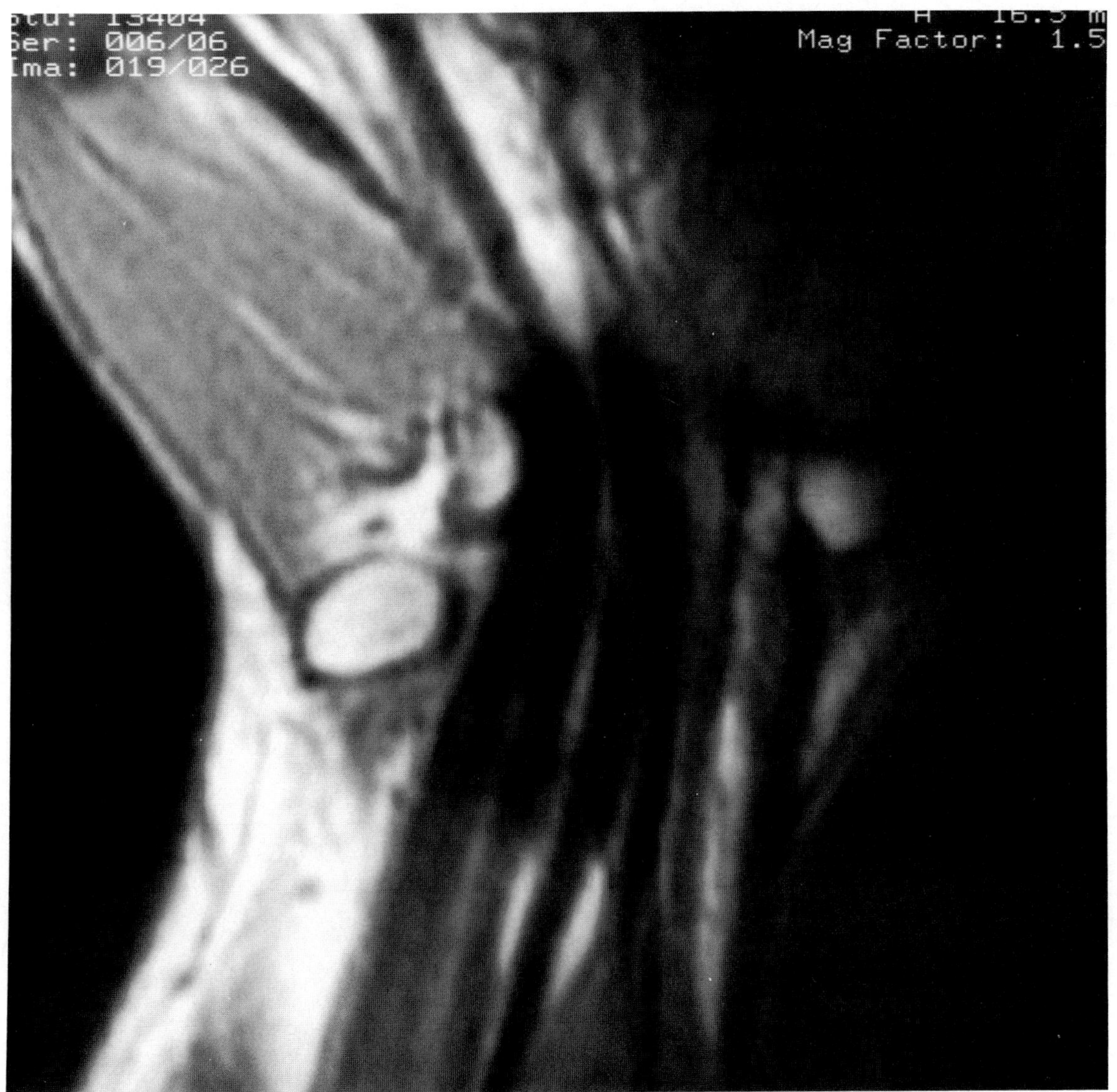

4-24 Wrist, coronal view (TR 2000; TE 20).

Wrist, Coronal

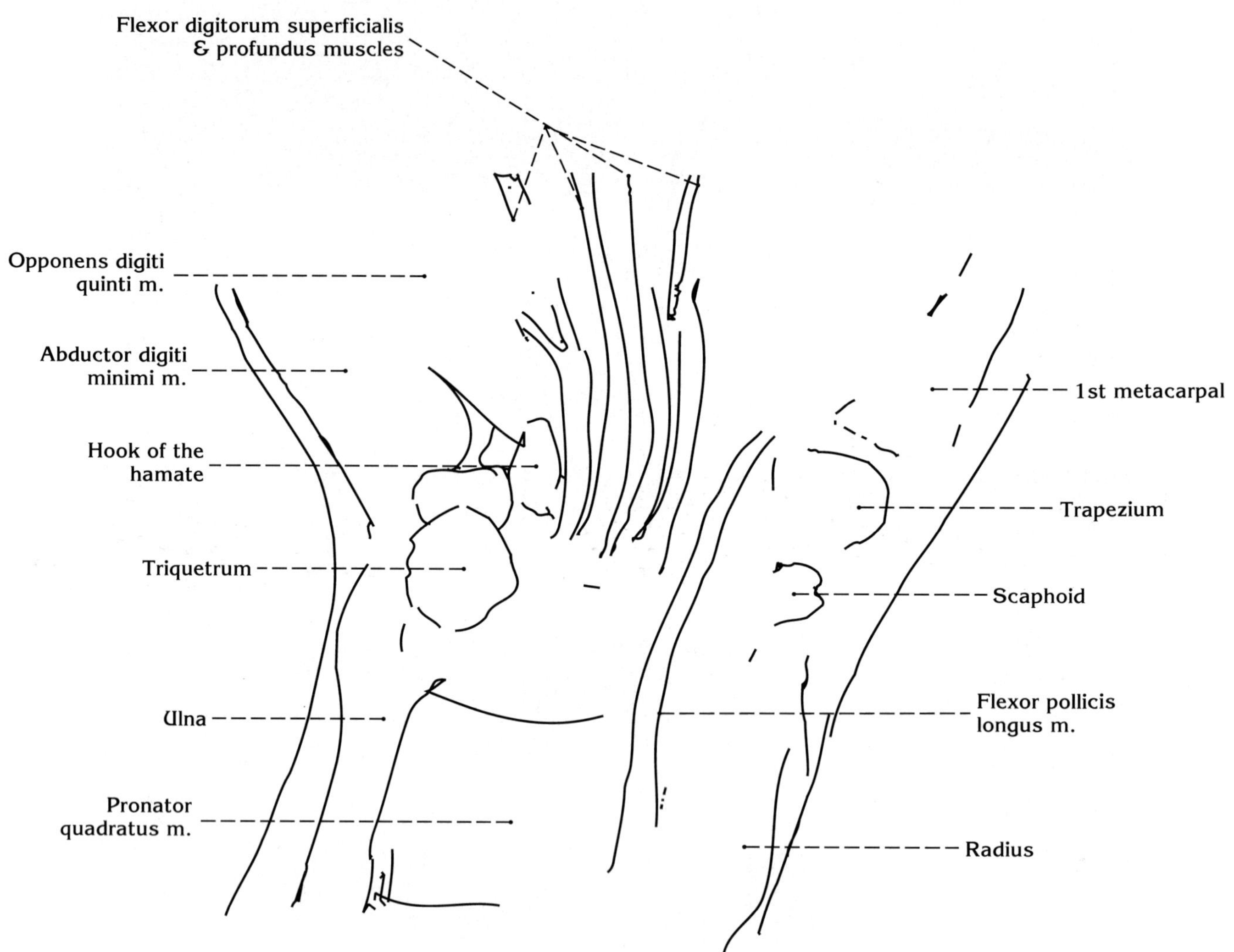

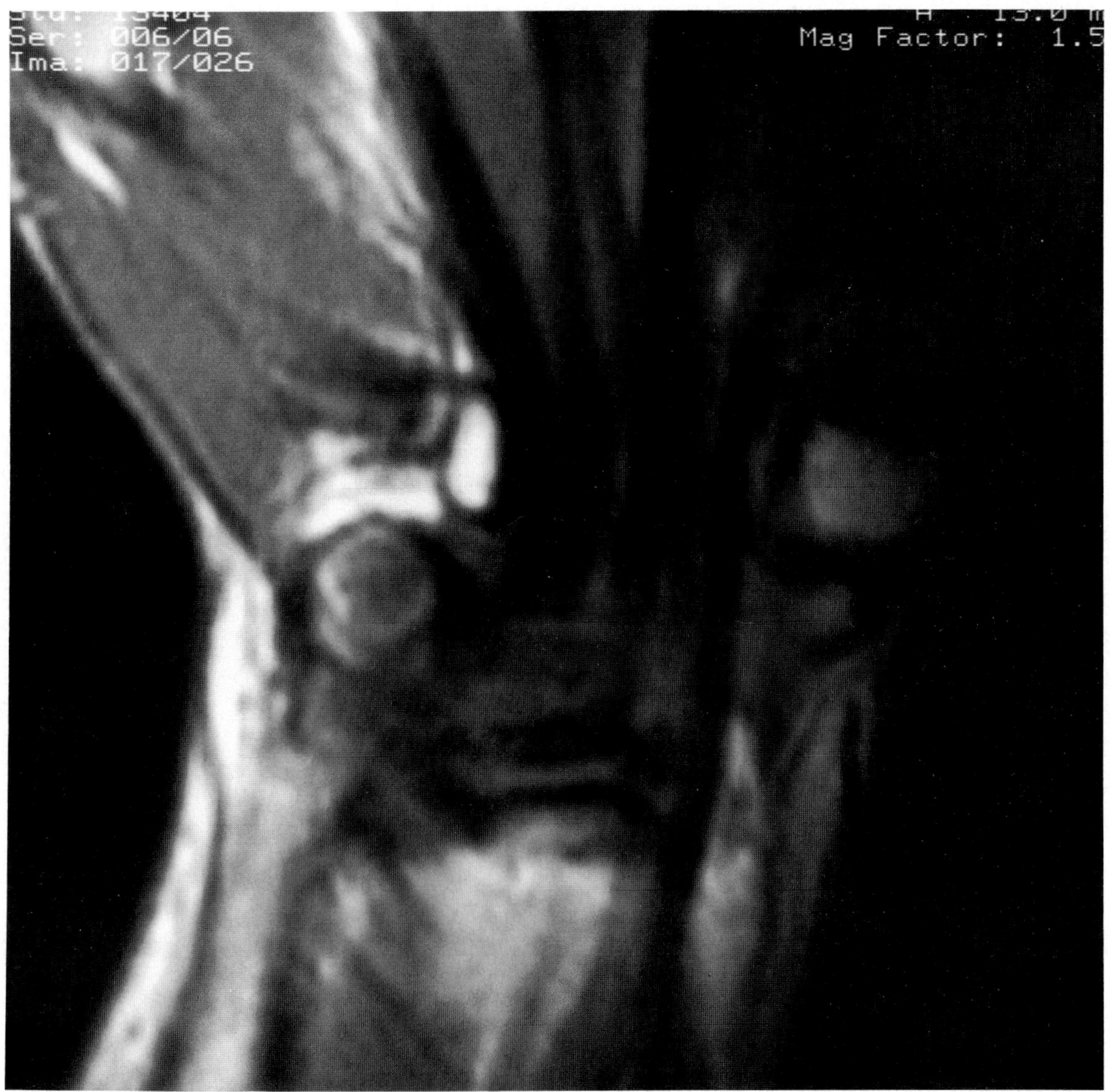

4-25 Wrist, coronal view (TR 2000; TE 20).

Wrist, Coronal

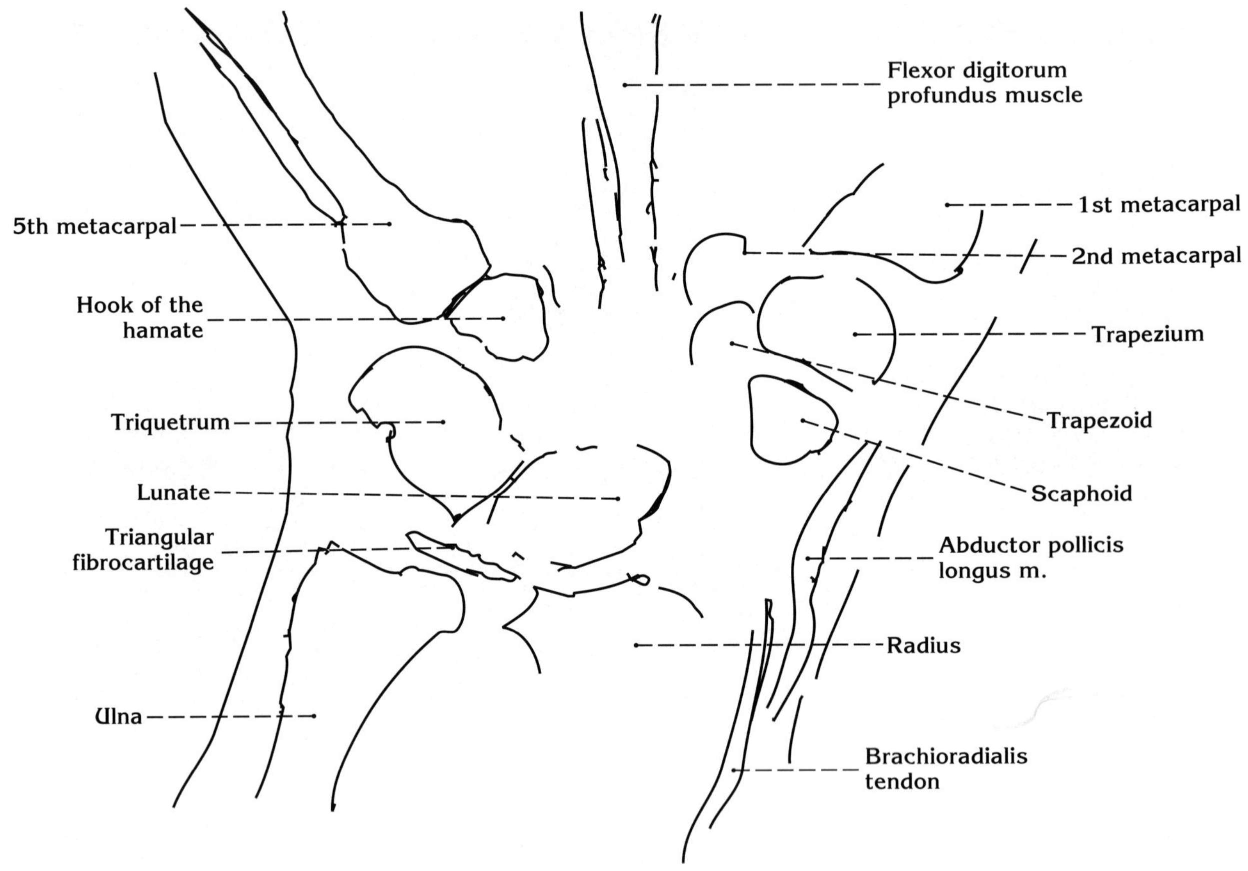

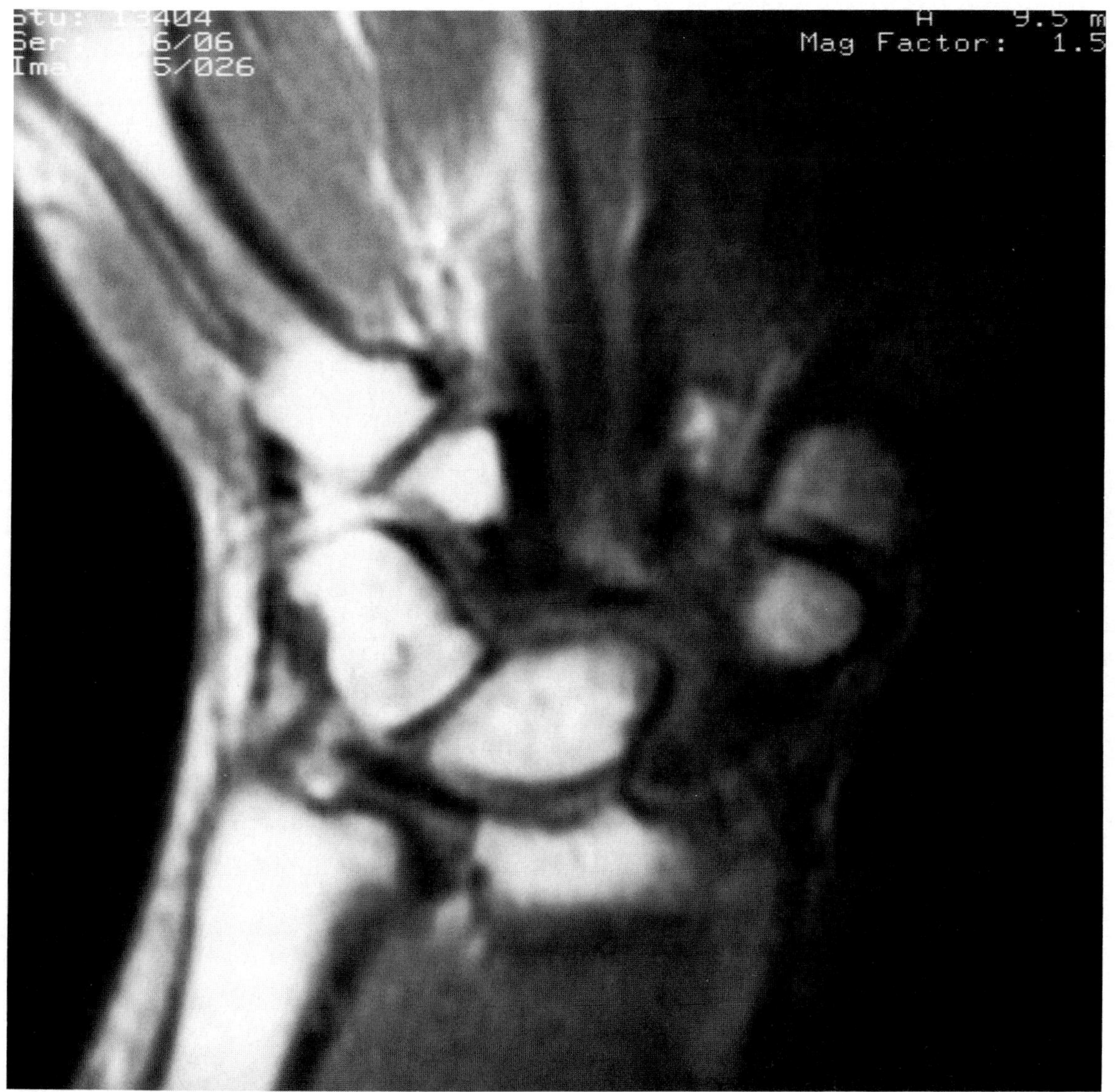

4-26 Wrist, coronal view (TR 2000; TE 20).

Wrist, Coronal

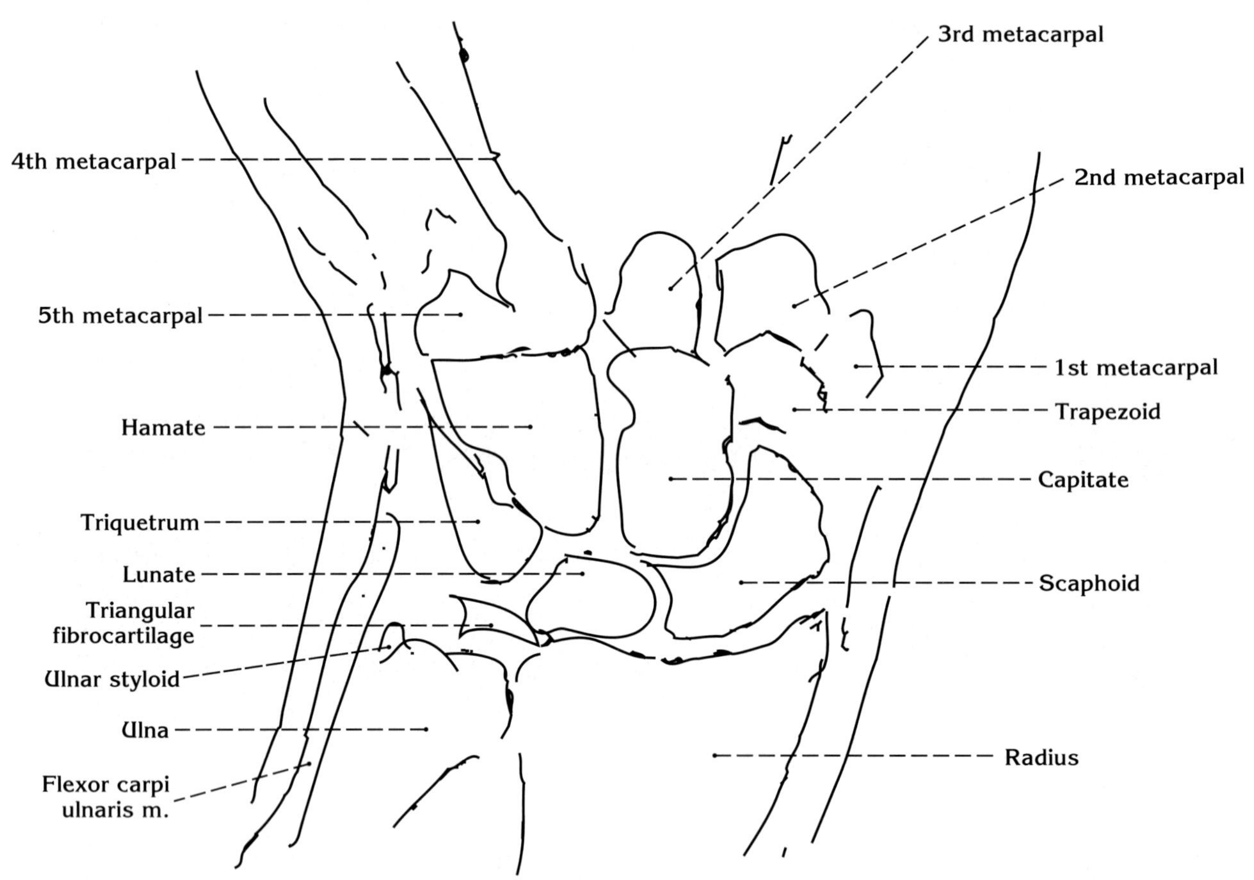

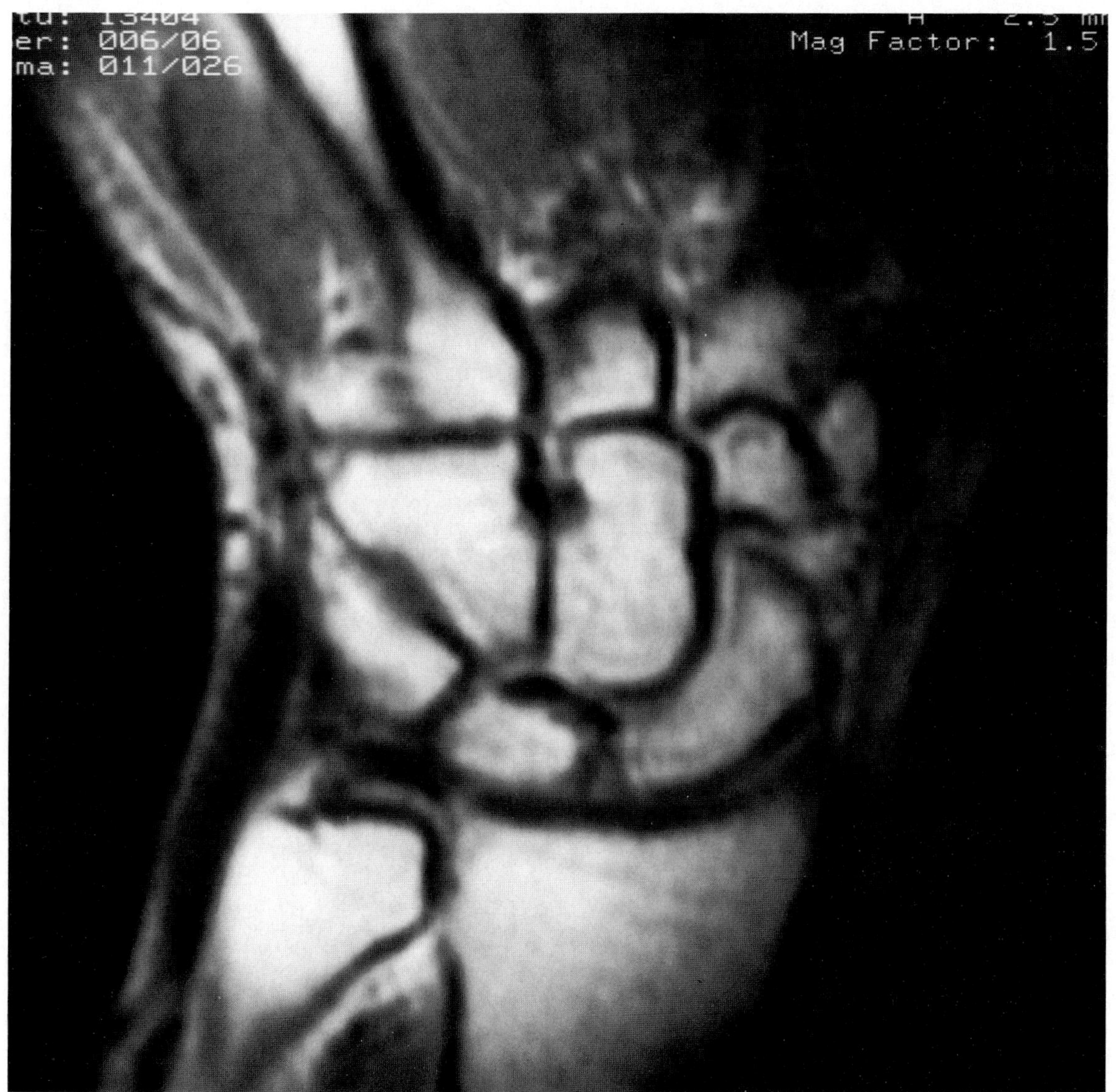

4-27 Wrist, coronal view (TR 2000; TE 20).

Forearm and Wrist, Axial

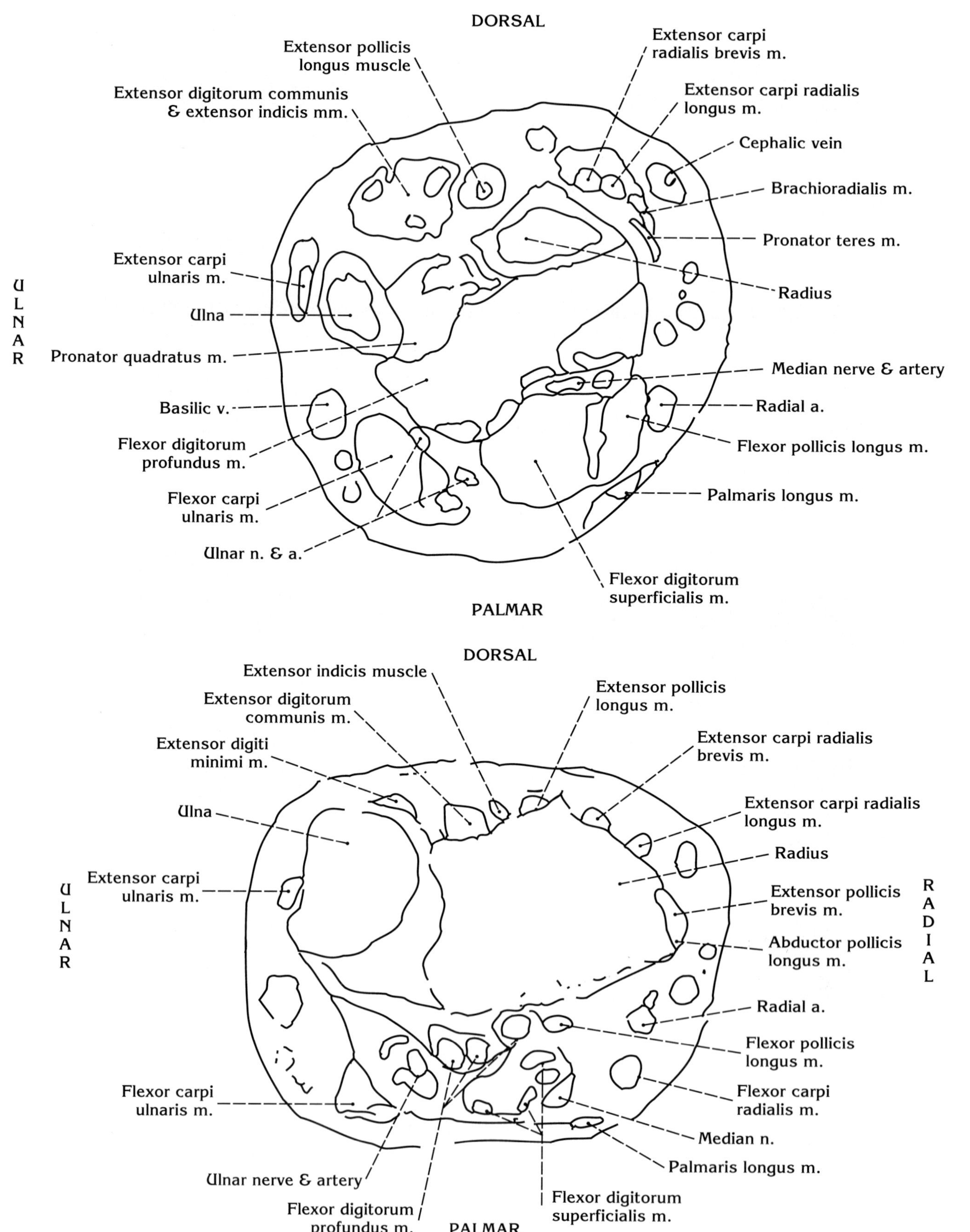

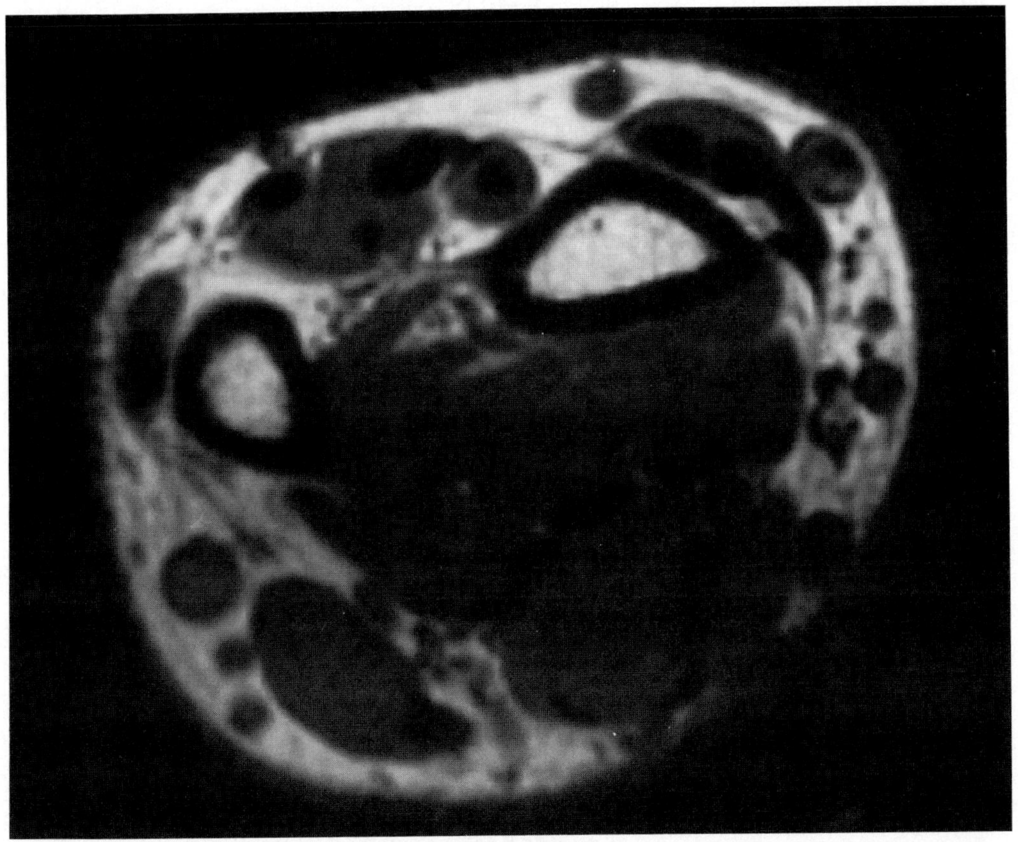

4-28 Distal forearm, axial view (TR 600; TE 20).

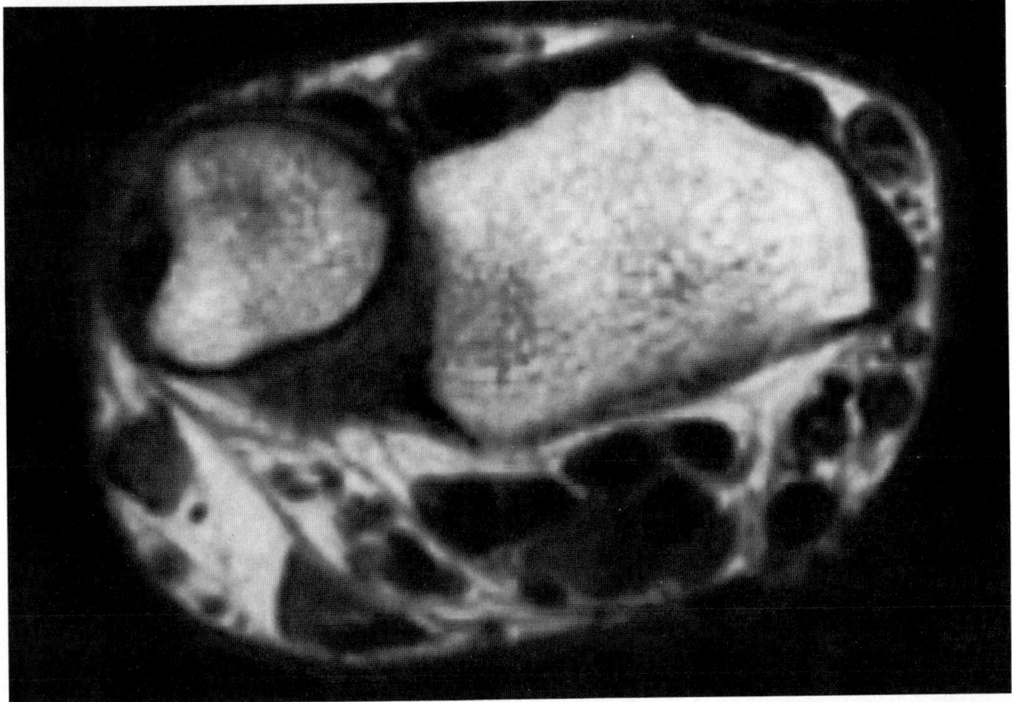

4-29 Wrist, axial view (TR 600; TE 20).

Wrist, Axial

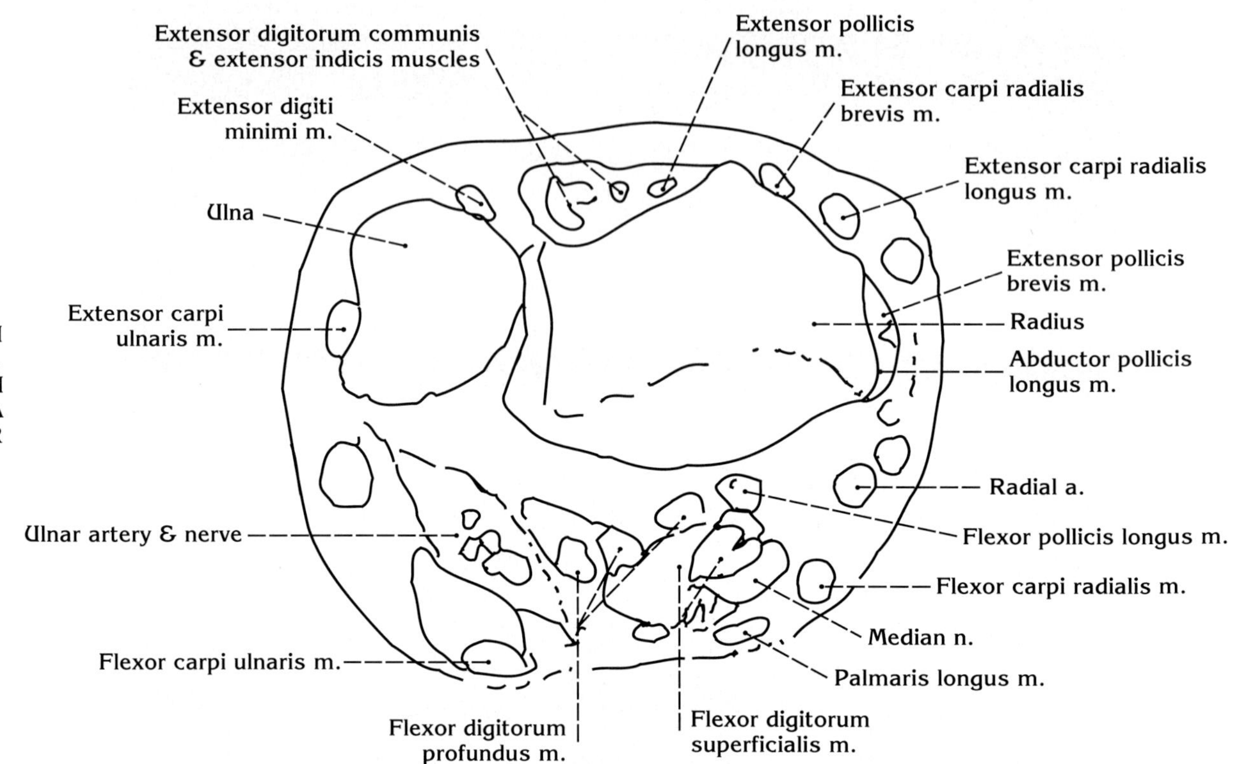
DORSAL
Extensor digitorum communis & extensor indicis muscles
Extensor pollicis longus m.
Extensor carpi radialis brevis m.
Extensor digiti minimi m.
Extensor carpi radialis longus m.
Ulna
Extensor pollicis brevis m.
Extensor carpi ulnaris m.
Radius
Abductor pollicis longus m.
ULNAR
RADIAL
Radial a.
Flexor pollicis longus m.
Ulnar artery & nerve
Flexor carpi radialis m.
Median n.
Flexor carpi ulnaris m.
Palmaris longus m.
Flexor digitorum profundus m.
Flexor digitorum superficialis m.
PALMAR

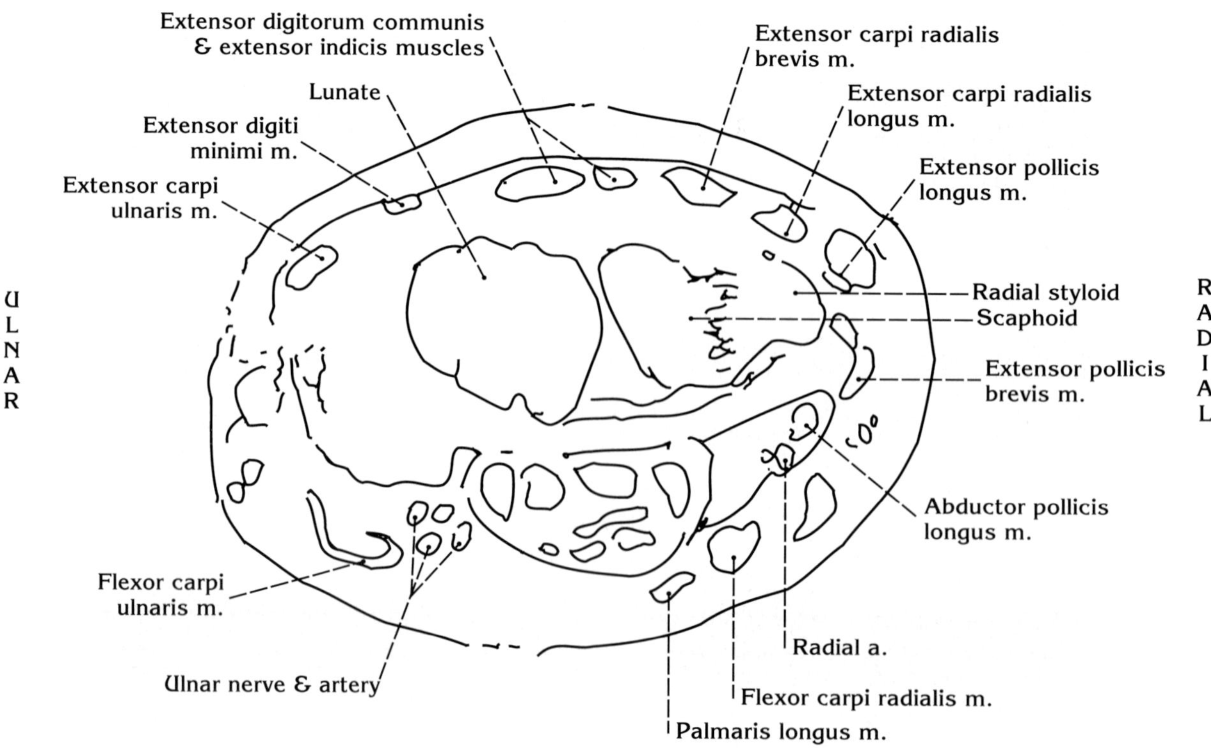
Extensor digitorum communis & extensor indicis muscles
Extensor carpi radialis brevis m.
Lunate
Extensor carpi radialis longus m.
Extensor digiti minimi m.
Extensor pollicis longus m.
Extensor carpi ulnaris m.
Radial styloid
Scaphoid
ULNAR
RADIAL
Extensor pollicis brevis m.
Abductor pollicis longus m.
Flexor carpi ulnaris m.
Radial a.
Ulnar nerve & artery
Flexor carpi radialis m.
Palmaris longus m.

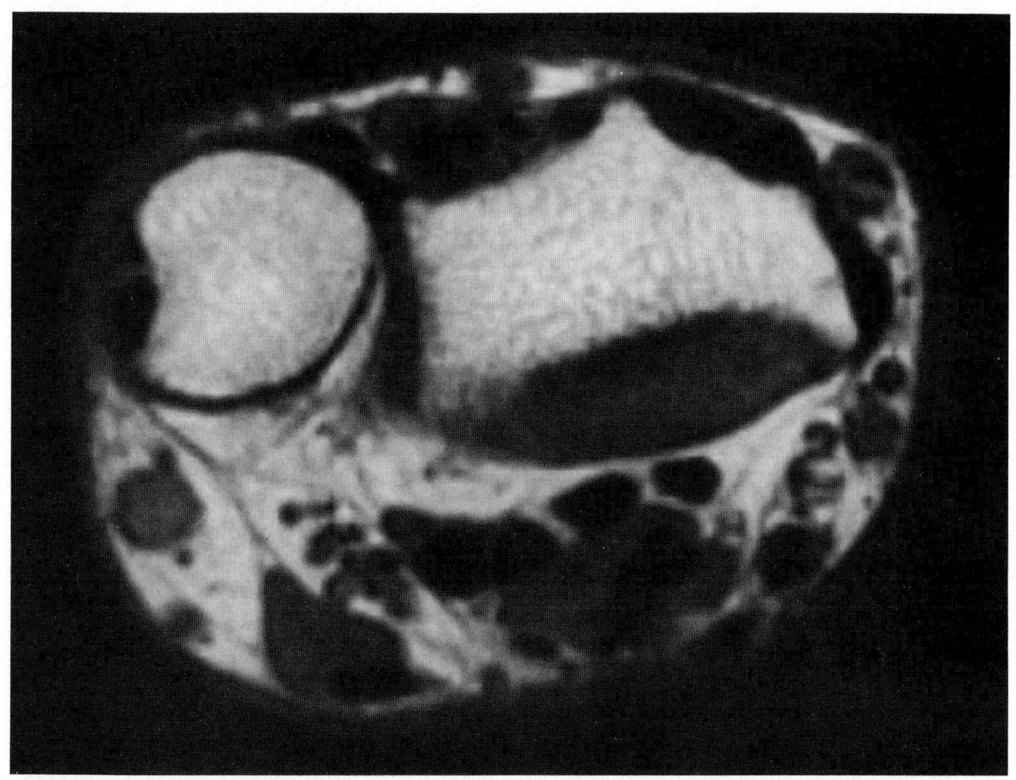

4-30 Wrist, axial view (TR 600; TE 20).

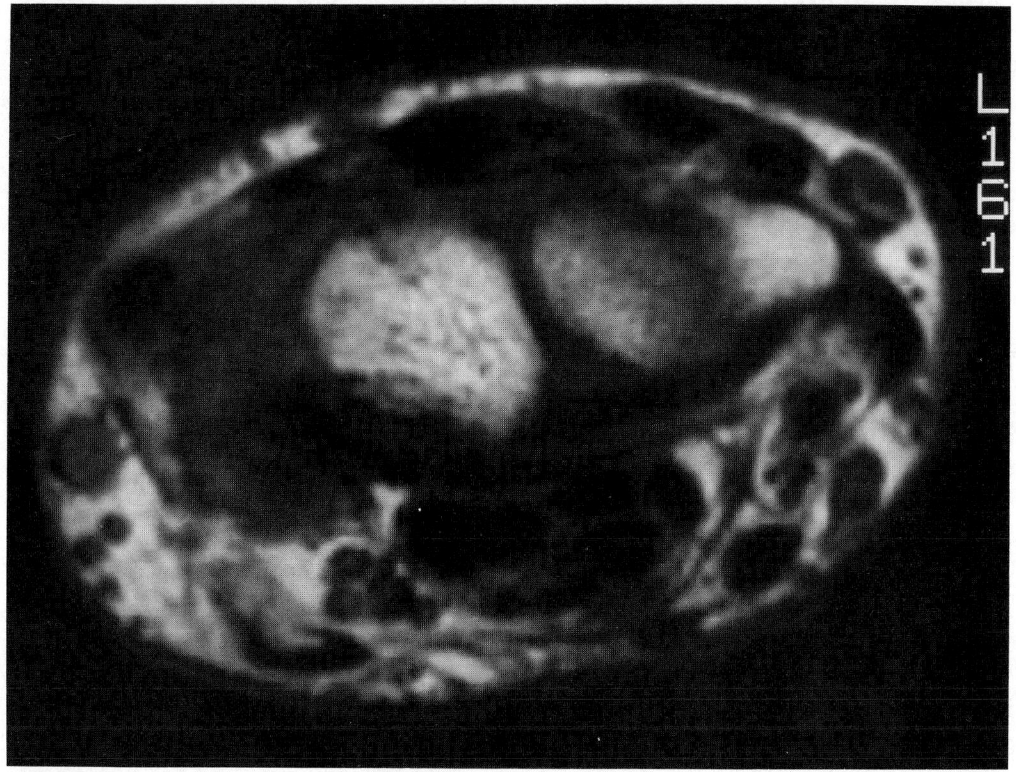

4-31 Wrist, axial view (TR 600; TE 20).

Wrist, Axial

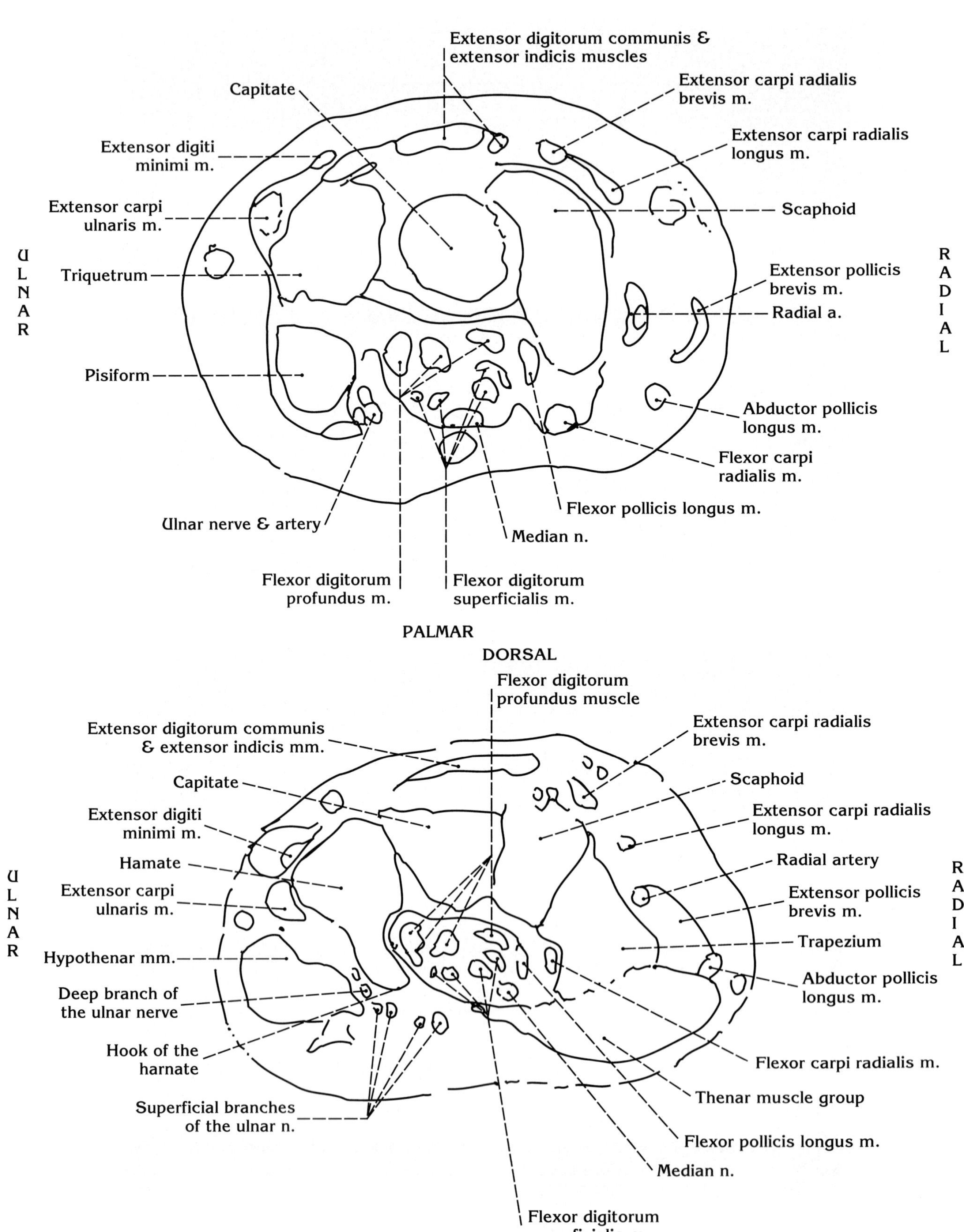
DORSAL
Extensor digitorum communis & extensor indicis muscles
Capitate
Extensor carpi radialis brevis m.
Extensor digiti minimi m.
Extensor carpi radialis longus m.
Extensor carpi ulnaris m.
Scaphoid
ULNAR
Triquetrum
RADIAL
Extensor pollicis brevis m.
Radial a.
Pisiform
Abductor pollicis longus m.
Flexor carpi radialis m.
Flexor pollicis longus m.
Ulnar nerve & artery
Median n.
Flexor digitorum profundus m.
Flexor digitorum superficialis m.
PALMAR
DORSAL
Flexor digitorum profundus muscle
Extensor digitorum communis & extensor indicis mm.
Extensor carpi radialis brevis m.
Scaphoid
Capitate
Extensor digiti minimi m.
Extensor carpi radialis longus m.
Hamate
Radial artery
ULNAR
RADIAL
Extensor carpi ulnaris m.
Extensor pollicis brevis m.
Trapezium
Hypothenar mm.
Abductor pollicis longus m.
Deep branch of the ulnar nerve
Hook of the harnate
Flexor carpi radialis m.
Thenar muscle group
Superficial branches of the ulnar n.
Flexor pollicis longus m.
Median n.
Flexor digitorum superficialis m.
PALMAR

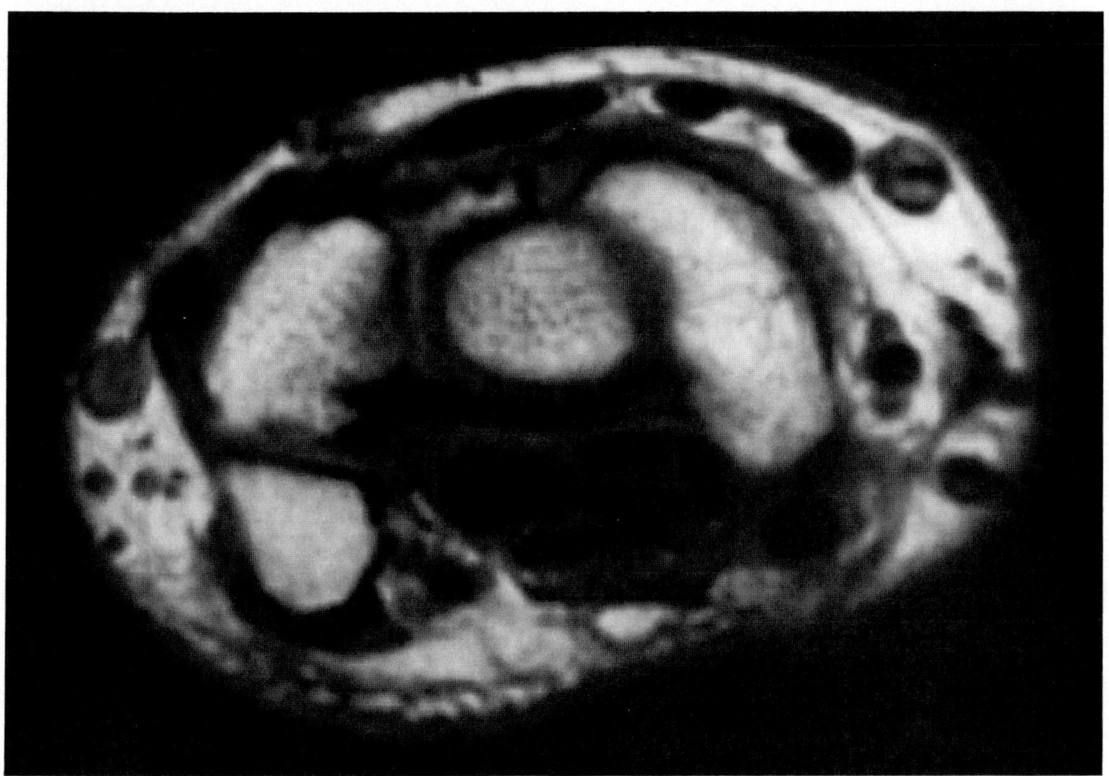

4-32 Wrist, axial view (TR 600; TE 20).

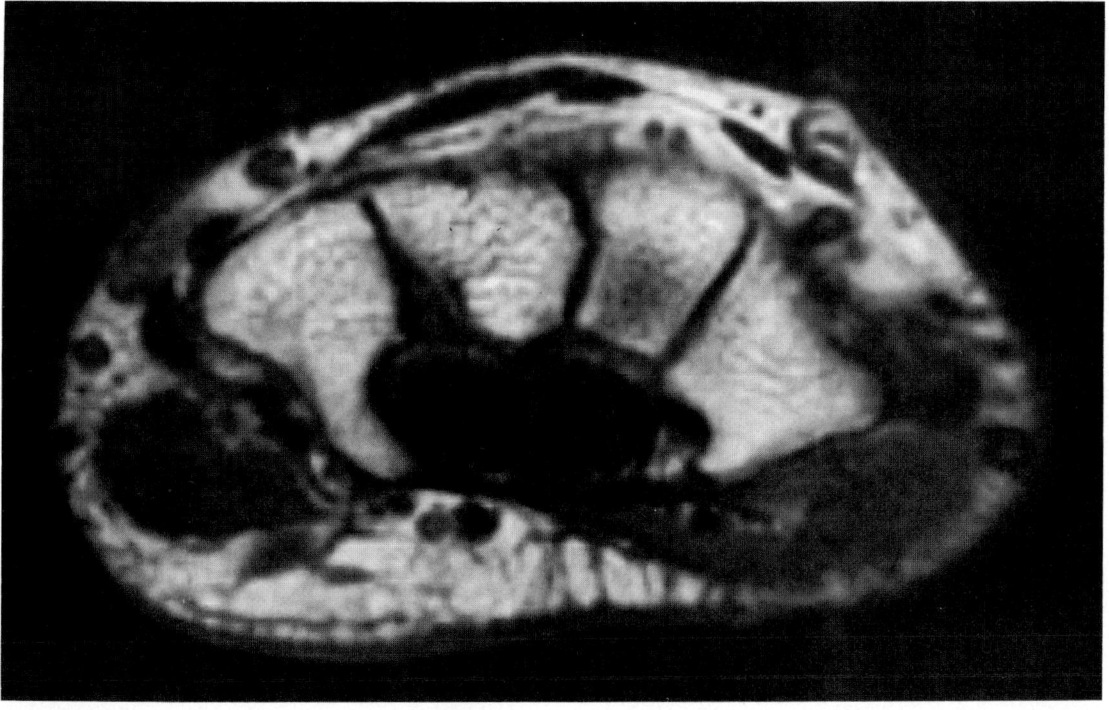

4-33 Wrist, axial view (TR 600; TE 20).

Hip and Thigh, Coronal

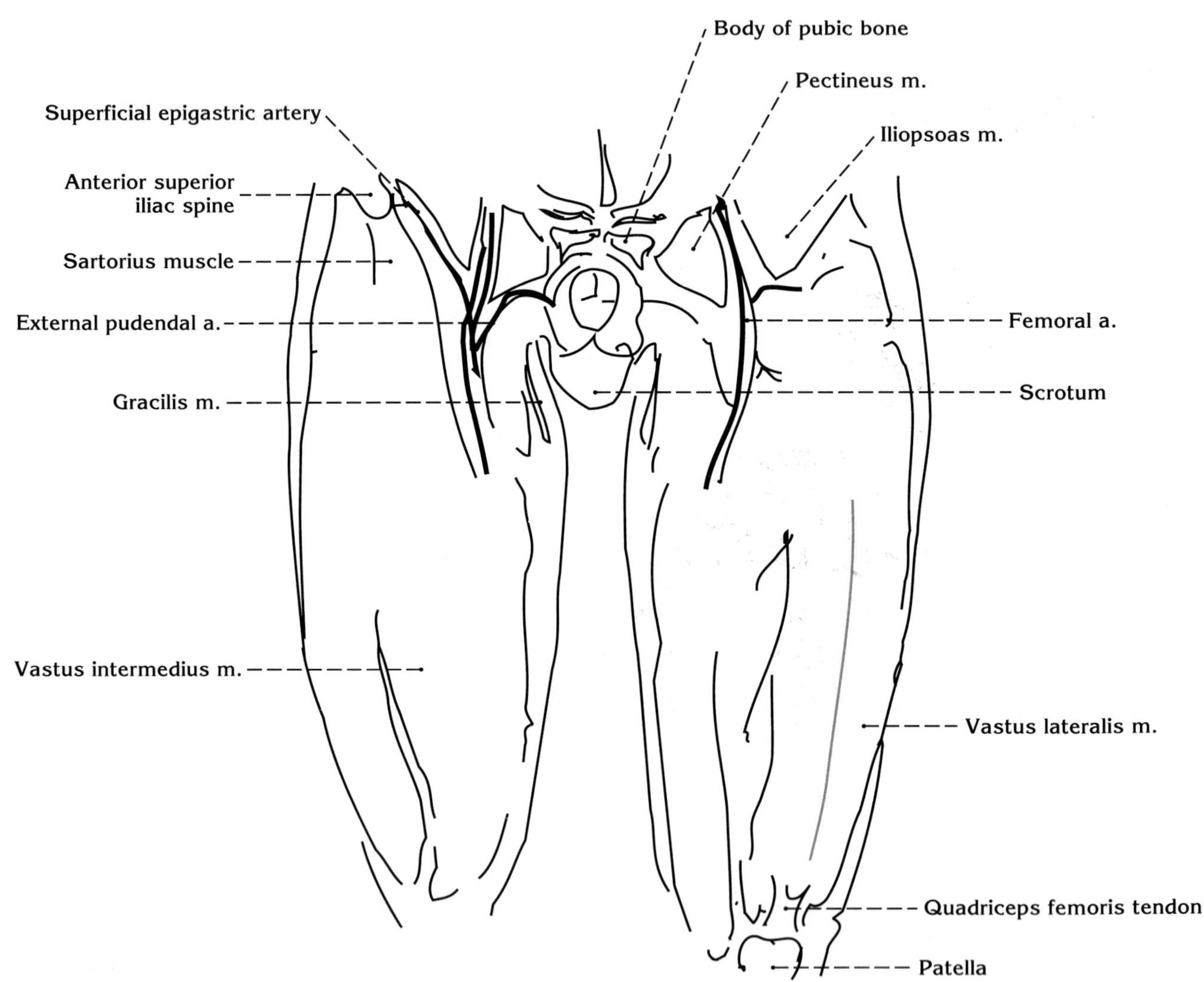

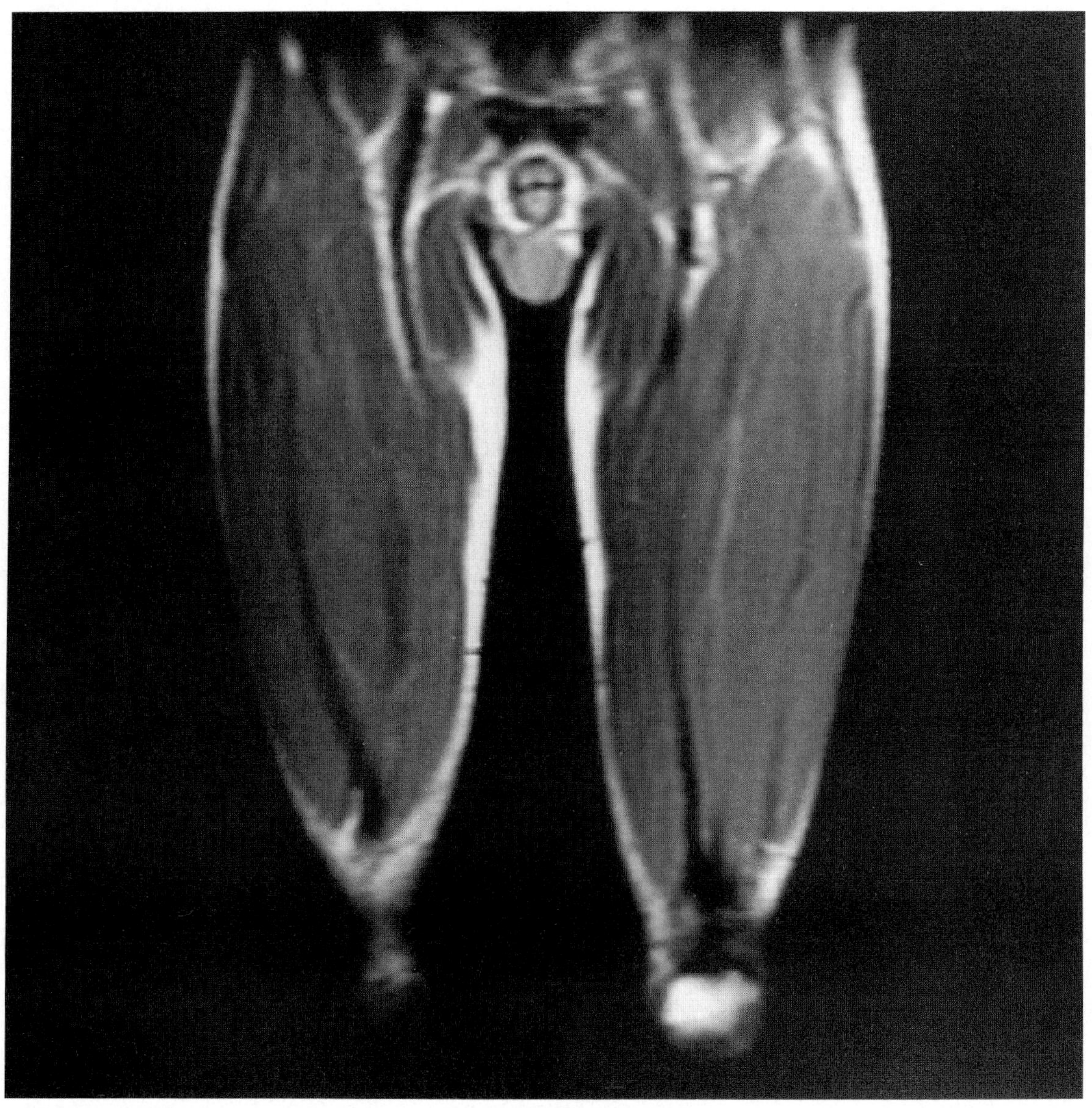

5-1 Hip and thigh (male), coronal view (TR 2000; TE 20).

Hip and Thigh, Coronal

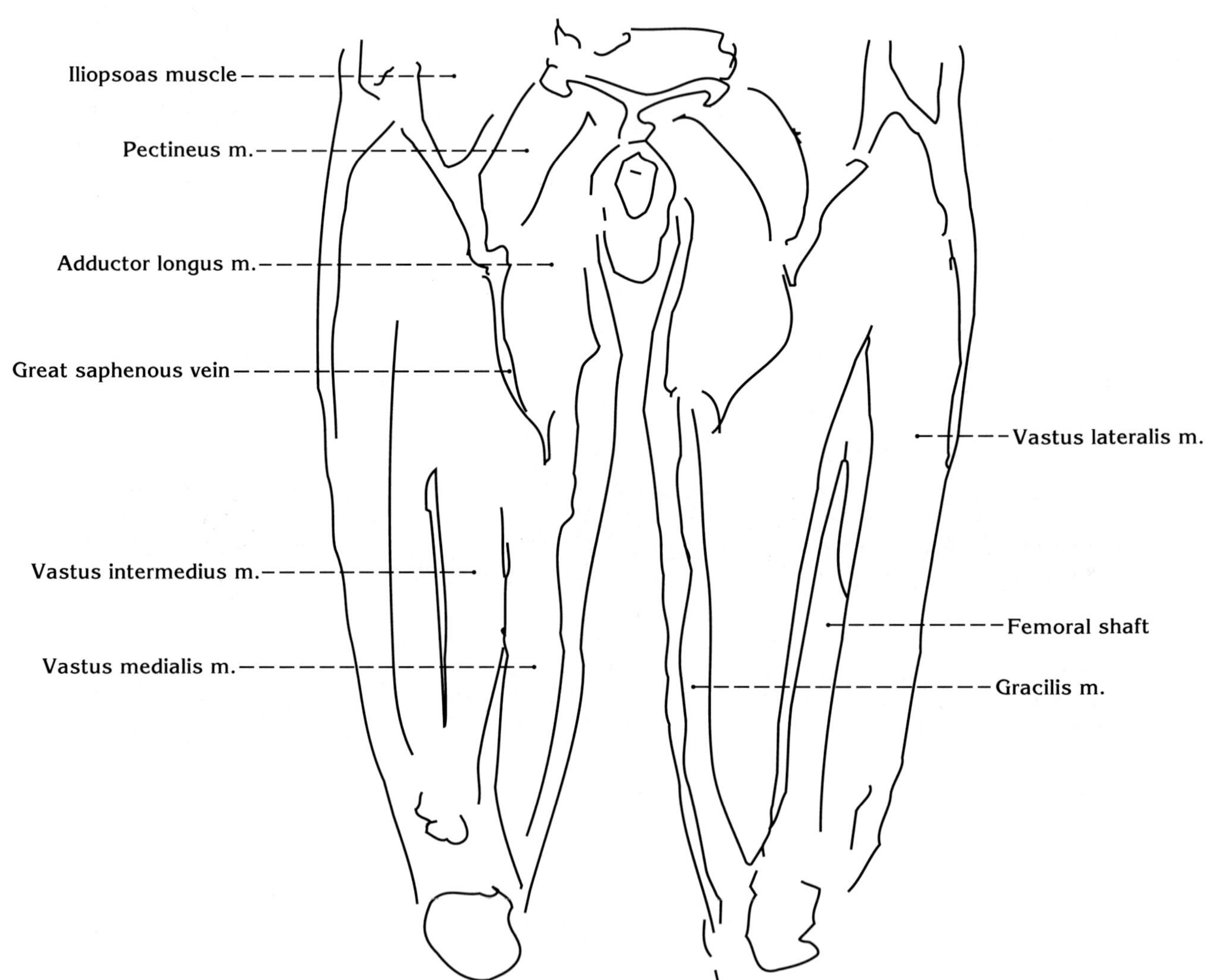

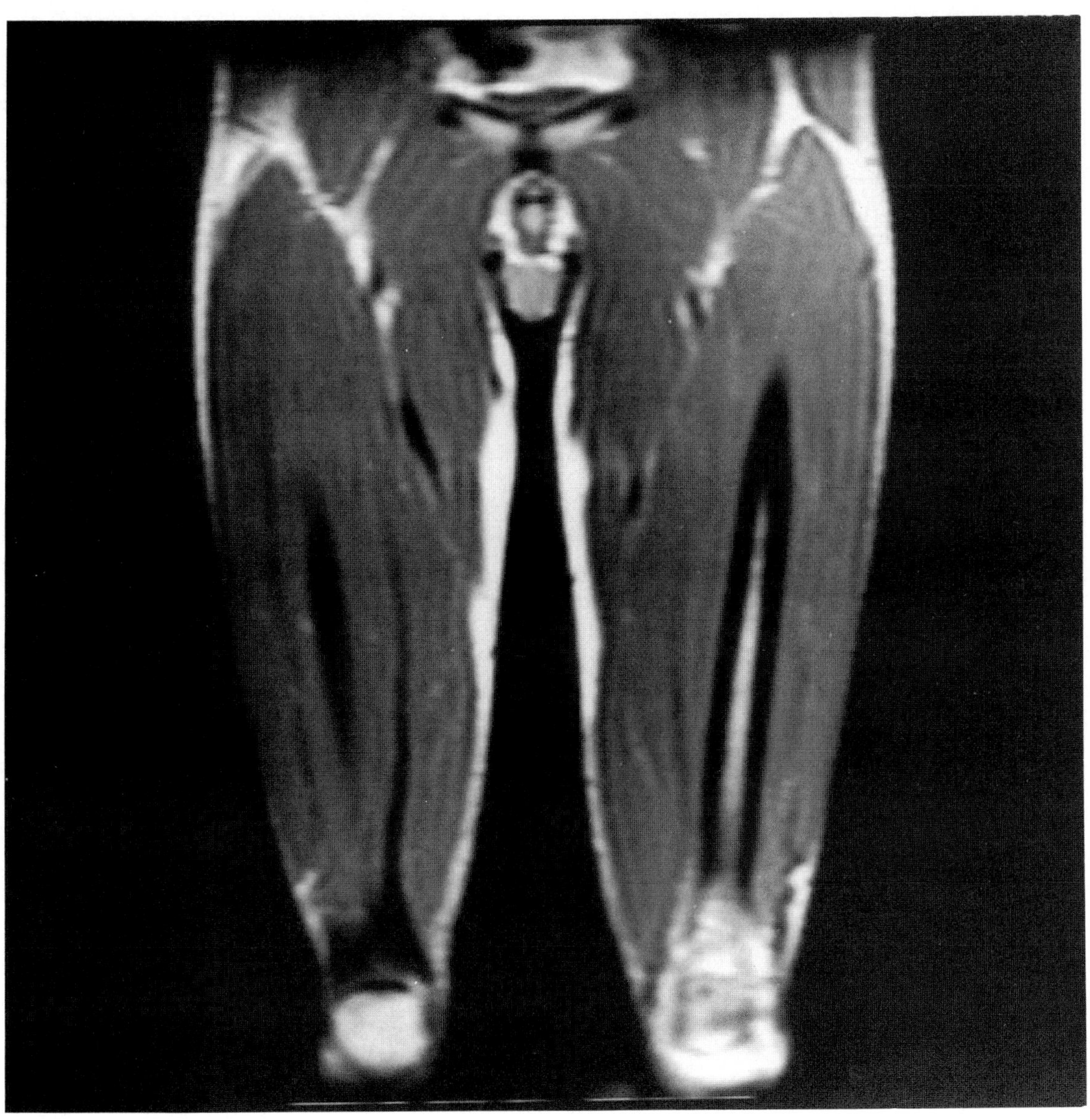

5-2 Hip and thigh (male), coronal view (TR 2000; TE 20).

Hip and Thigh, Coronal

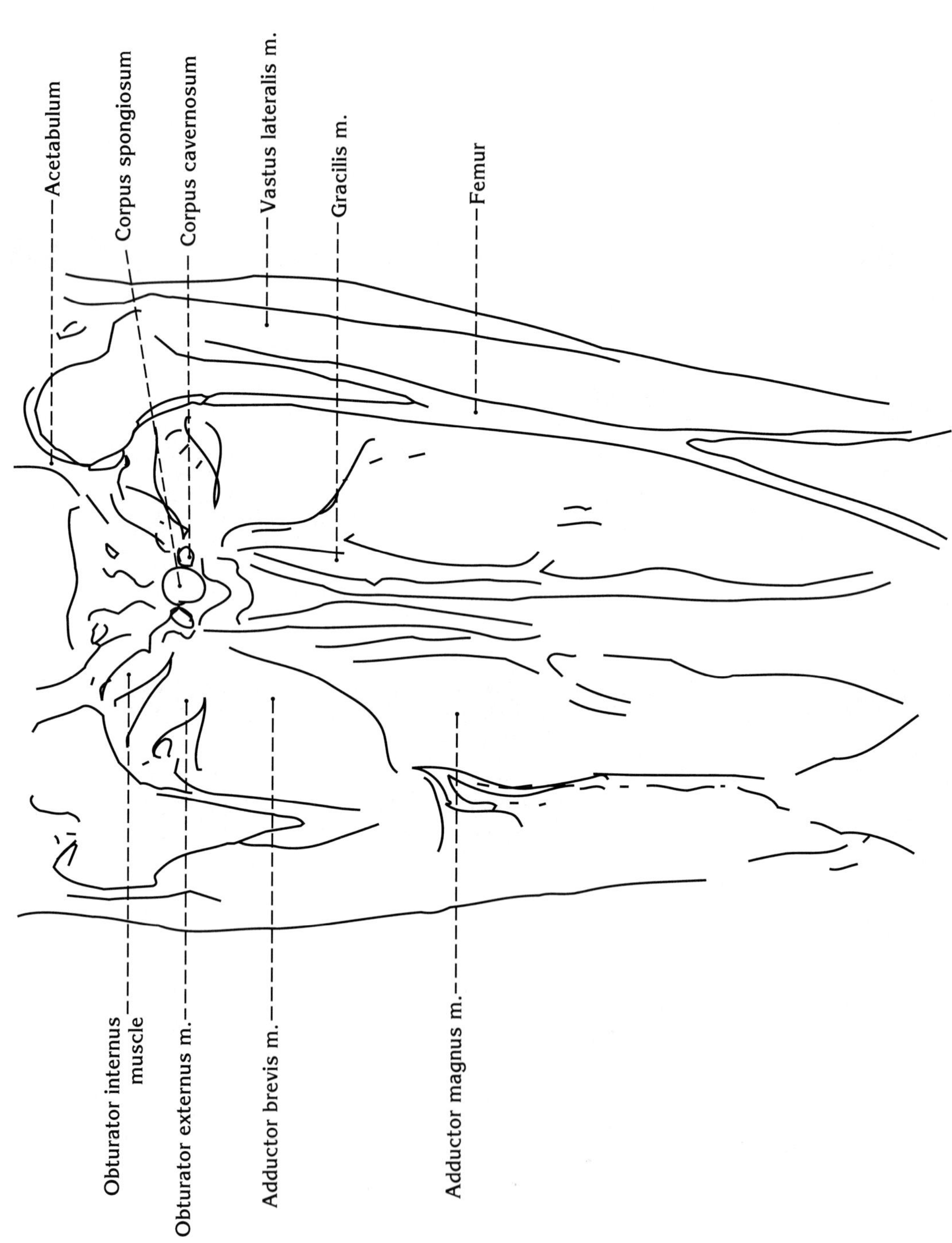

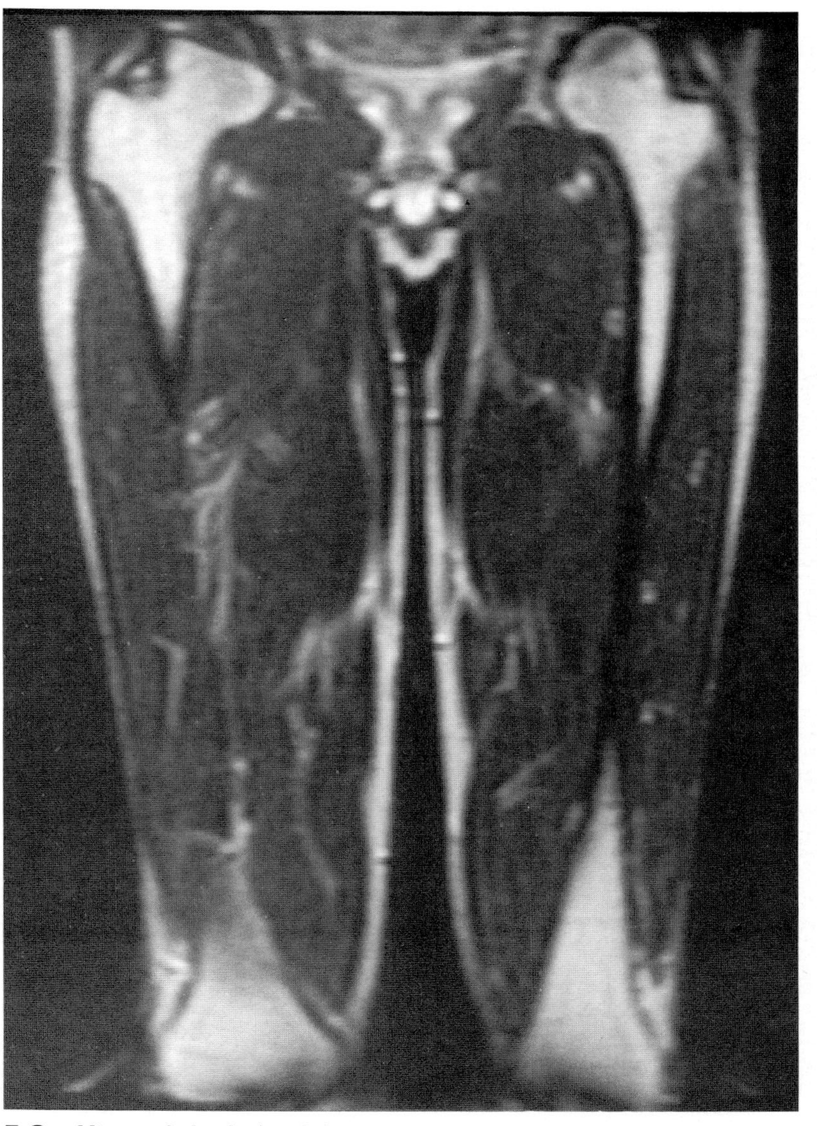

5-3a Hip and thigh (male), coronal view (TR 2000; TE 20).

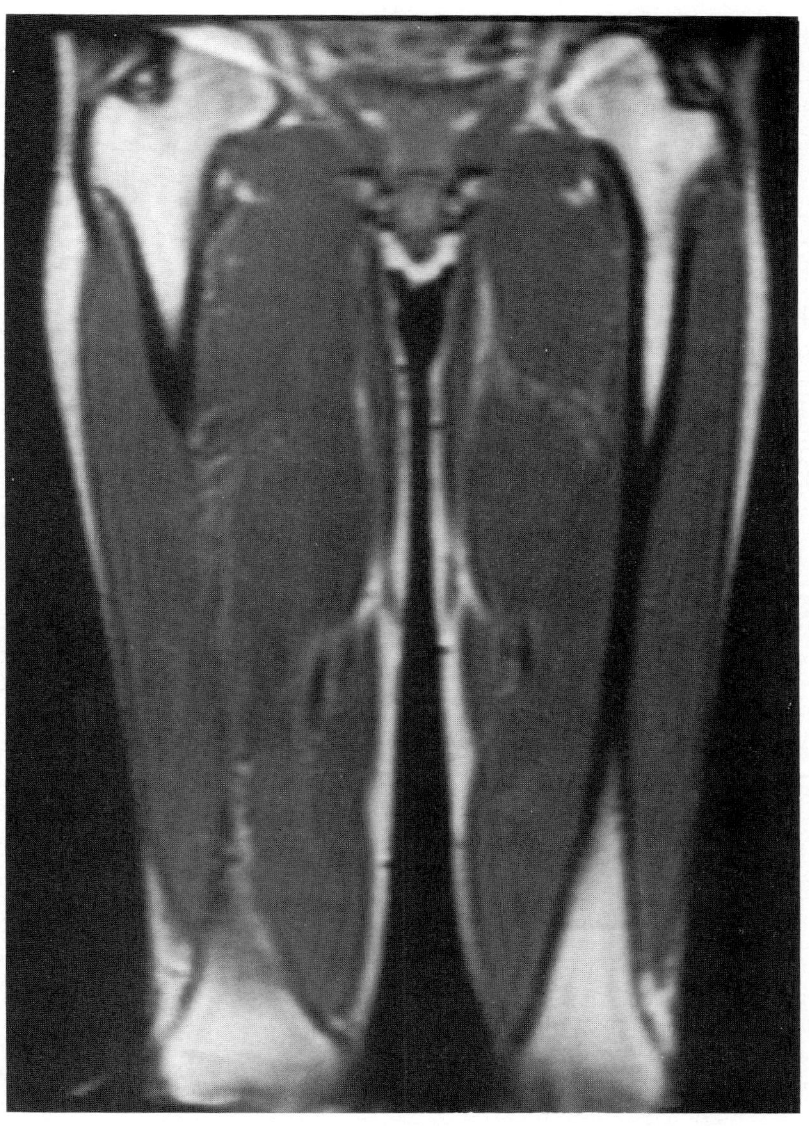

5-3b Hip and thigh (male), coronal view (TR 2000; TE 20).

Hip and Thigh, Coronal

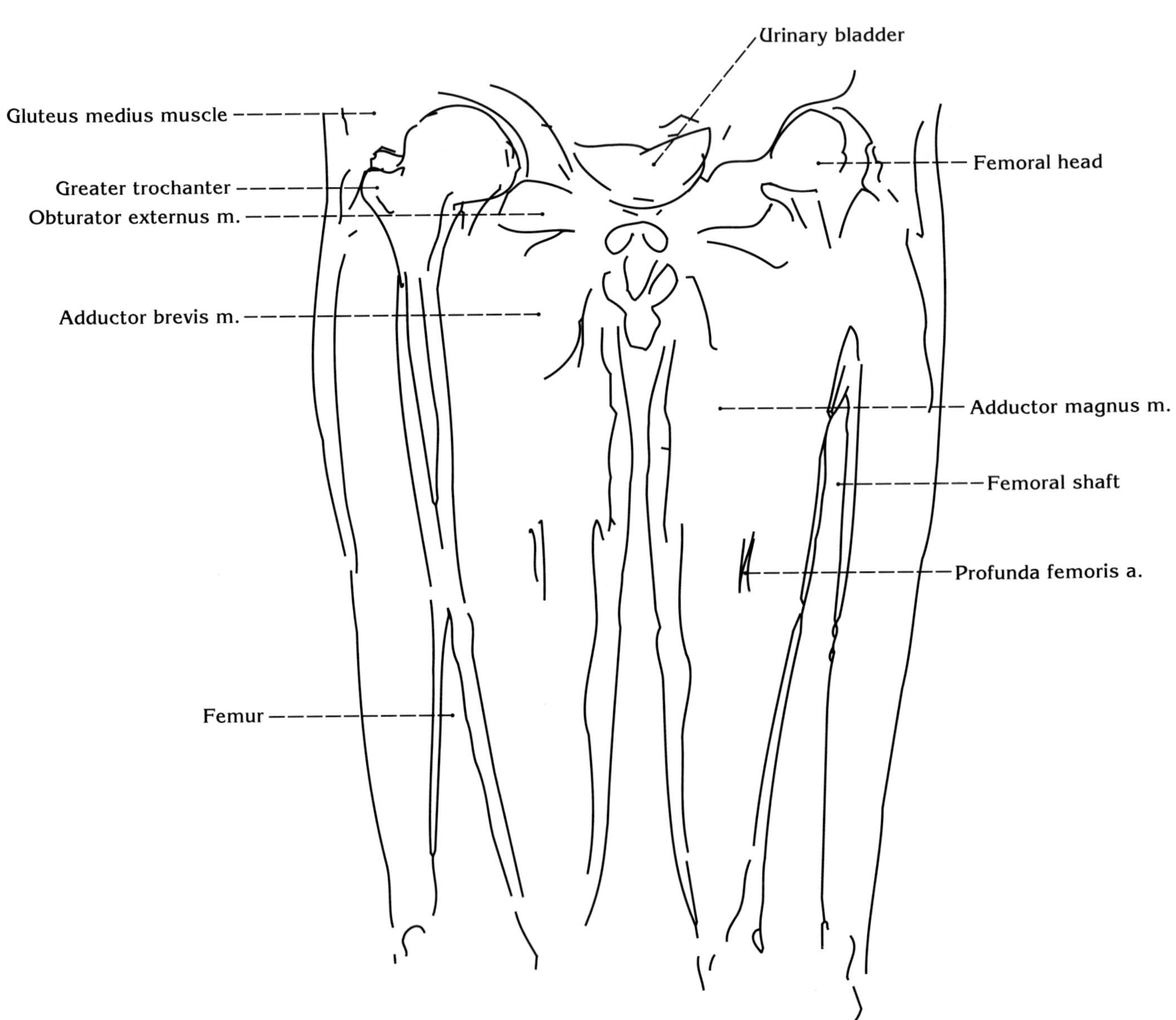

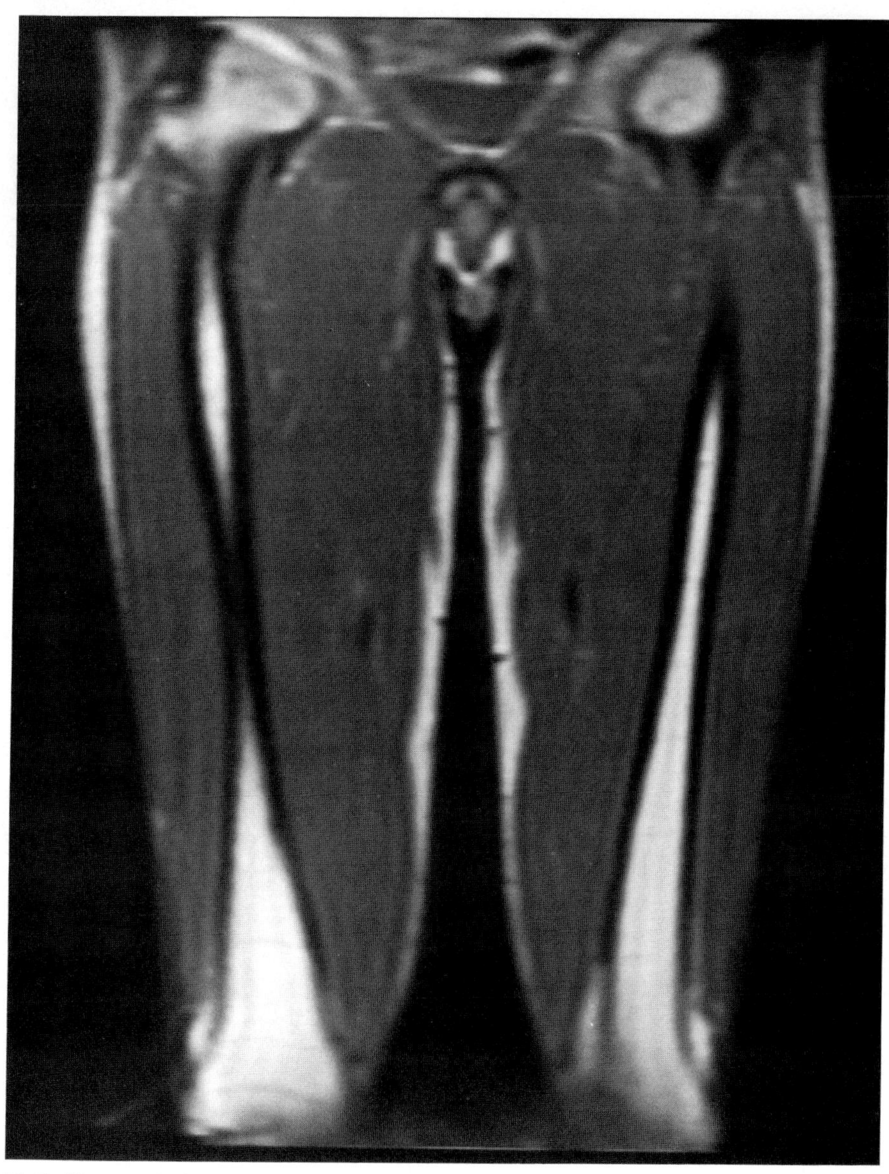

5-4 Hip and thigh (male), coronal view (TR 2000; TE 20).

Hip and Thigh, Coronal

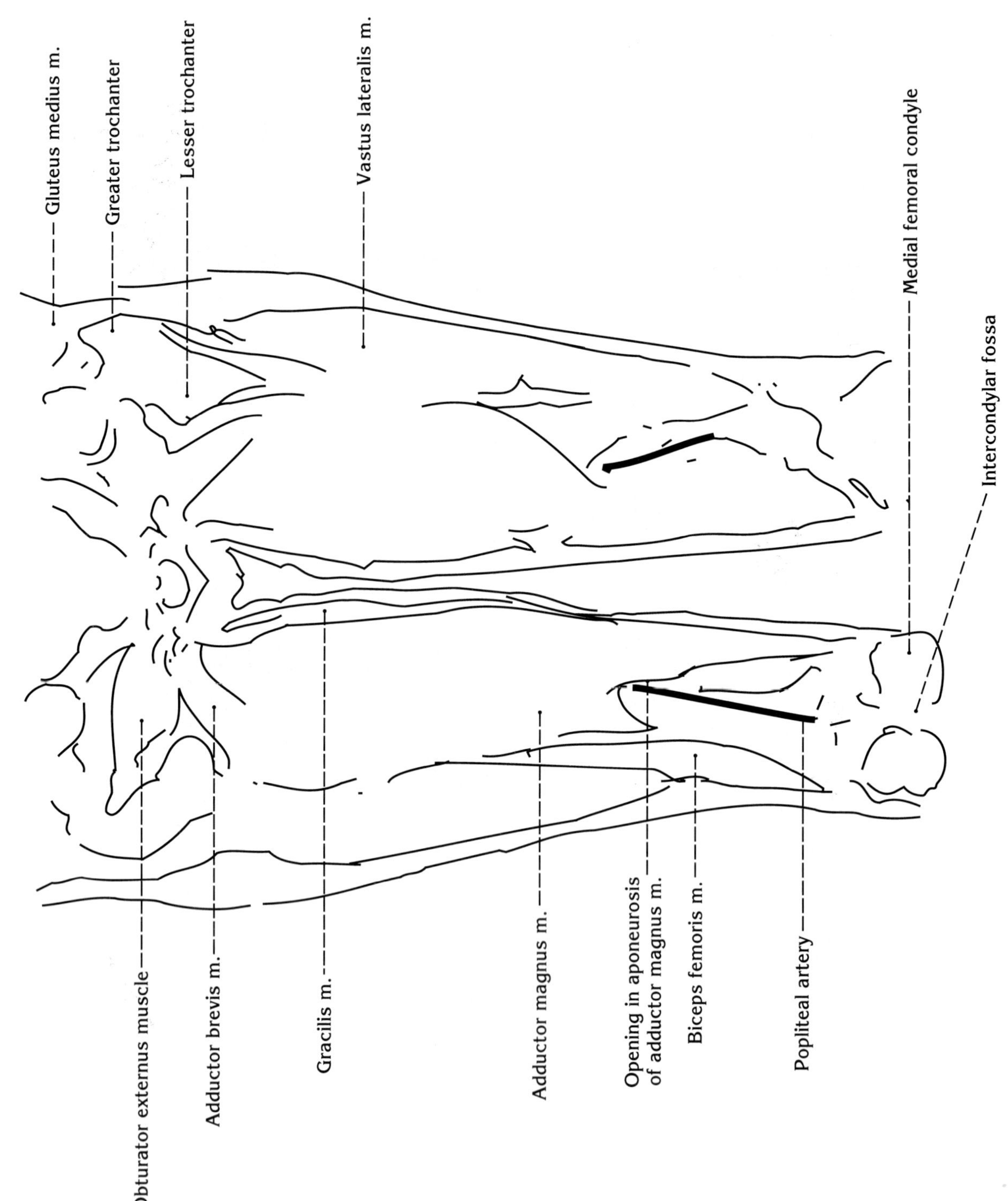

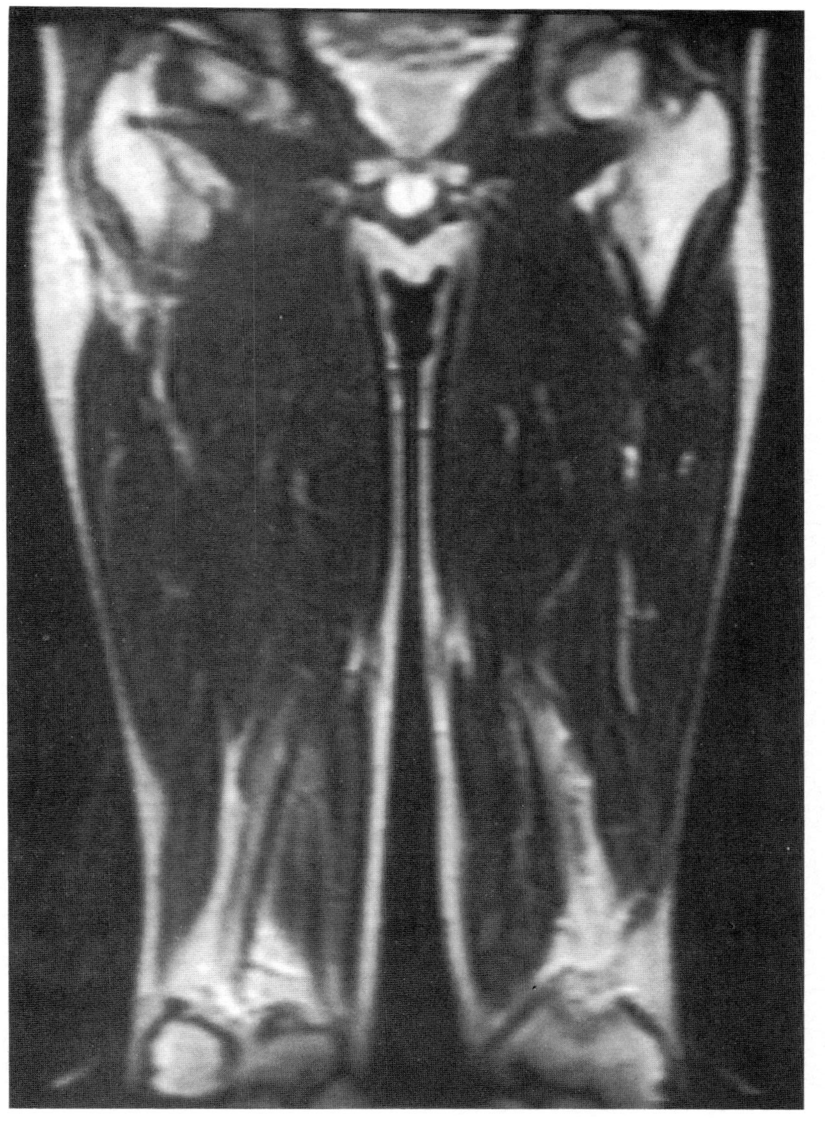

5-5a Hip and thigh, coronal view (TR 2000; TE 20).

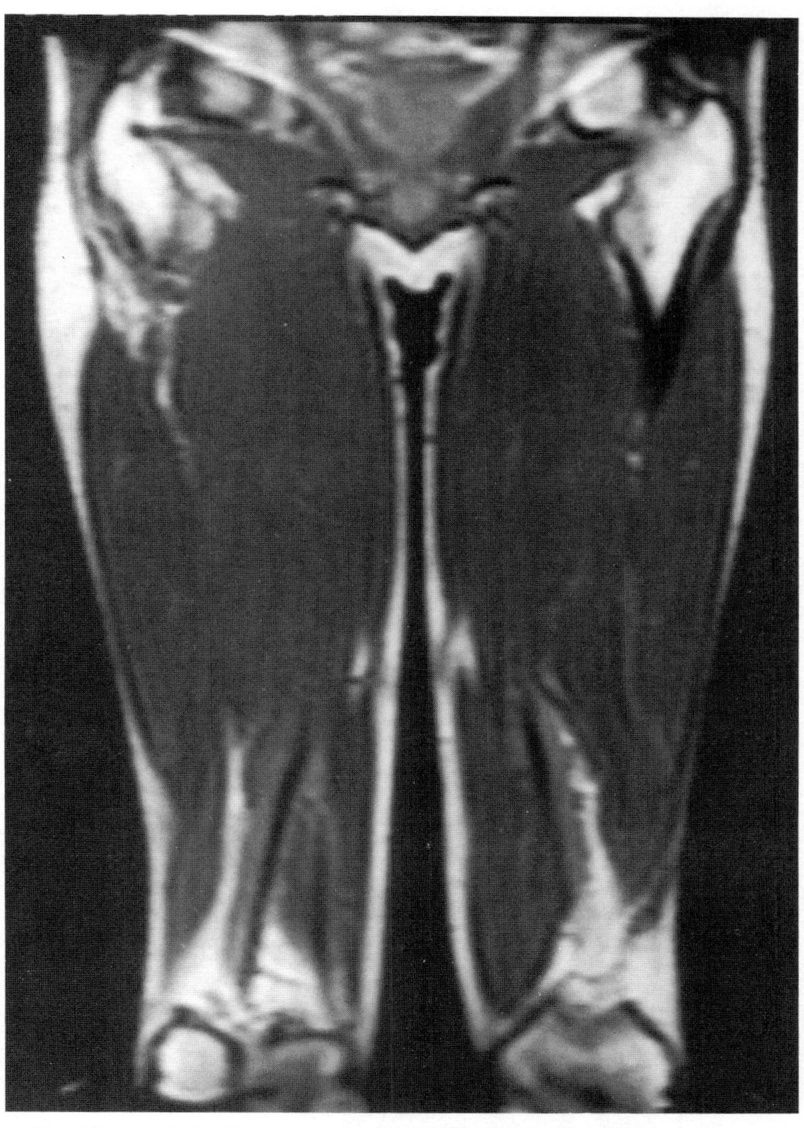

5-5b Hip and thigh, coronal view (TR 2000; TE 20).

Hip and Thigh, Coronal

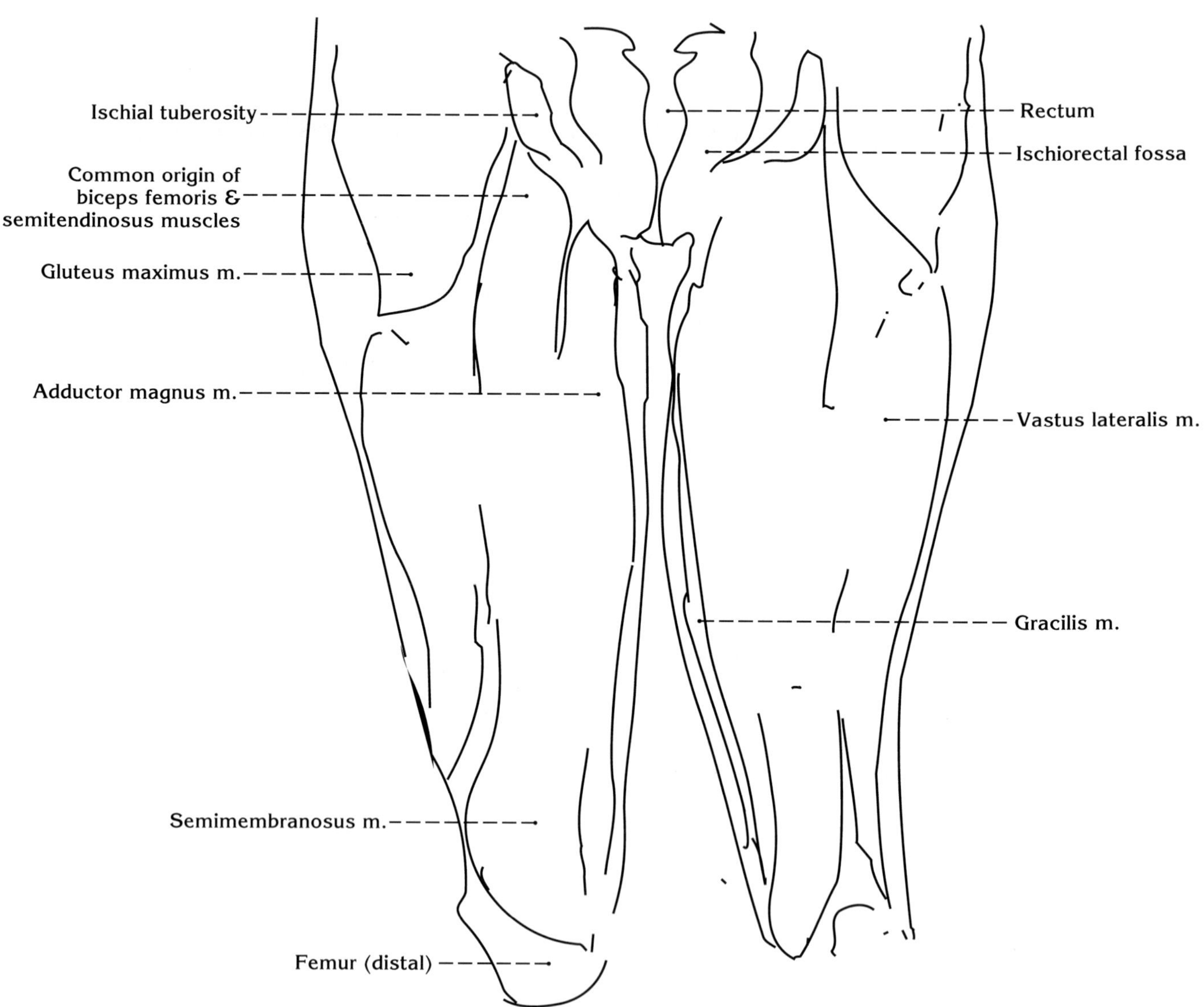

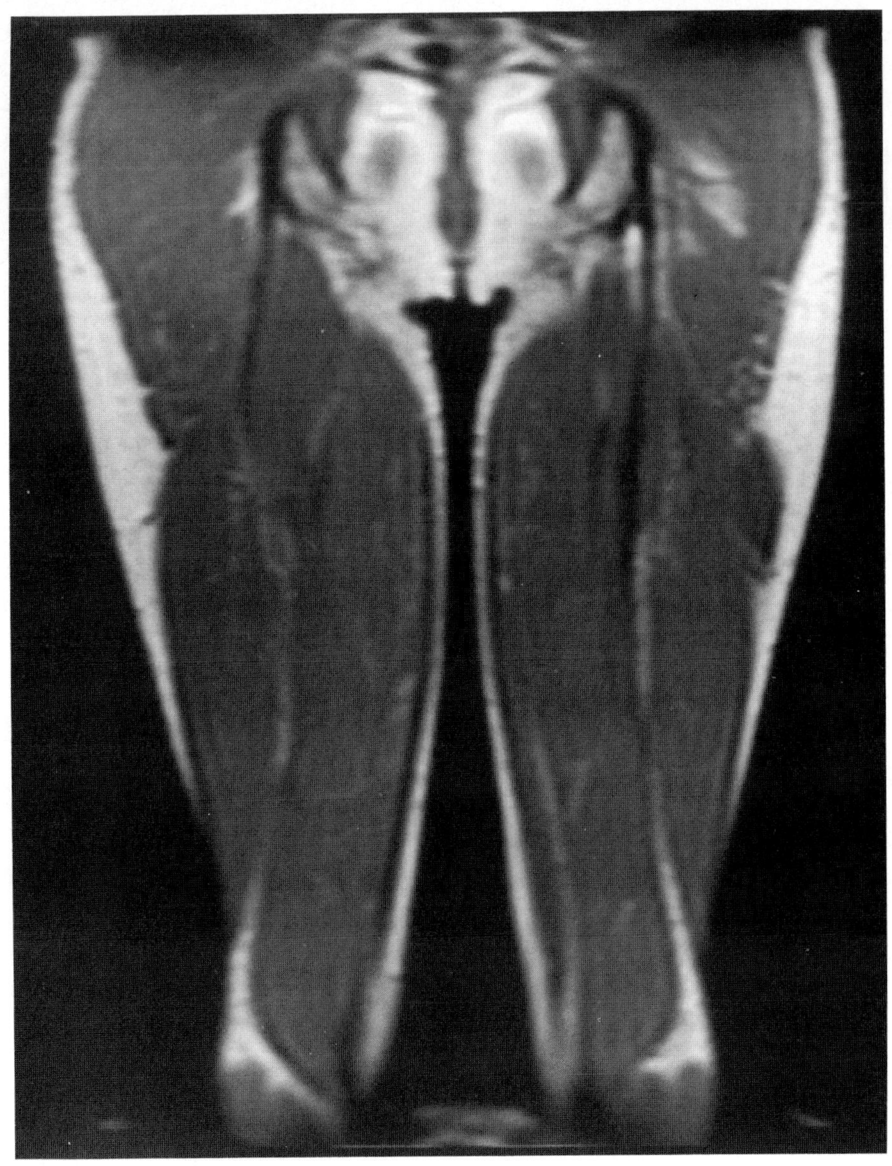

5-6 Hip and thigh, coronal view (TR 2000; TE 20).

Hip, Sagittal

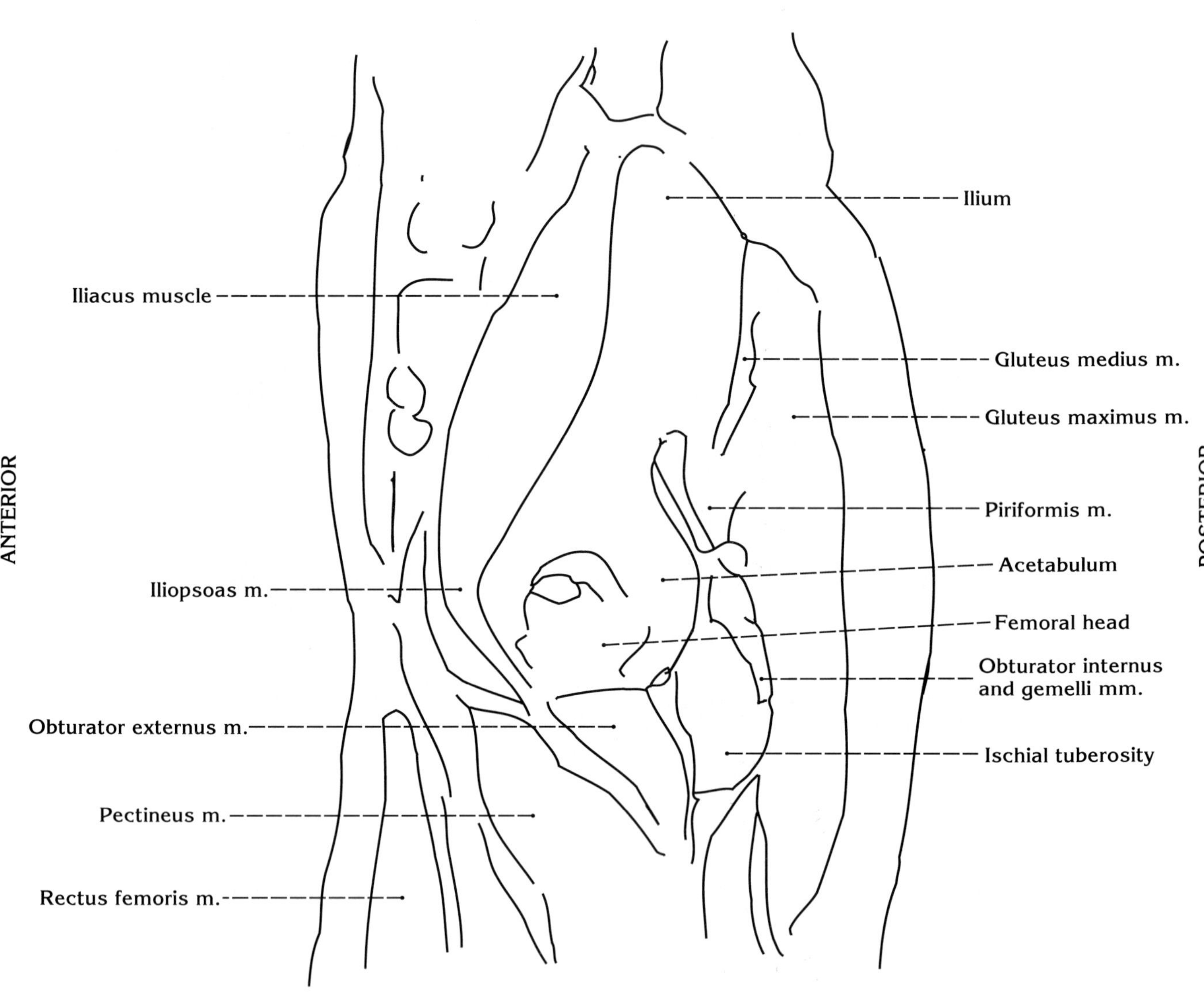

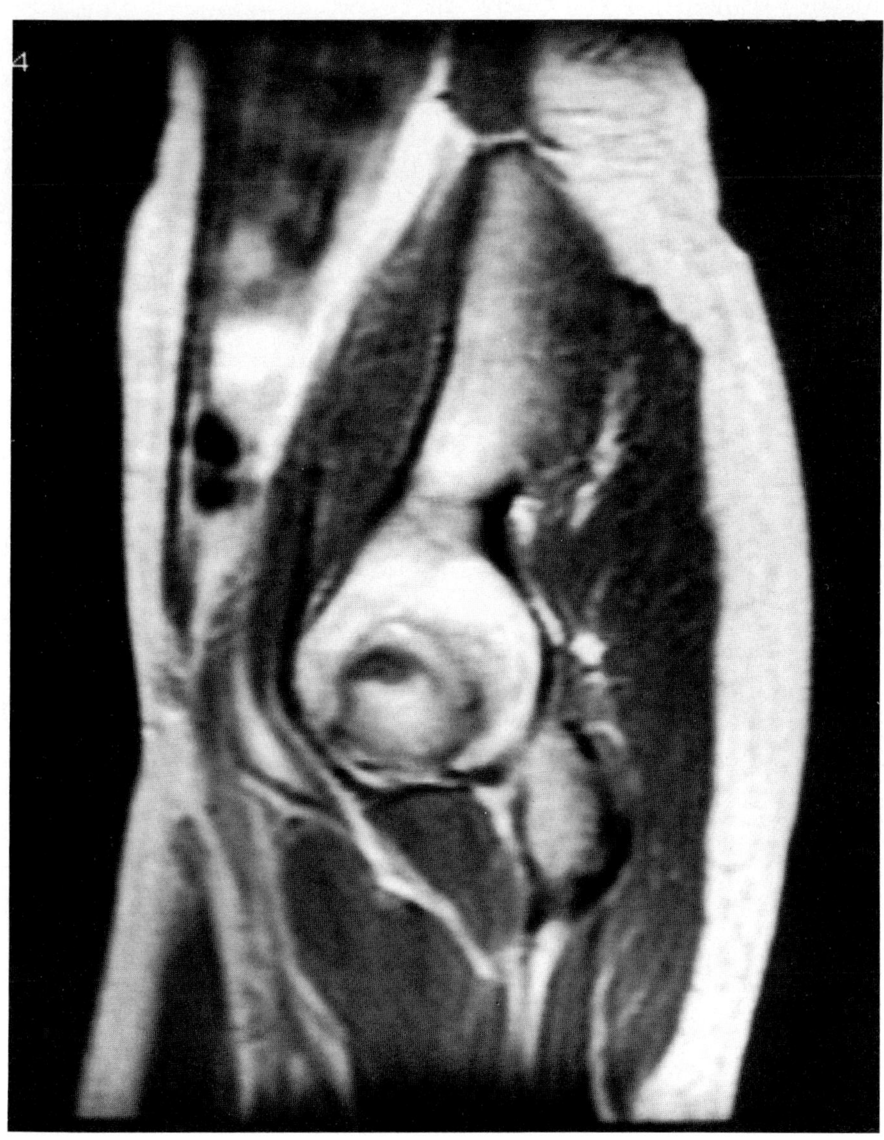

5-7 Hip, sagittal view (TR 2000; TE 30).

Hip, Sagittal

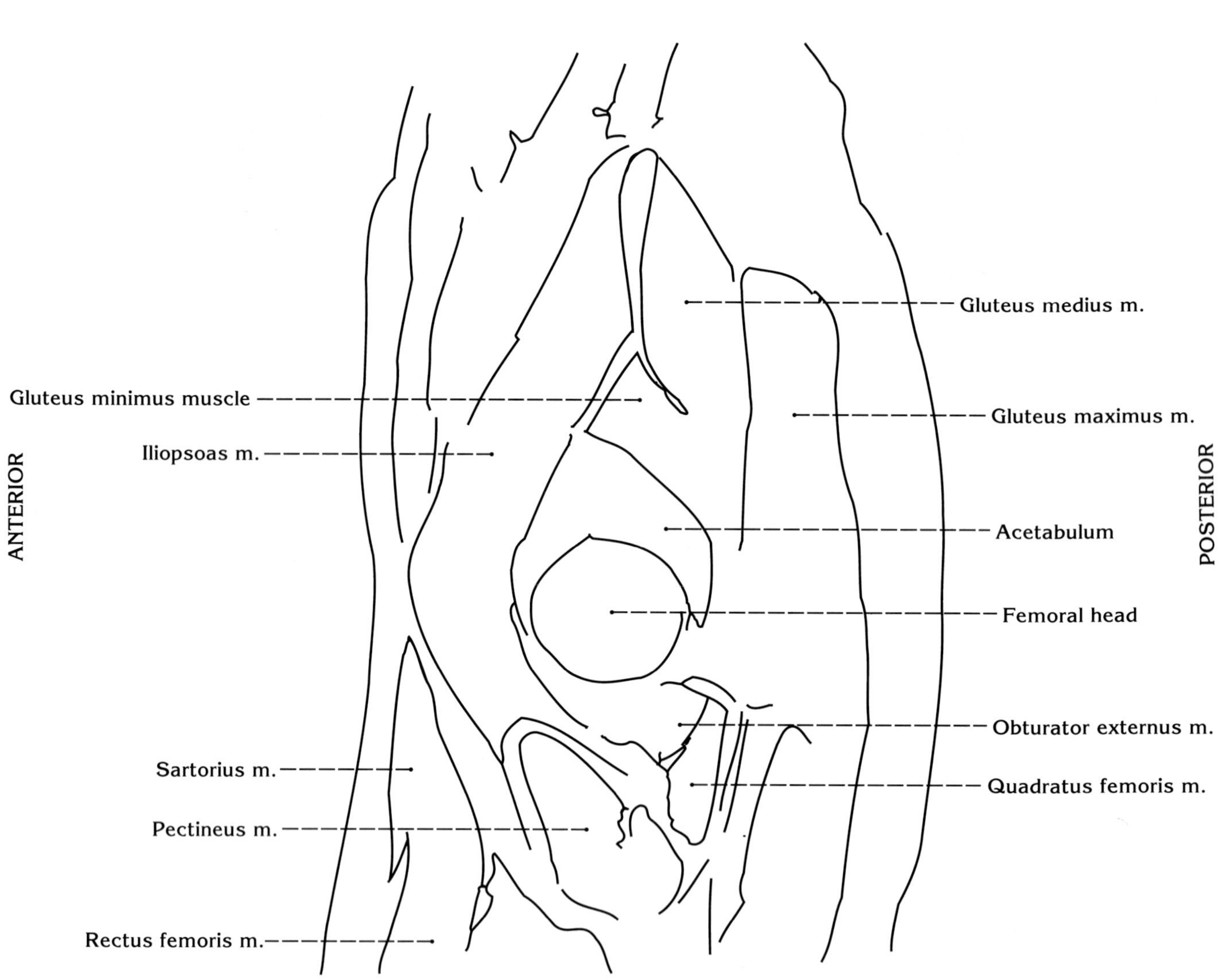

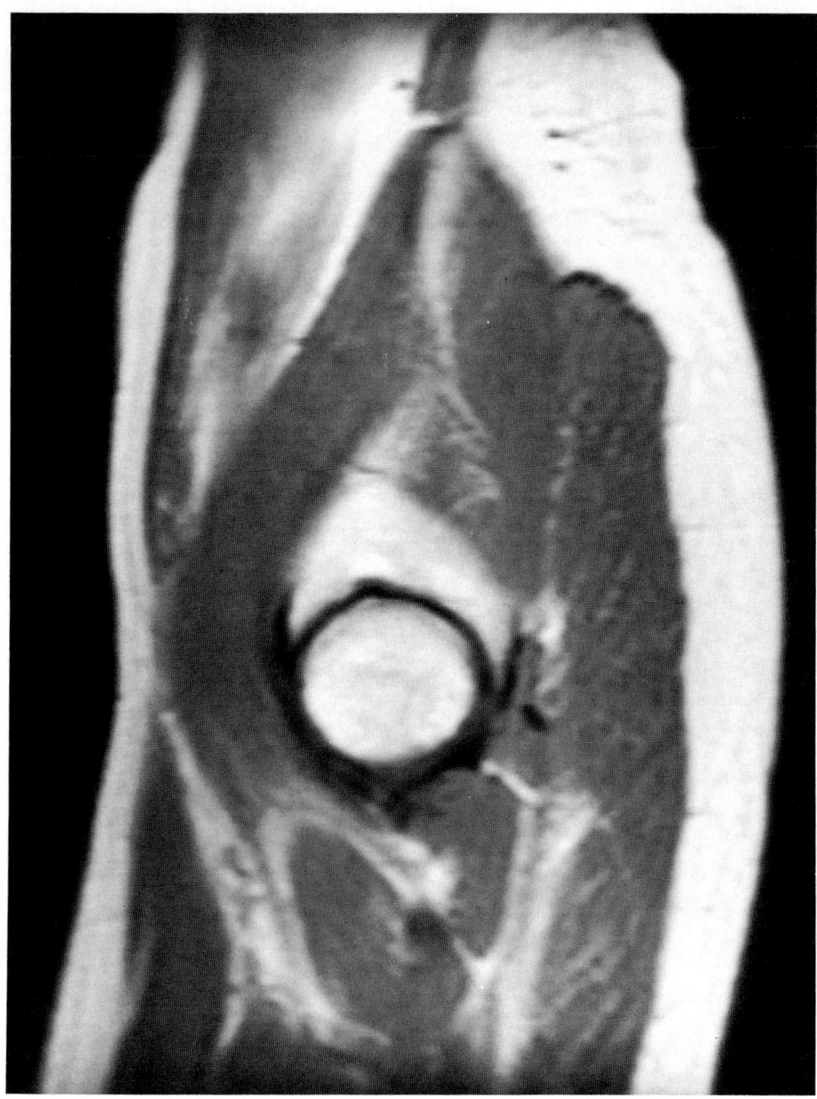

5-8 Hip, sagittal view (TR 2000; TE 30).

Hip, Sagittal

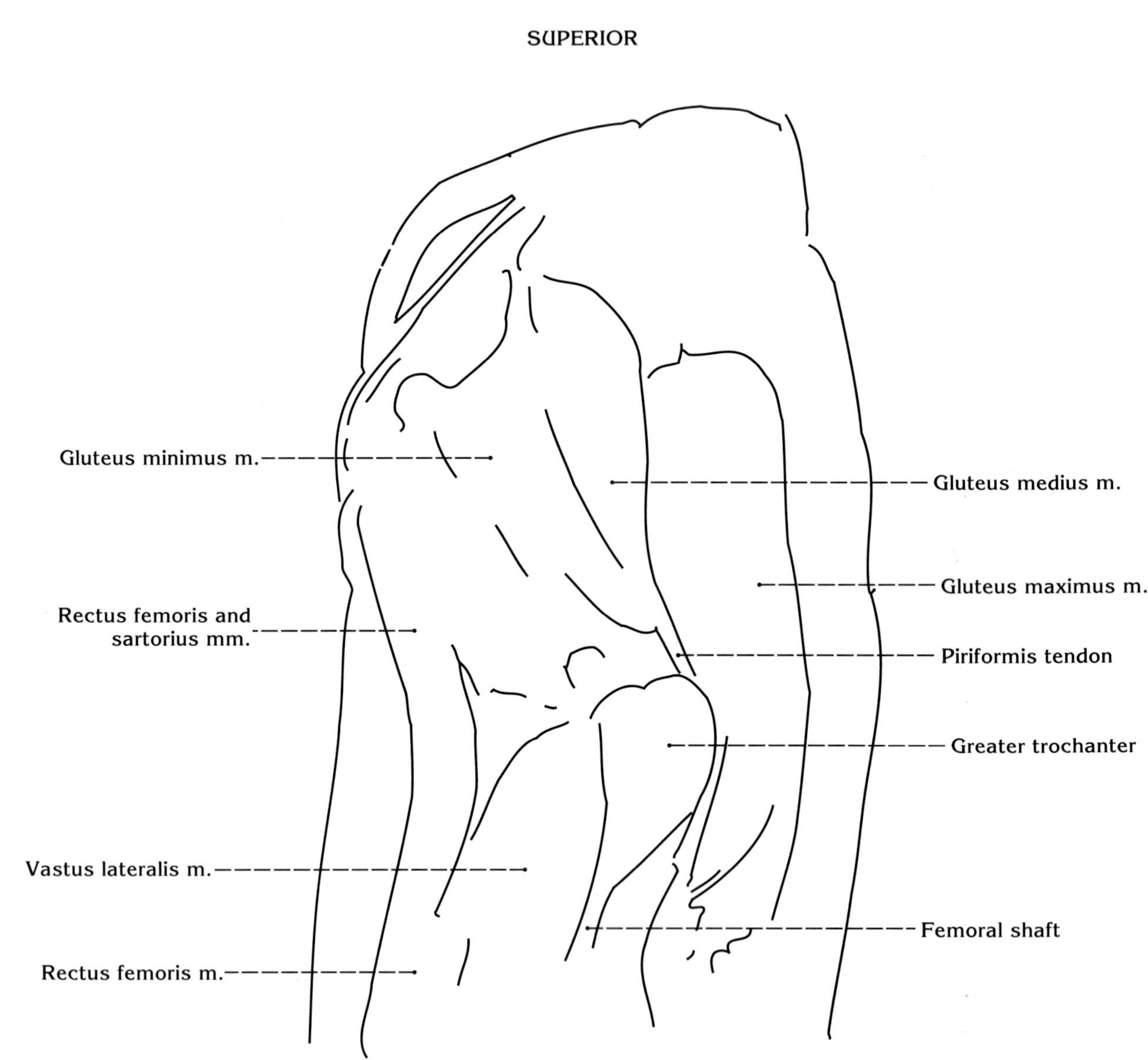

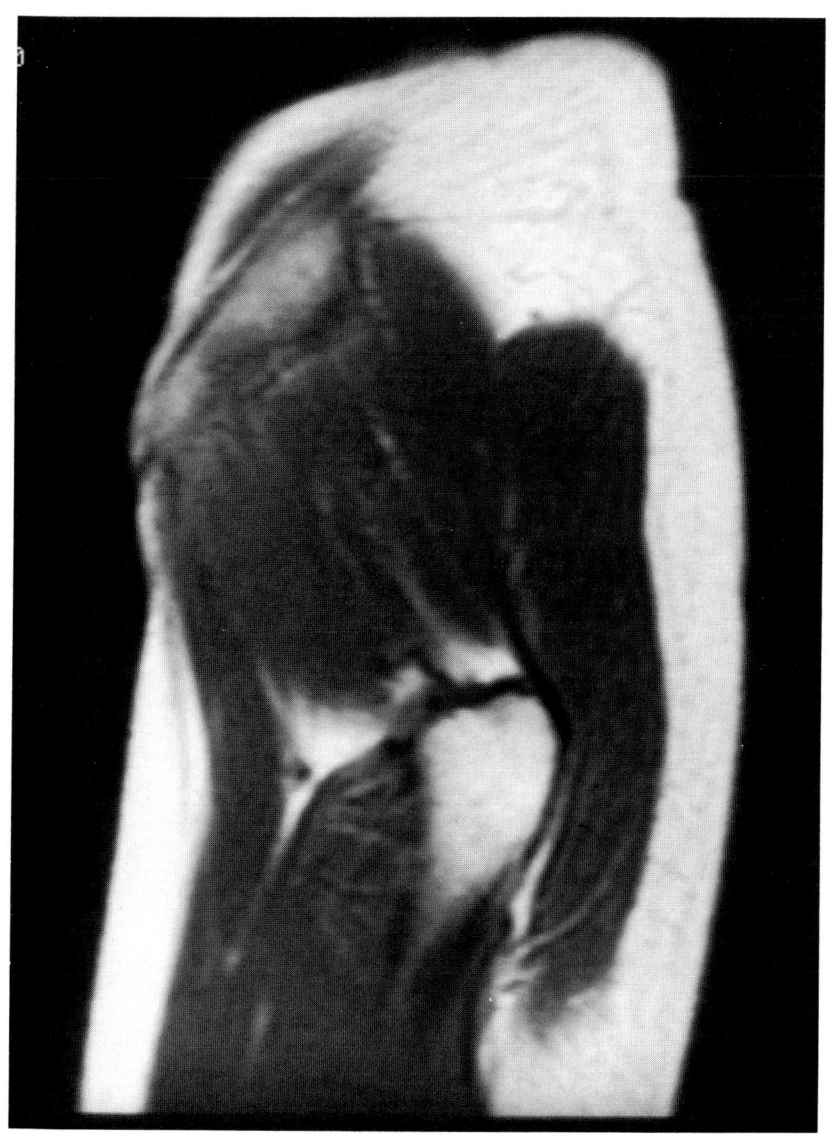

5-9 Hip, sagittal view (TR 2000; TE 30).

Thigh, Axial

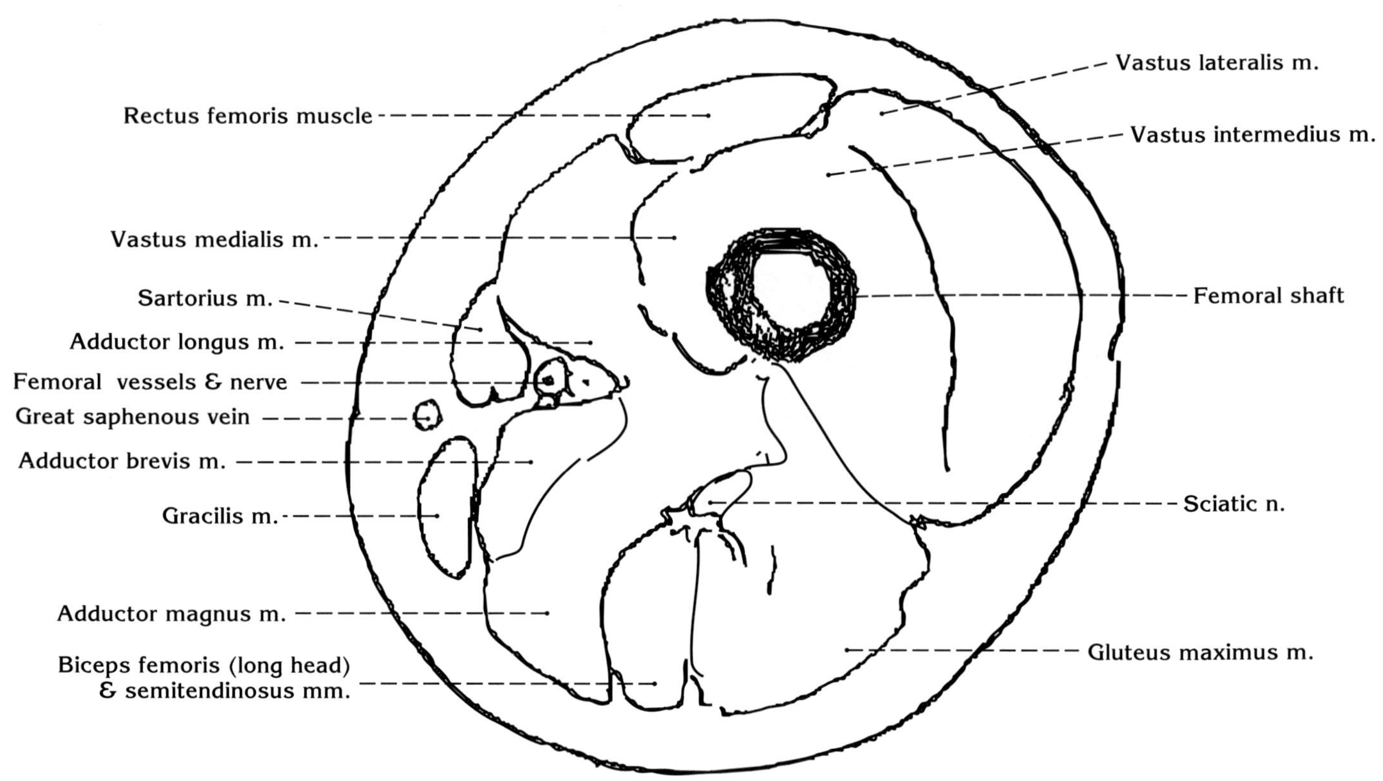
Rectus femoris muscle
Vastus lateralis m.
Vastus intermedius m.
Vastus medialis m.
Sartorius m.
Adductor longus m.
Femoral vessels & nerve
Great saphenous vein
Adductor brevis m.
Gracilis m.
Adductor magnus m.
Biceps femoris (long head)
& semitendinosus mm.
Femoral shaft
Sciatic n.
Gluteus maximus m.

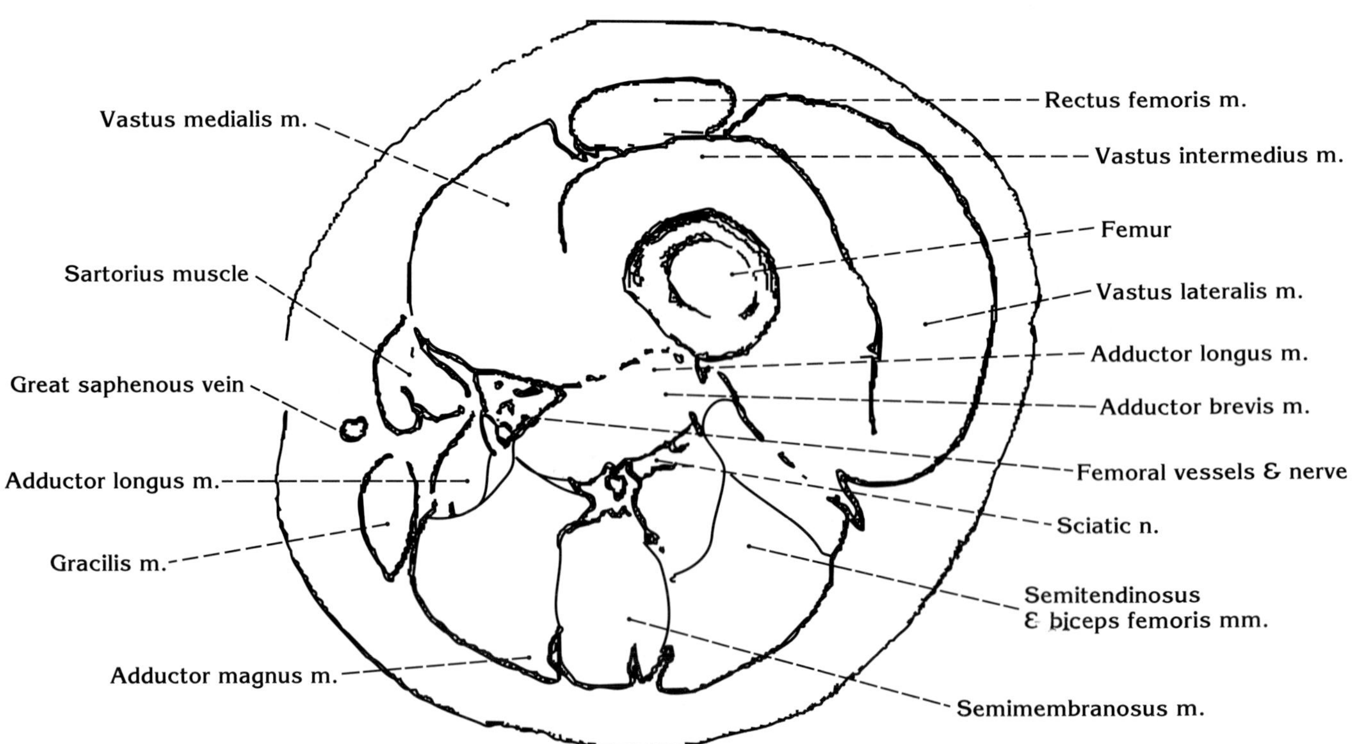
Vastus medialis m.
Sartorius muscle
Great saphenous vein
Adductor longus m.
Gracilis m.
Adductor magnus m.
Rectus femoris m.
Vastus intermedius m.
Femur
Vastus lateralis m.
Adductor longus m.
Adductor brevis m.
Femoral vessels & nerve
Sciatic n.
Semitendinosus
& biceps femoris mm.
Semimembranosus m.

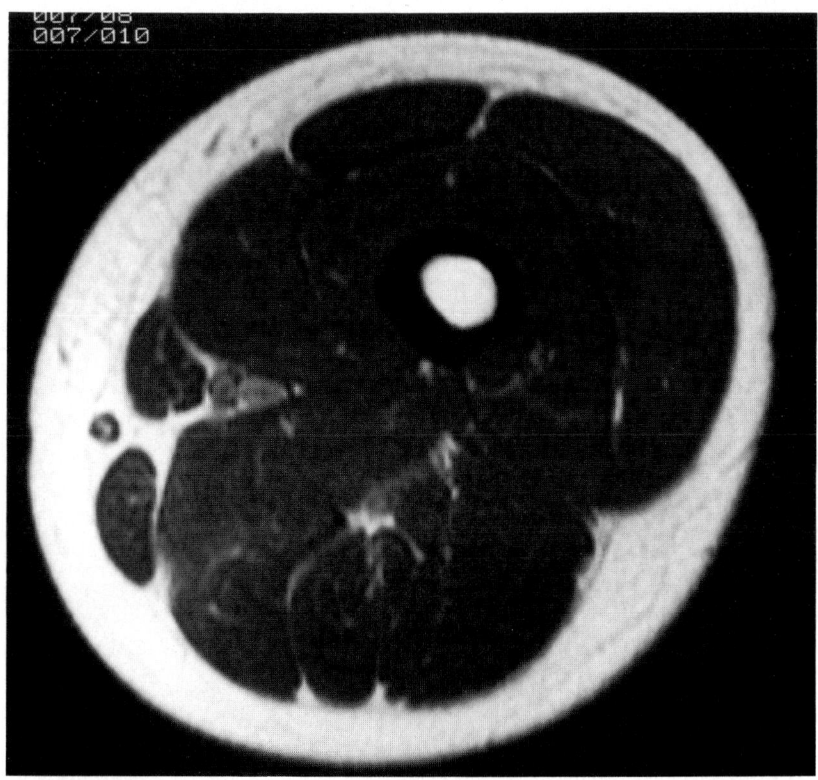

5-10 Thigh, axial view (TR 800; TE 30).

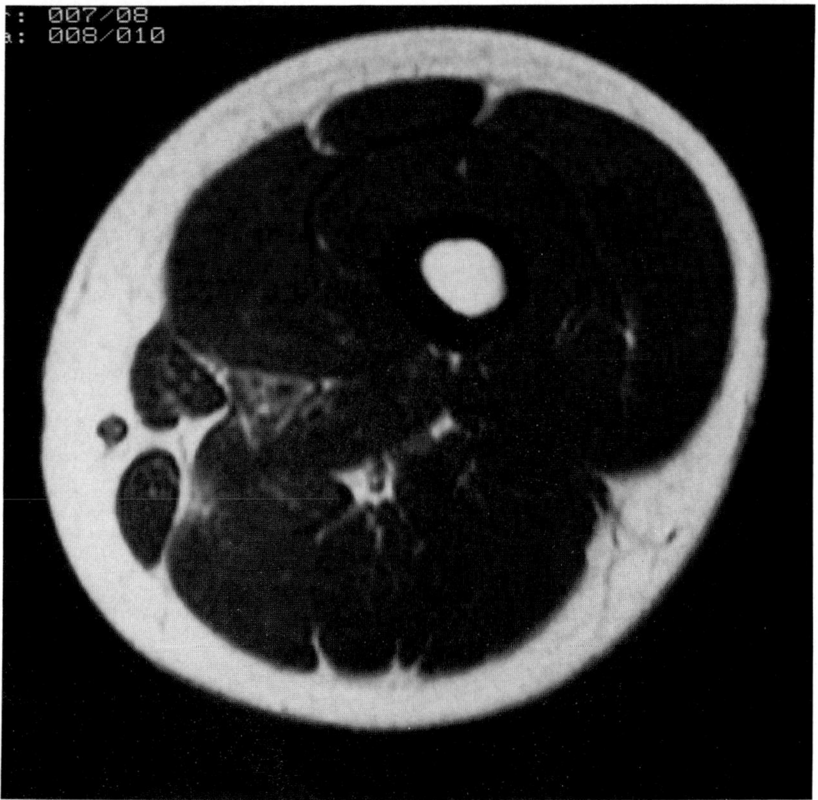

5-11 Thigh, axial view (TR 800; TE 30).

Thigh, Axial

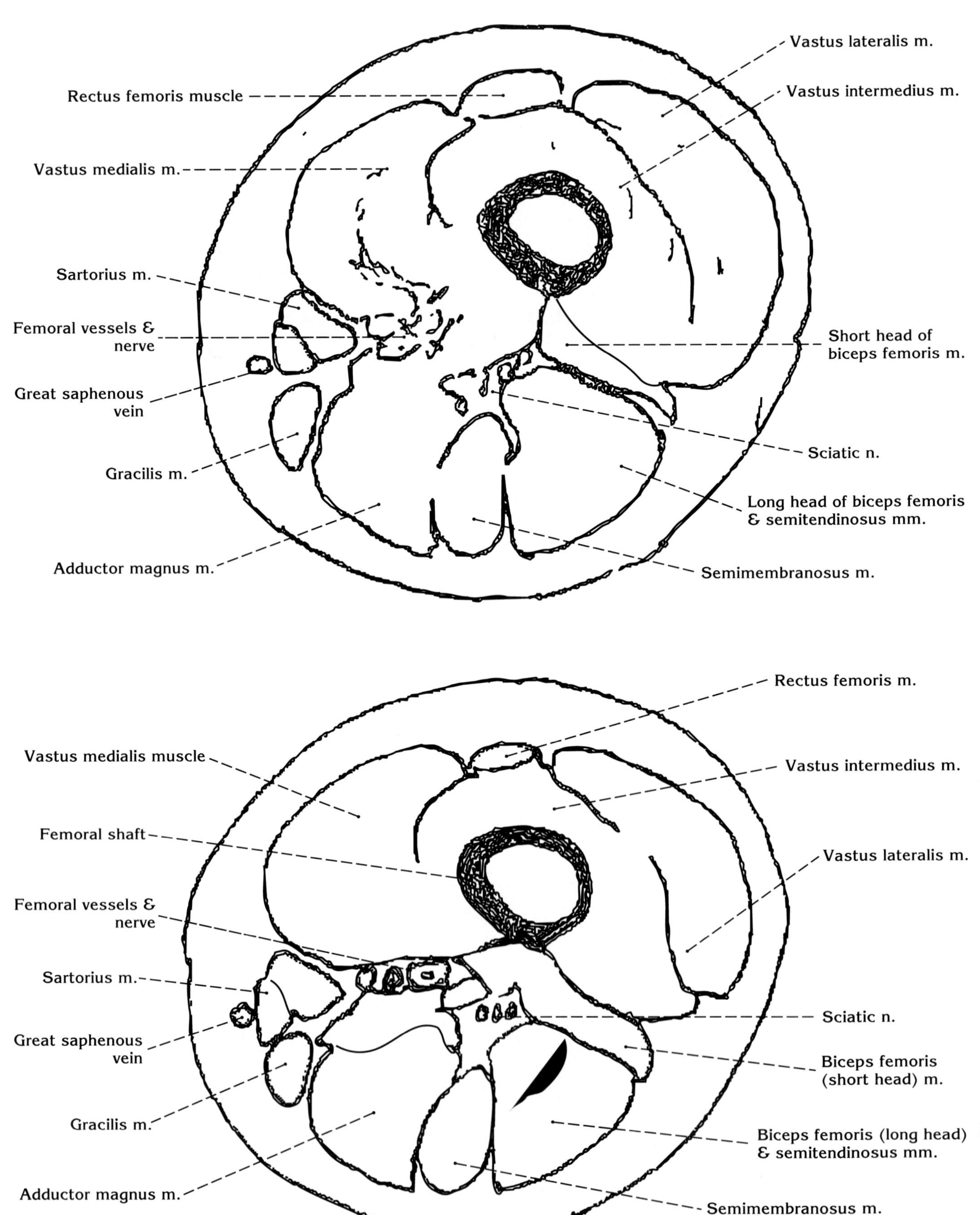
Rectus femoris muscle
Vastus medialis m.
Sartorius m.
Femoral vessels & nerve
Great saphenous vein
Gracilis m.
Adductor magnus m.
Vastus lateralis m.
Vastus intermedius m.
Short head of biceps femoris m.
Sciatic n.
Long head of biceps femoris & semitendinosus mm.
Semimembranosus m.
Rectus femoris m.
Vastus medialis muscle
Femoral shaft
Femoral vessels & nerve
Sartorius m.
Great saphenous vein
Gracilis m.
Adductor magnus m.
Vastus intermedius m.
Vastus lateralis m.
Sciatic n.
Biceps femoris (short head) m.
Biceps femoris (long head) & semitendinosus mm.
Semimembranosus m.

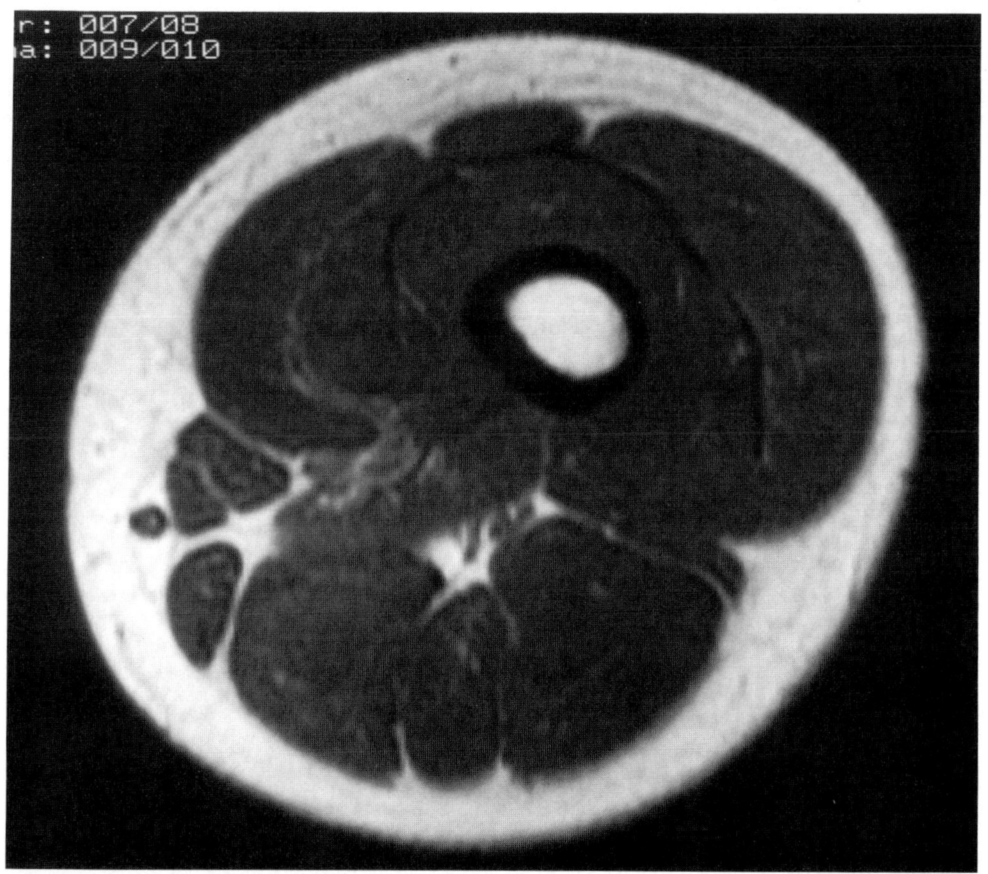

5-12 Thigh, axial view (TR 800; TE 30).

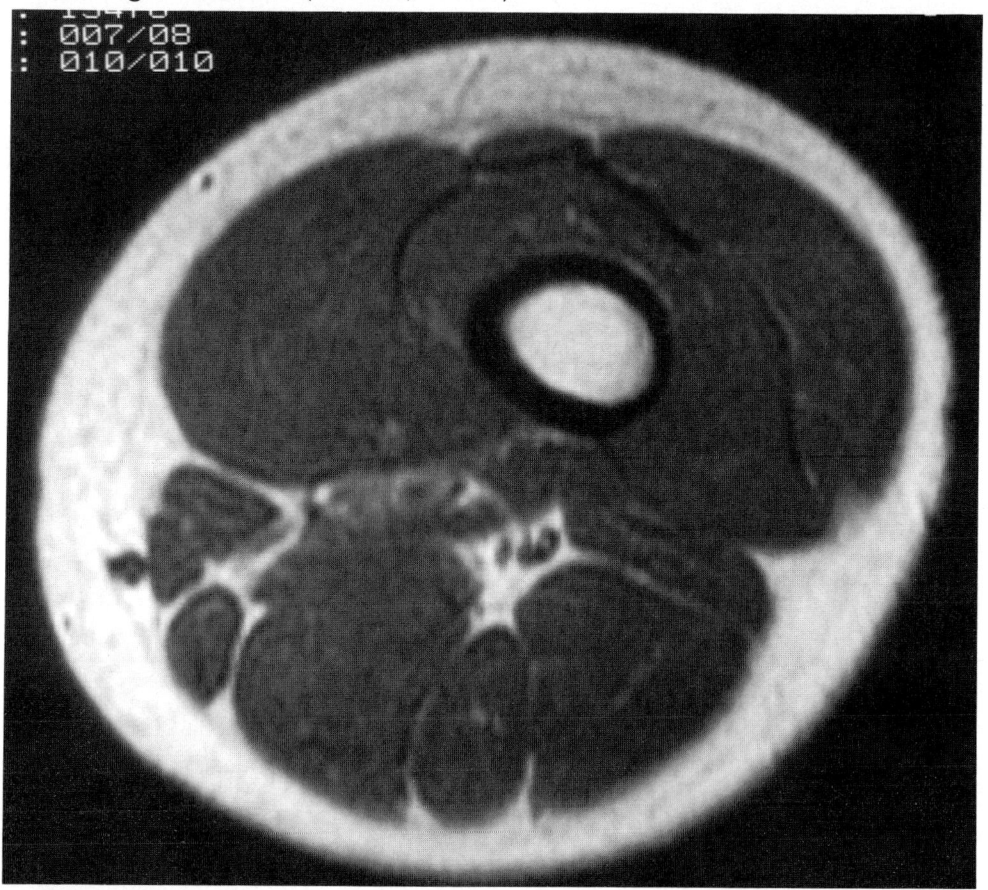

5-13 Thigh, axial view (TR 800; TE 30).

Knee, Coronal

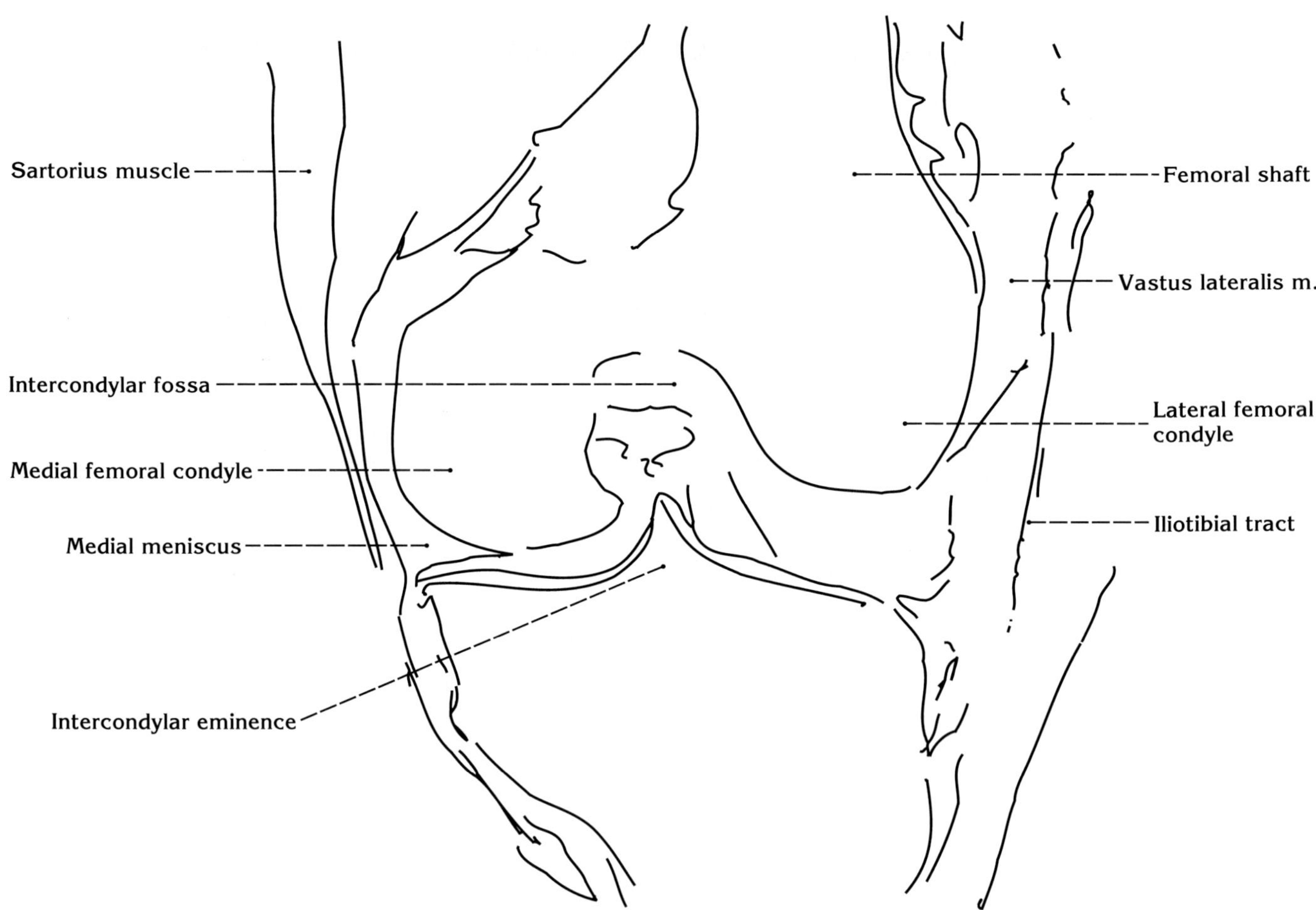

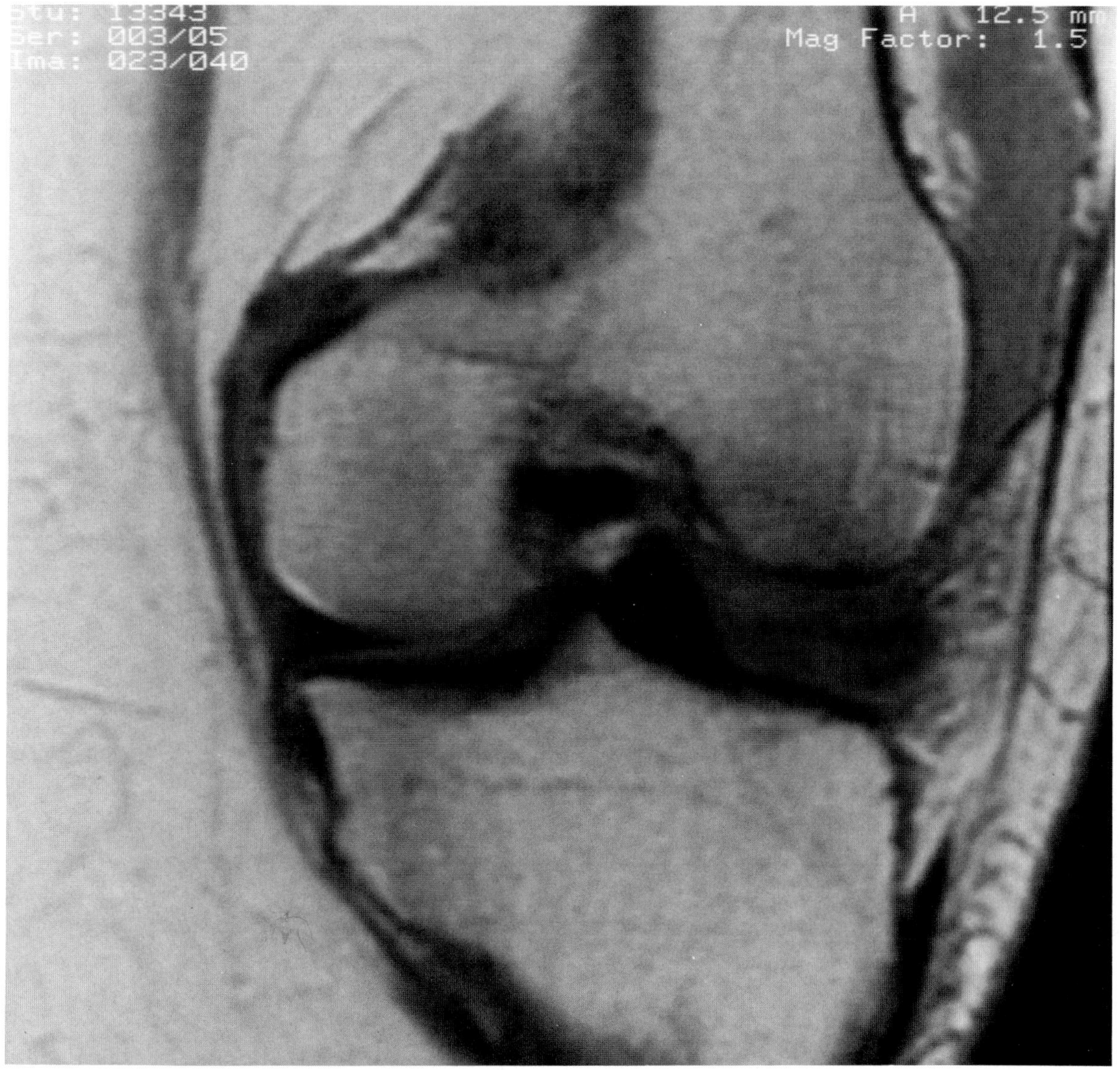

5-14 Knee, coronal view (TR 2000; TE 20). *Note:* This image, along with Figs. 5-15 through 5-21, has been obtained in a slightly oblique projection in order to demonstrate some of the structures around the knee joint to best advantage.

Knee, Coronal

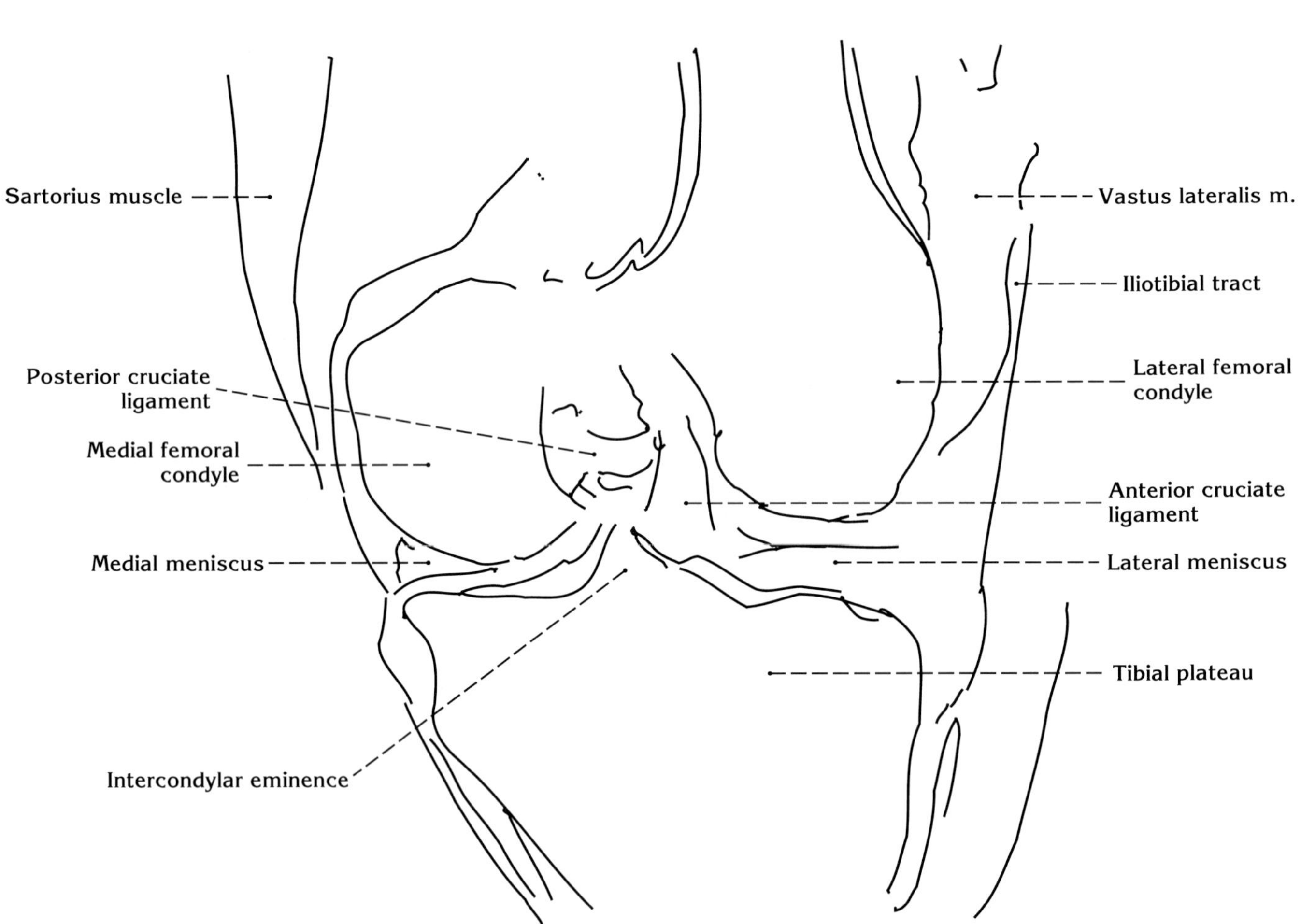

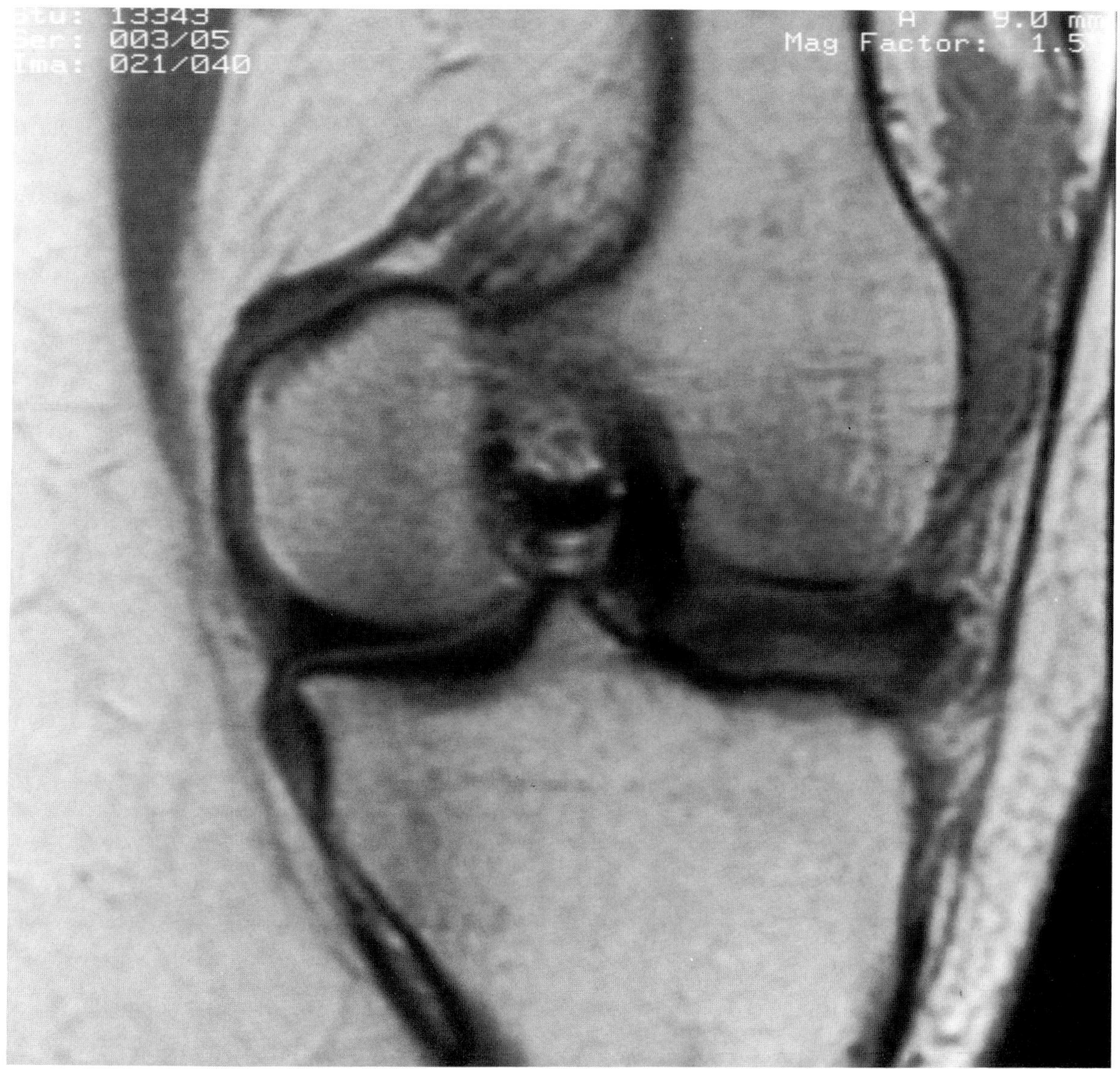

5-15 Knee, coronal view (TR 2000; TE 20). (See note to legend 5-14.)

Knee, Coronal

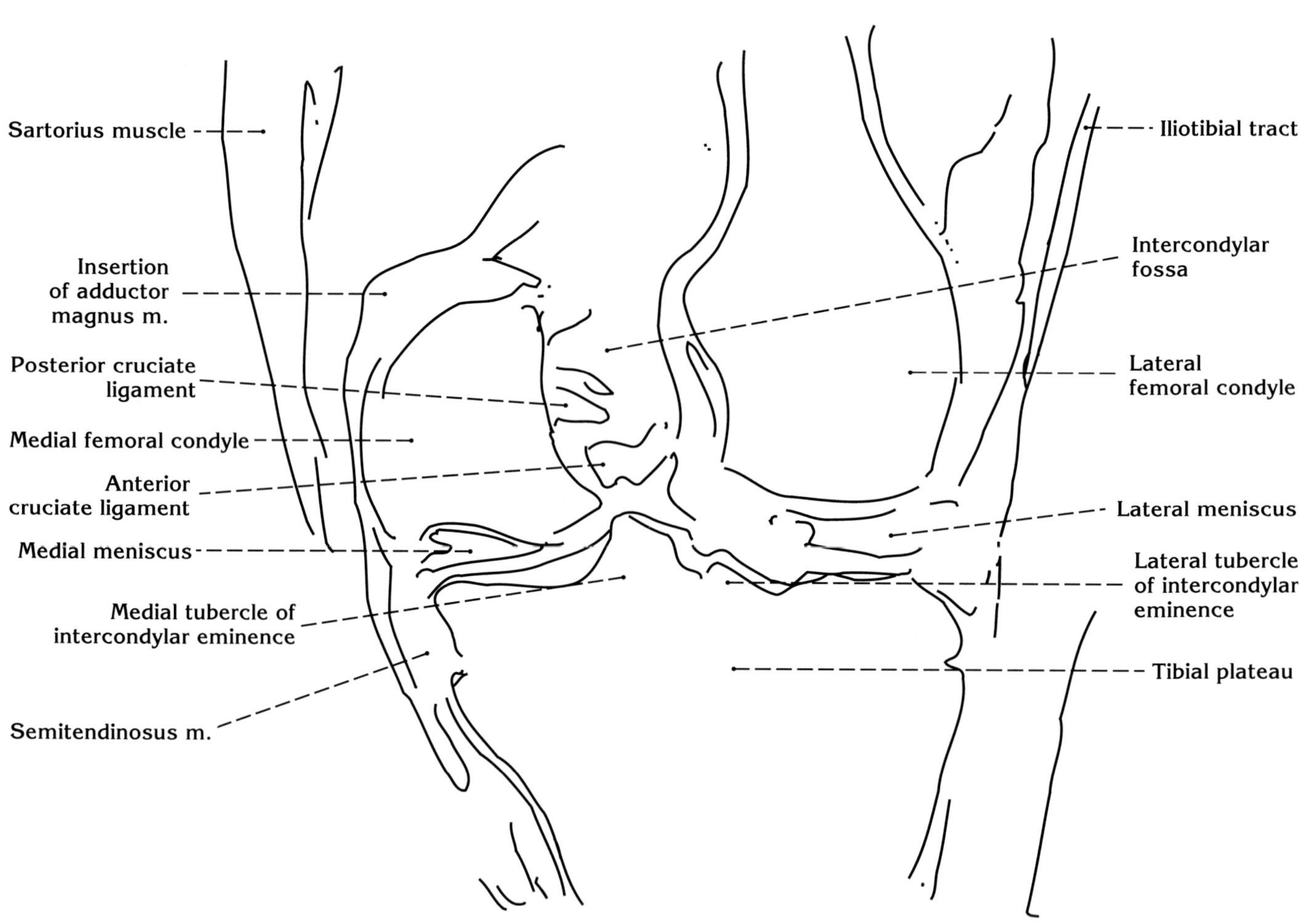

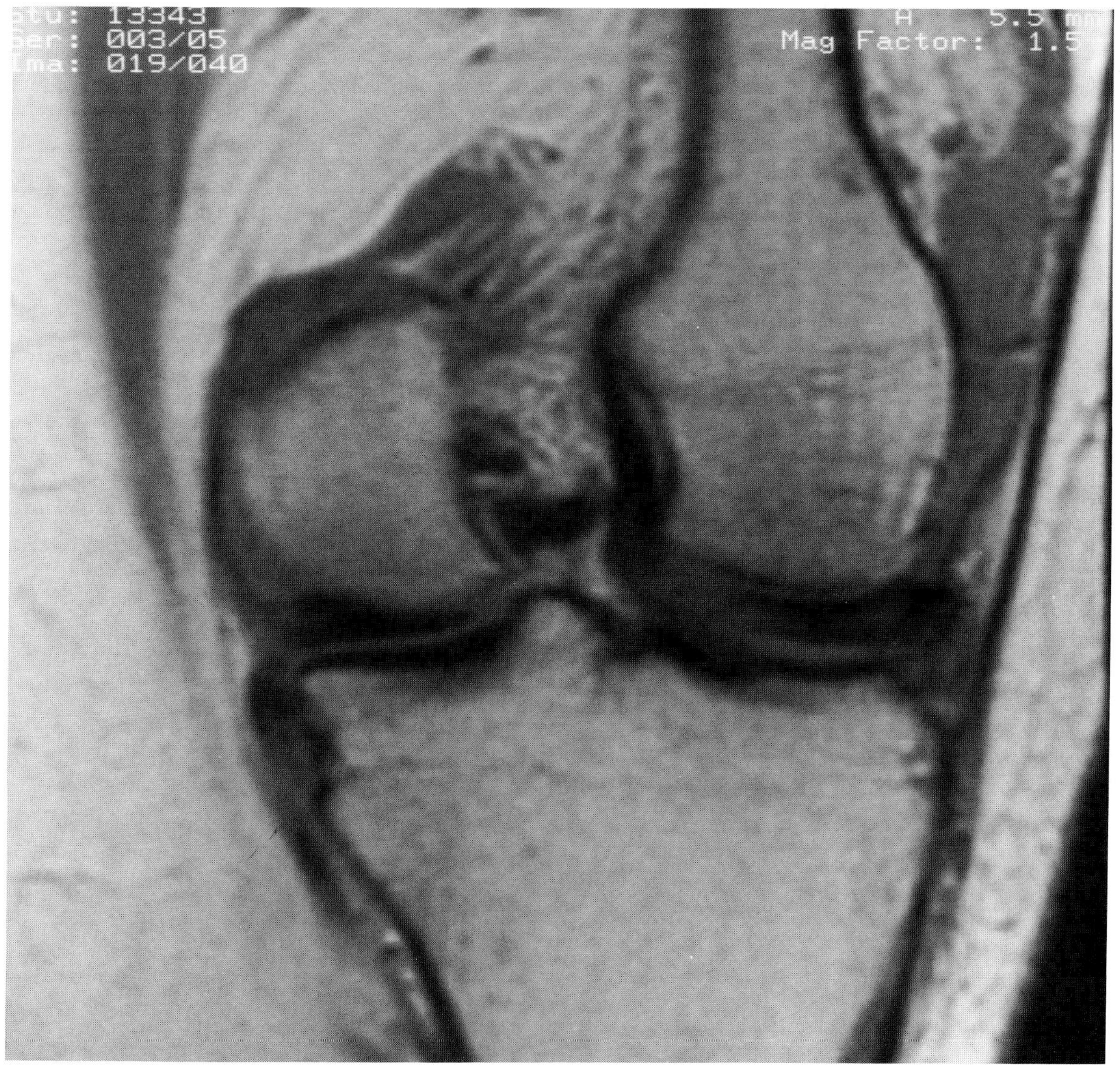

5-16 Knee, coronal view (TR 2000; TE 20). (See note to legend 5-14.)

Knee, Coronal

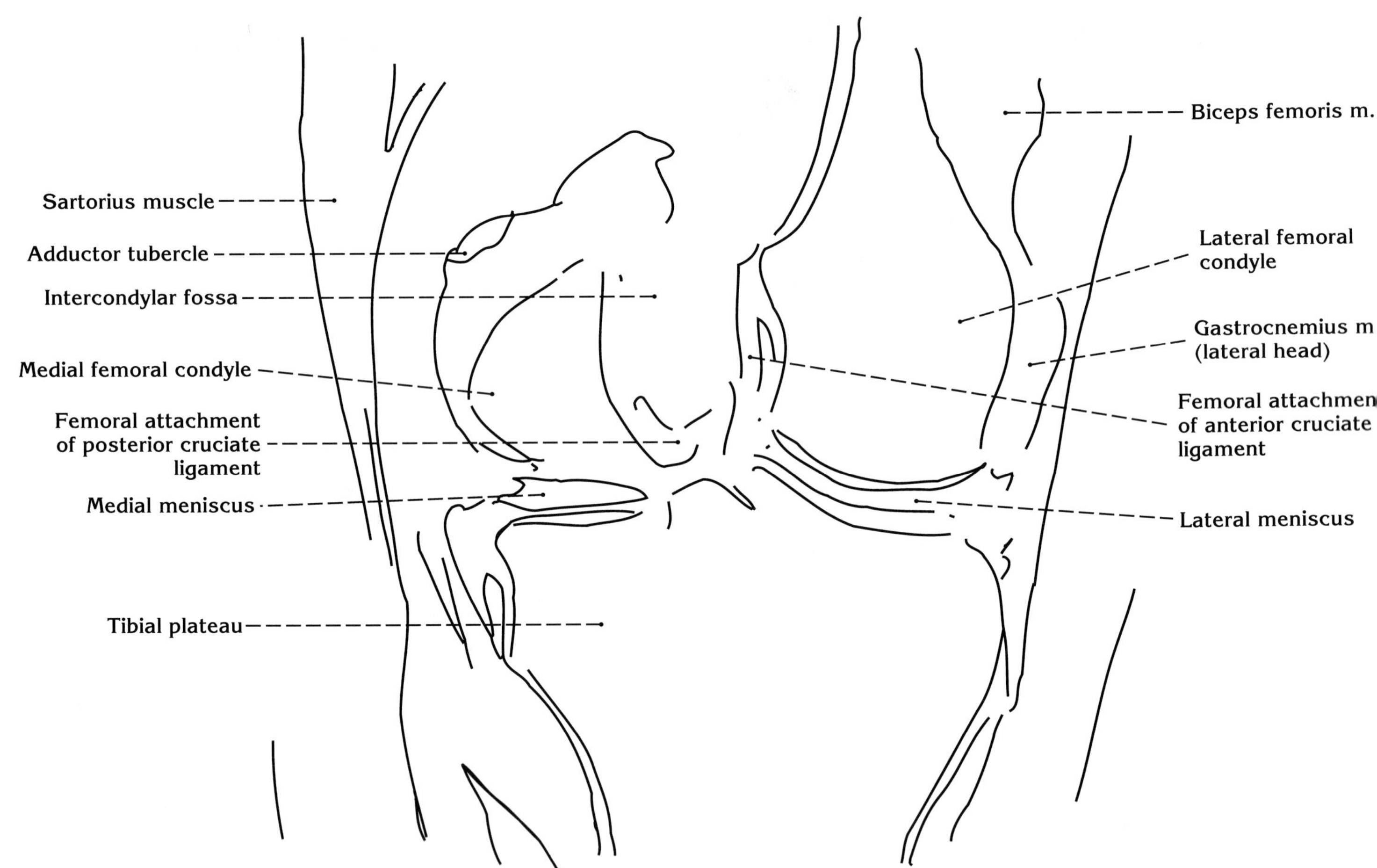

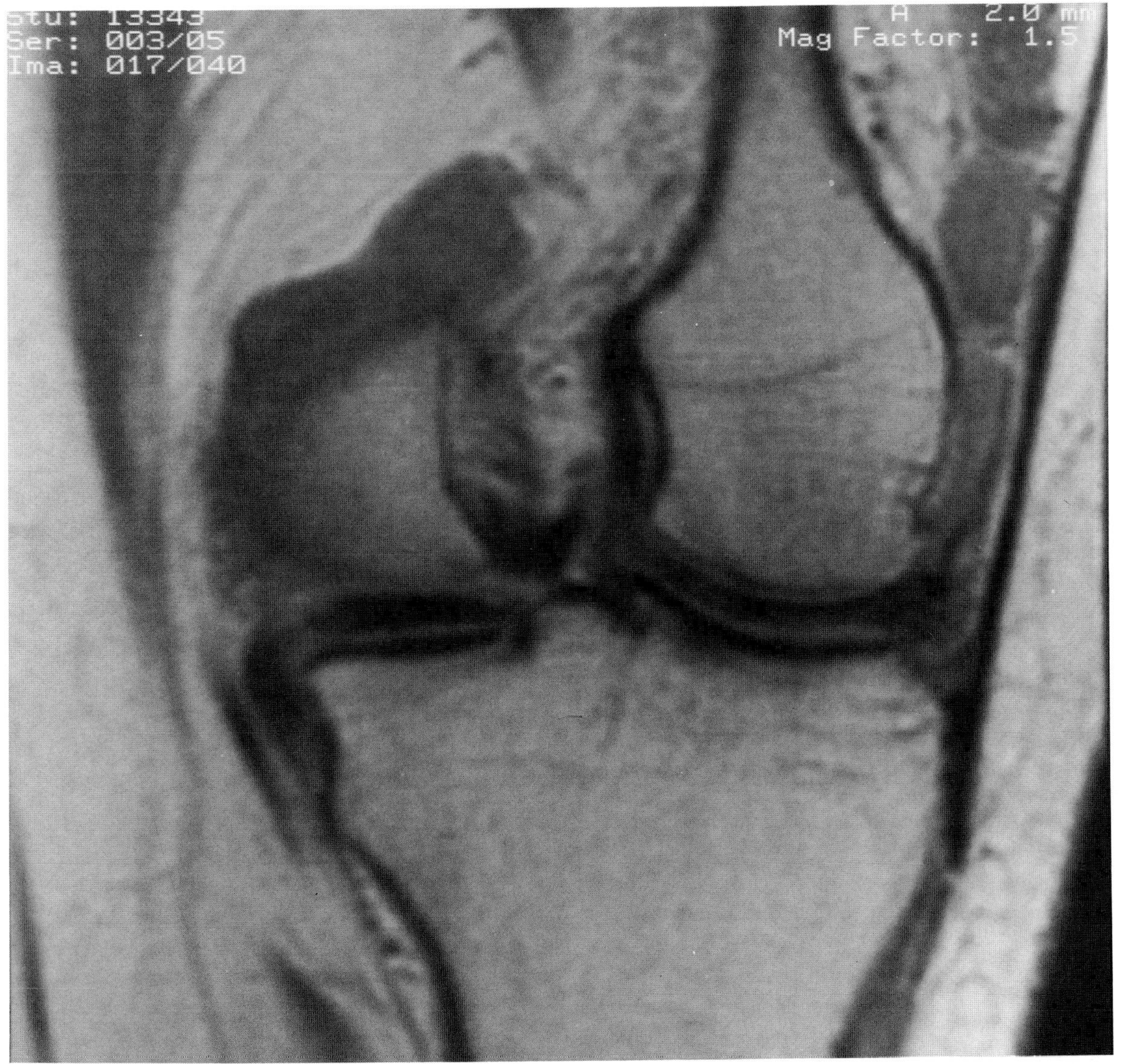

5-17 Knee, coronal view (TR 2000; TE 20). (See note to legend 5-14.)

Knee, Coronal

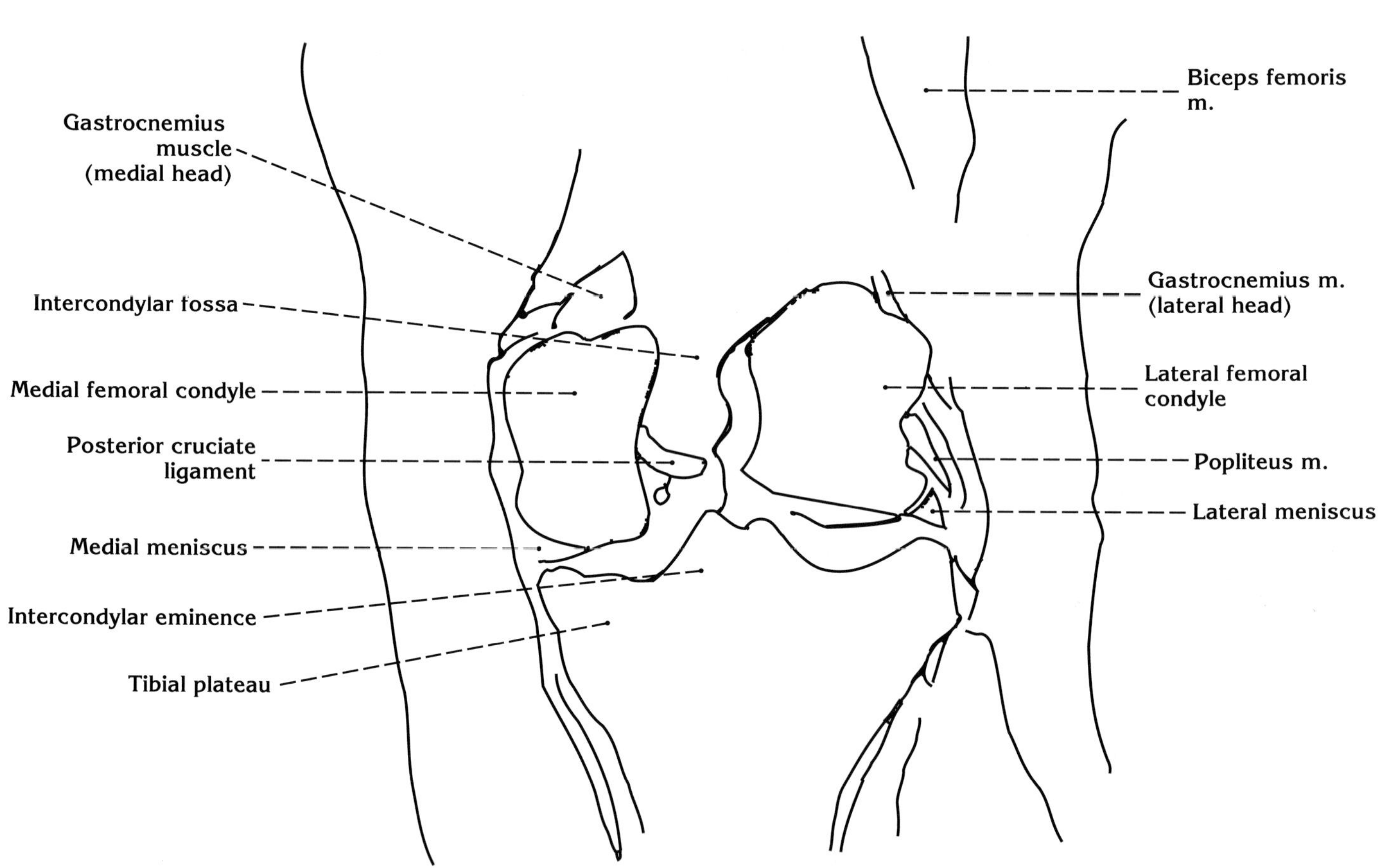

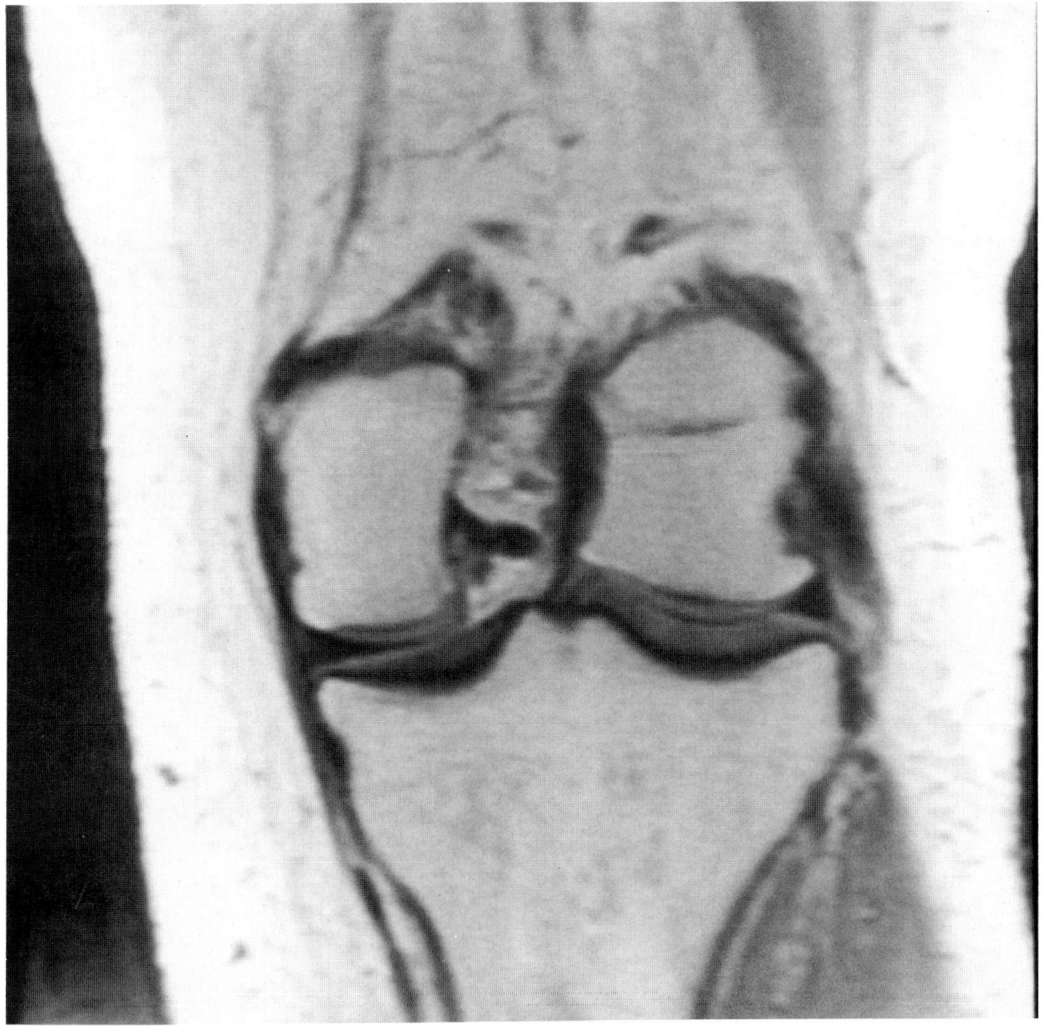

5-18 Knee, coronal view (TR 2000; TE 20). (See note to legend 5-14.)

Knee, Coronal

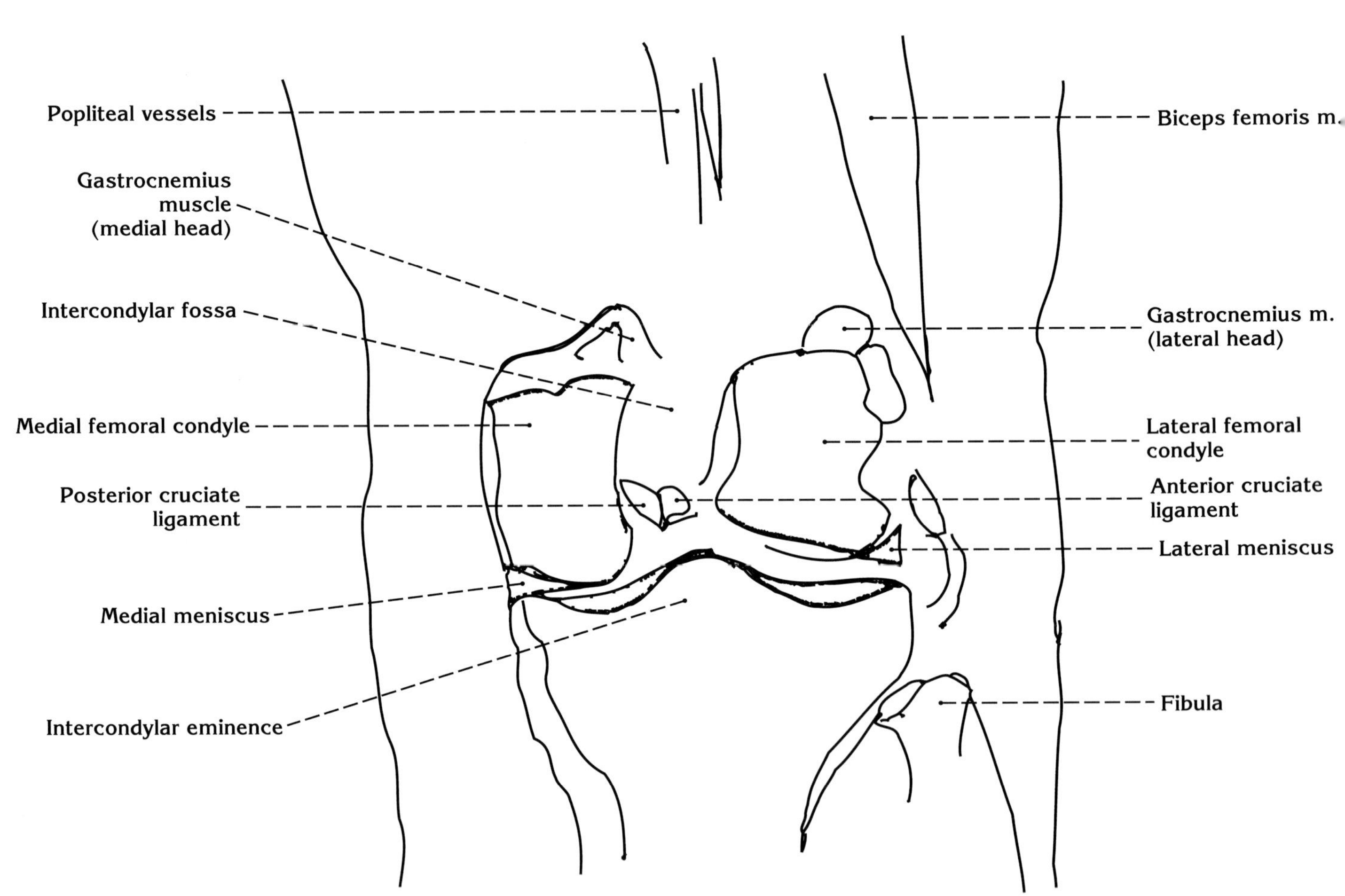

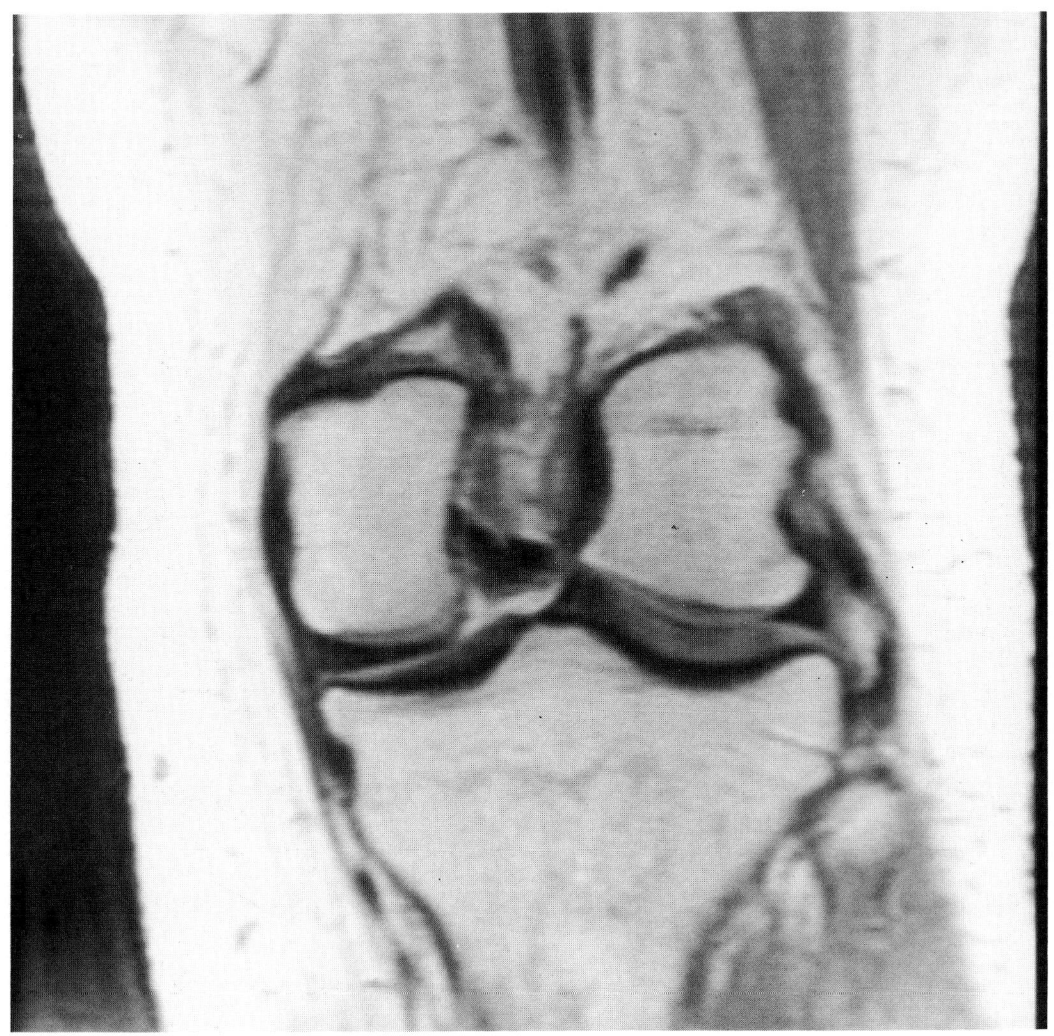

5-19 Knee, coronal view (TR 2000; TE 20). (See note to legend 5-14.)

Knee, Coronal

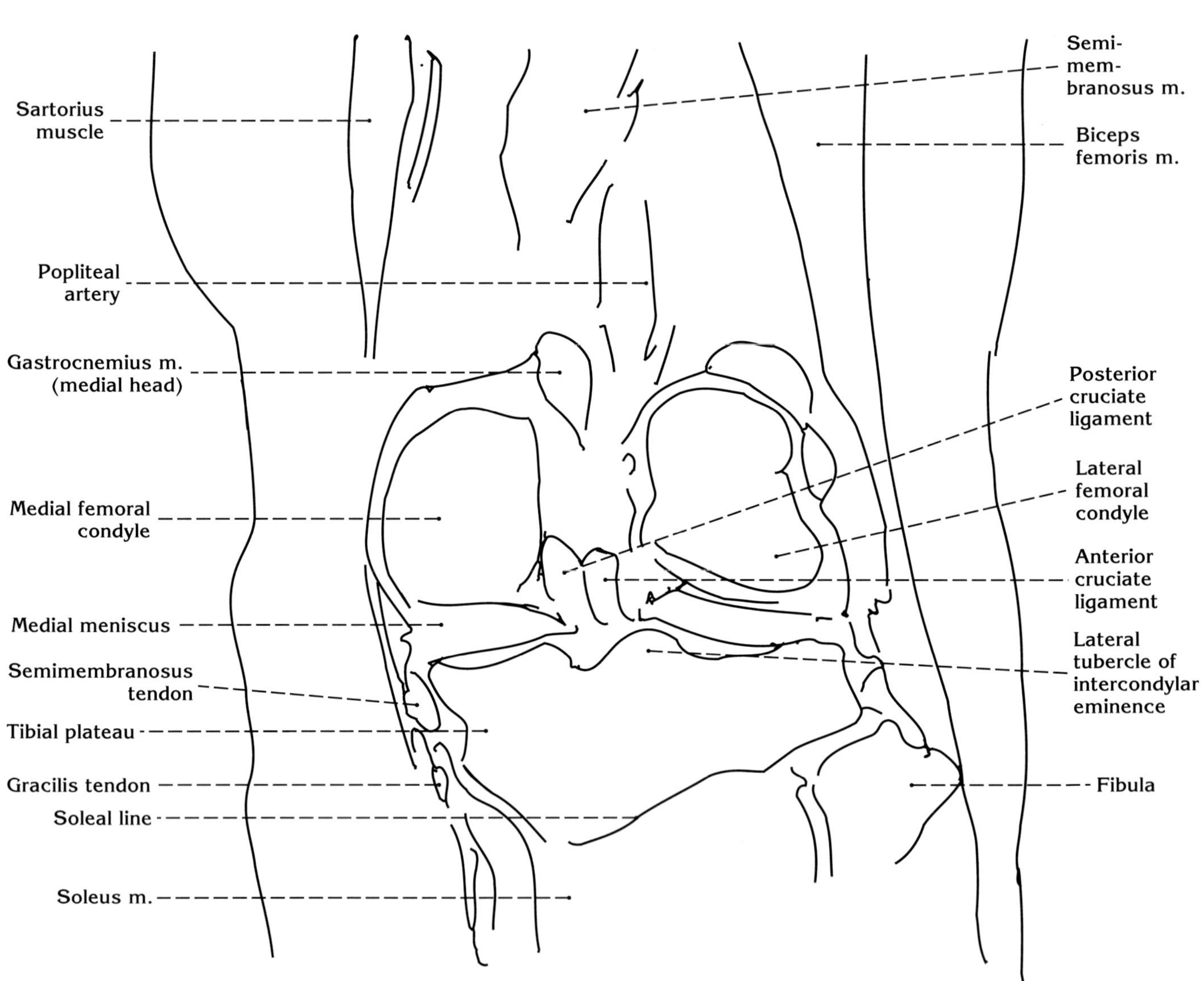

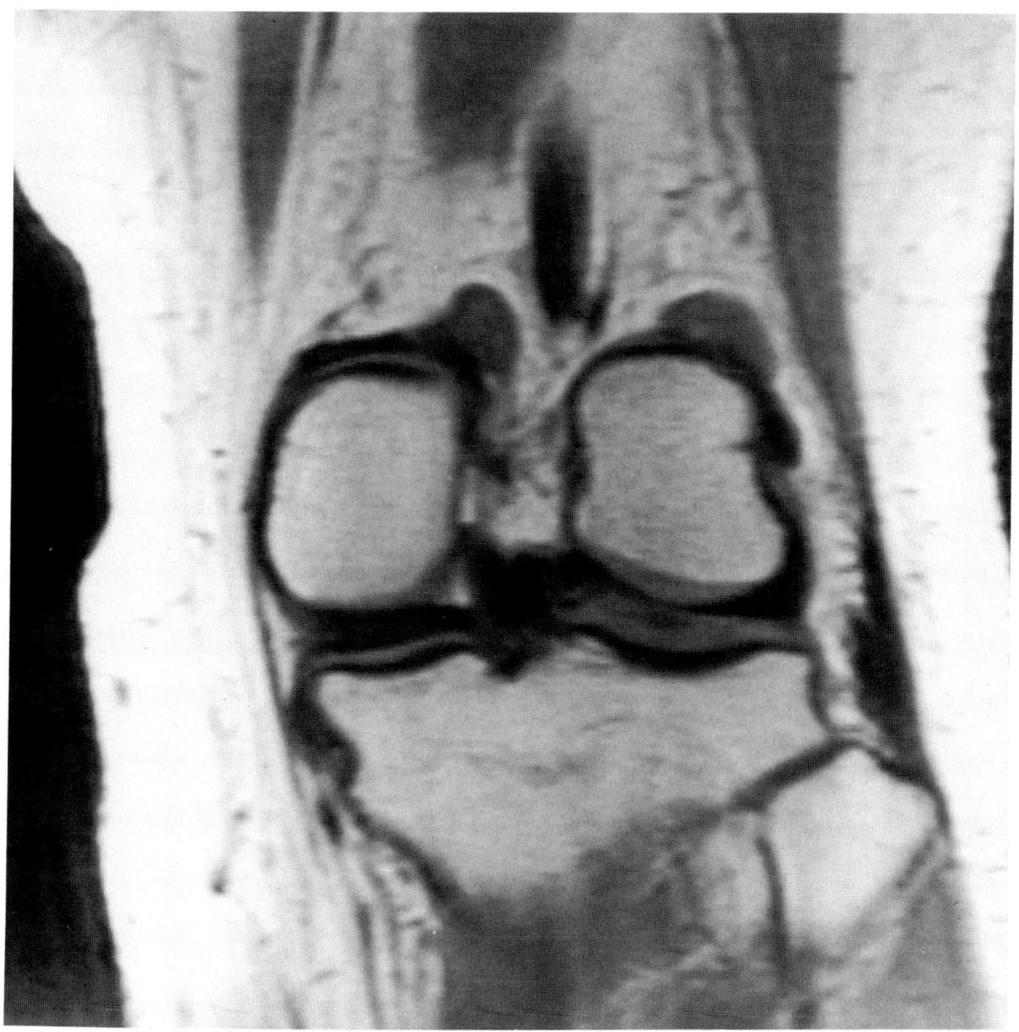

5-20 Knee, coronal view (TR 2000; TE 20). (See note to legend 5-14.)

Knee, Coronal

SUPERIOR

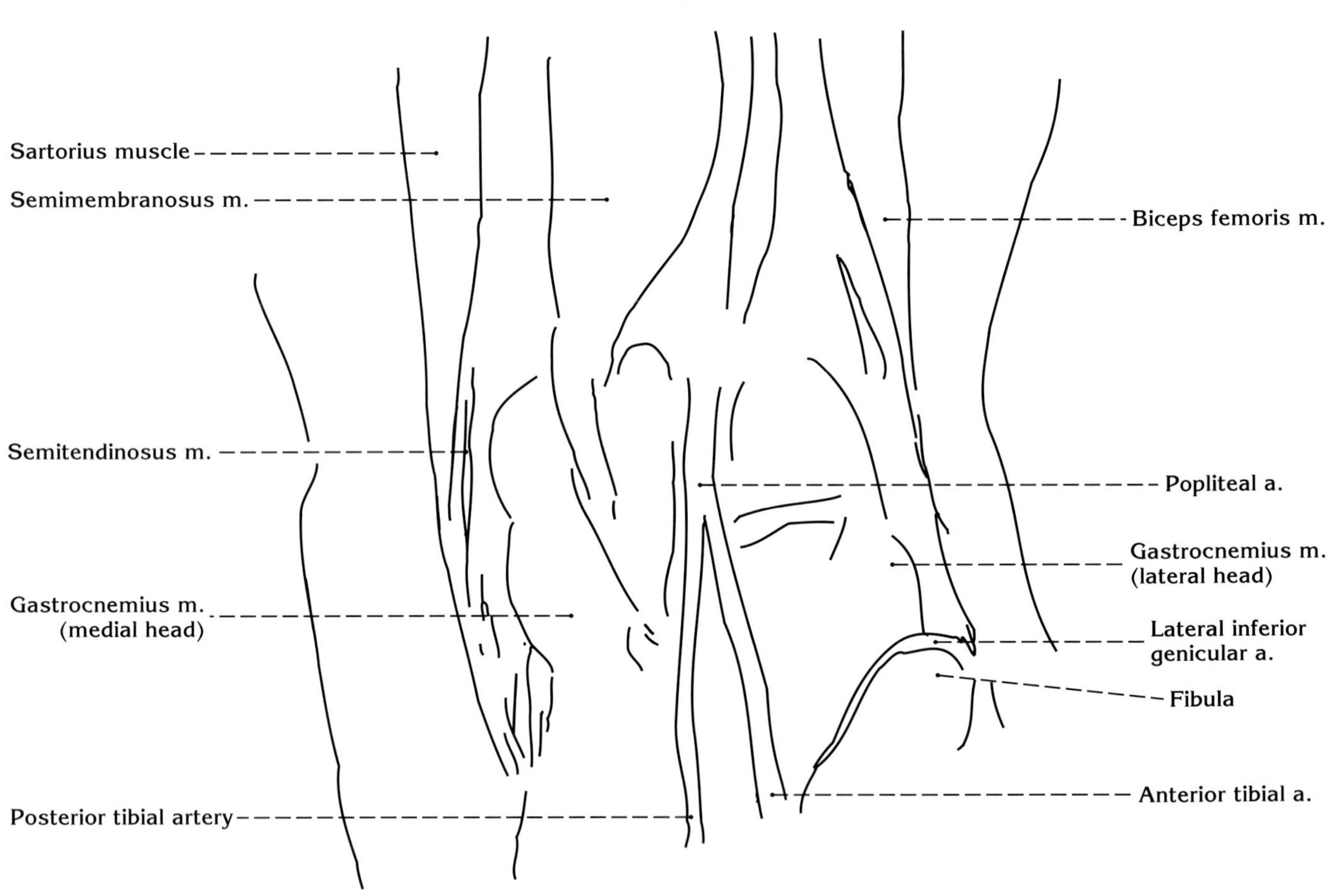

INFERIOR

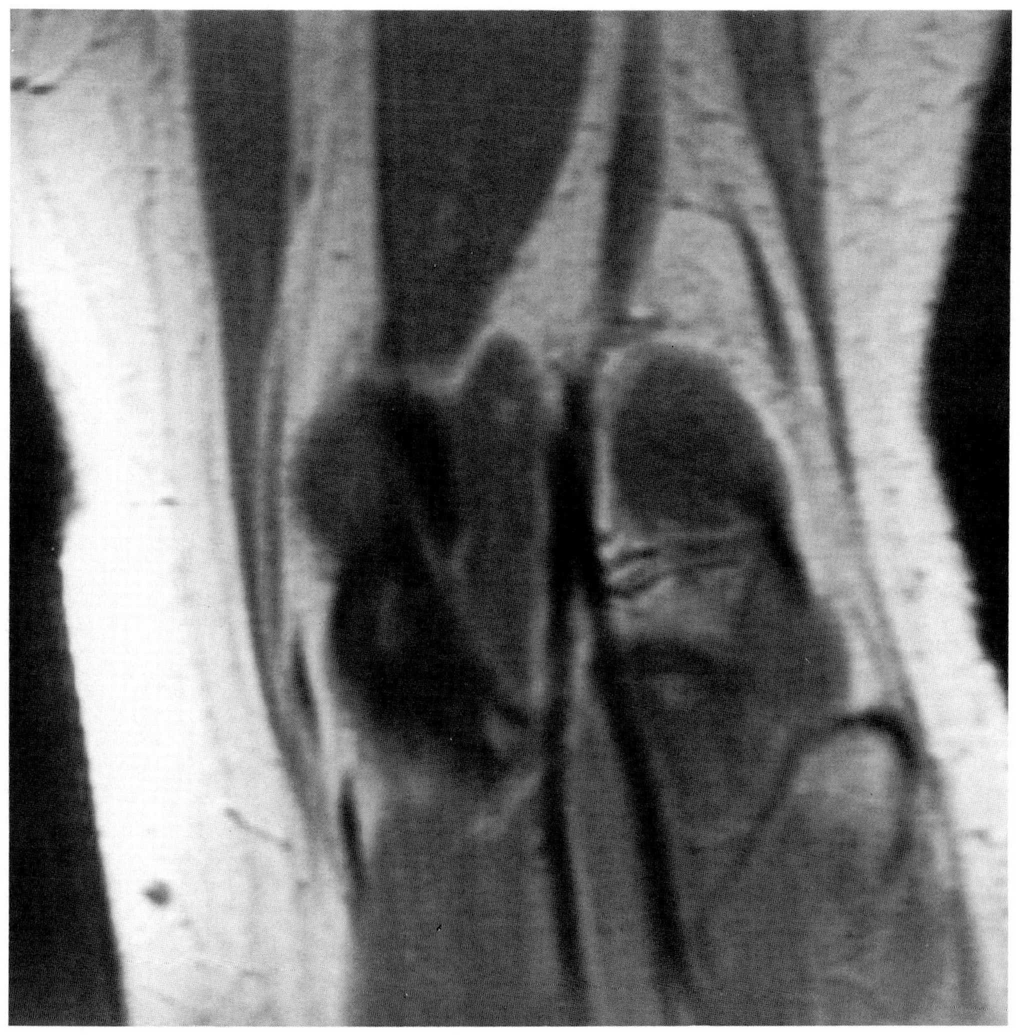

5-21 Knee, coronal view (TR 2000; TE 20).

Knee, Sagittal

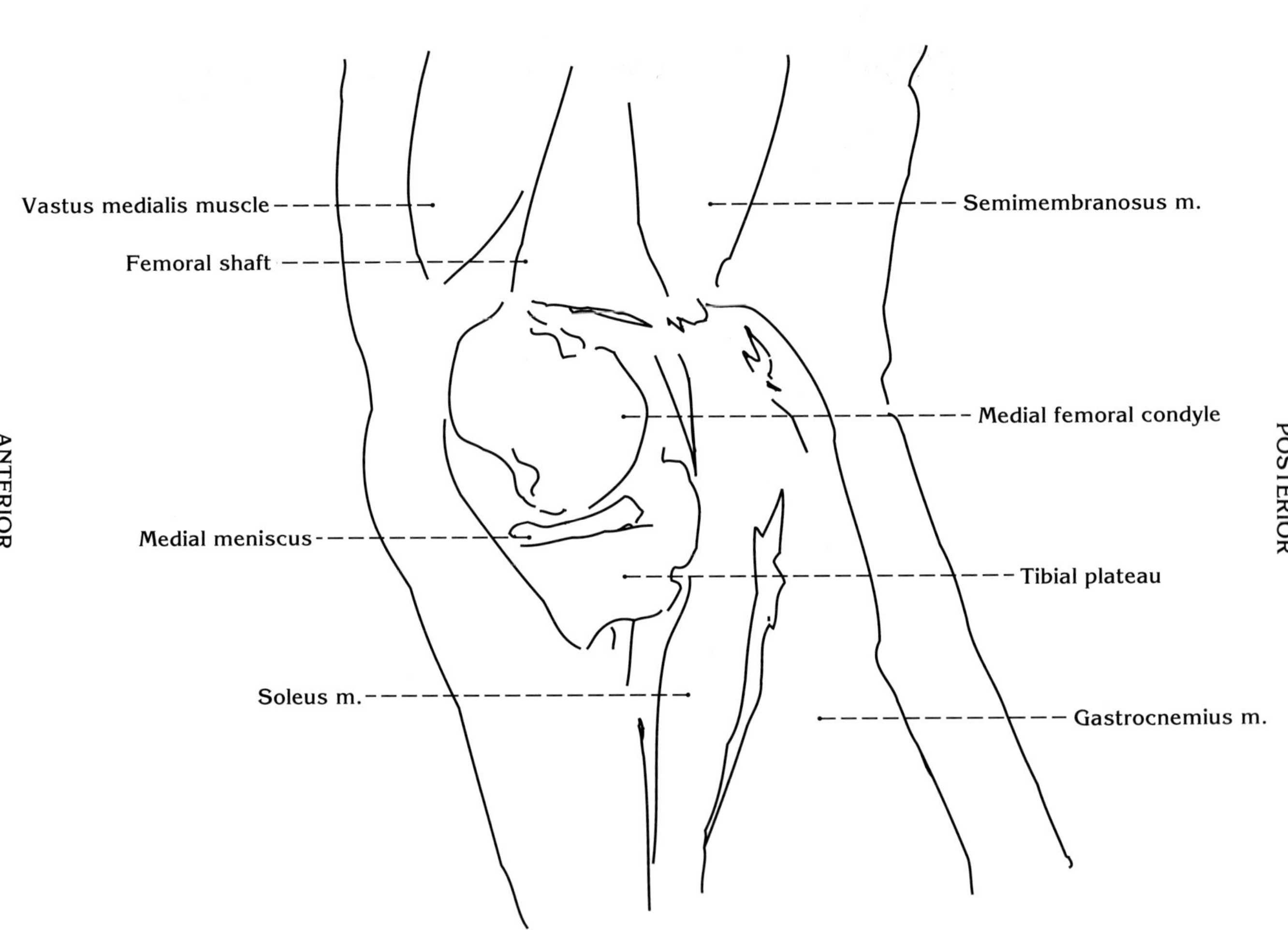

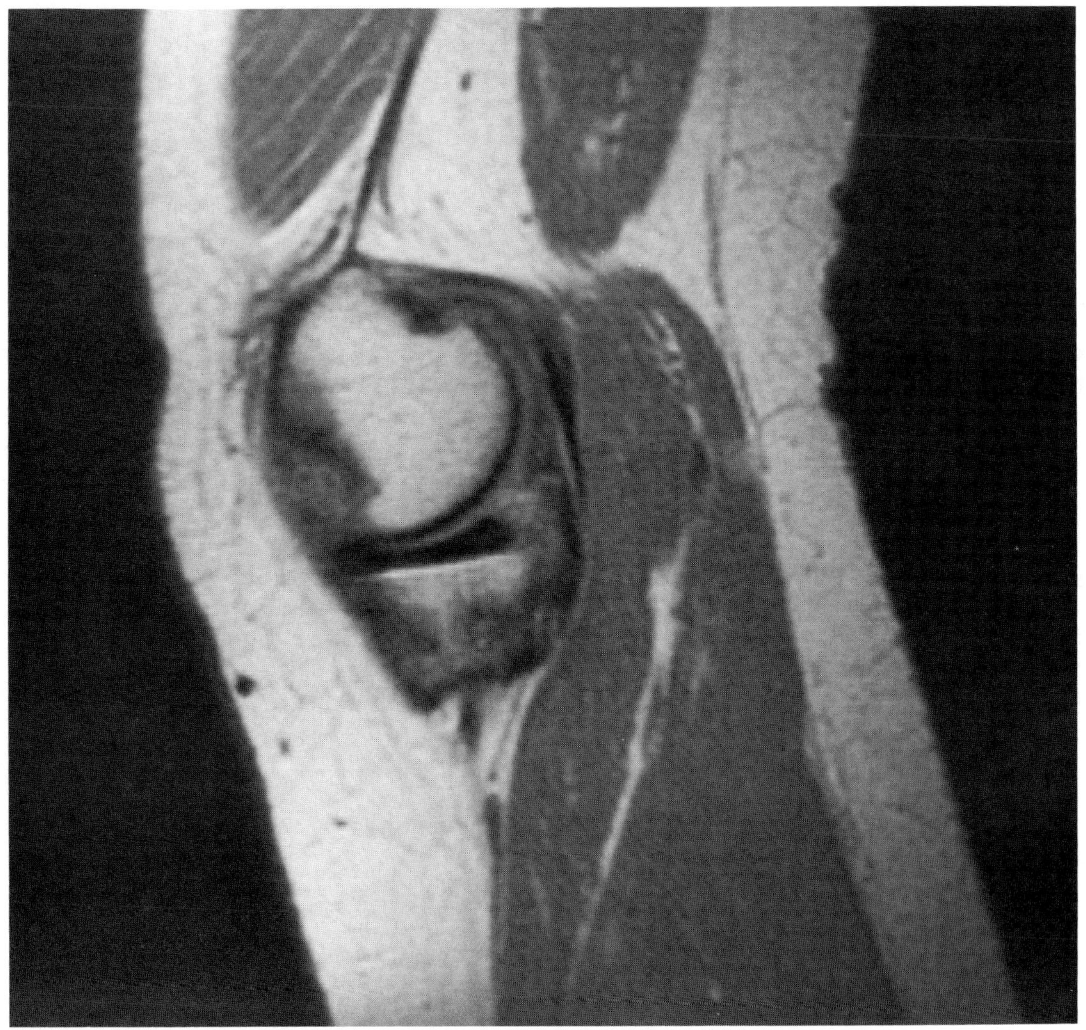

5-22 Knee, sagittal view (TR 2000; TE 20).

Knee, Sagittal

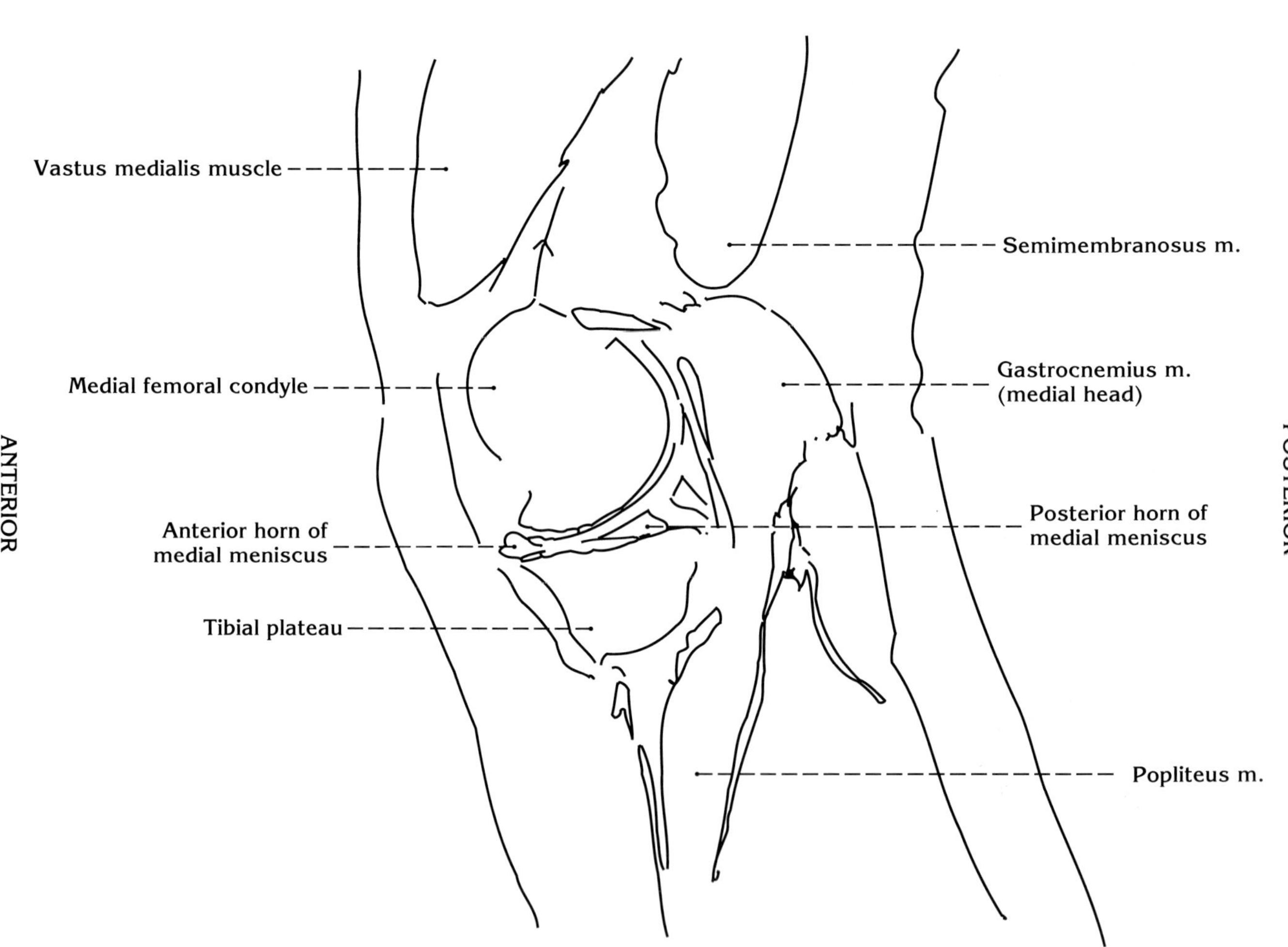

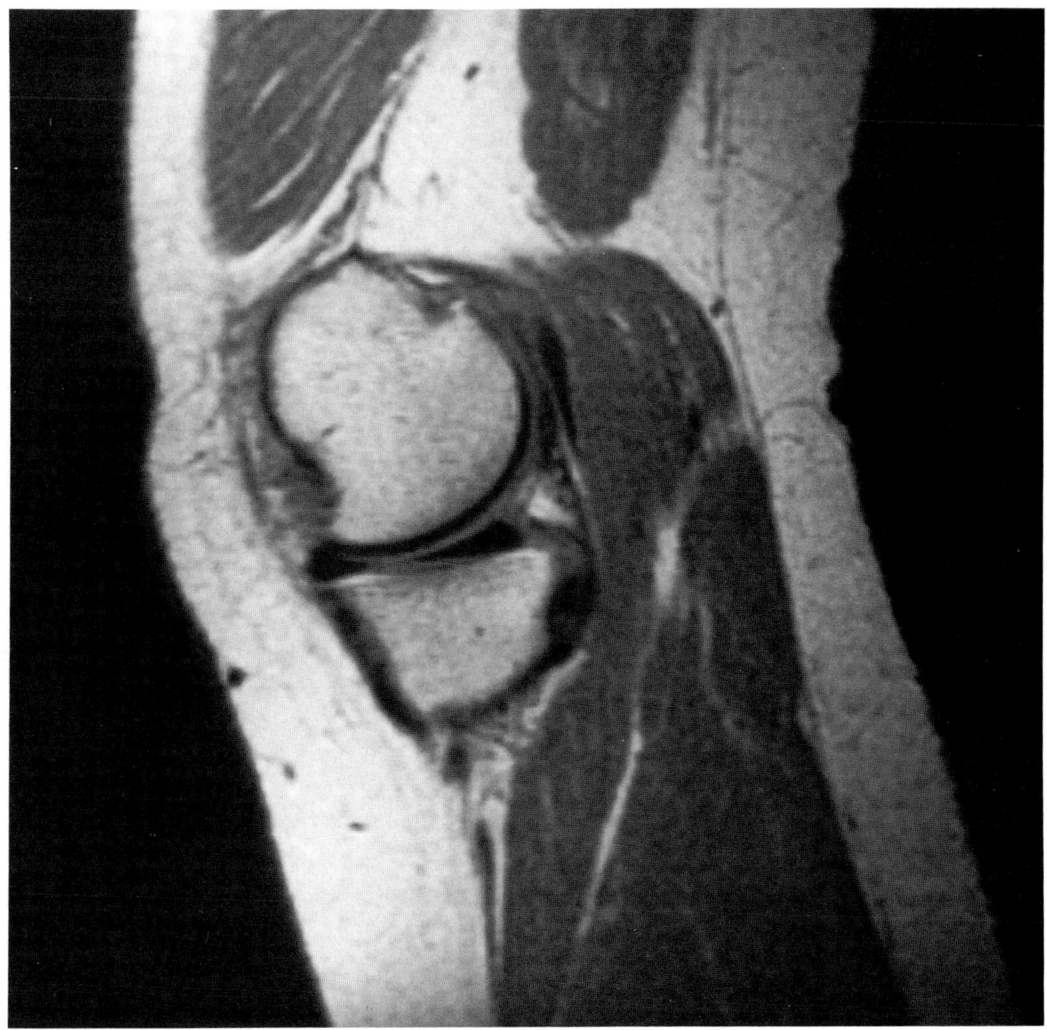

5-23 Knee, sagittal view (TR 2000; TE 20).

Knee, Sagittal

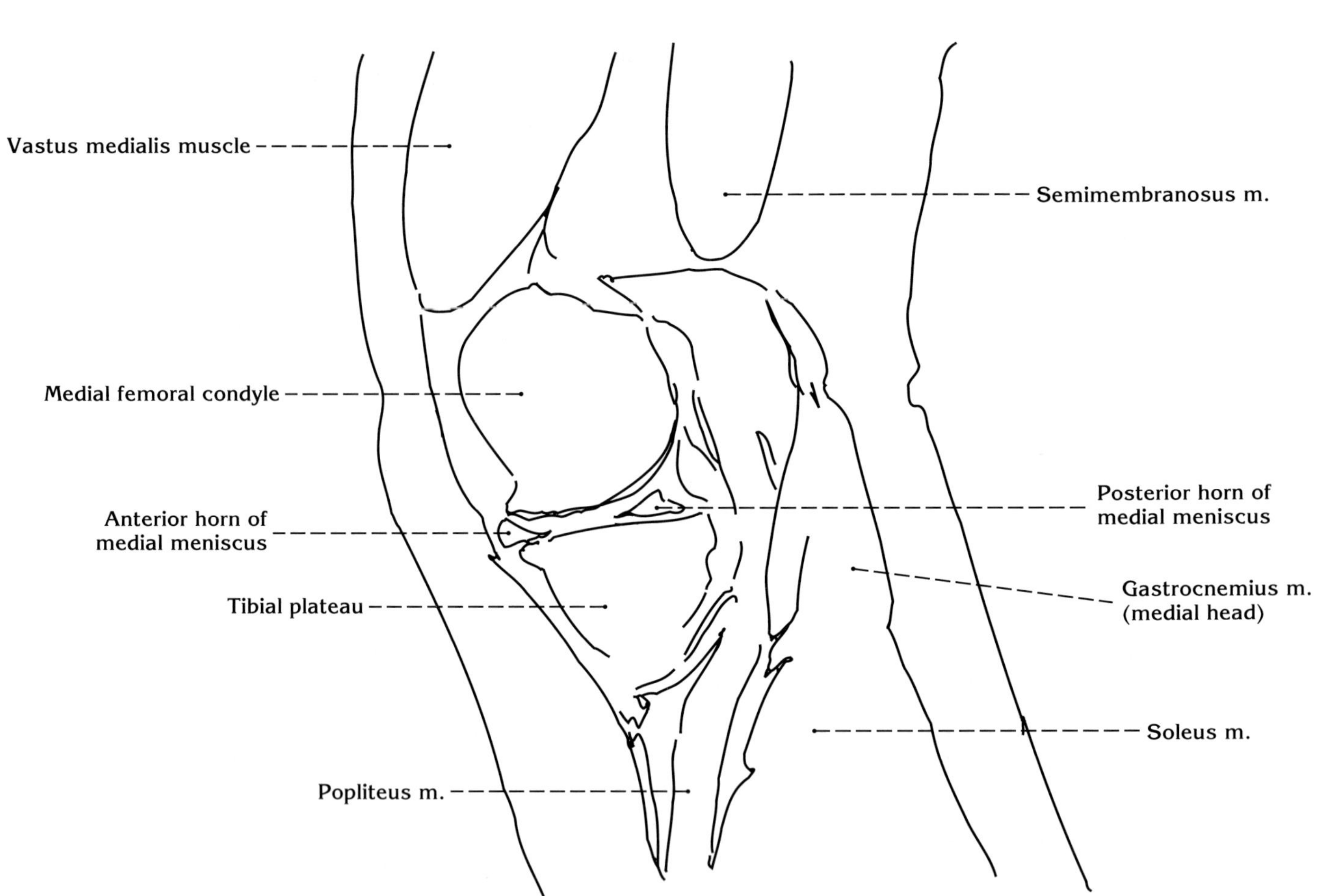

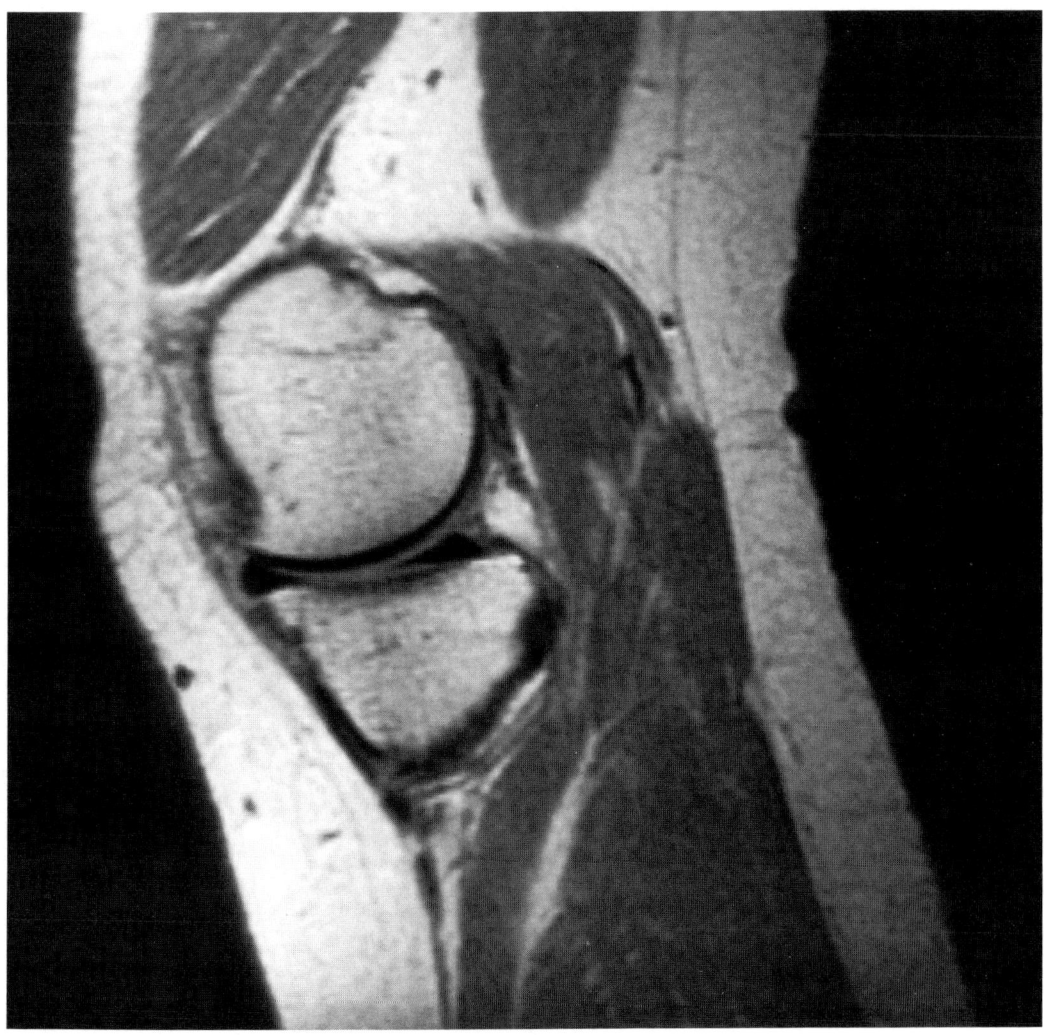

5-24 Knee, sagittal view (TR 2000; TE 20).

Knee, Sagittal

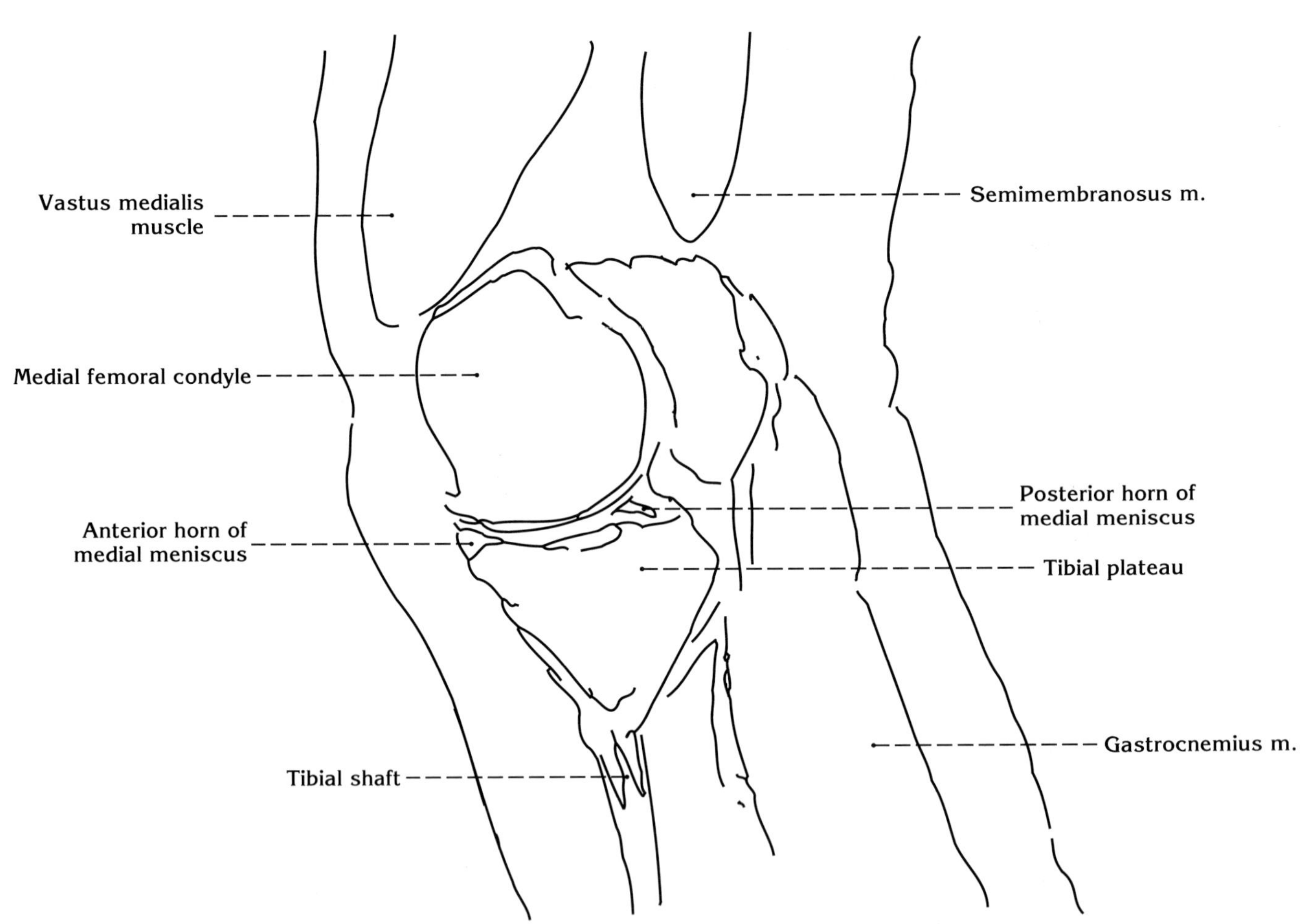

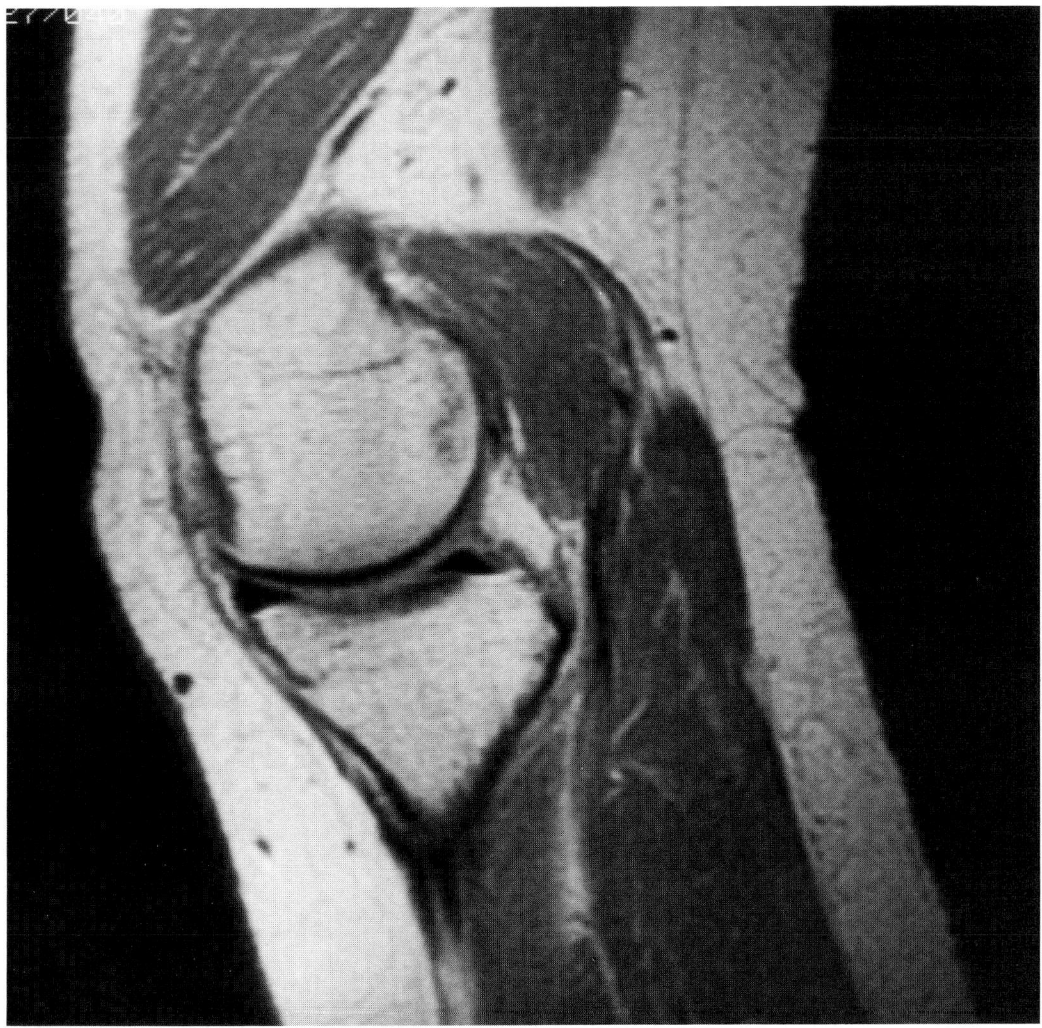

5-25 Knee, sagittal view (TR 2000; TE 20).

Knee, Sagittal

SUPERIOR

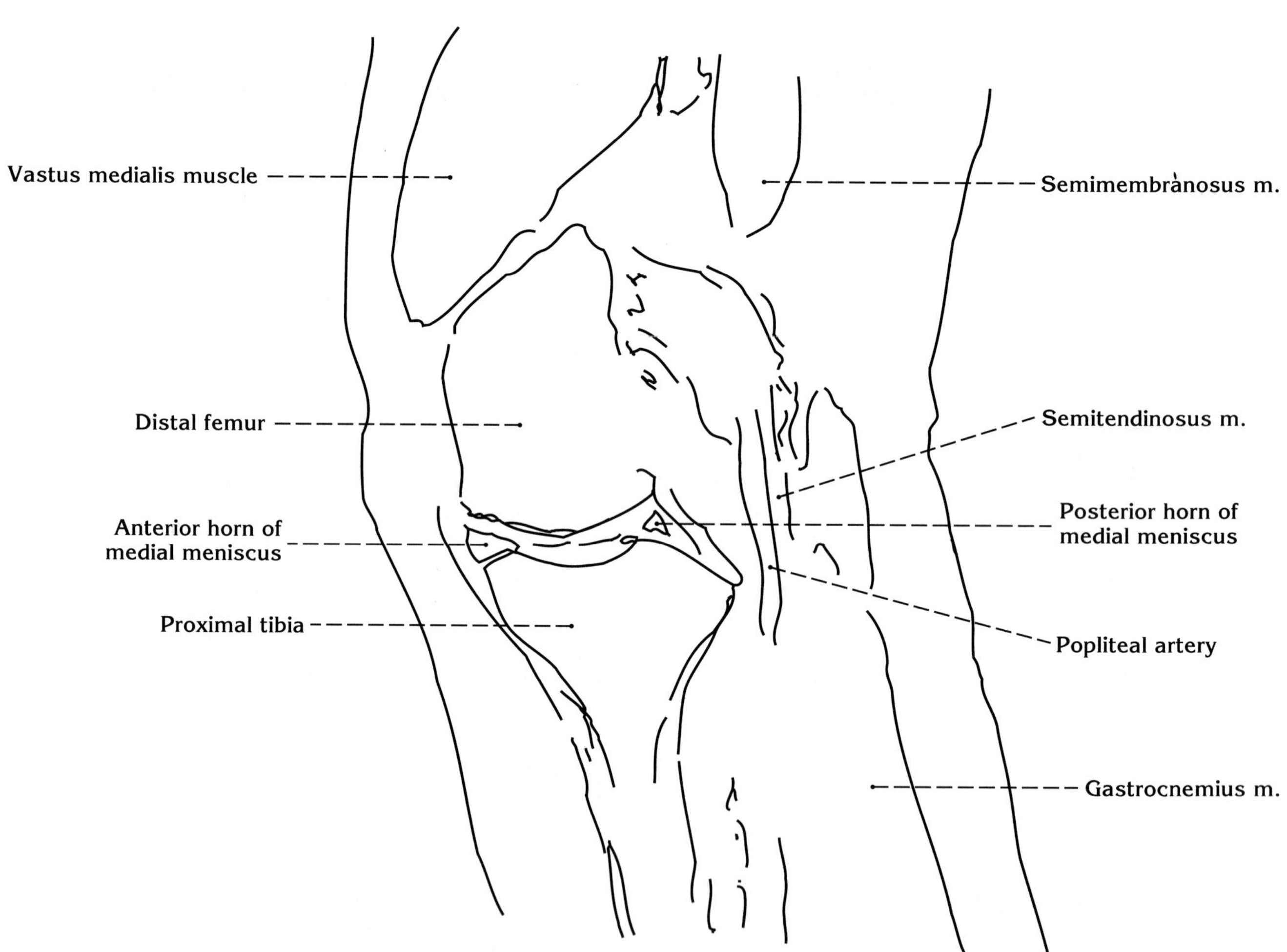

INFERIOR

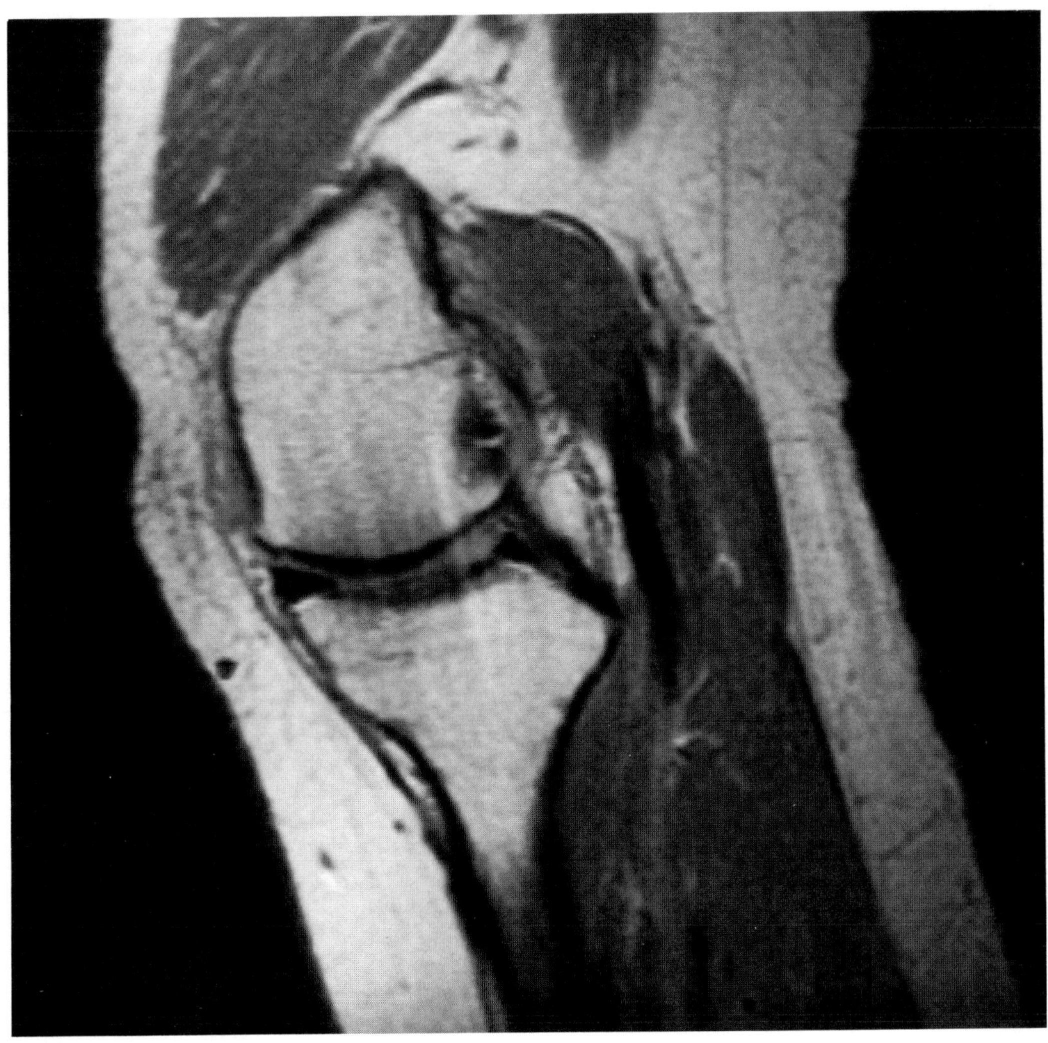

5-26 Knee, sagittal view (TR 2000; TE 20).

Knee, Sagittal

SUPERIOR

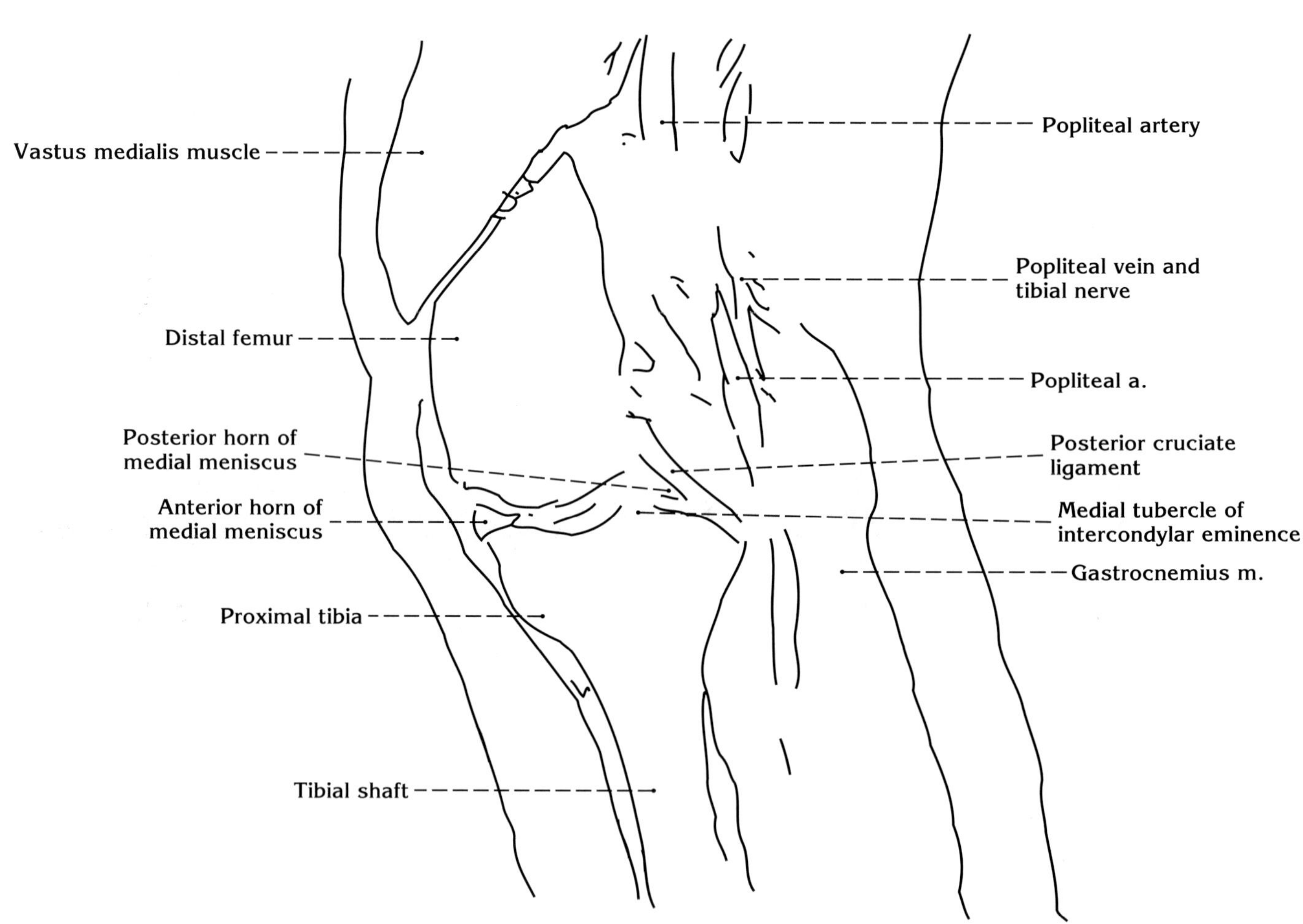

INFERIOR

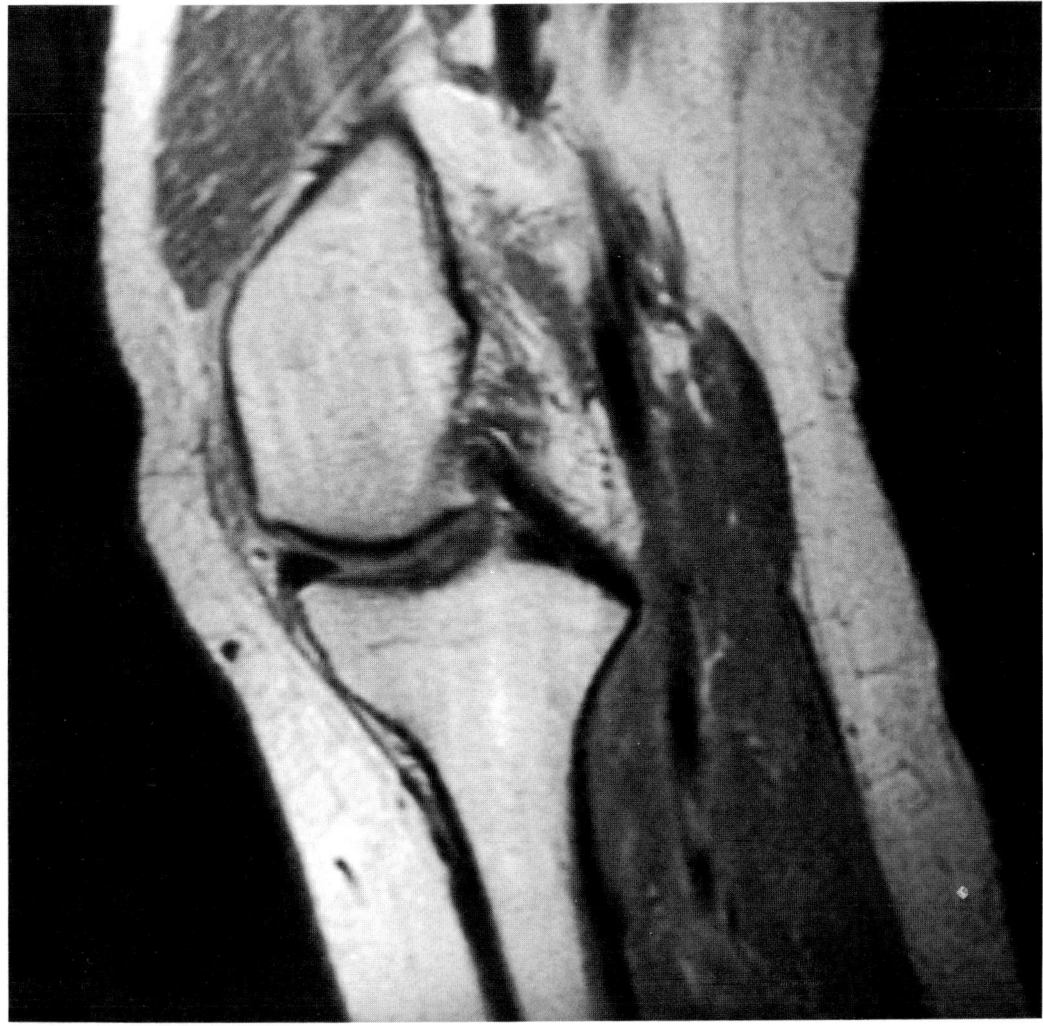

5-27 Knee, sagittal view (TR 2000; TE 20).

Knee, Sagittal

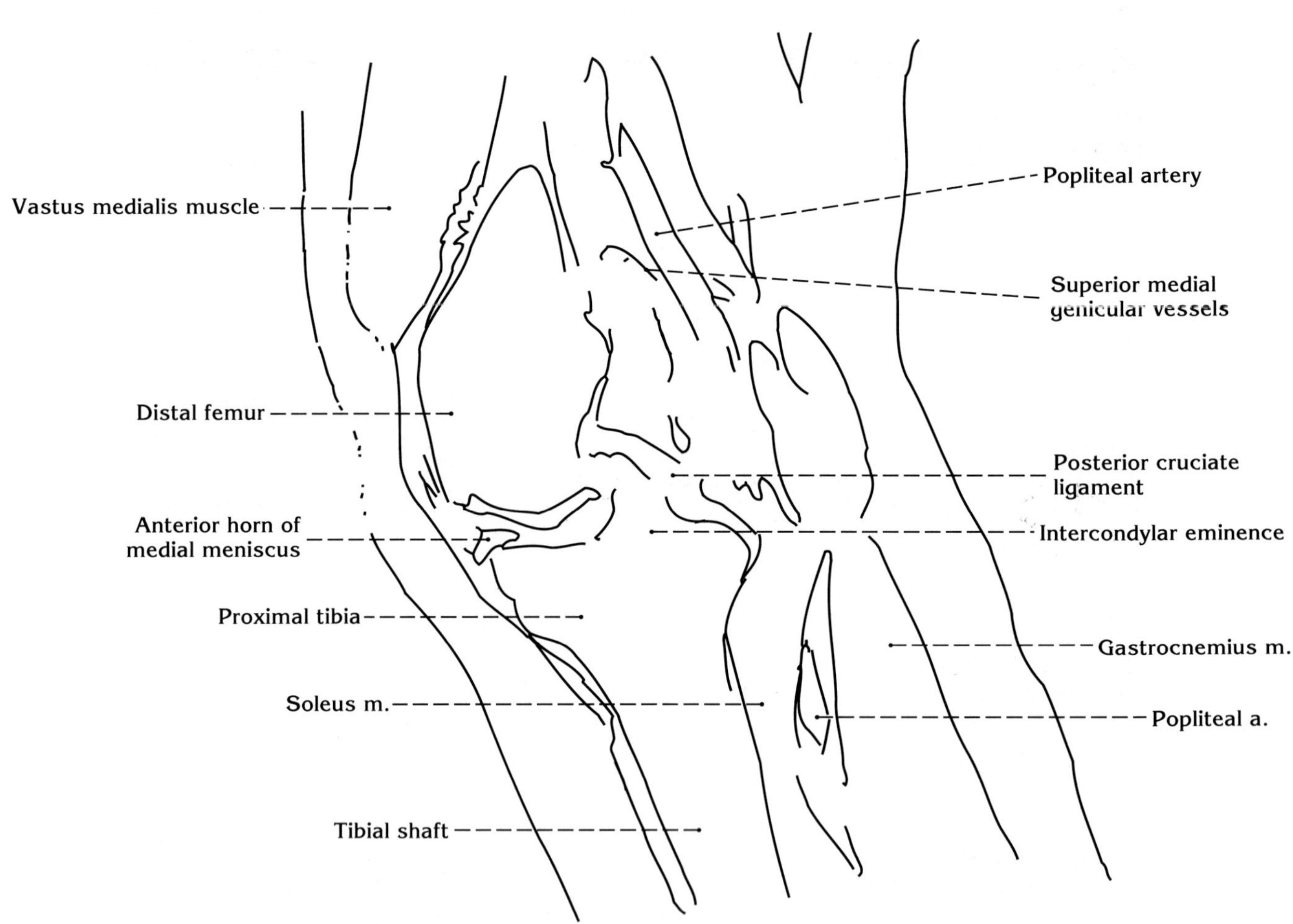

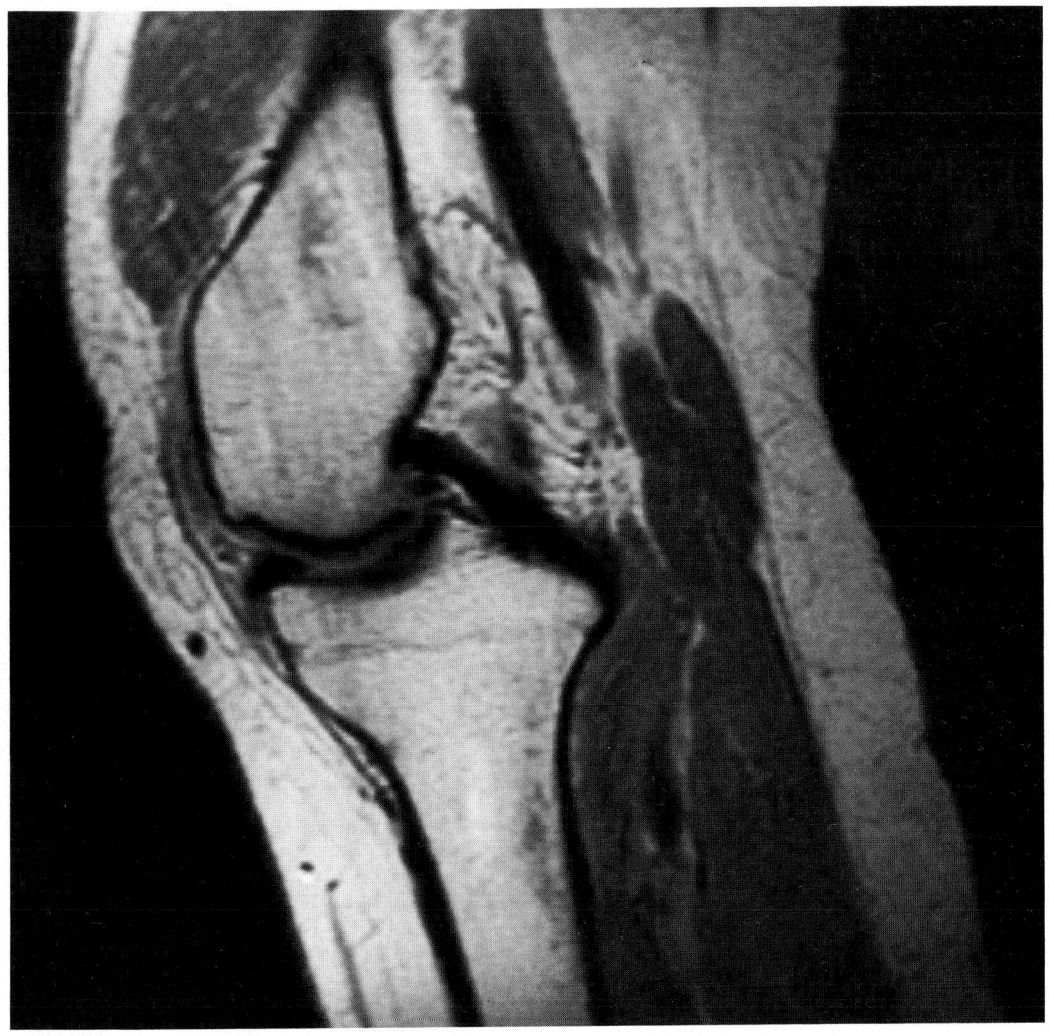

5-28 Knee, sagittal view (TR 2000; TE 20).

Knee, Sagittal

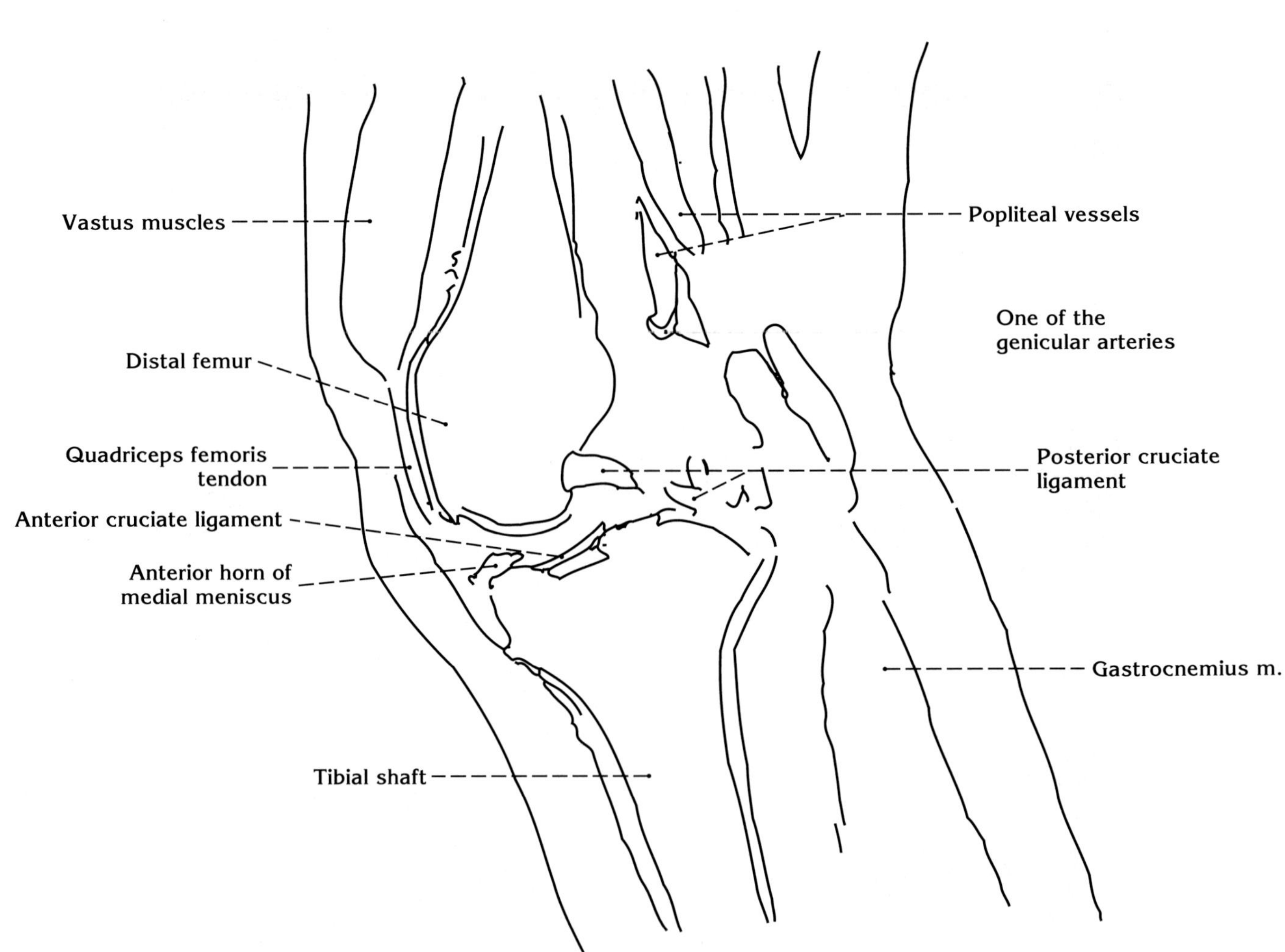

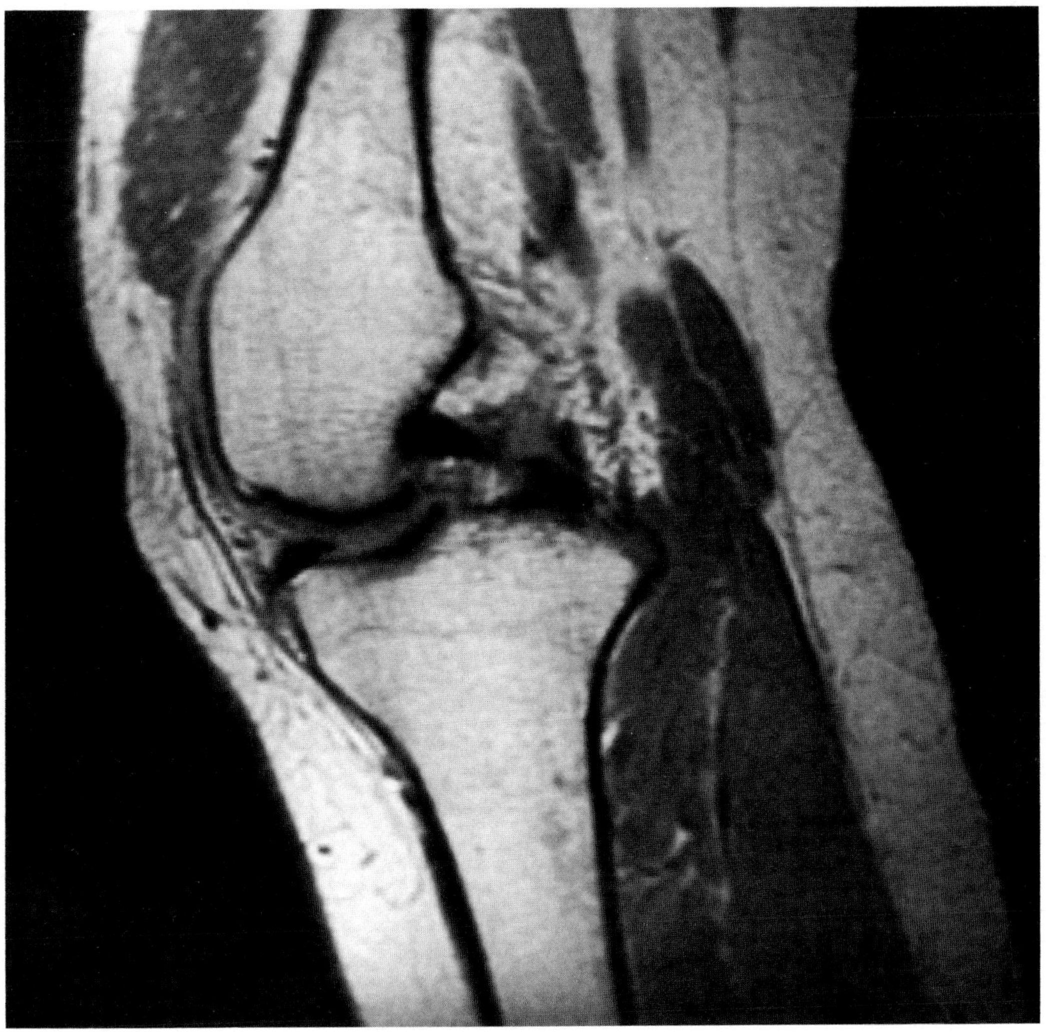

5-29 Knee, sagittal view (TR 2000; TE 20).

Knee, Sagittal

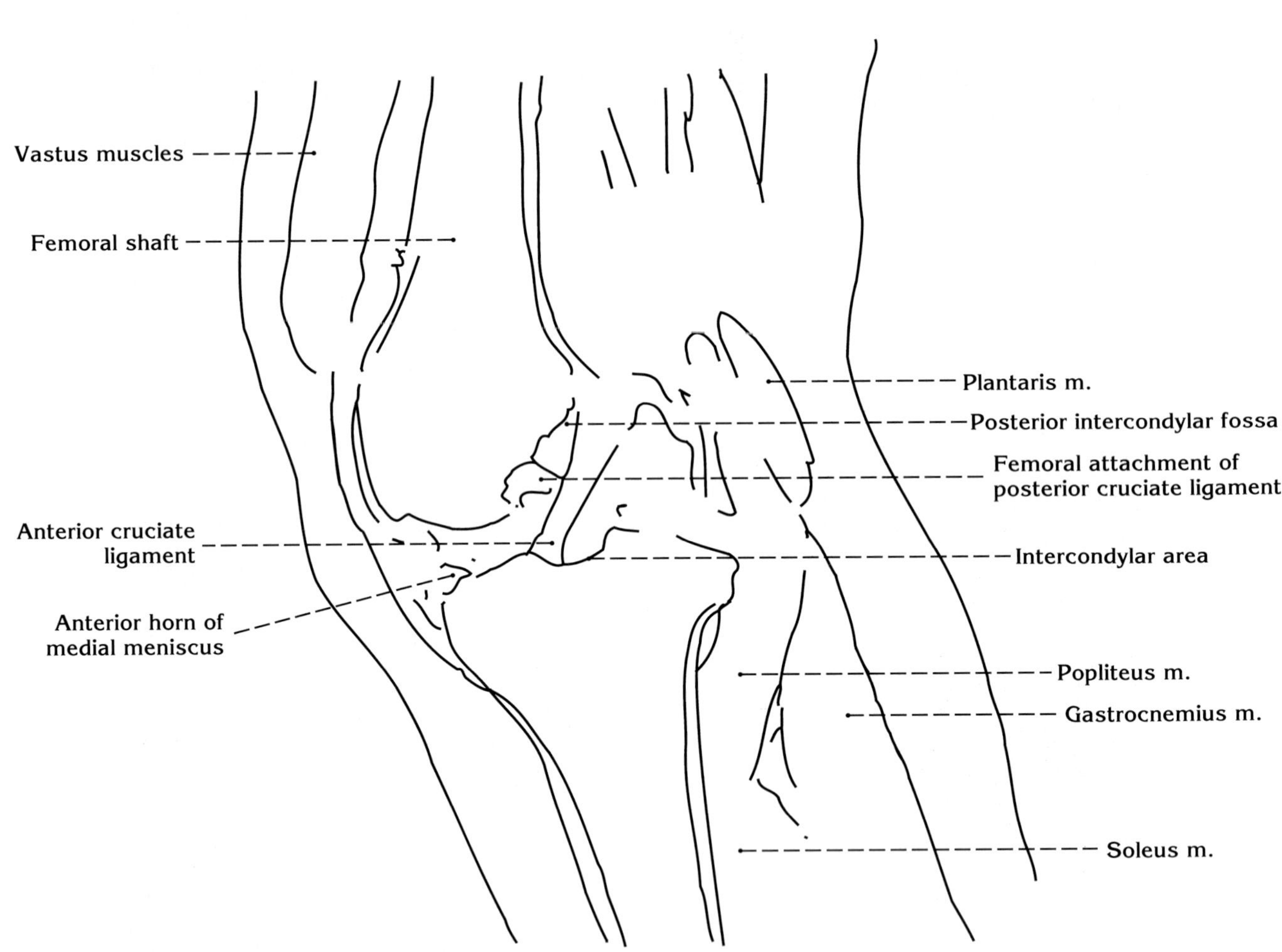

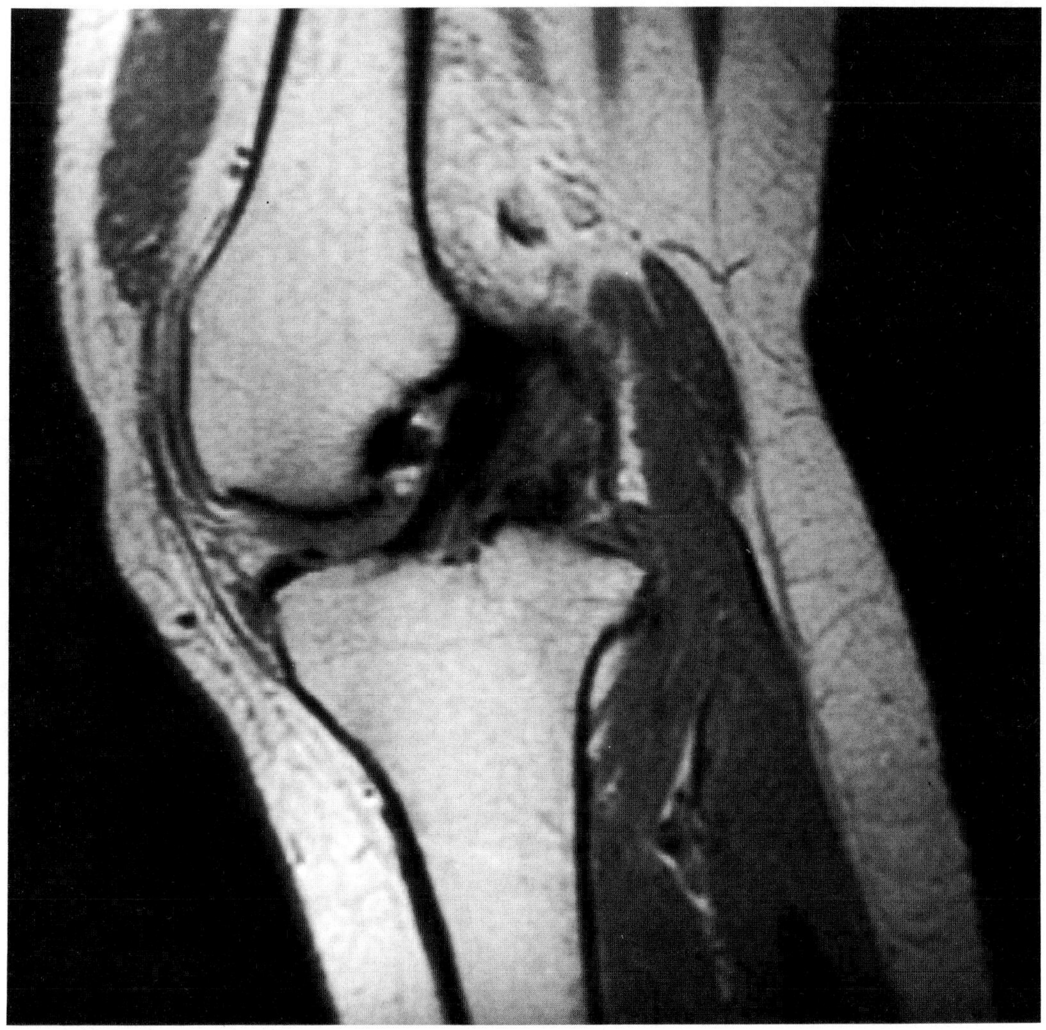

5-30 Knee, sagittal view (TR 2000; TE 20).

Knee, Sagittal

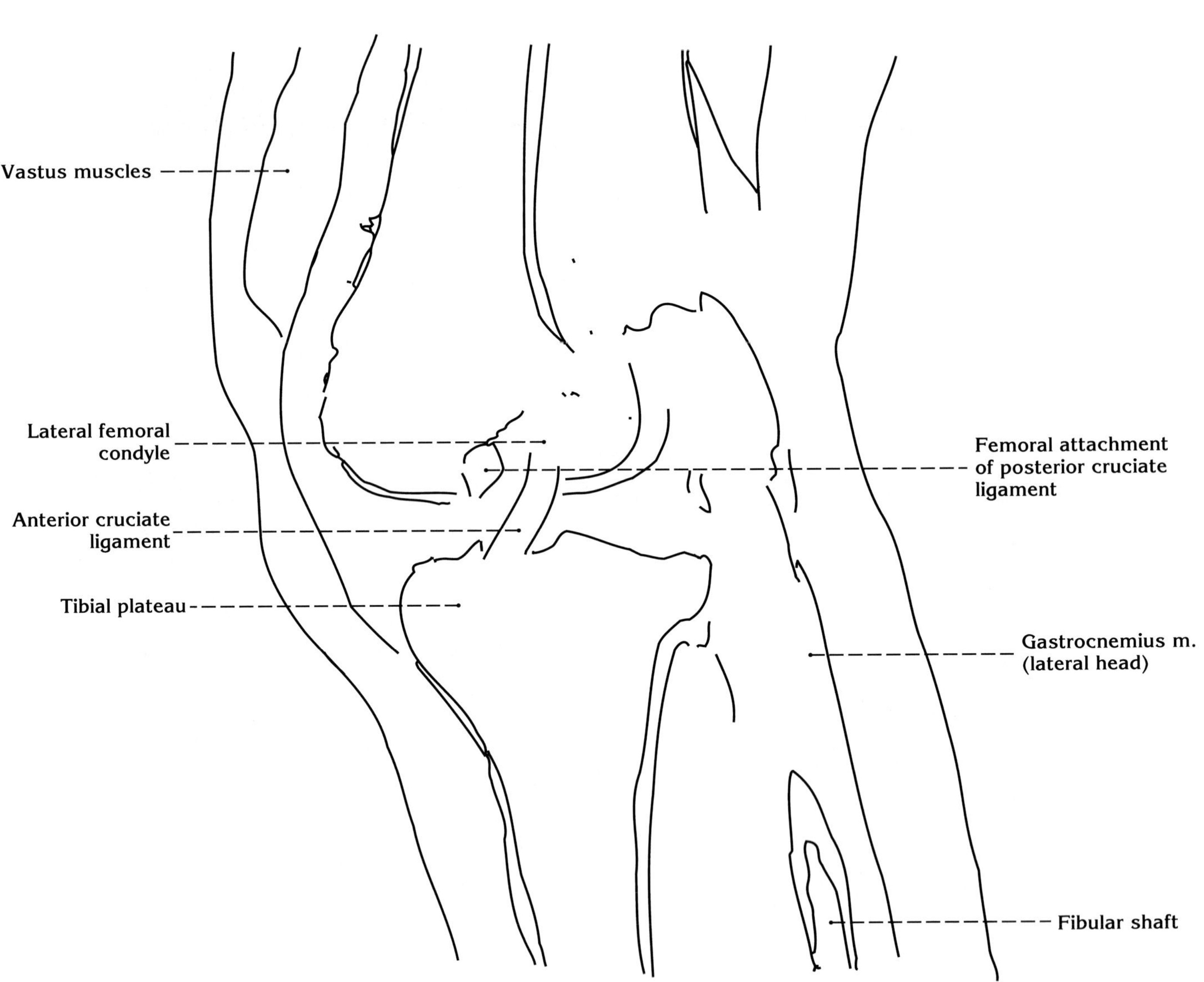

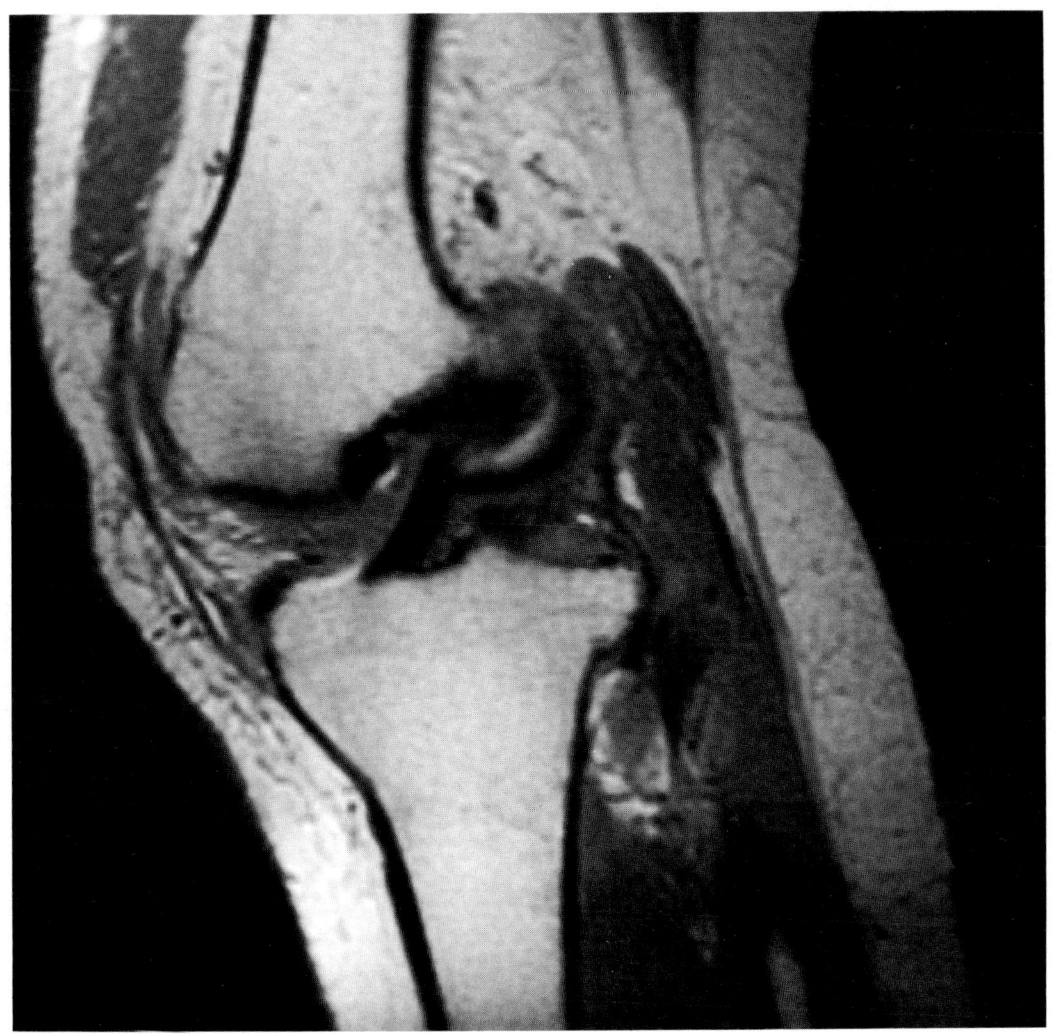

5-31 Knee, sagittal view (TR 2000; TE 20).

Knee, Sagittal

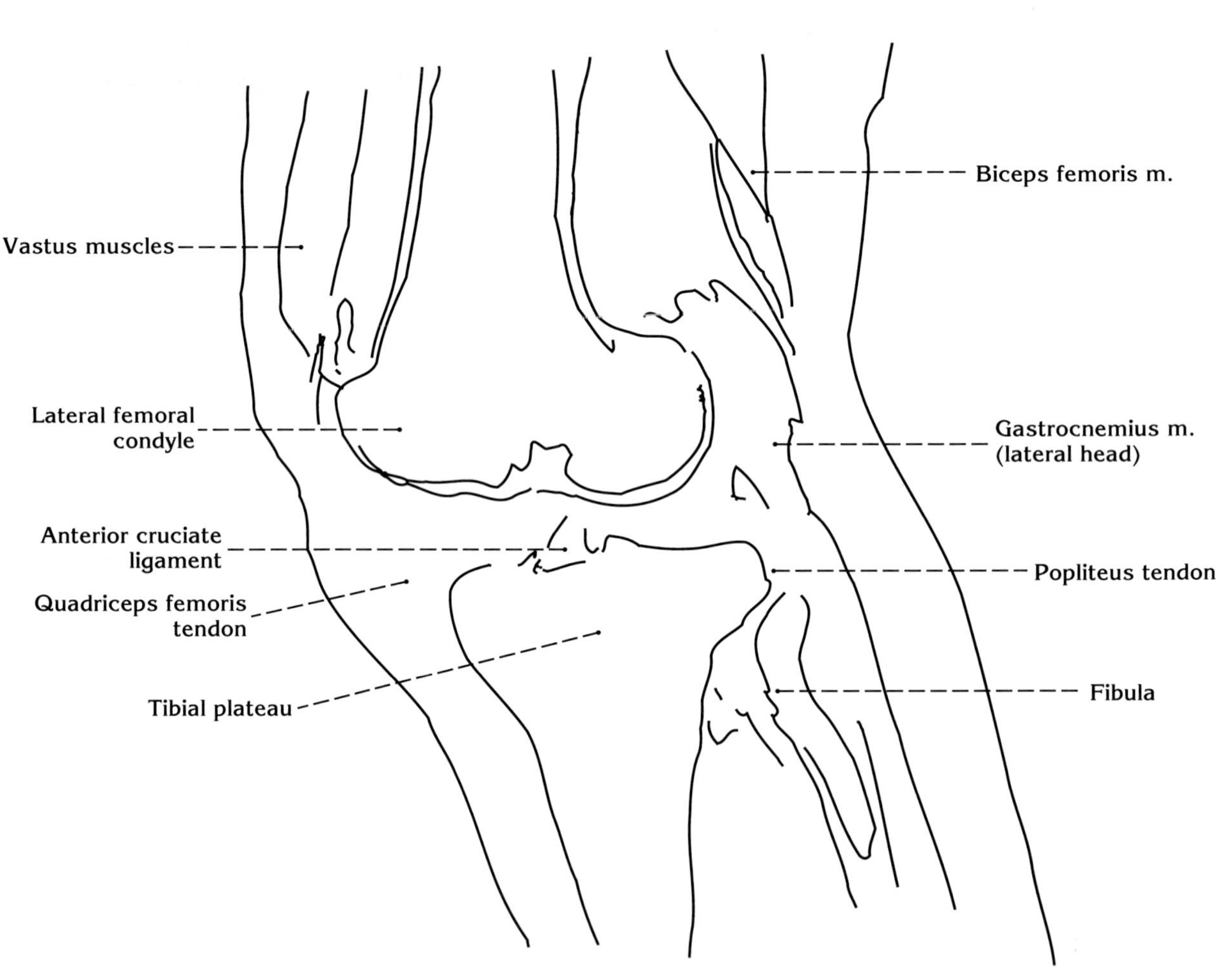

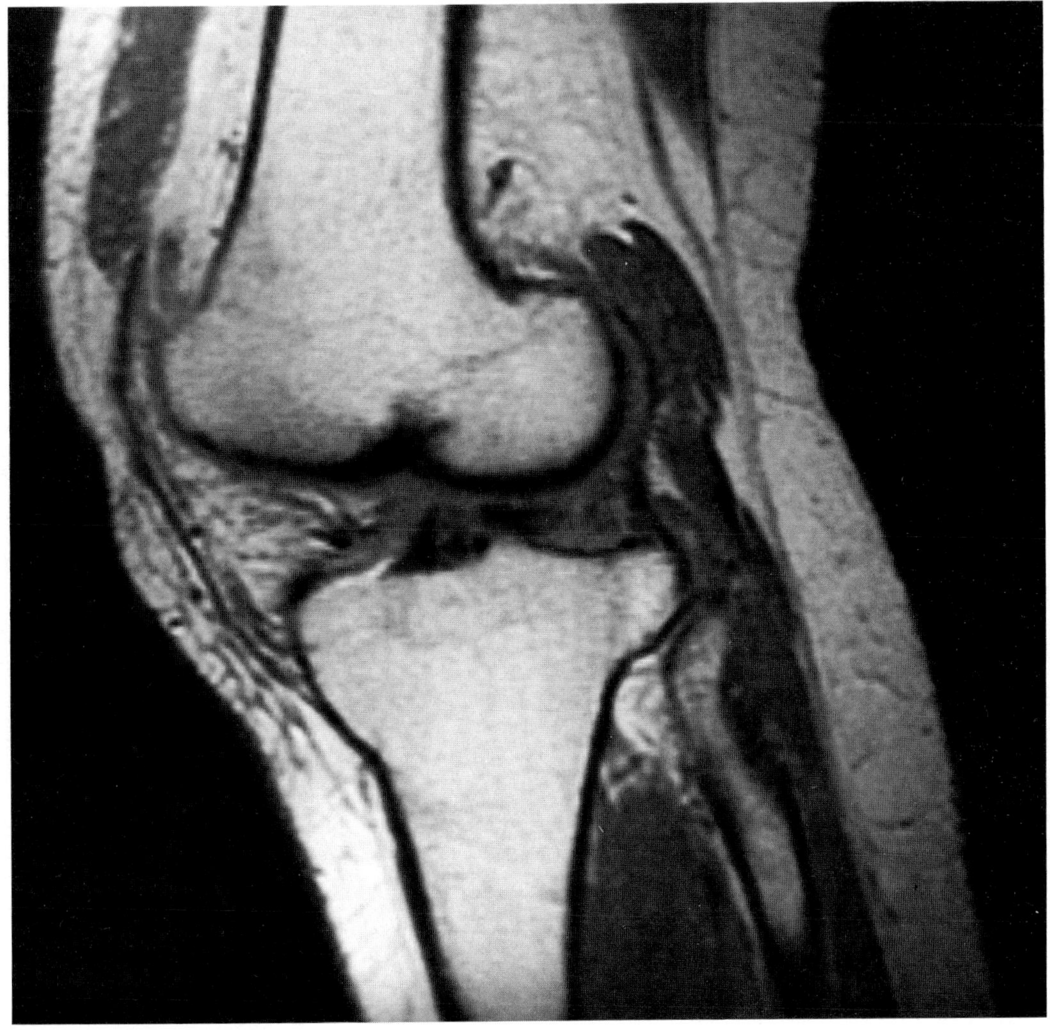

5-32 Knee, sagittal view (TR 2000; TE 20).

Knee, Sagittal

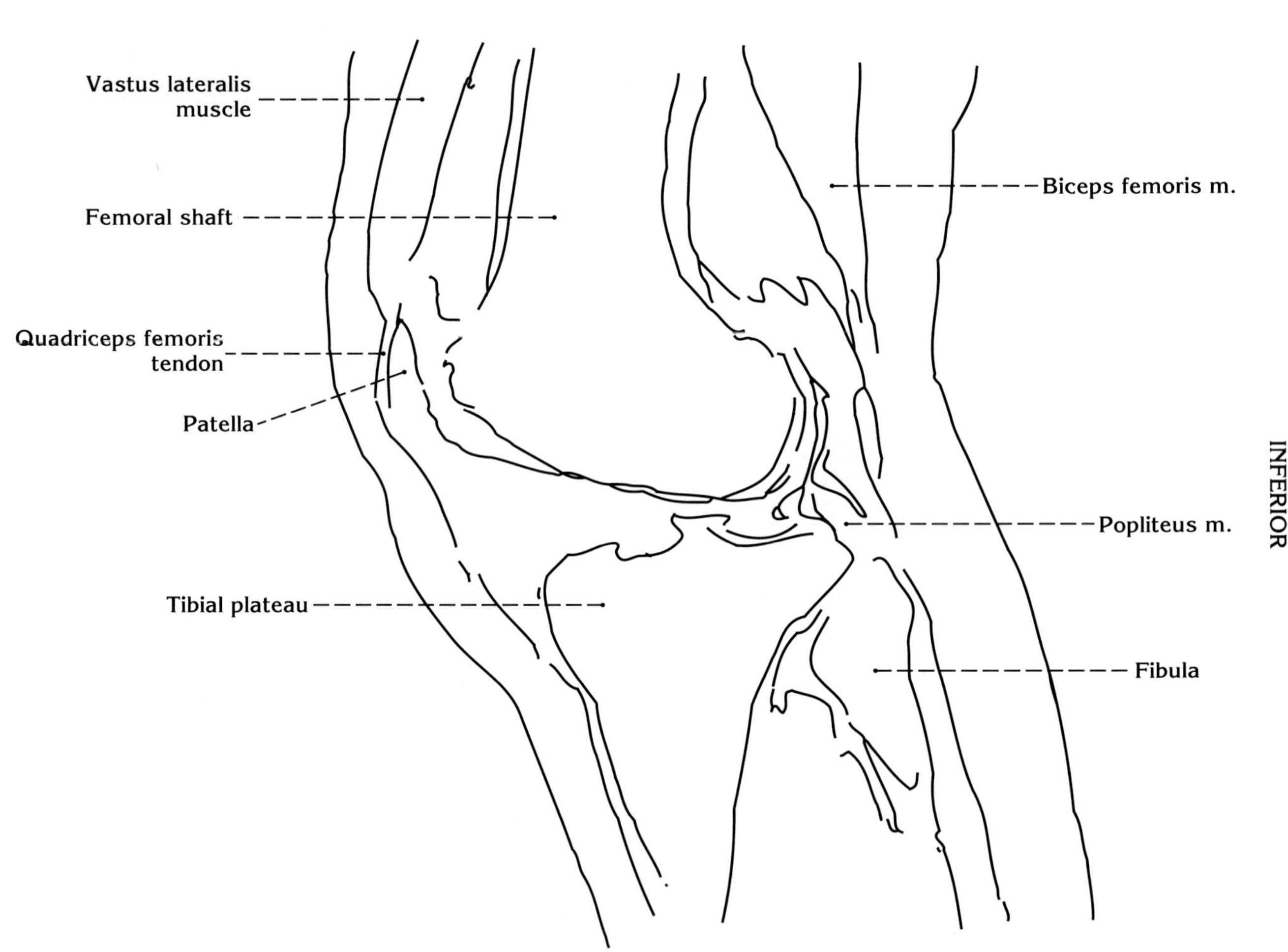

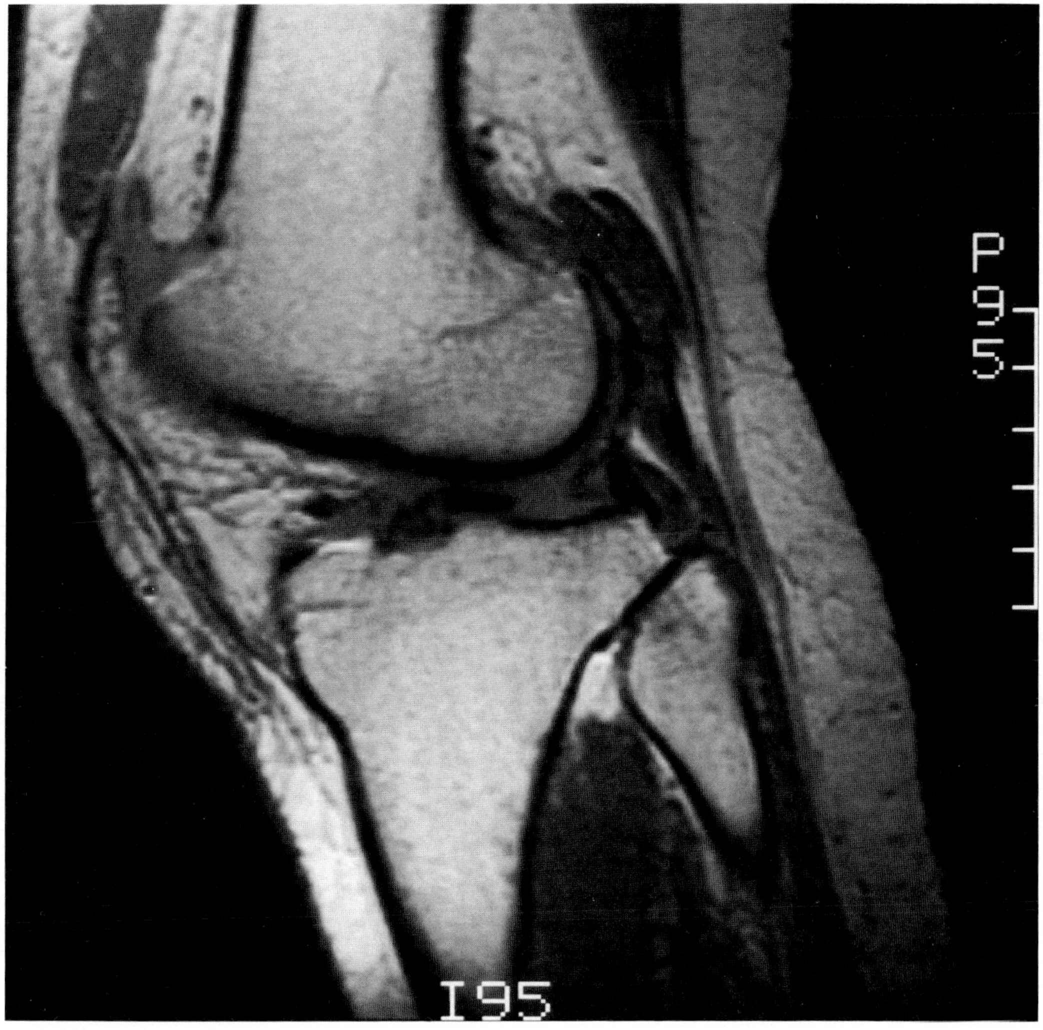

5-33 Knee, sagittal view (TR 2000; TE 20).

Knee, Sagittal

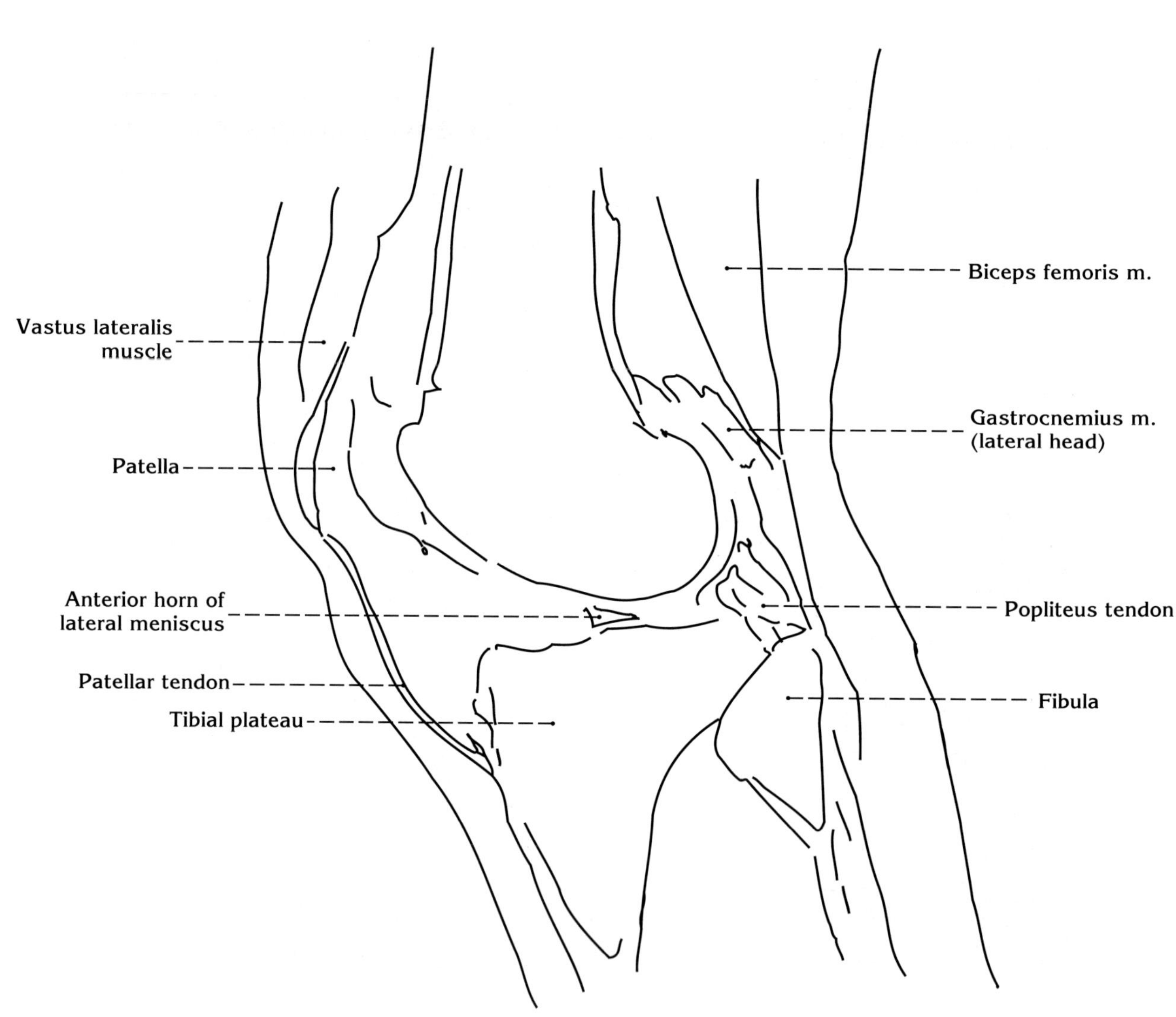

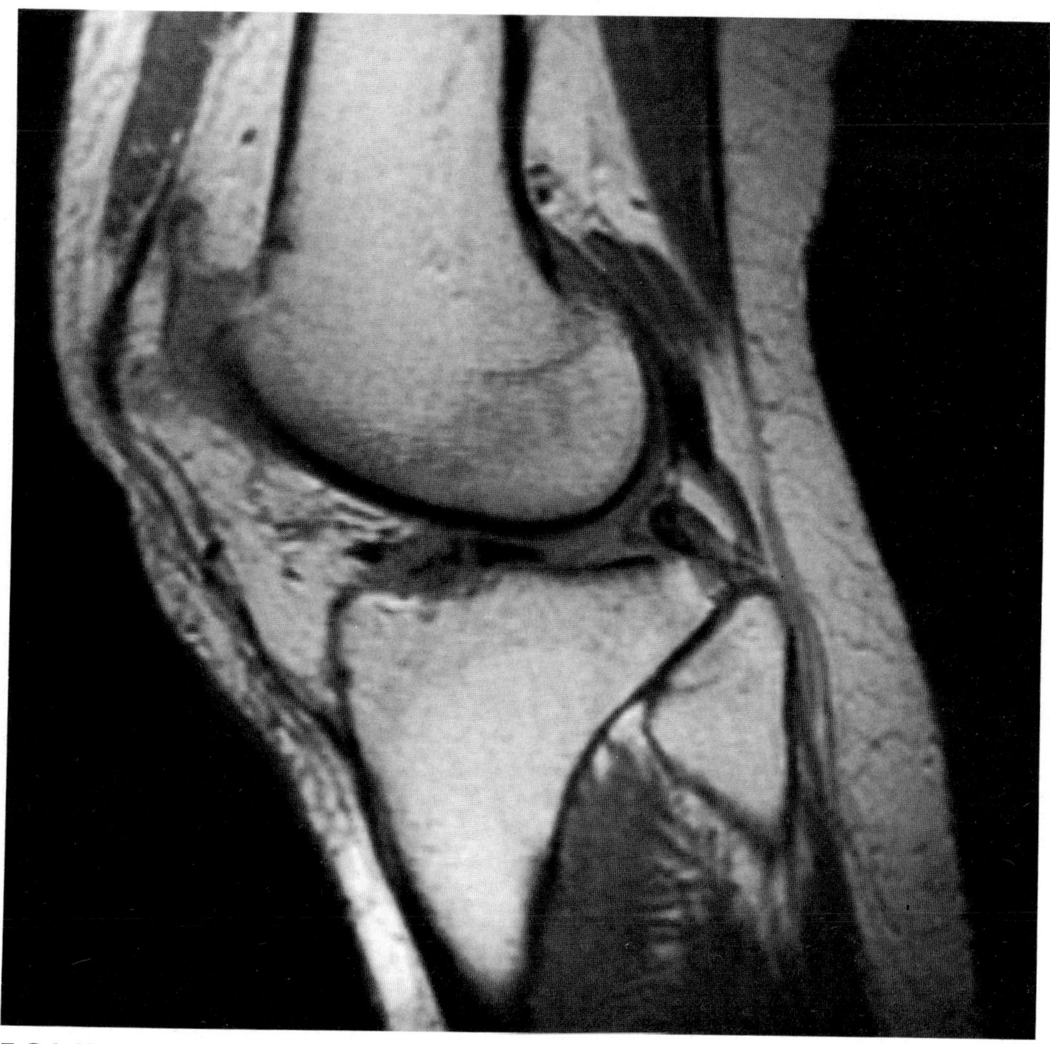

5-34 Knee, sagittal view (TR 2000; TE 20).

Knee, Sagittal

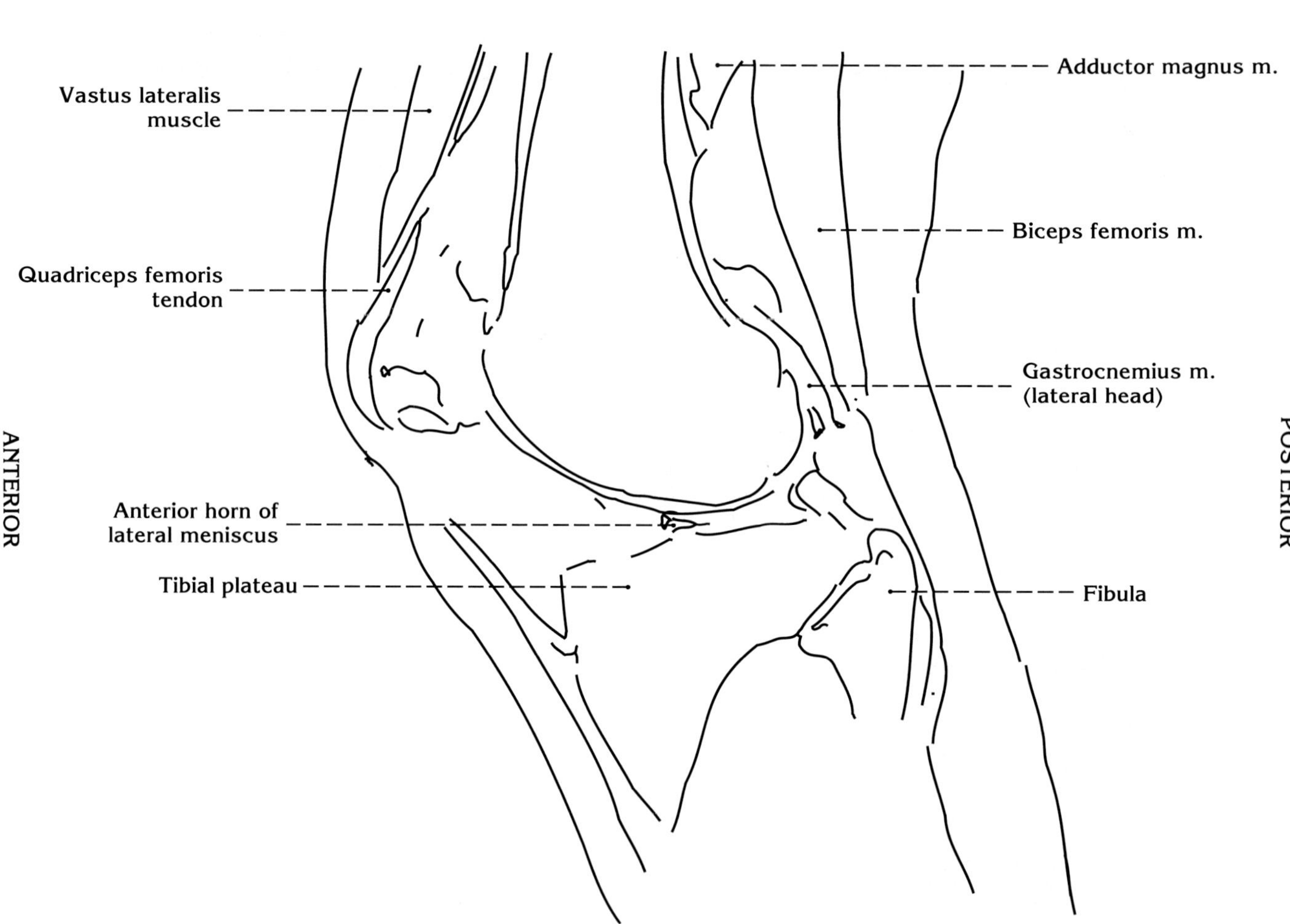

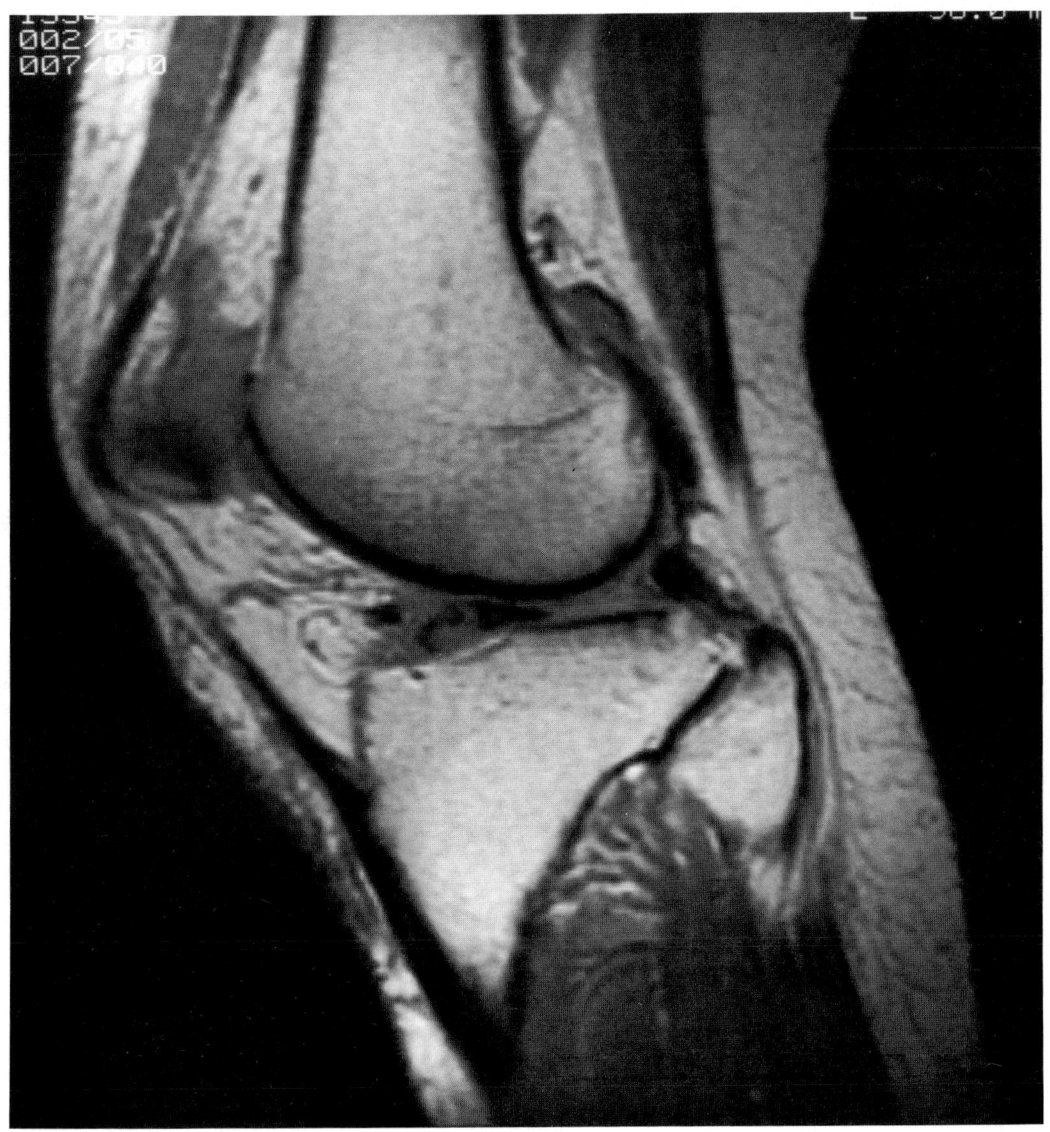

5-35 Knee, sagittal view (TR 2000; TE 20).

Knee, Sagittal

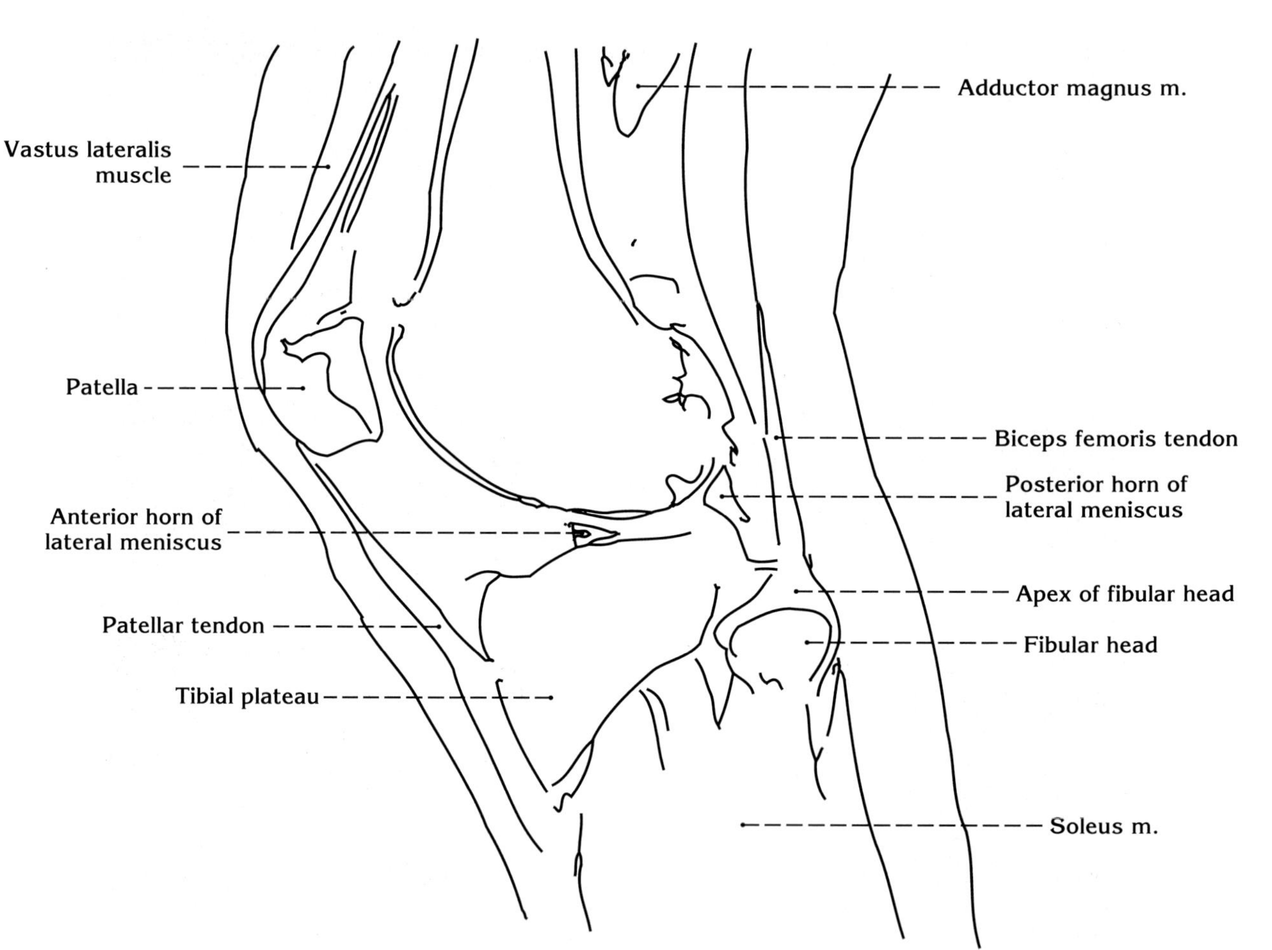

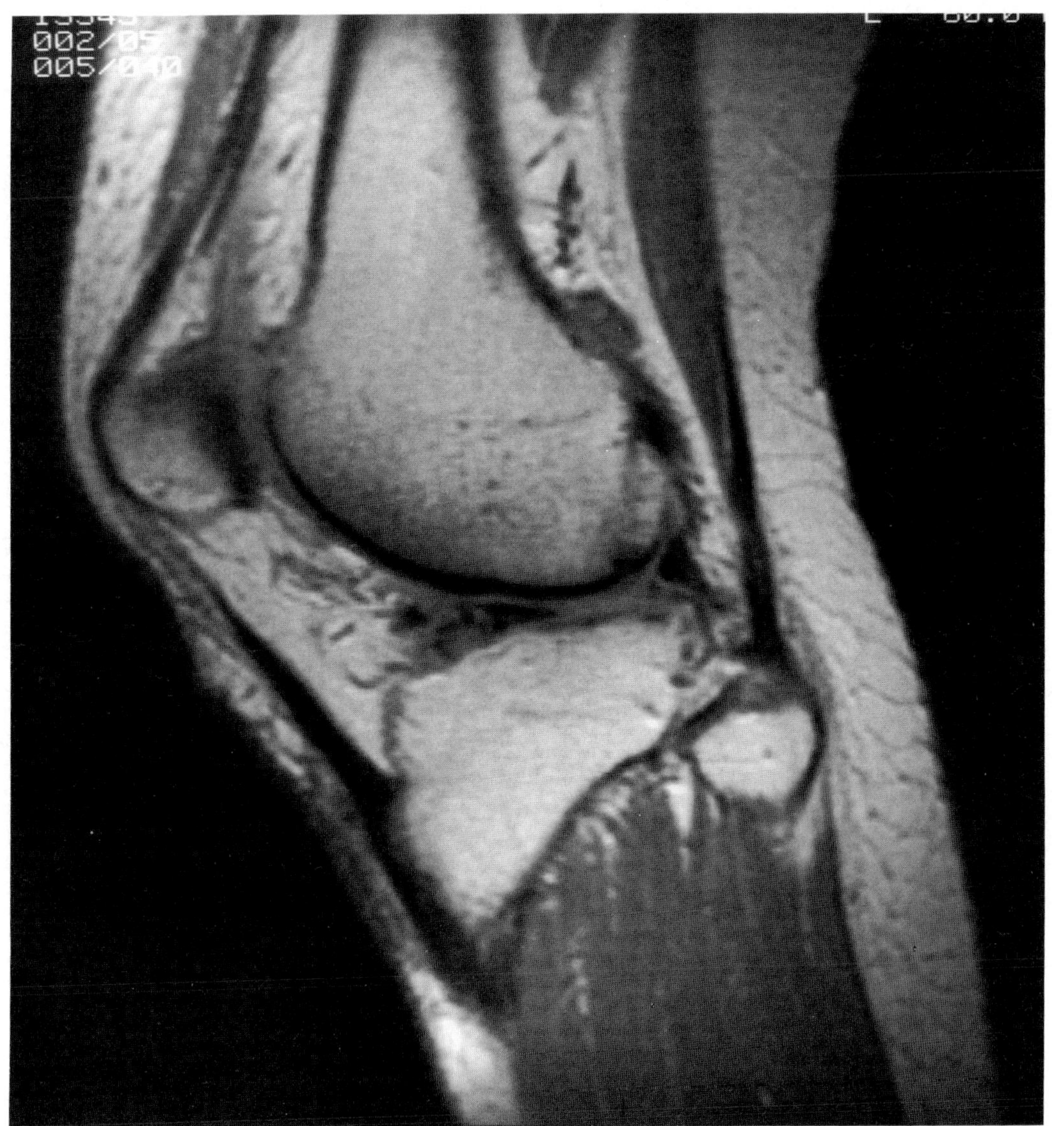

5-36 Knee, sagittal view (TR 2000; TE 20).

Knee, Sagittal

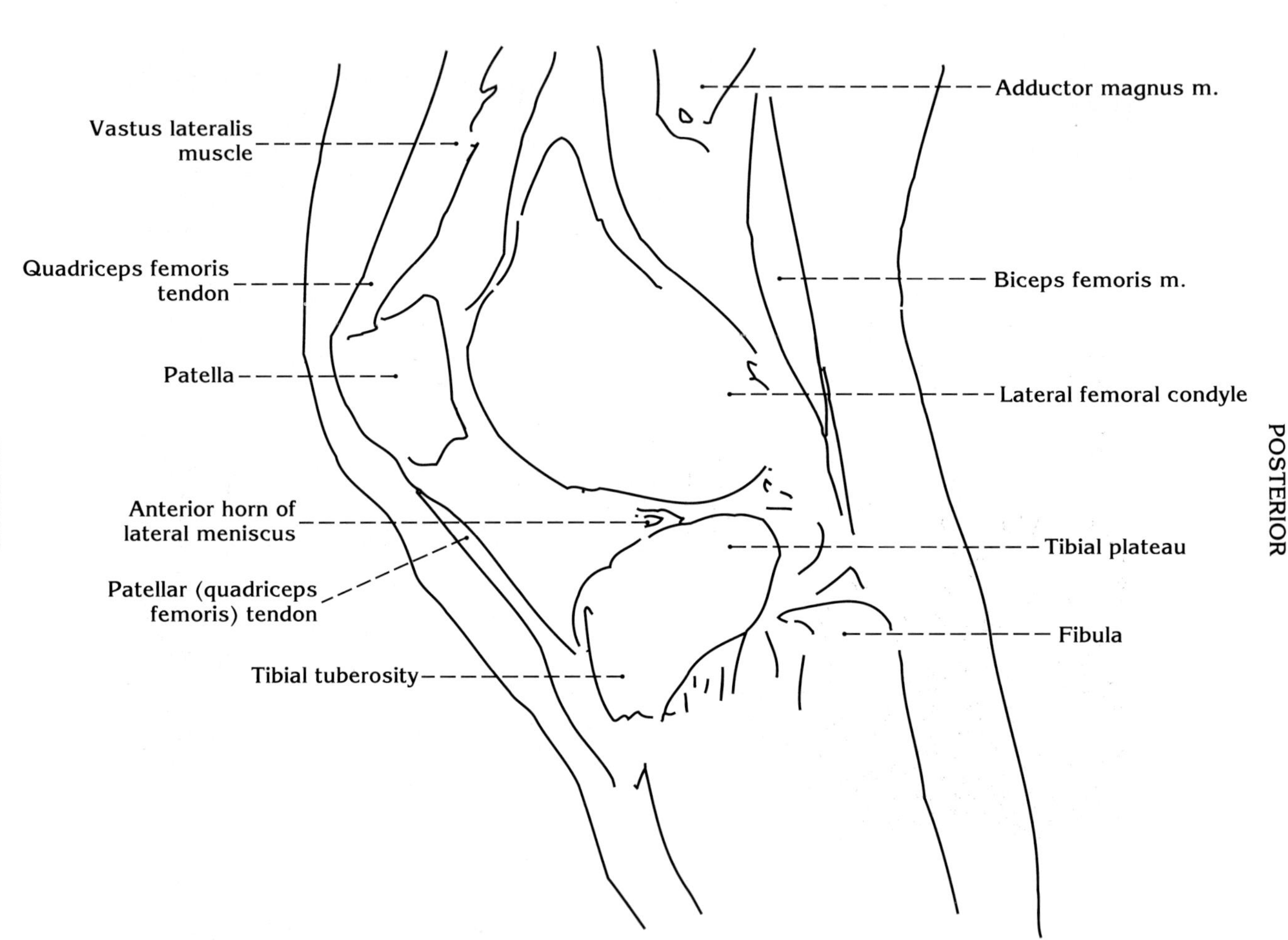

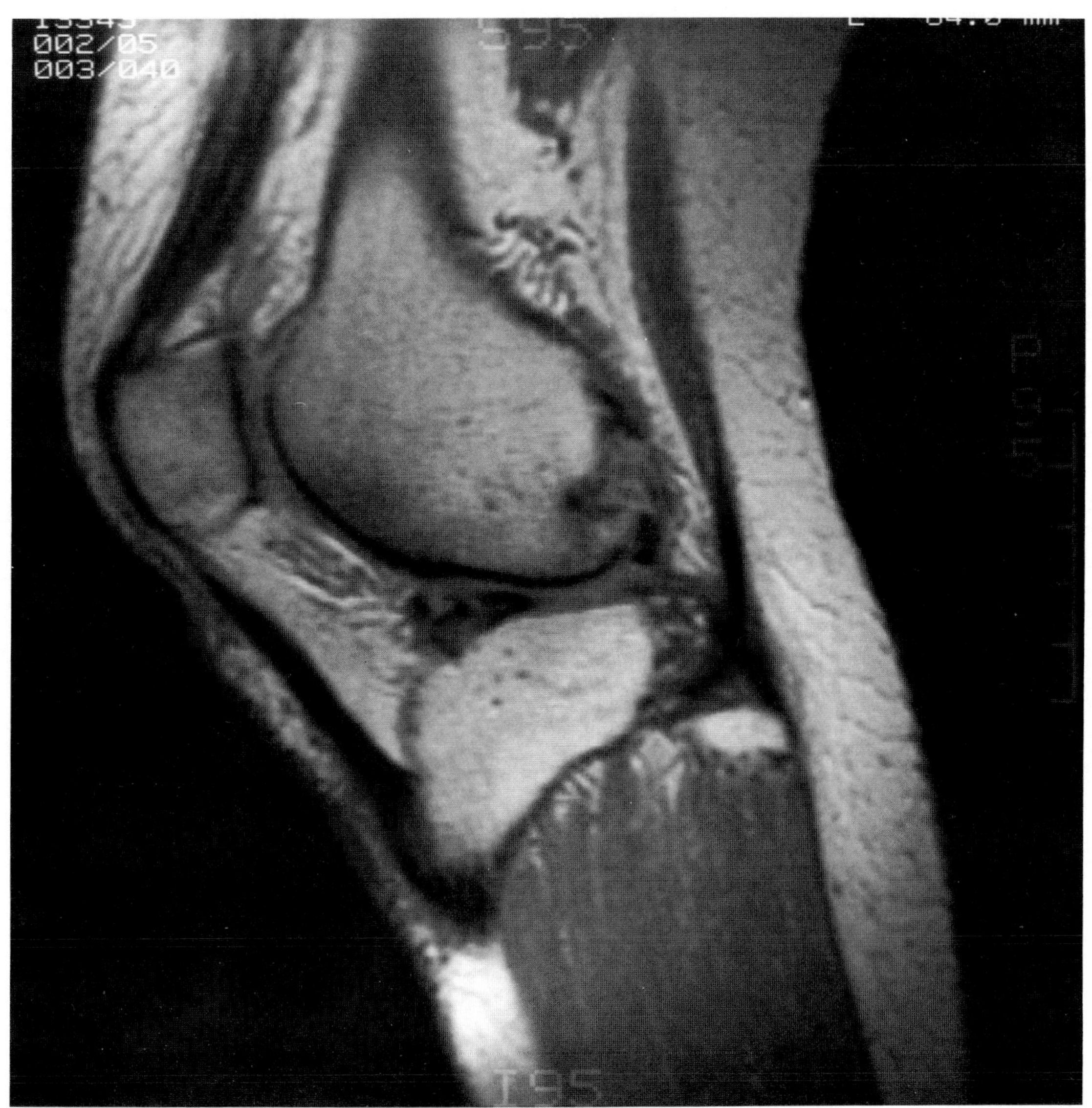

5-37 Knee, sagittal view (TR 2000; TE 20).

Knee, Sagittal

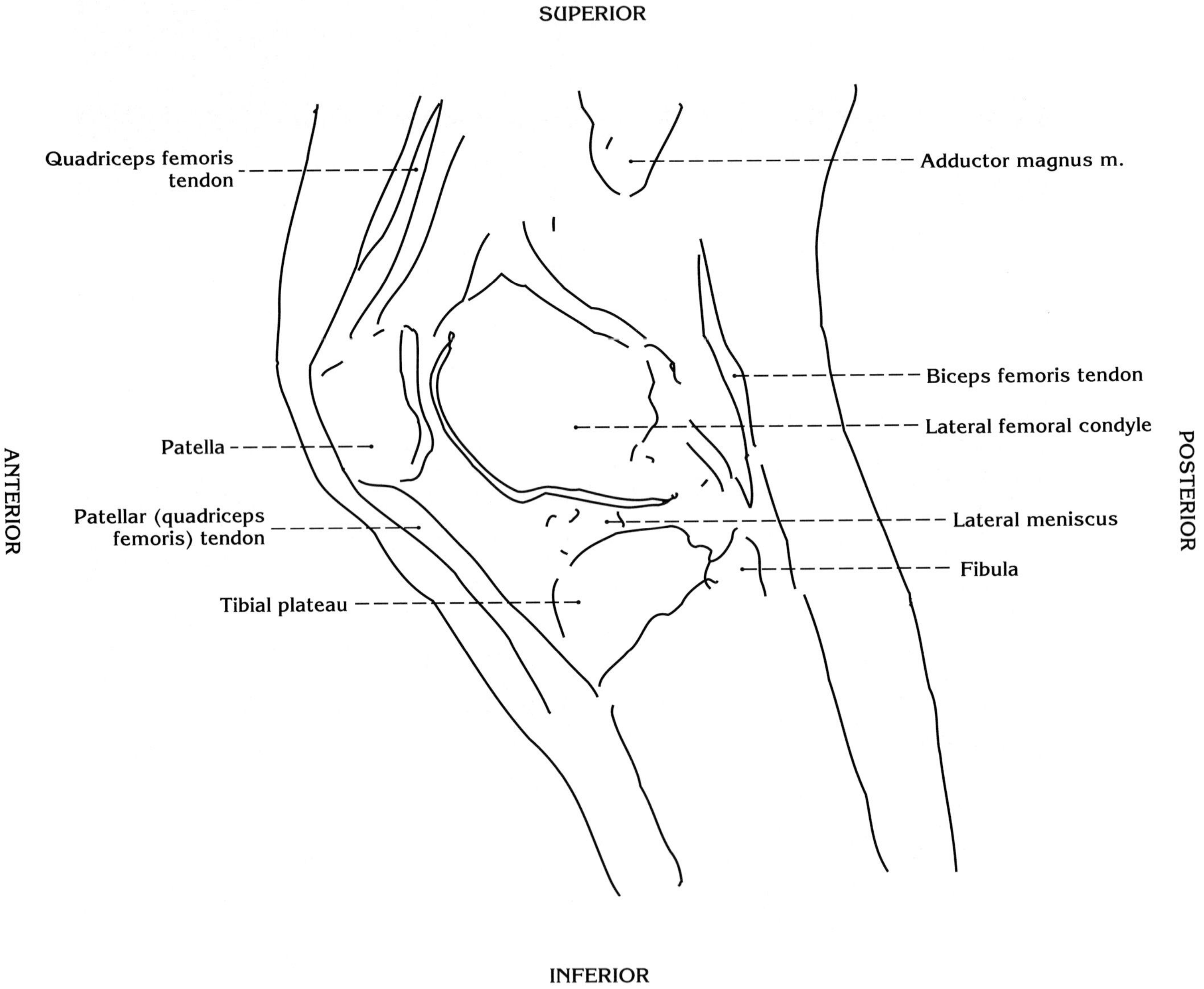

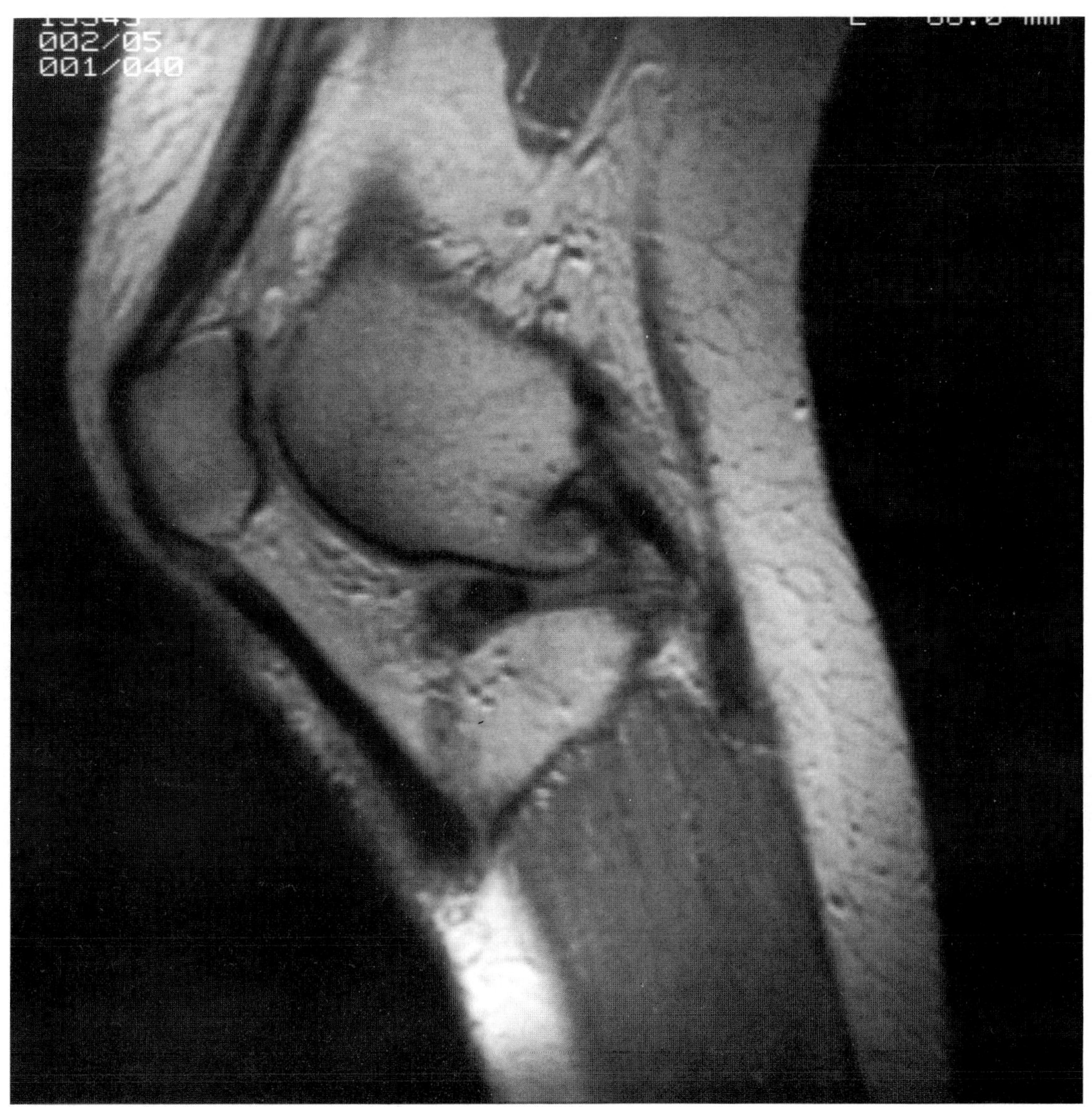

5-38 Knee, sagittal view (TR 2000; TE 20).

Lower Leg, Coronal

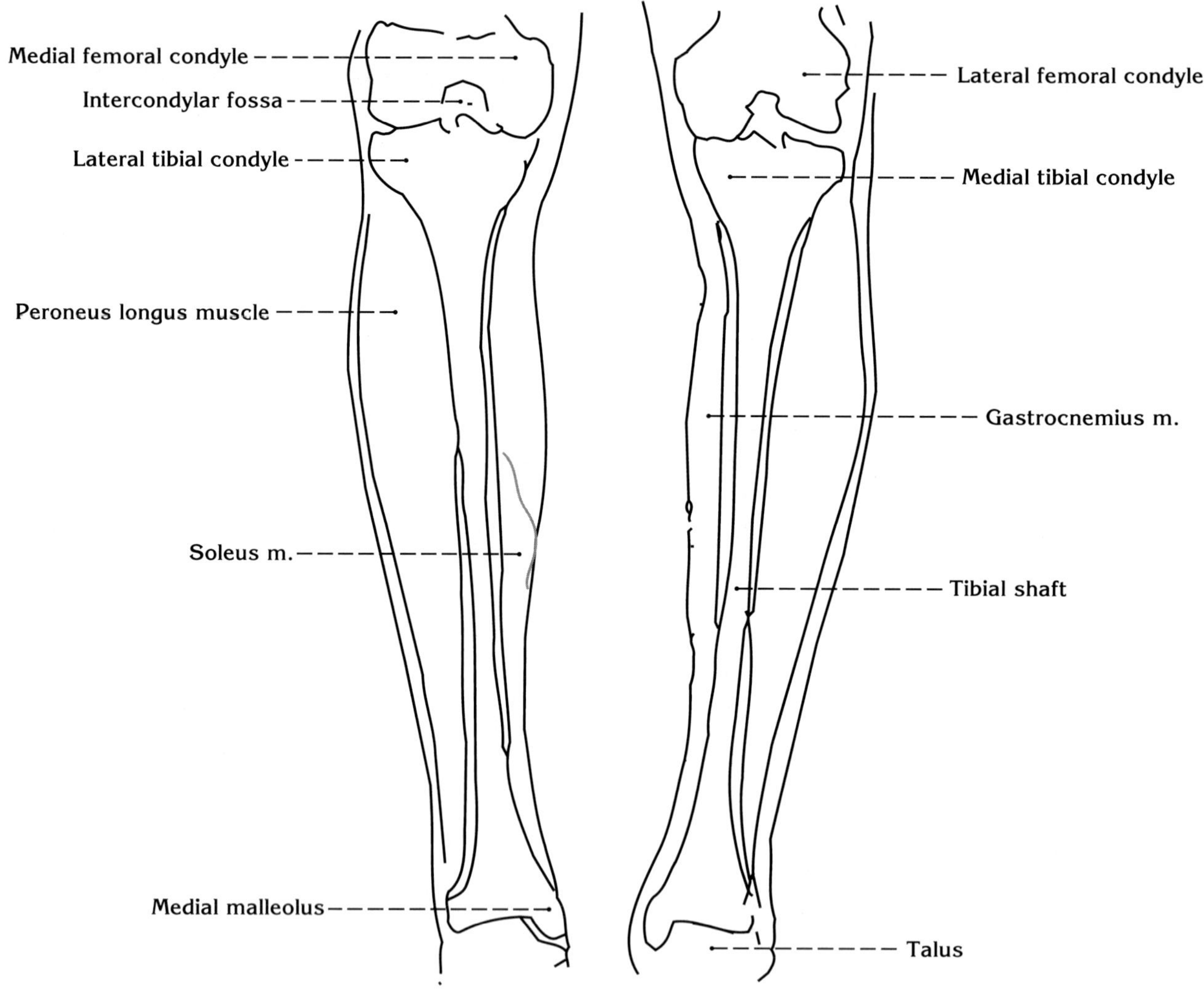

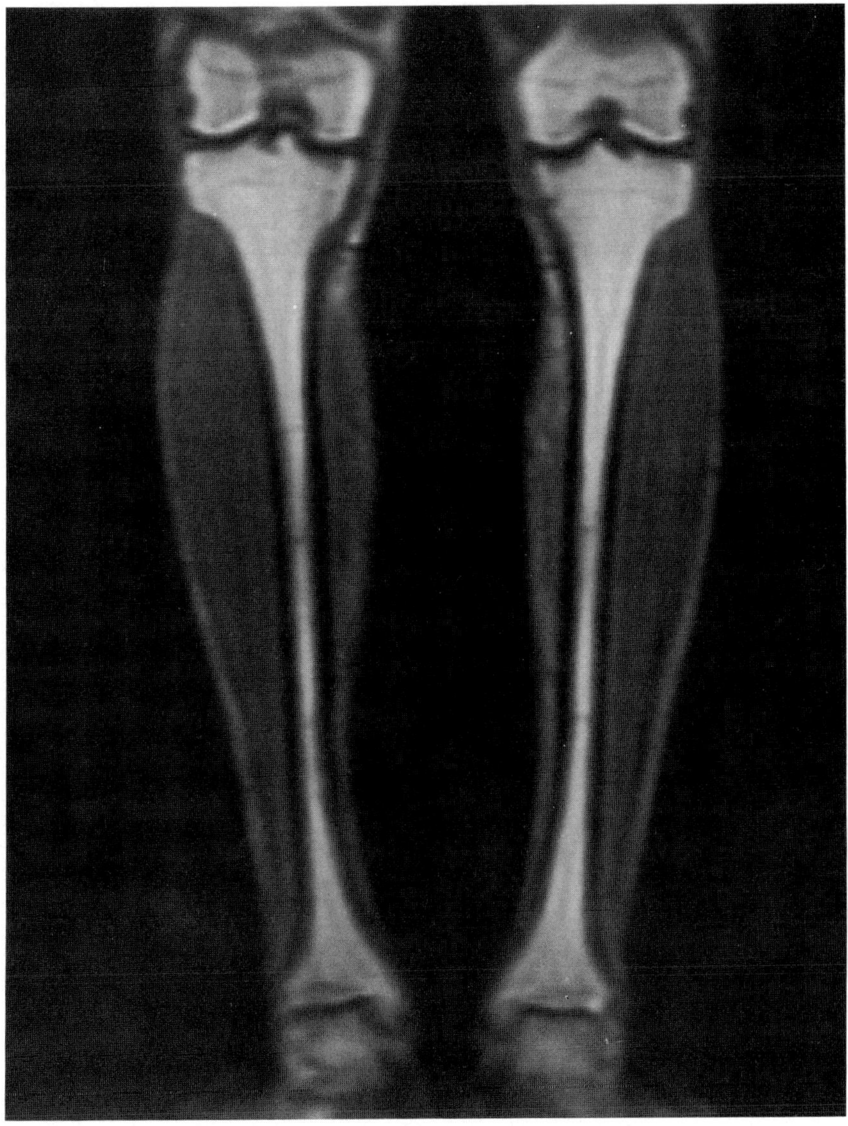

5-39 Lower Leg, coronal view (TR 2000; TE 20).

Lower Leg, Coronal

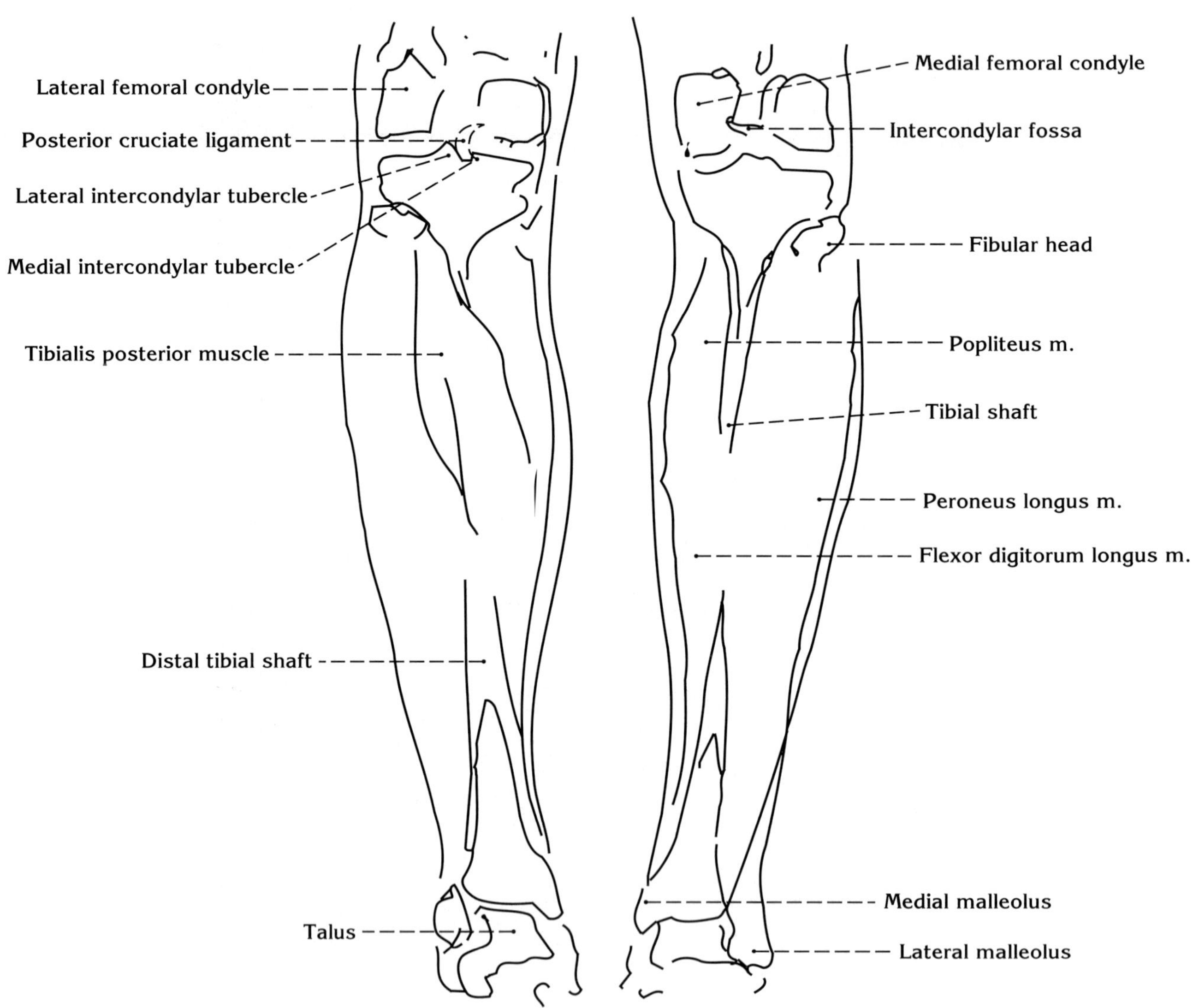

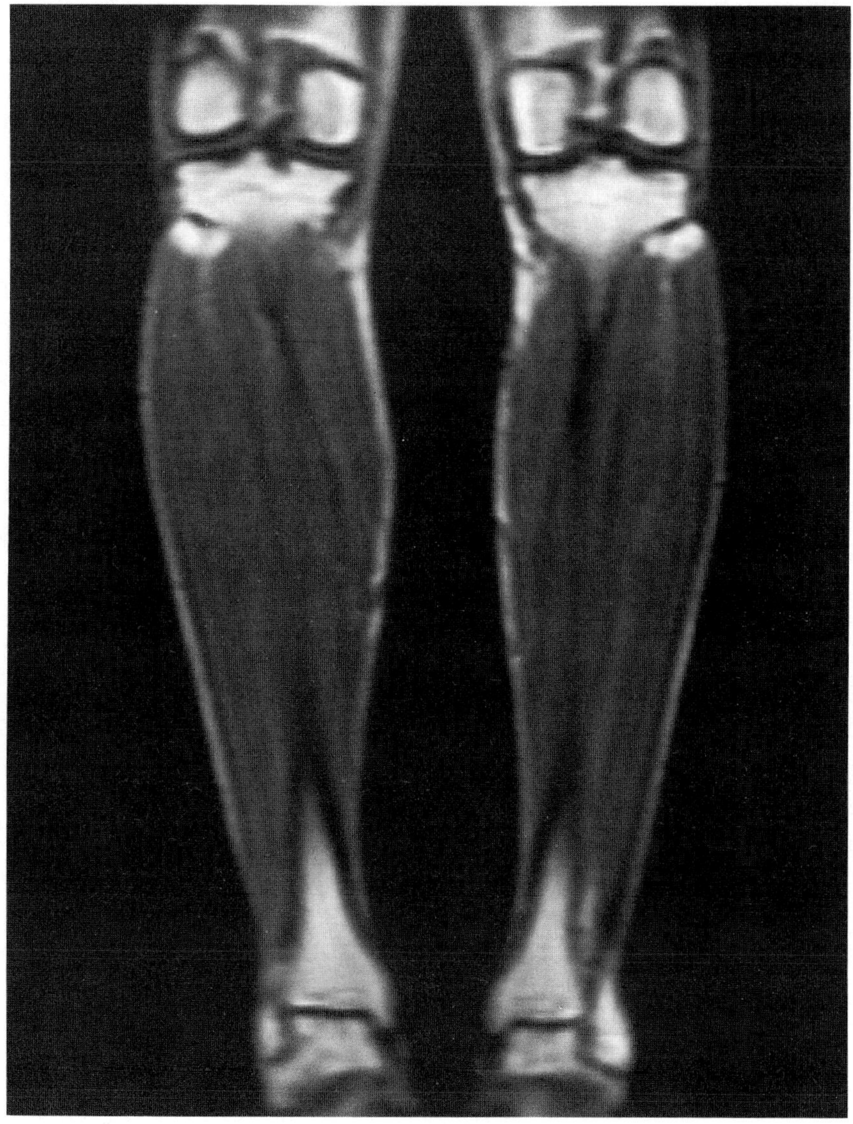

5-40 Lower Leg, coronal view (TR 2000; TE 20).

Lower Leg, Coronal

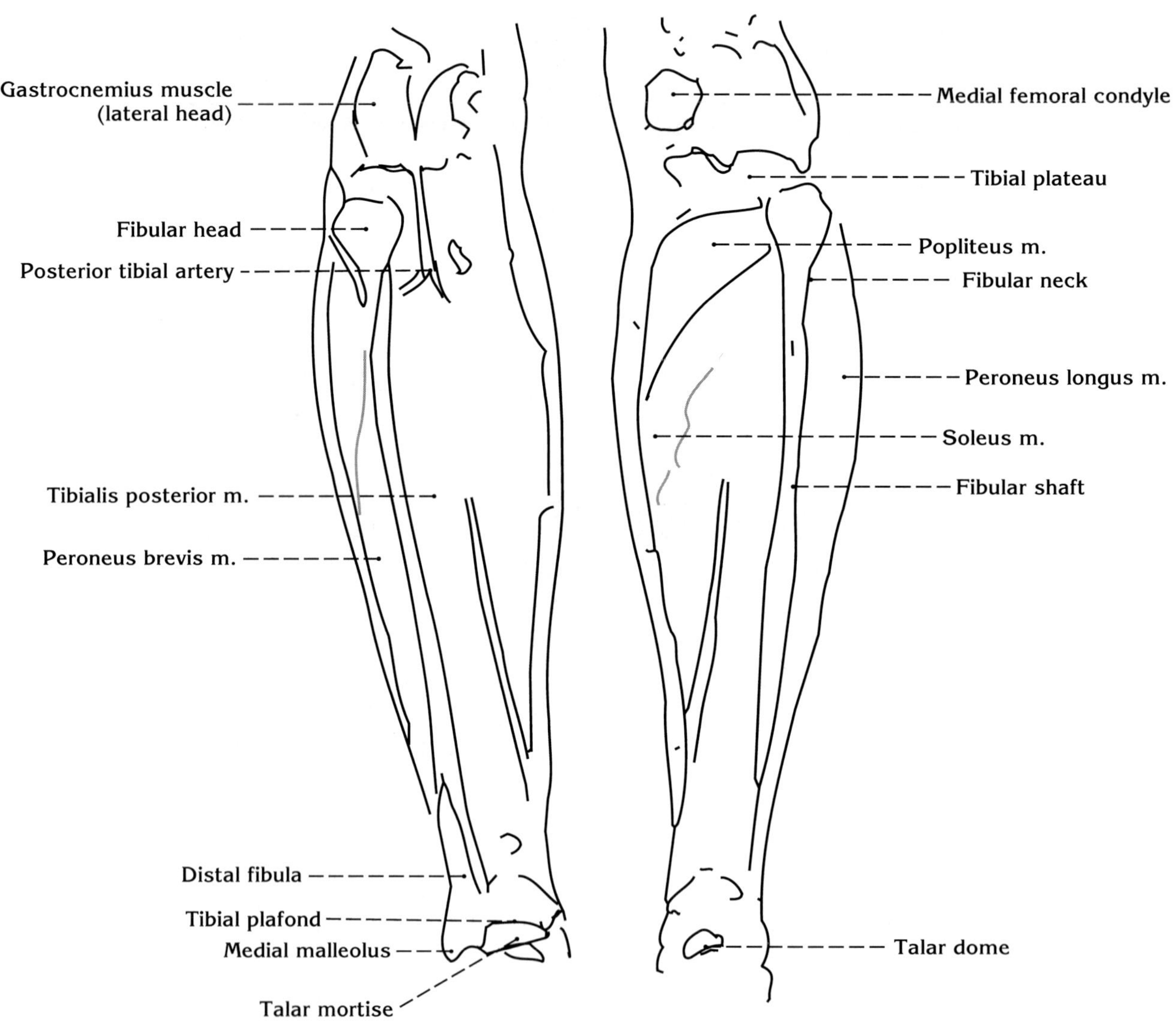

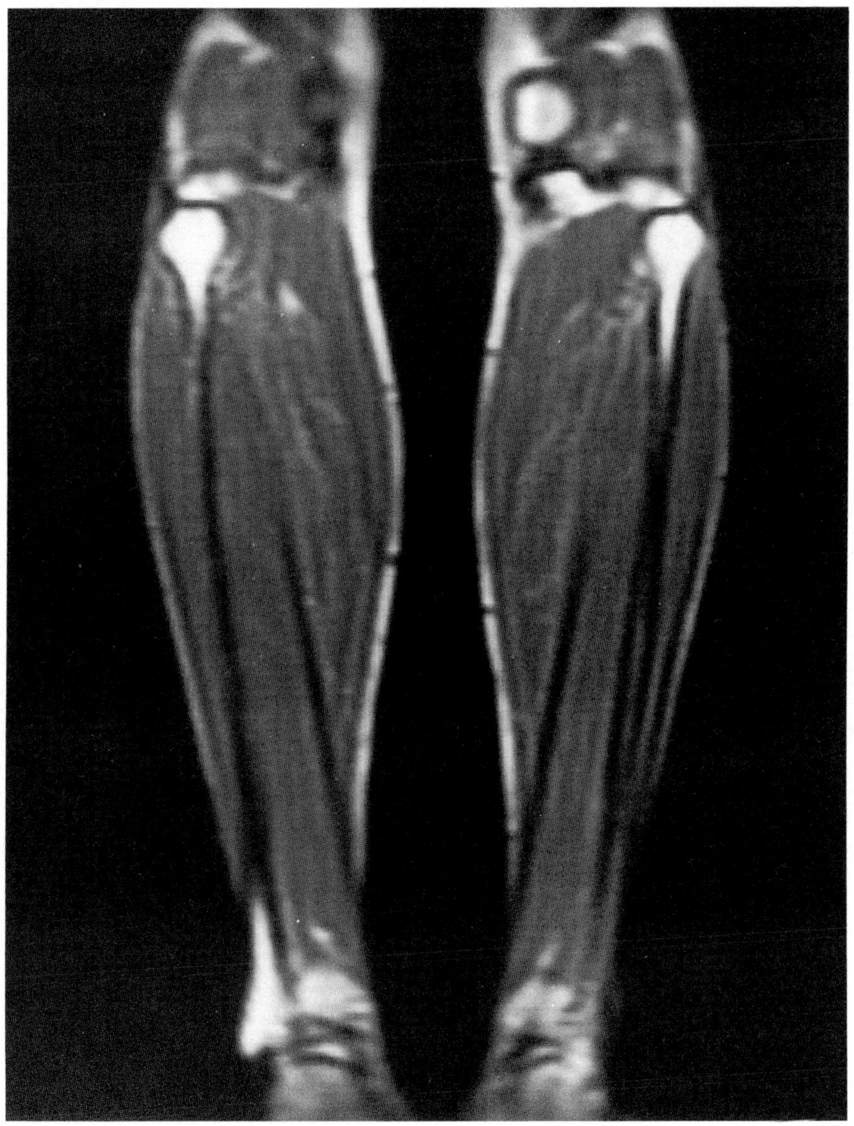

5-41 Lower Leg, coronal view (TR 2000; TE 20).

Lower Leg, Axial

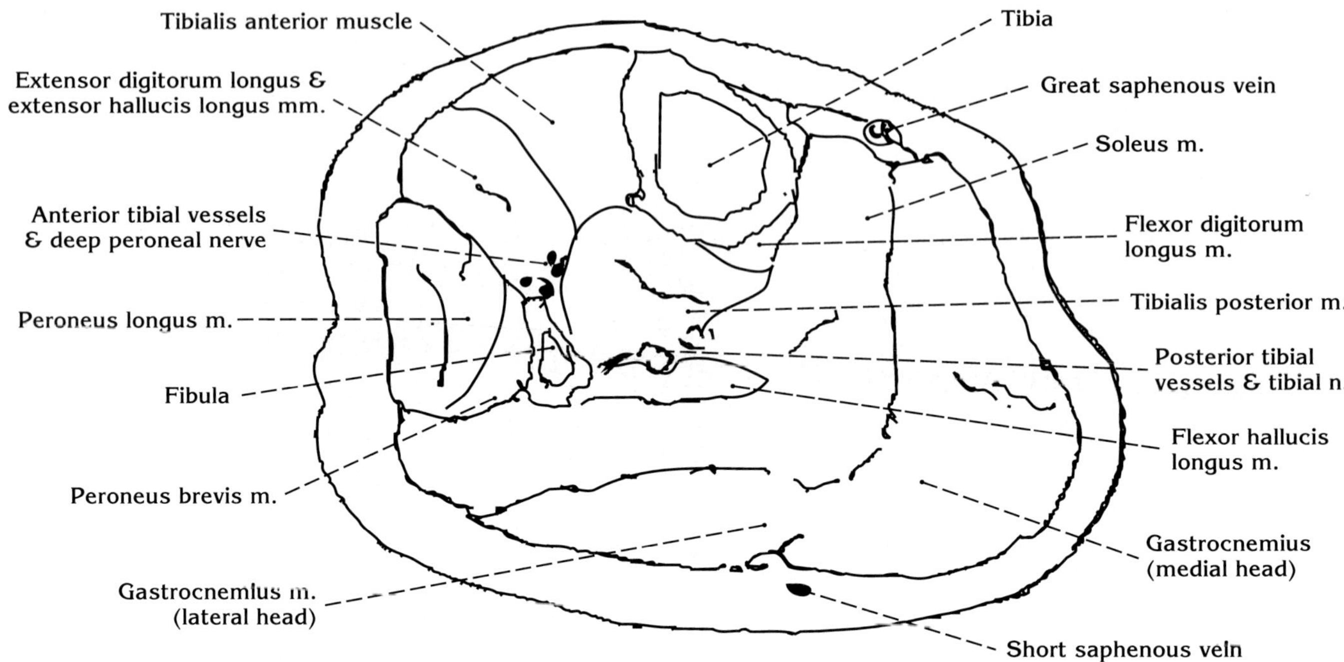

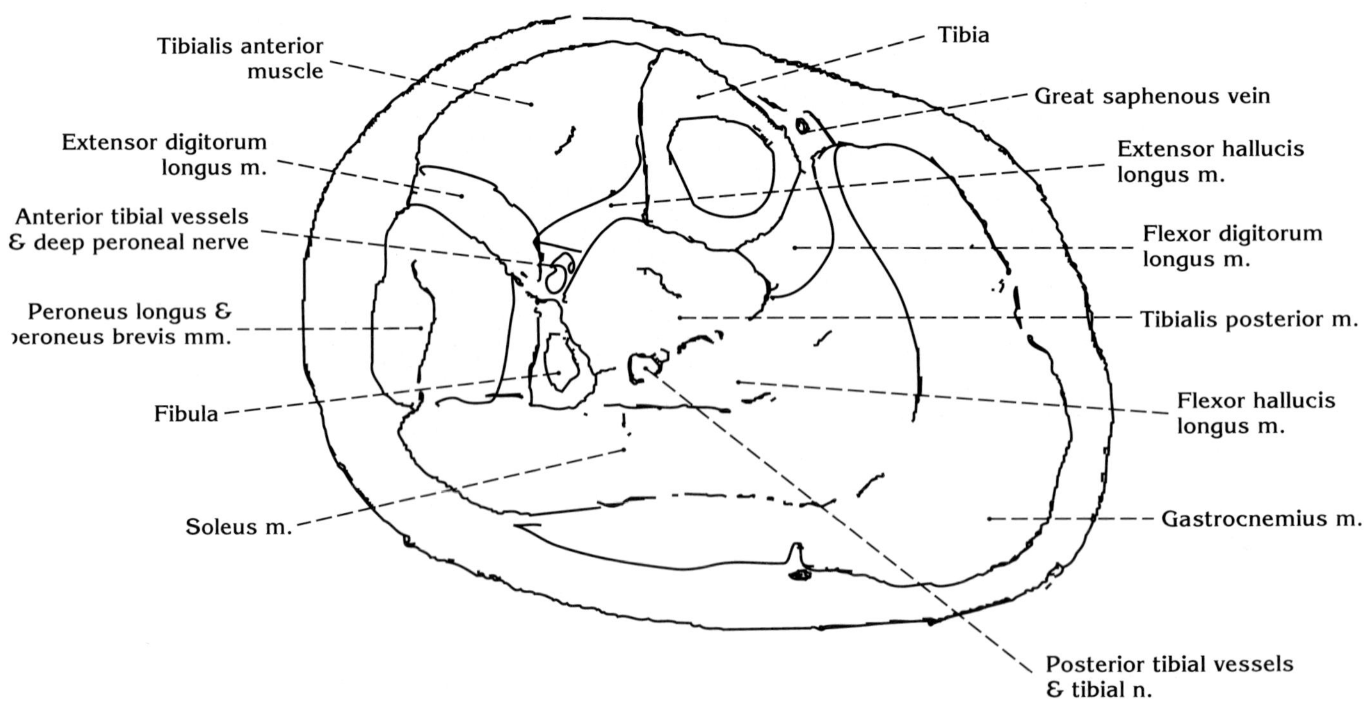

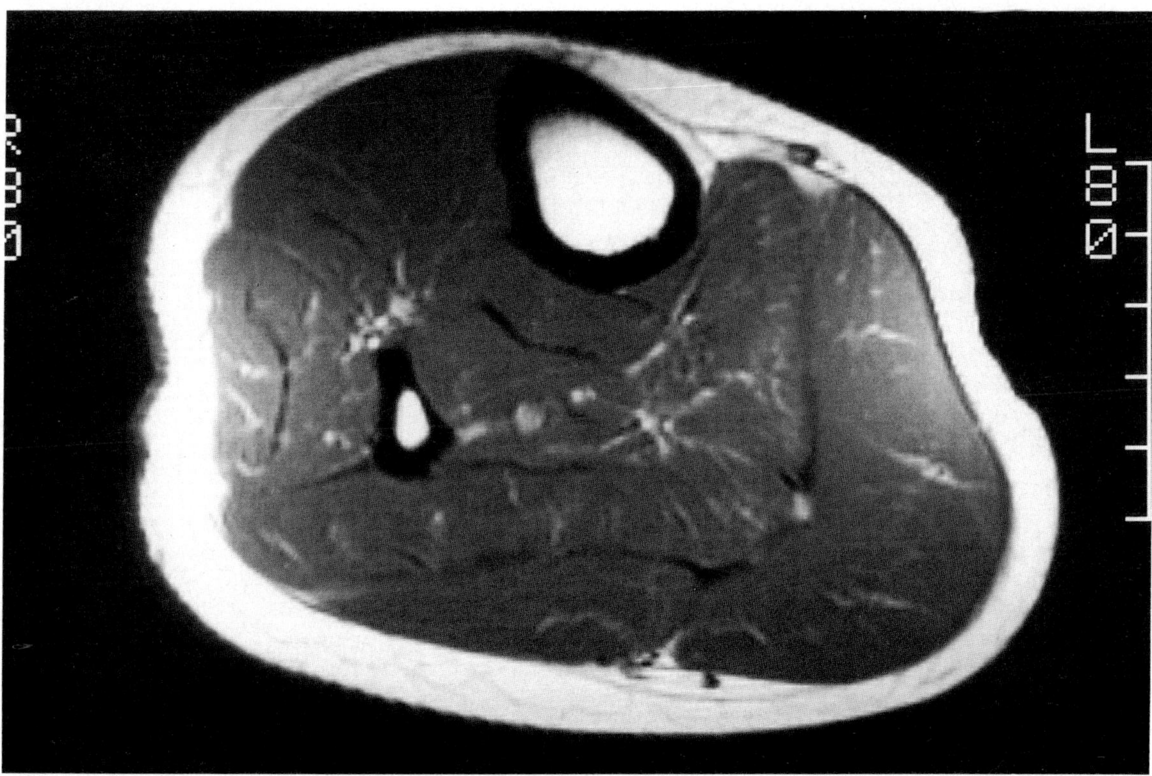

5-42 Lower Leg, axial view (TR 800; TE 30).

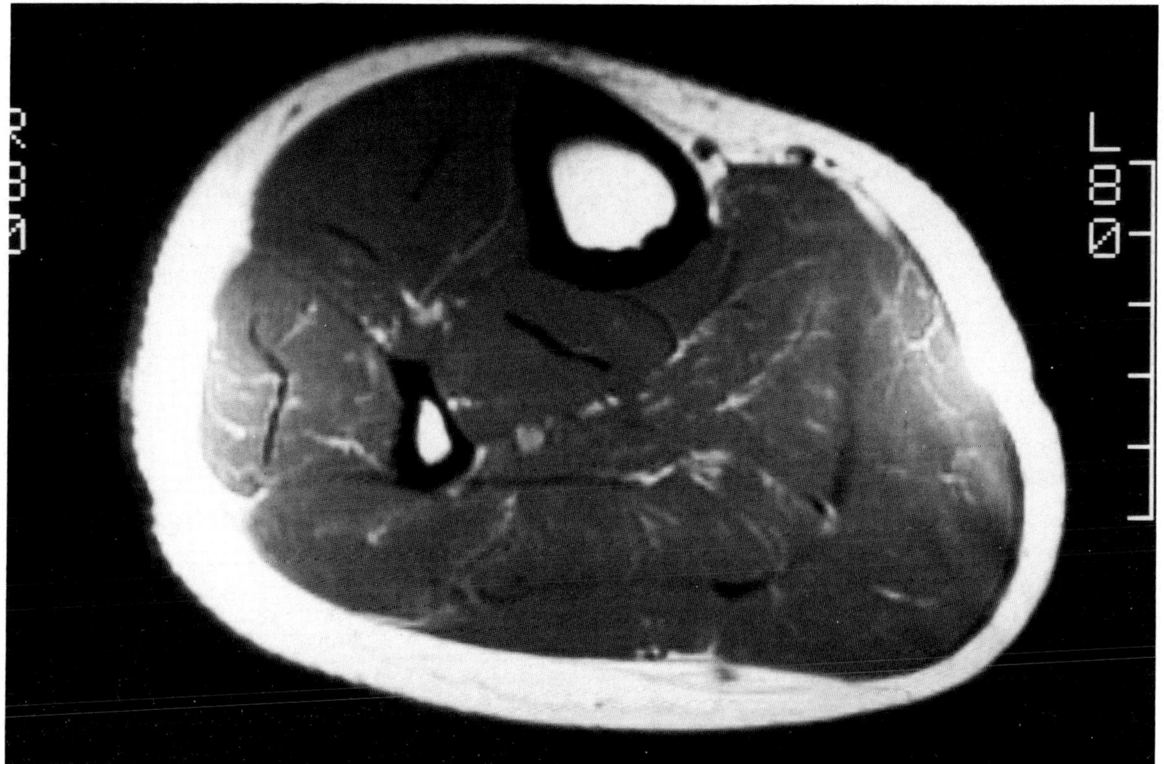

5-43 Lower Leg, axial view (TR 800; TE 30).

Lower Leg, Axial

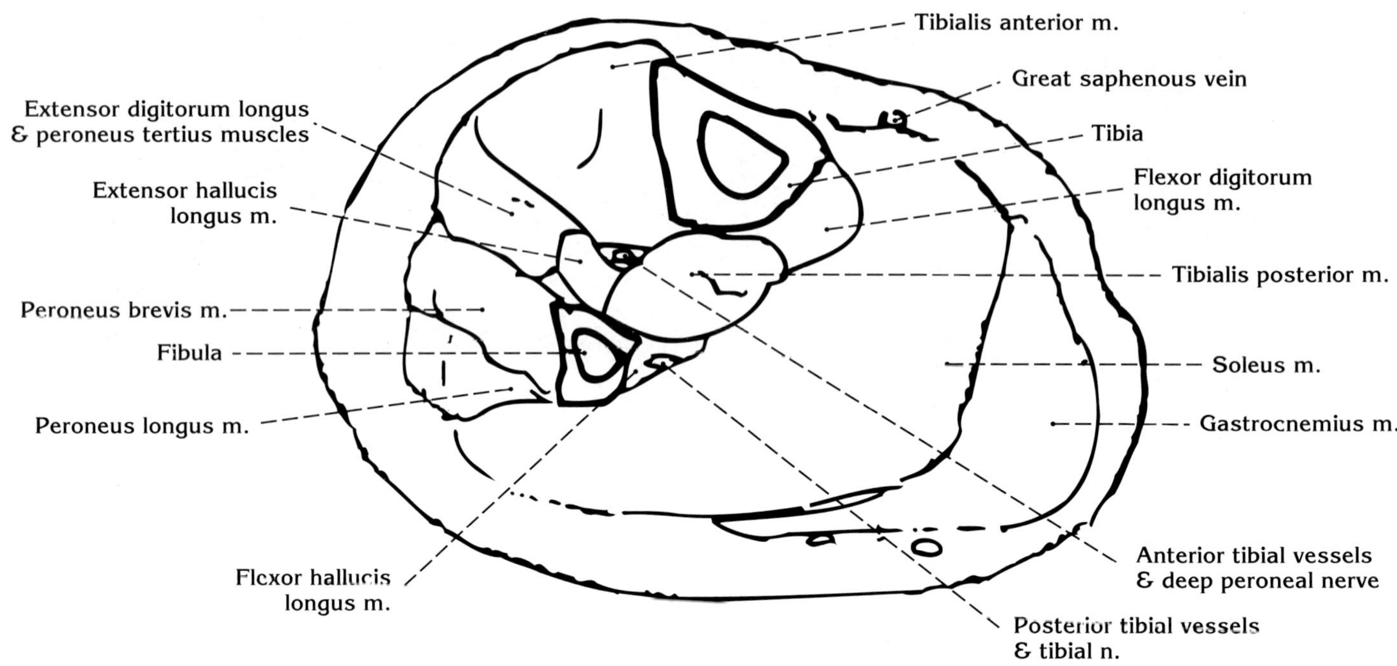

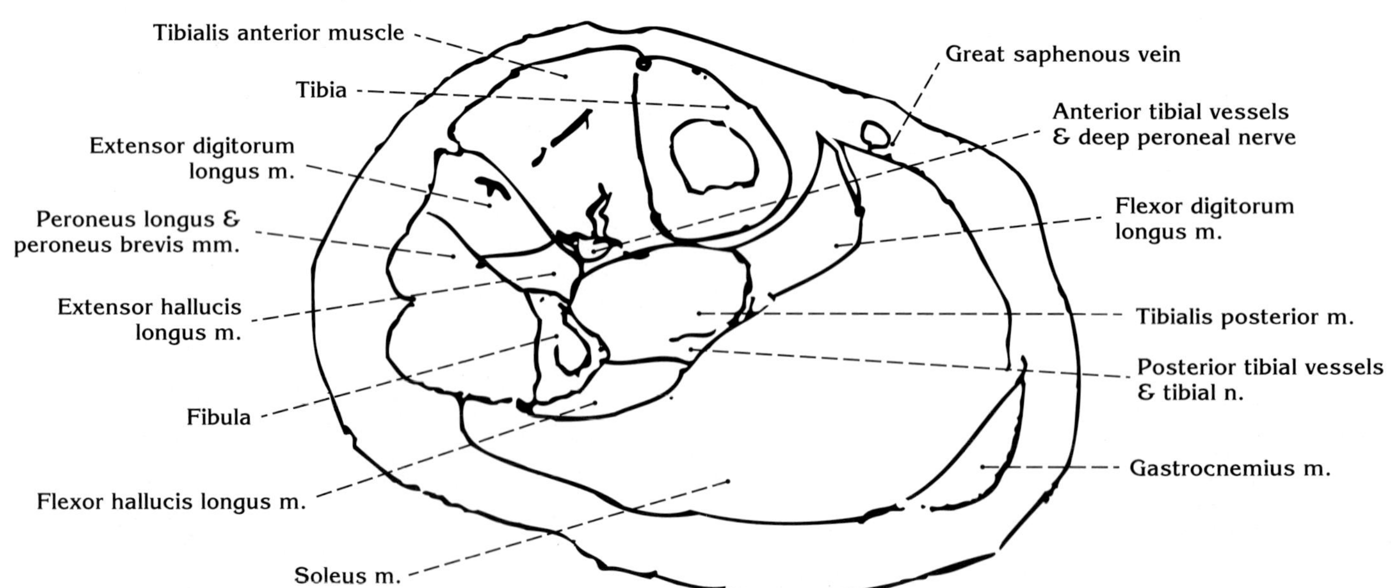

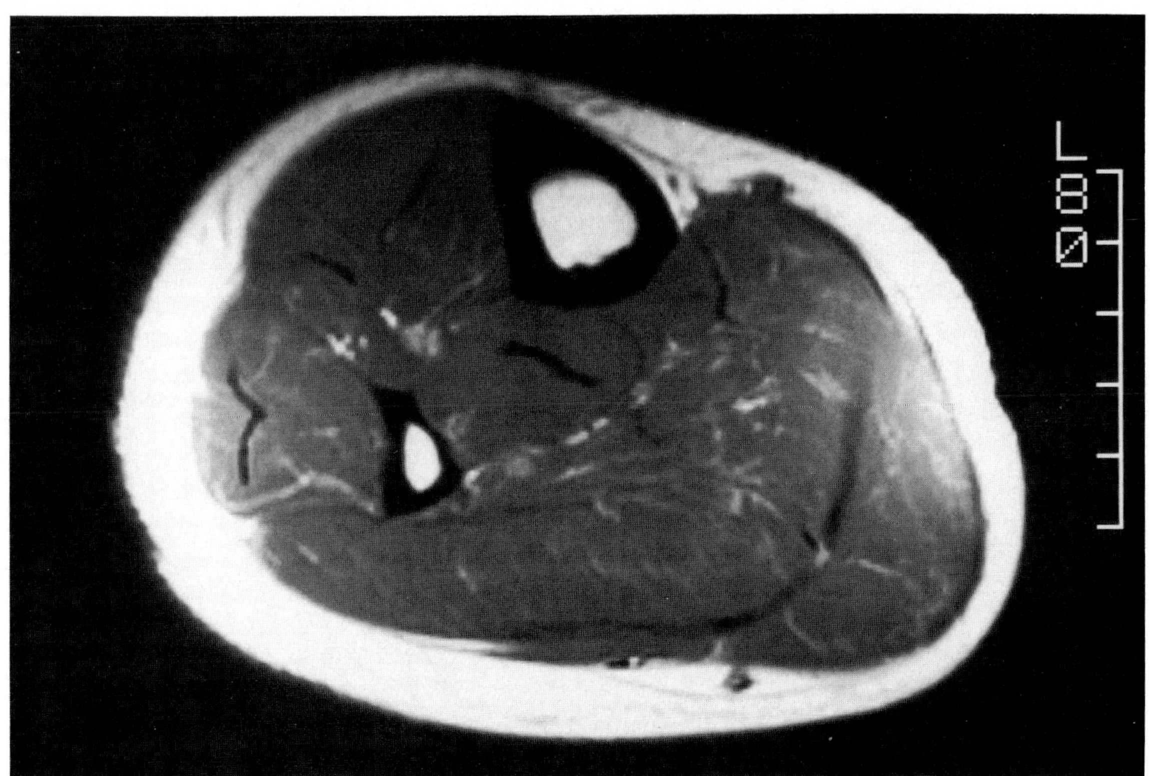

5-44 Lower Leg, axial view (TR 800; TE 30).

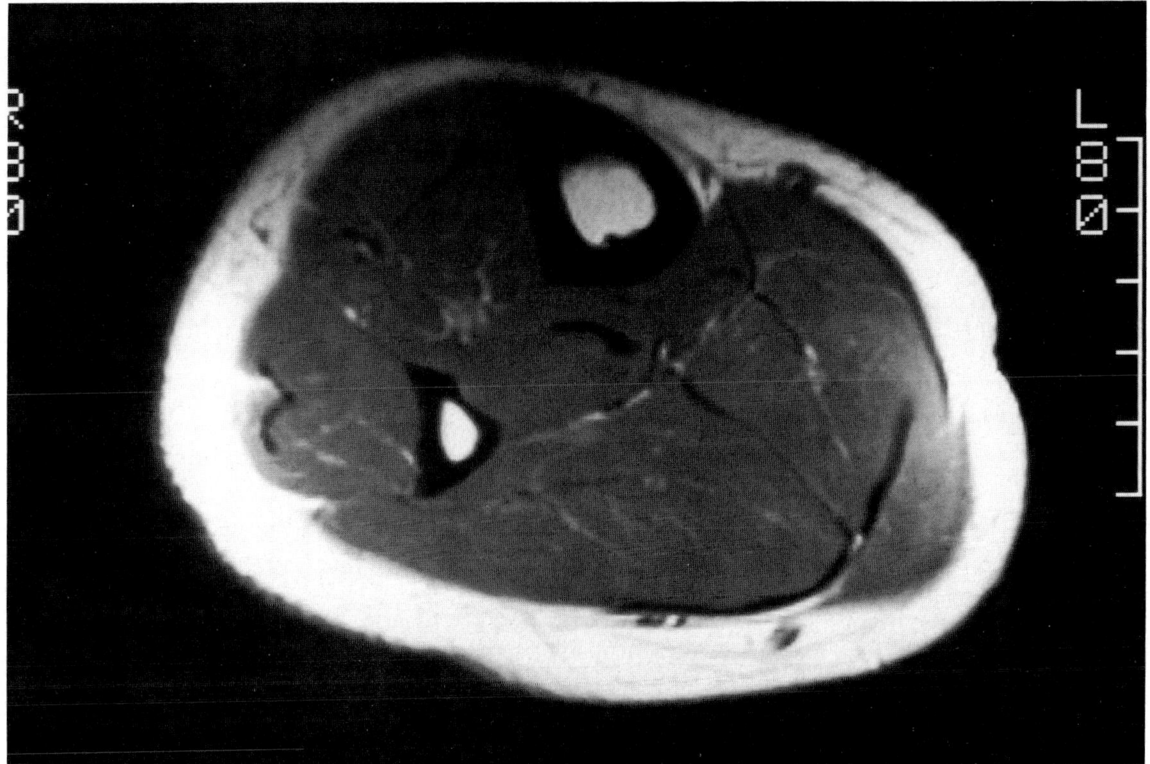

5-45 Lower Leg, axial view (TR 800; TE 30).

Lower Leg and Ankle, Axial

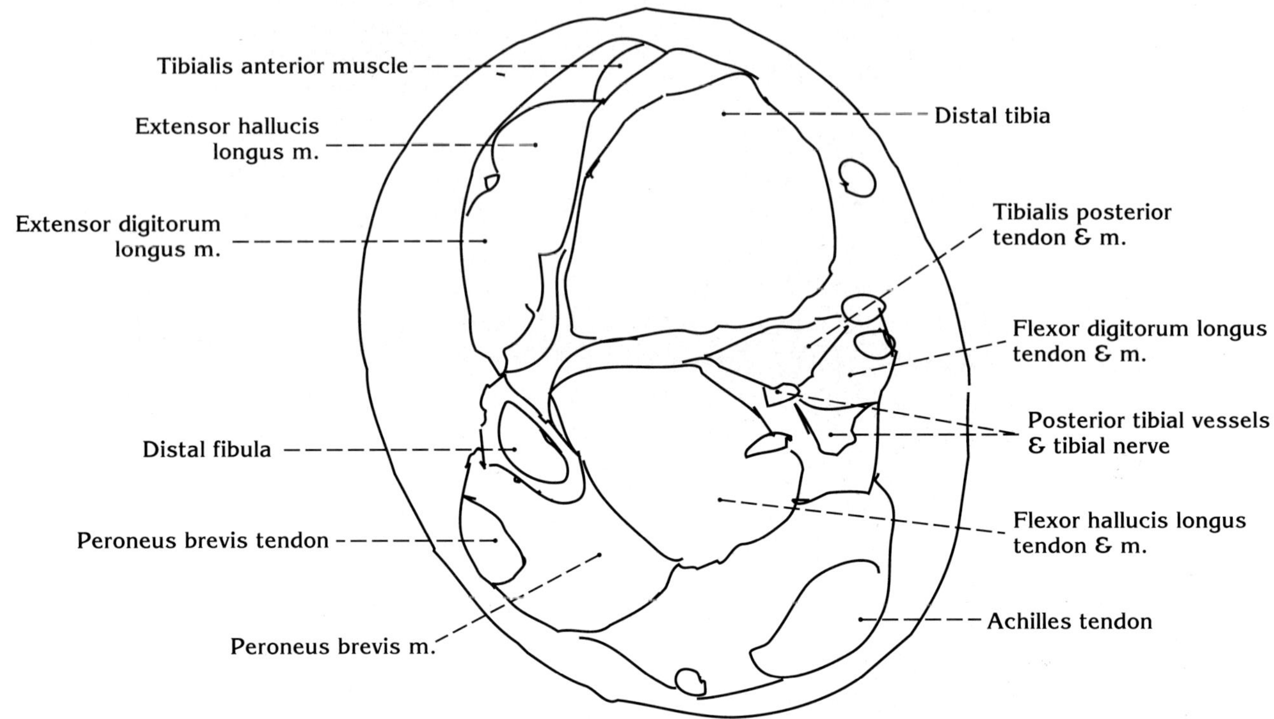

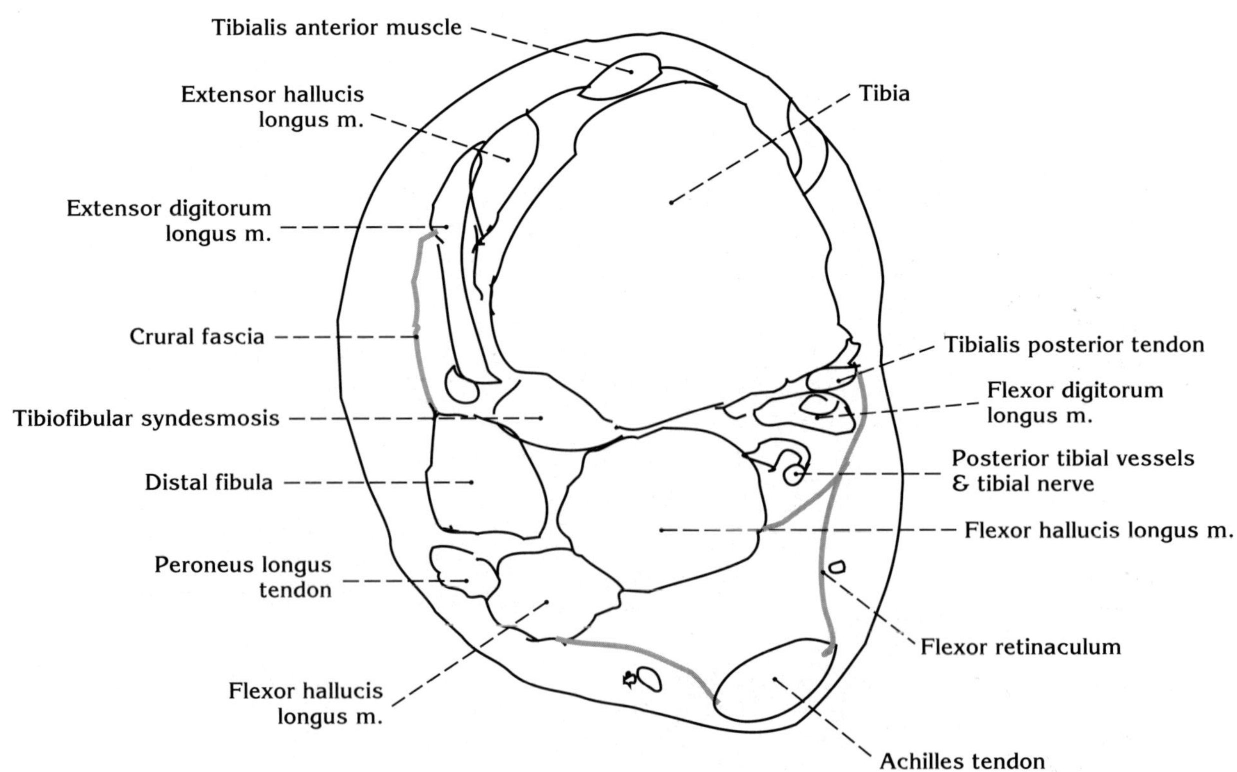

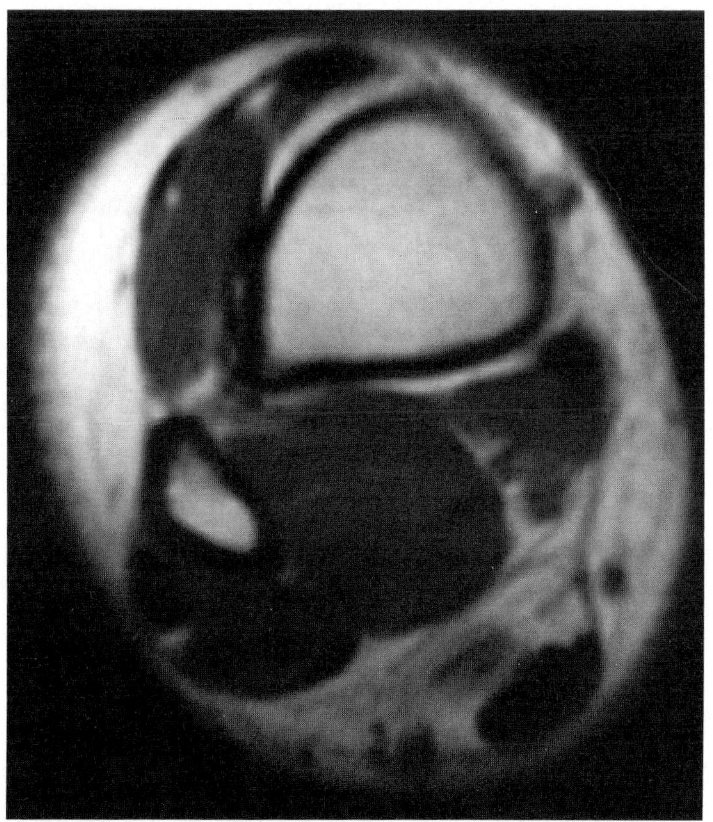

5-46 Lower Leg (distal third), axial view (TR 800; TE 30).

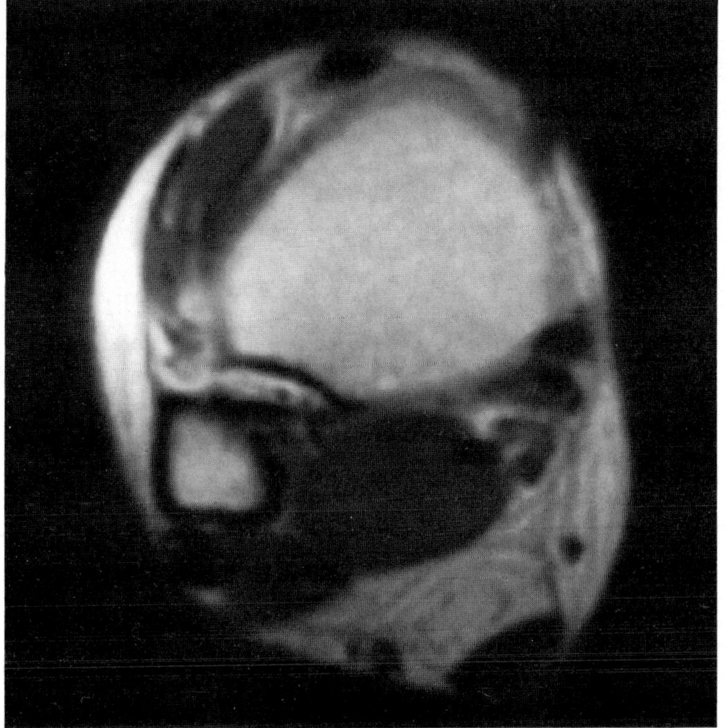

5-47 Ankle, axial view (TR 800; TE 30).

Ankle, Axial

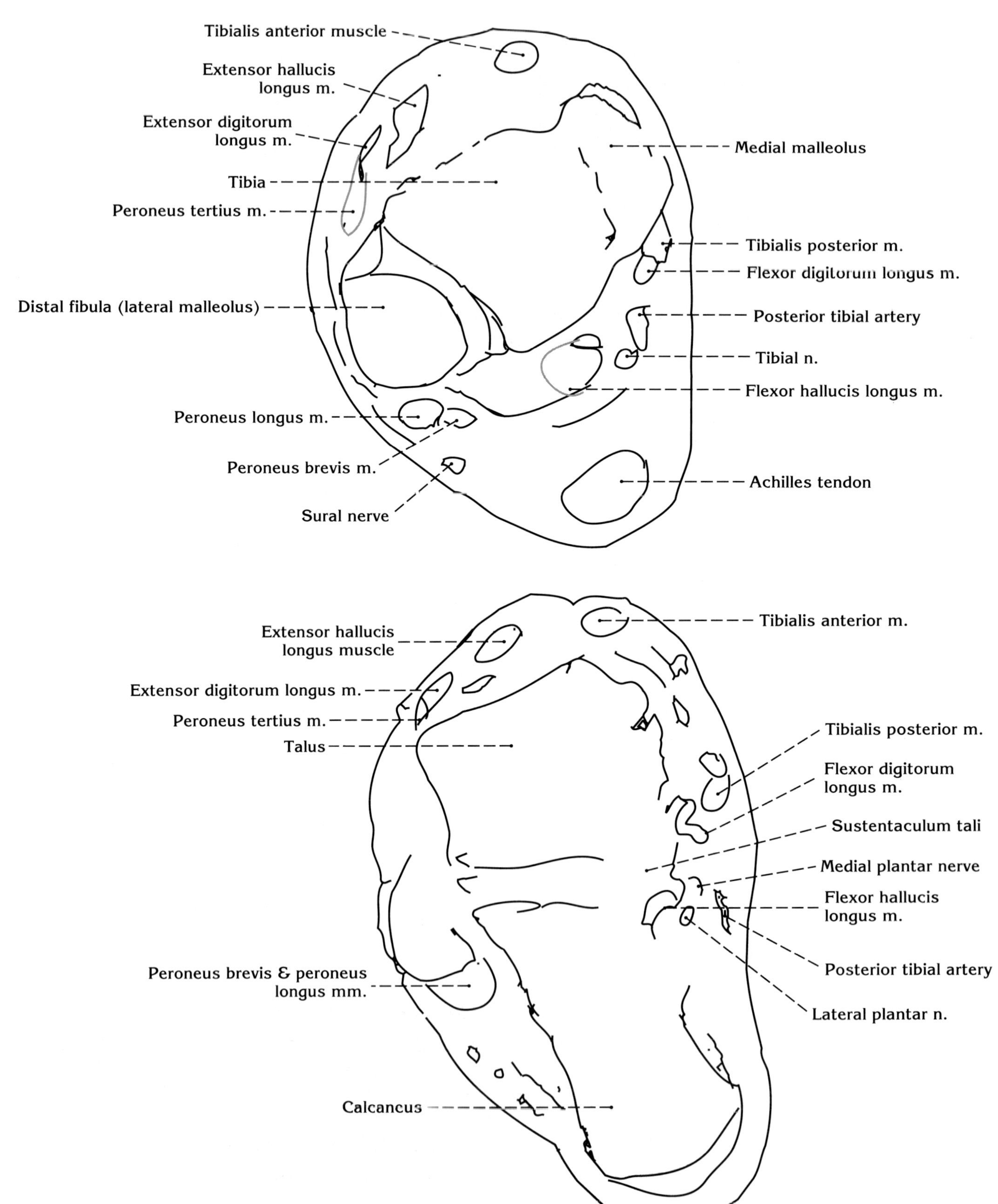
Tibialis anterior muscle
Extensor hallucis longus m.
Extensor digitorum longus m.
Tibia
Peroneus tertius m.
Distal fibula (lateral malleolus)
Peroneus longus m.
Peroneus brevis m.
Sural nerve
Medial malleolus
Tibialis posterior m.
Flexor digitorum longus m.
Posterior tibial artery
Tibial n.
Flexor hallucis longus m.
Achilles tendon
Extensor hallucis longus muscle
Extensor digitorum longus m.
Peroneus tertius m.
Talus
Peroneus brevis & peroneus longus mm.
Calcaneus
Tibialis anterior m.
Tibialis posterior m.
Flexor digitorum longus m.
Sustentaculum tali
Medial plantar nerve
Flexor hallucis longus m.
Posterior tibial artery
Lateral plantar n.

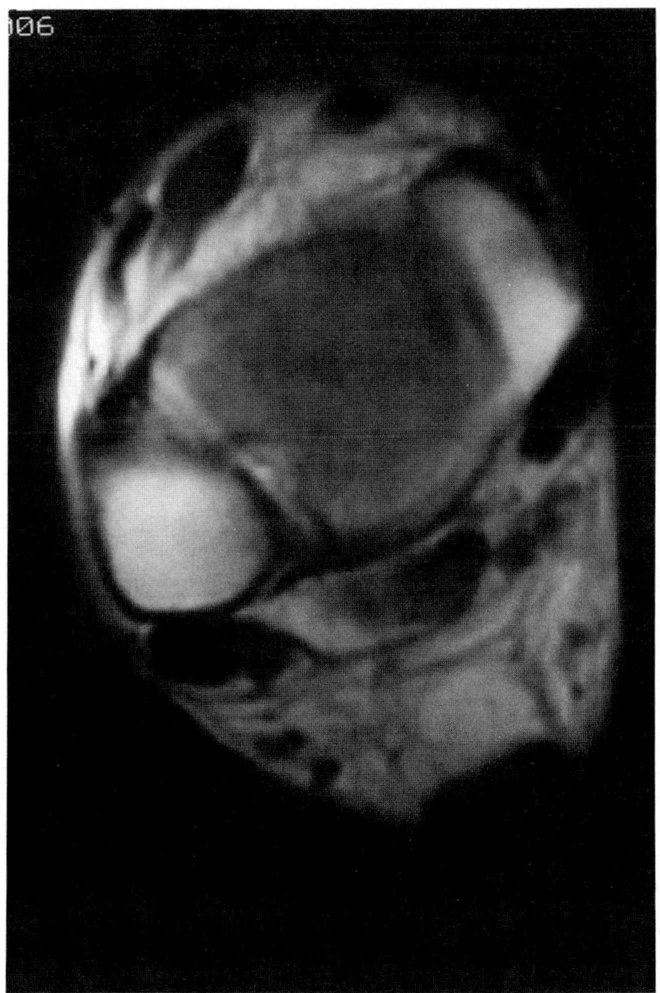

5-48 Ankle, axial view (TR 800; TE 30).

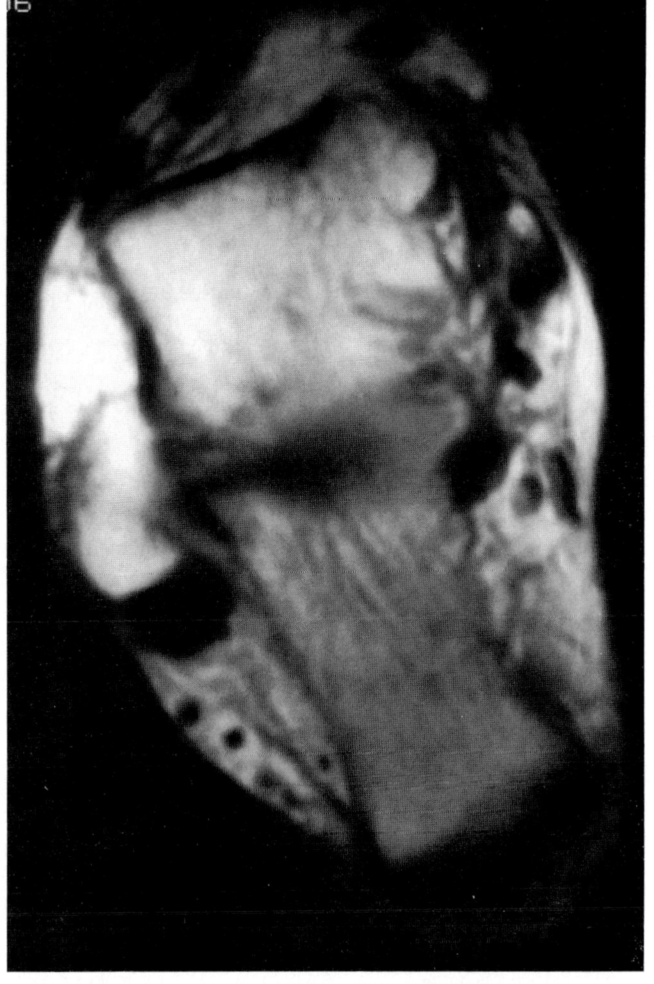

5-49 Ankle, axial view (TR 800; TE 30).

Ankle (Coronal) and Tarsus (Axial)

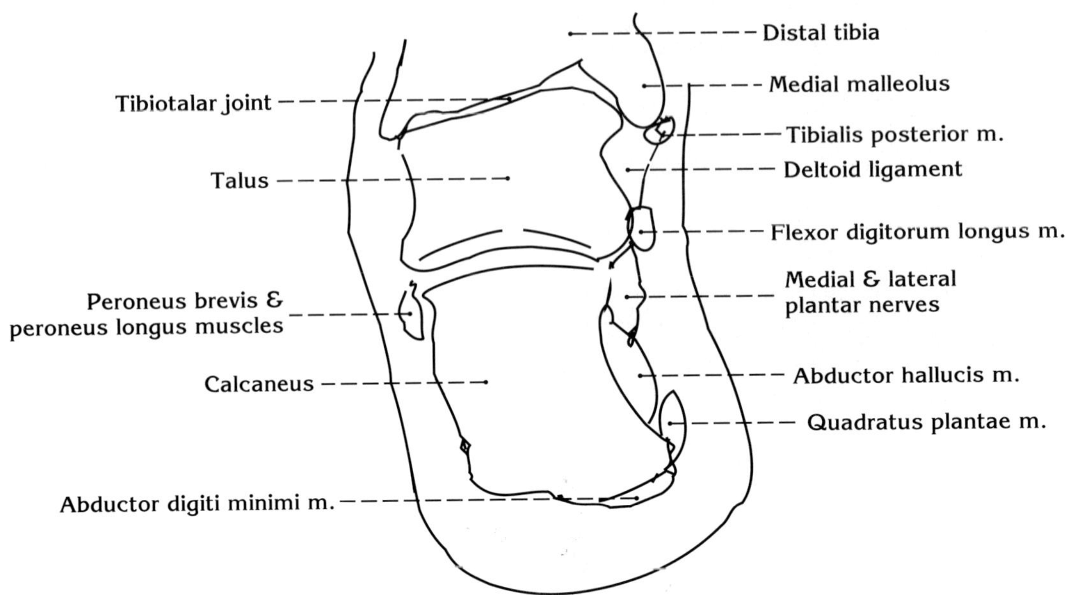

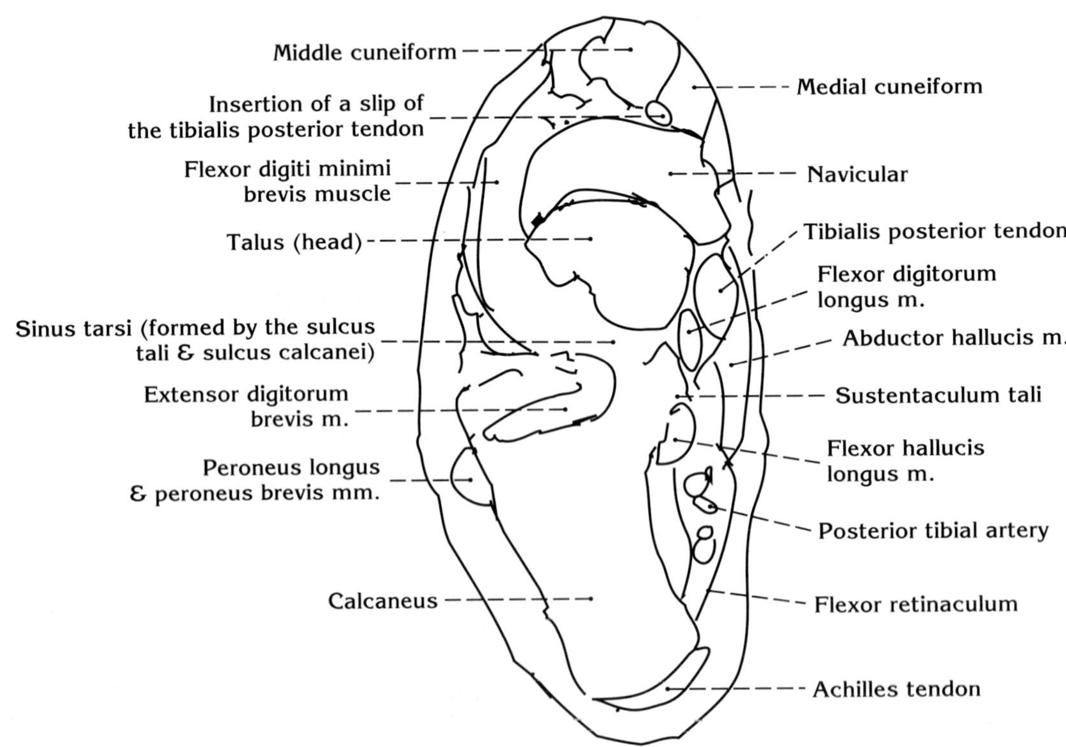

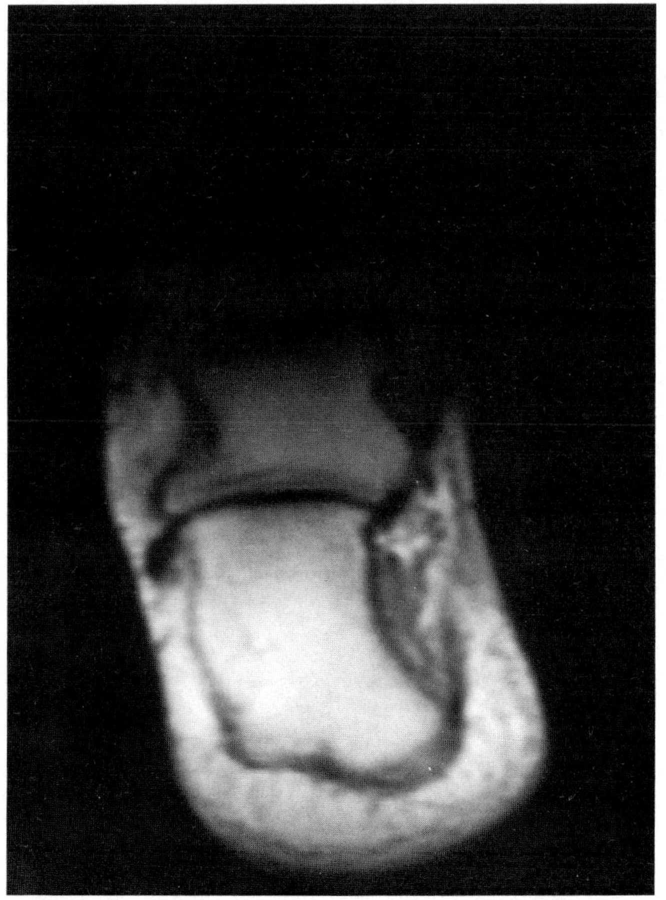

5-50 Ankle, coronal view (TR 800; TE 20).

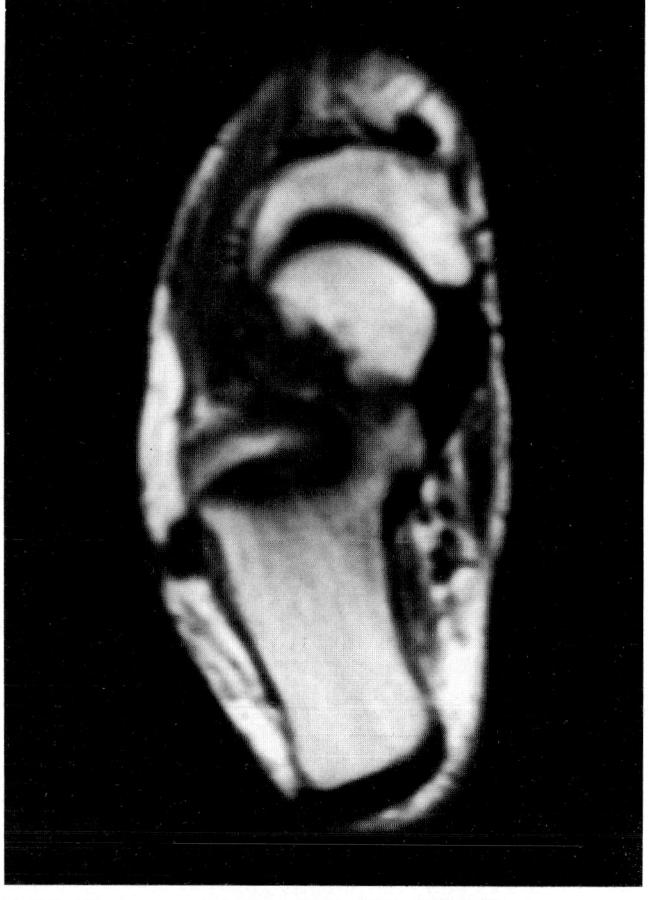

5-51 Tarsus, axial view (TR 800; TE 20).

Tarsus, Axial

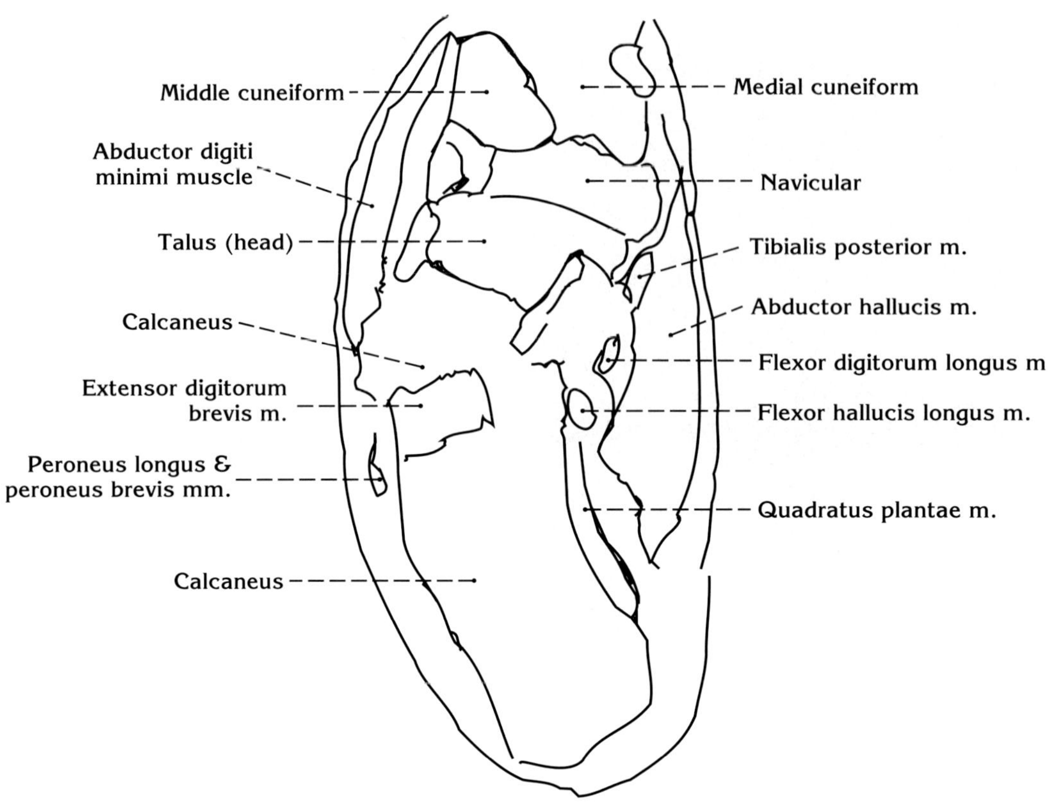

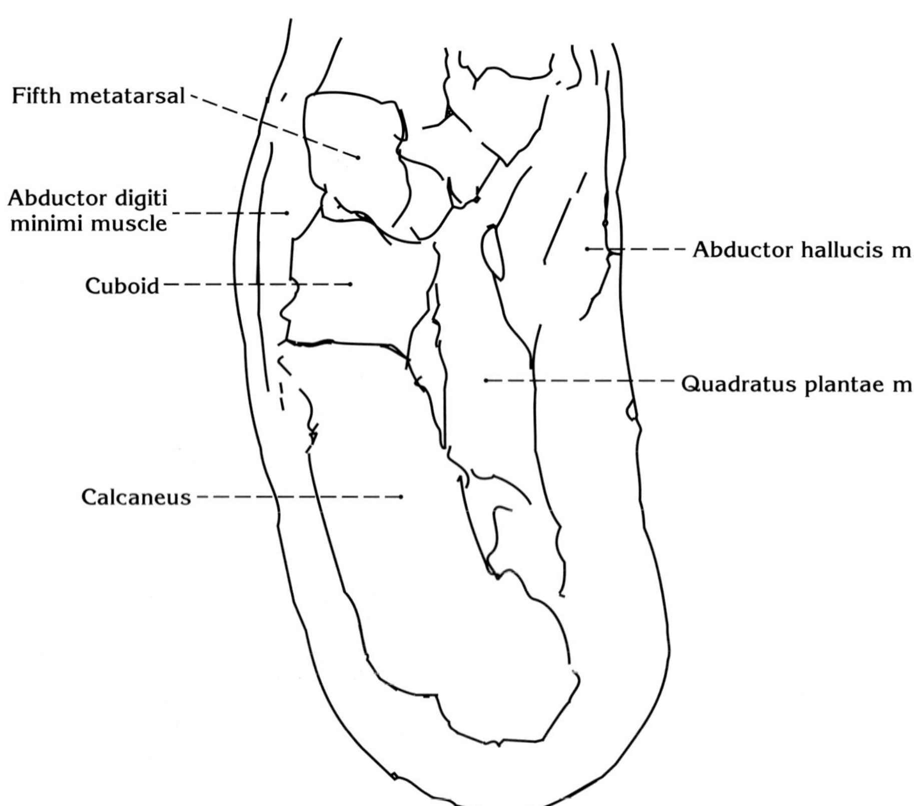

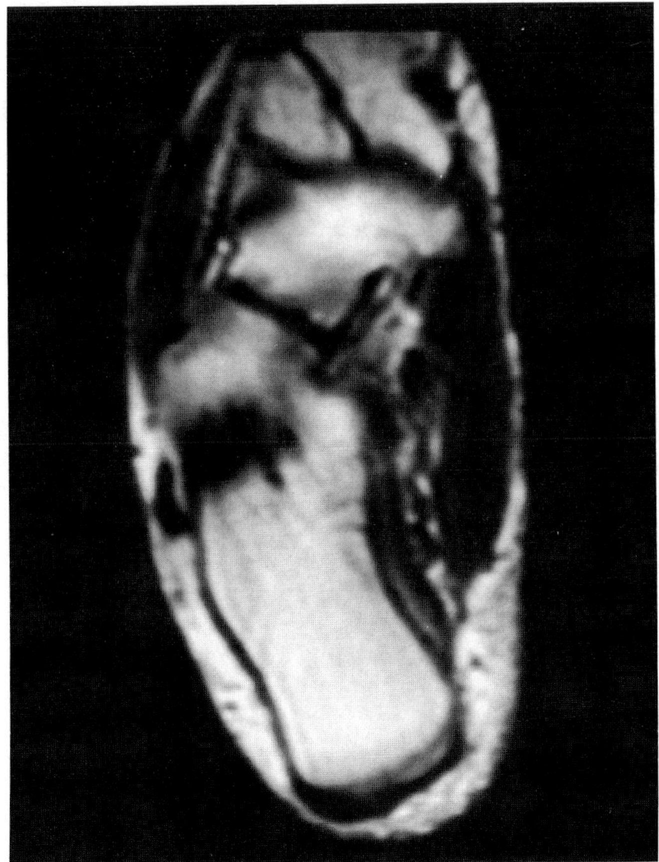

5-52 Tarsus, axial view (TR 800; TE 20).

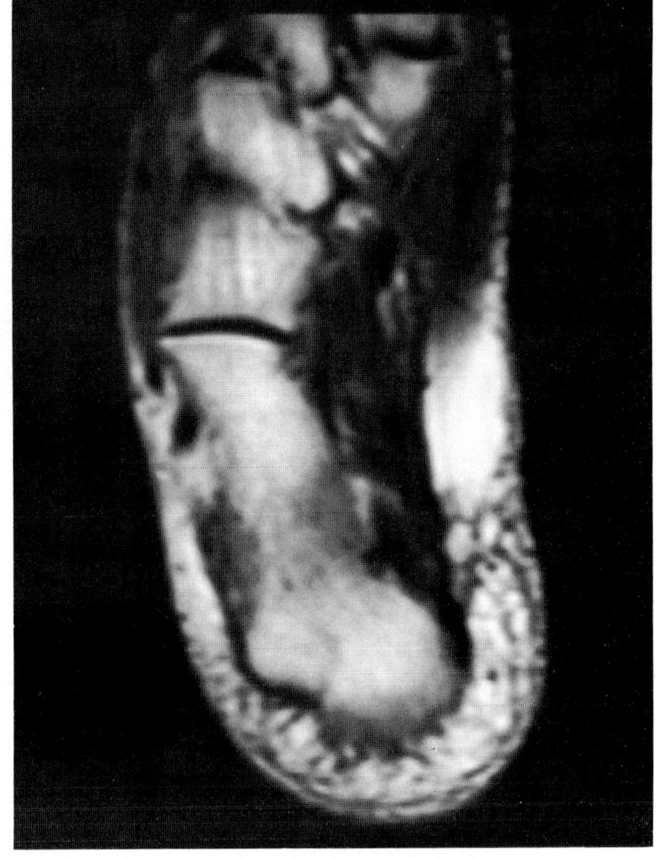

5-53 Tarsus, axial view (TR 800; TE 20).

Tarsus, Coronal

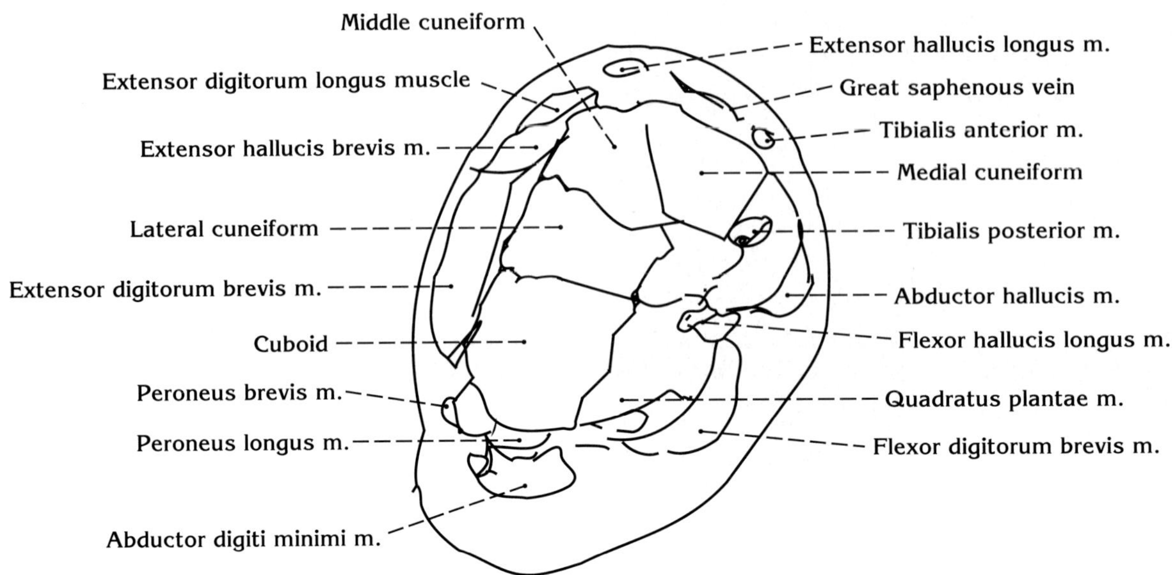

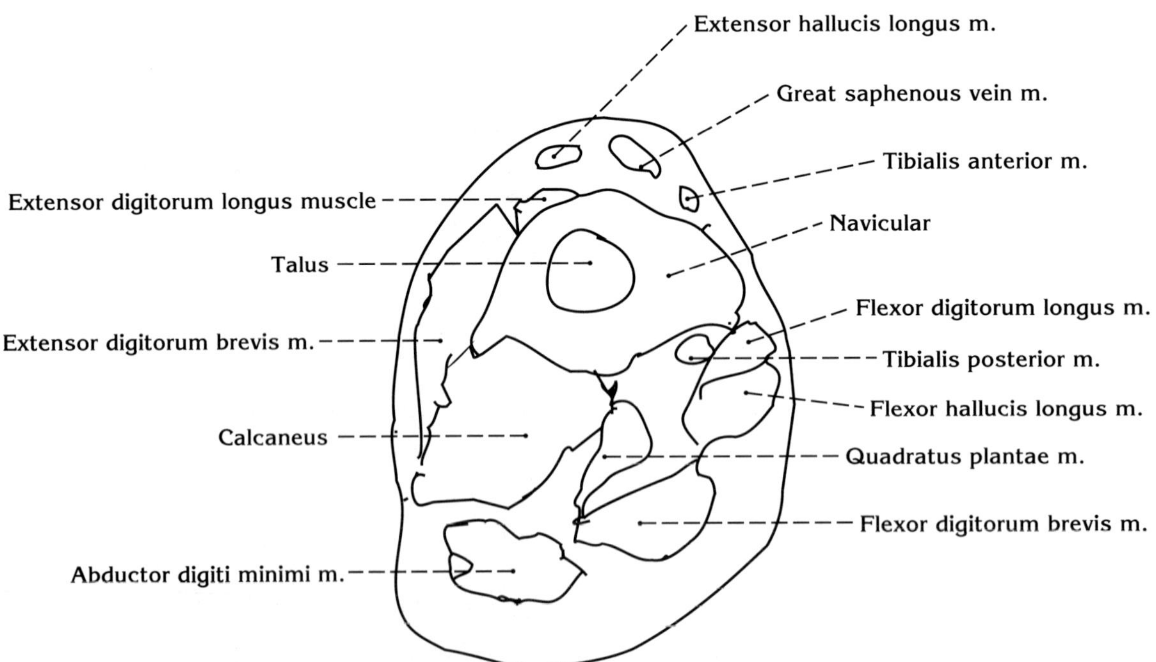

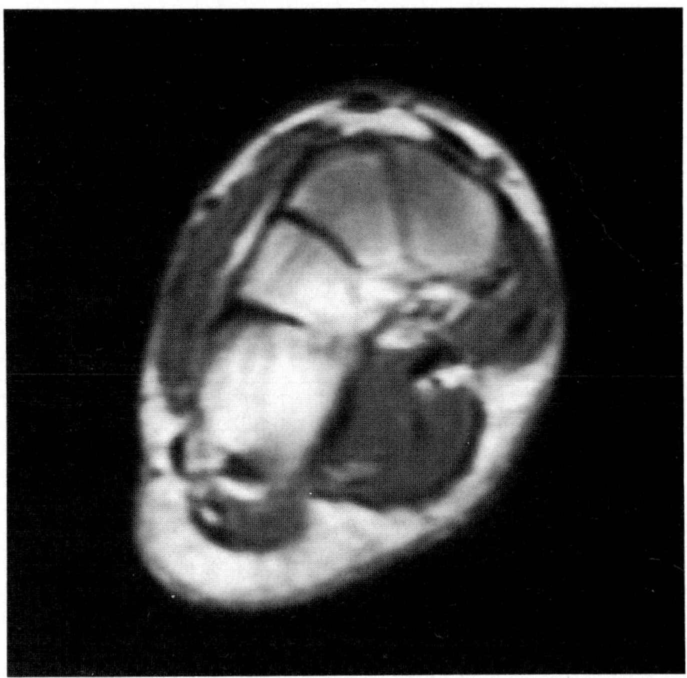

5-54 Tarsus, coronal view (TR 800; TE 20).

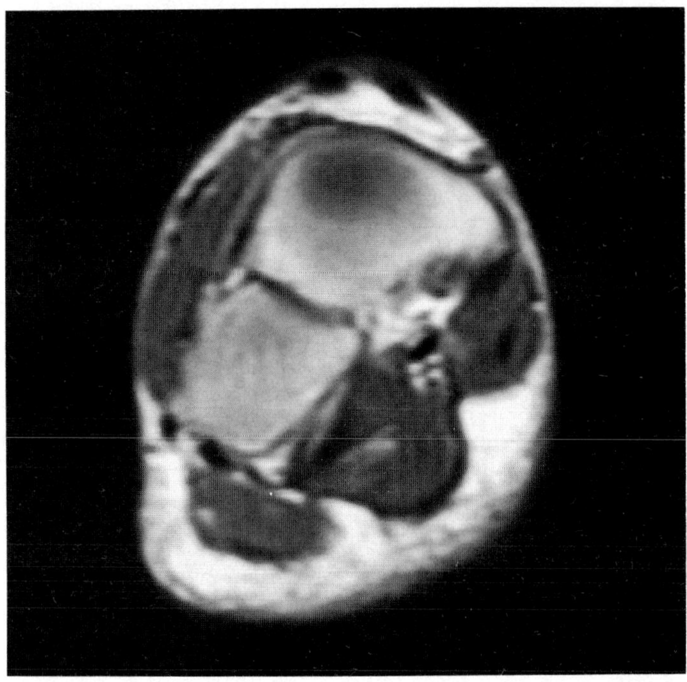

5-55 Tarsus, coronal view (TR 800; TE 20).

Foot, Axial

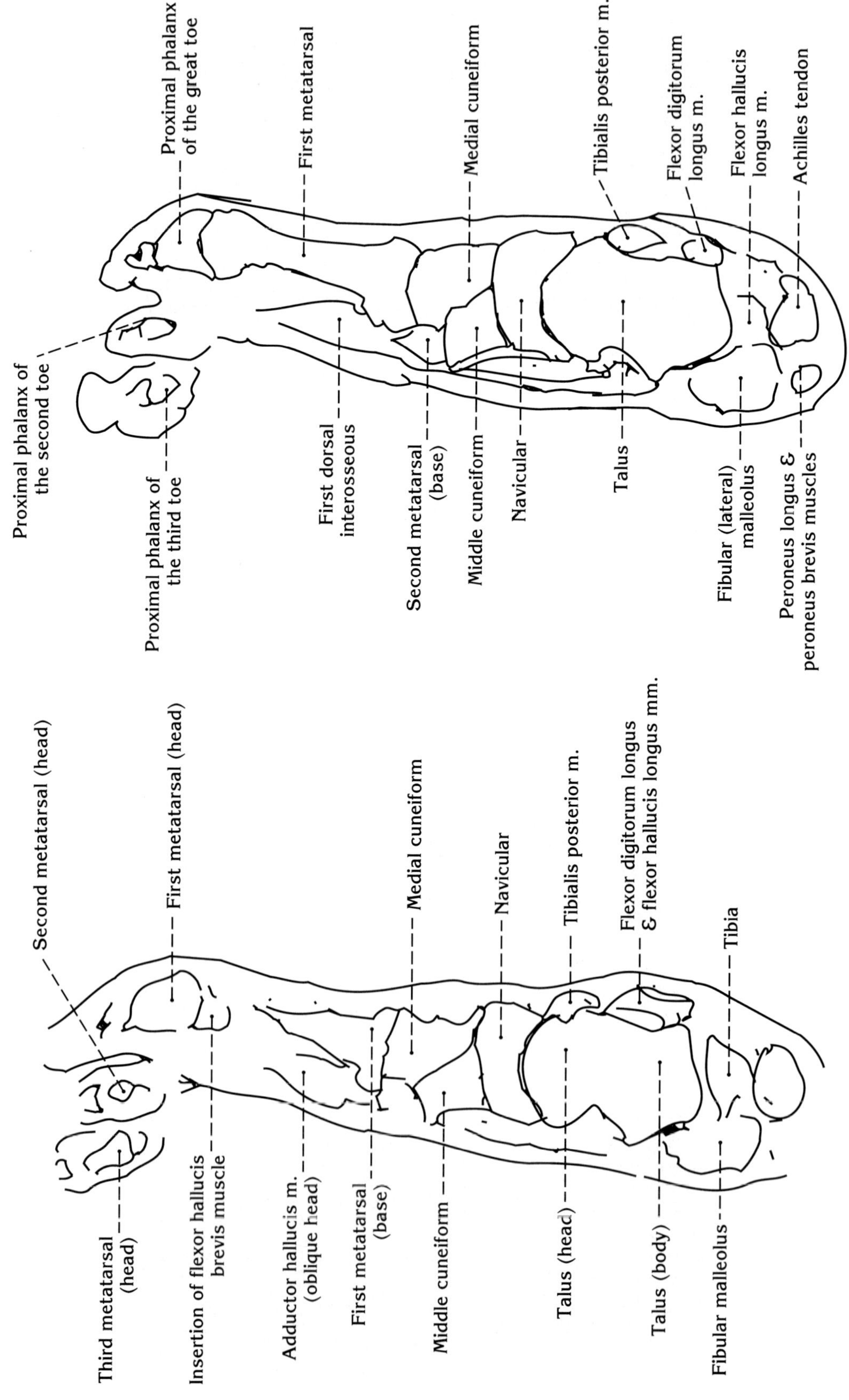
Proximal phalanx of the great toe
First metatarsal
Medial cuneiform
Tibialis posterior m.
Flexor digitorum longus m.
Flexor hallucis longus m.
Achilles tendon
Proximal phalanx of the second toe
Proximal phalanx of the third toe
First dorsal interosseous
Second metatarsal (base)
Middle cuneiform
Navicular
Talus
Fibular (lateral) malleolus
Peroneus longus & peroneus brevis muscles
Second metatarsal (head)
First metatarsal (head)
Medial cuneiform
Navicular
Tibialis posterior m.
Flexor digitorum longus & flexor hallucis longus mm.
Tibia
Third metatarsal (head)
Insertion of flexor hallucis brevis muscle
Adductor hallucis m. (oblique head)
First metatarsal (base)
Middle cuneiform
Talus (head)
Talus (body)
Fibular malleolus

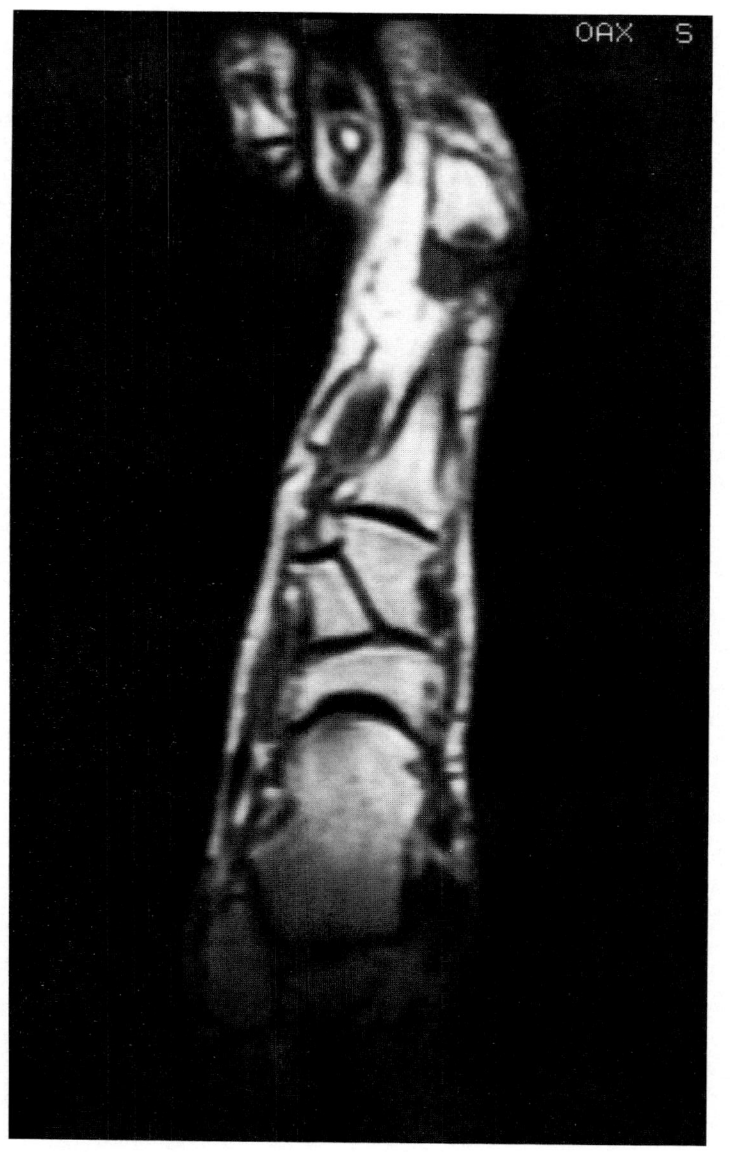

5-56 Foot, axial view (TR 800; TE 20).

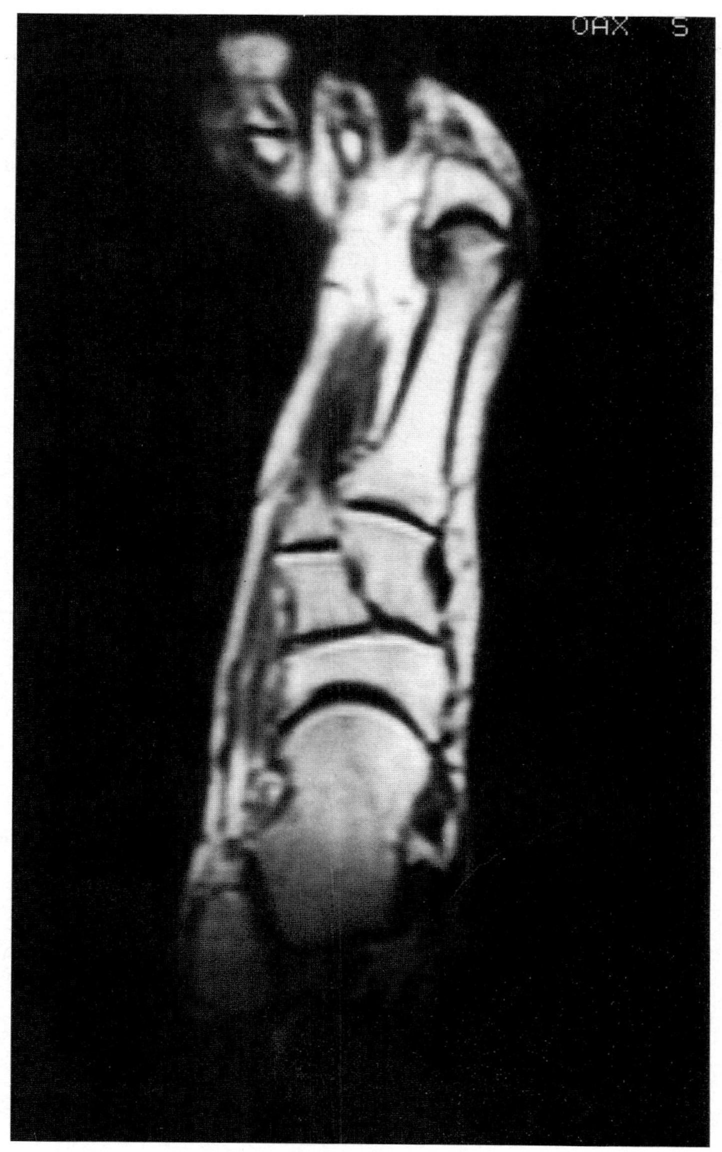

5-57 Foot, axial view (TR 800; TE 20).

Foot, Axial

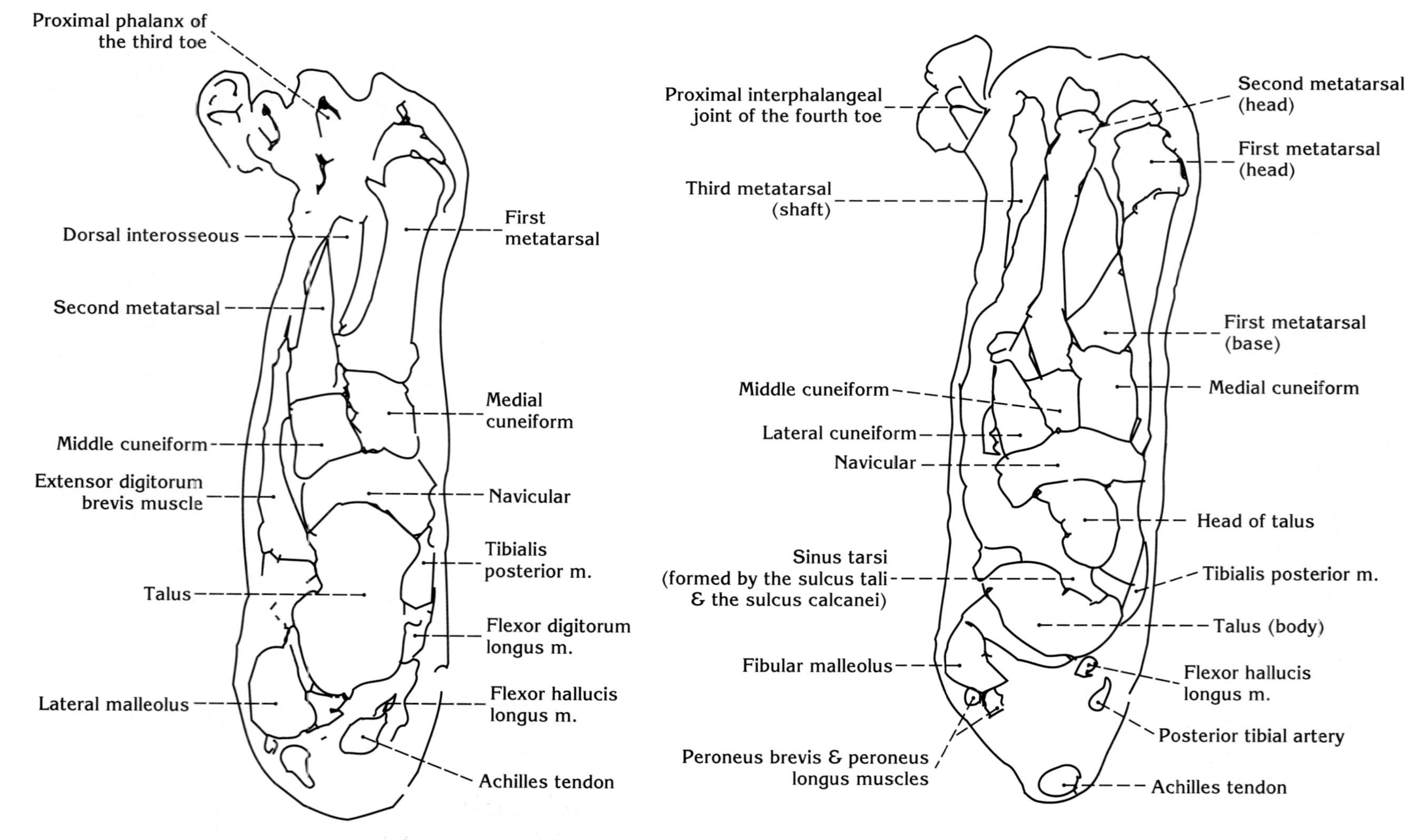
Proximal phalanx of the third toe
Dorsal interosseous
First metatarsal
Second metatarsal
Medial cuneiform
Middle cuneiform
Extensor digitorum brevis muscle
Navicular
Tibialis posterior m.
Talus
Flexor digitorum longus m.
Lateral malleolus
Flexor hallucis longus m.
Achilles tendon
Proximal interphalangeal joint of the fourth toe
Second metatarsal (head)
First metatarsal (head)
Third metatarsal (shaft)
First metatarsal (base)
Middle cuneiform
Medial cuneiform
Lateral cuneiform
Navicular
Head of talus
Sinus tarsi (formed by the sulcus tali & the sulcus calcanei)
Tibialis posterior m.
Talus (body)
Fibular malleolus
Flexor hallucis longus m.
Posterior tibial artery
Peroneus brevis & peroneus longus muscles
Achilles tendon

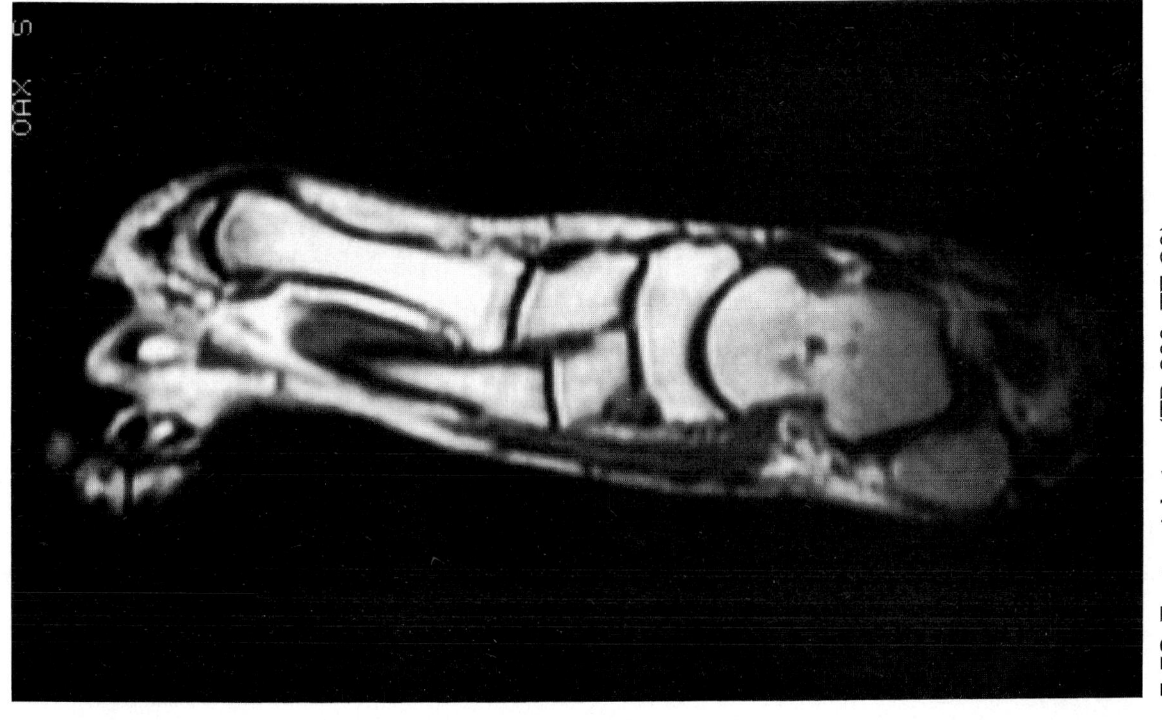

5-58 Foot, axial view (TR 800; TE 20).

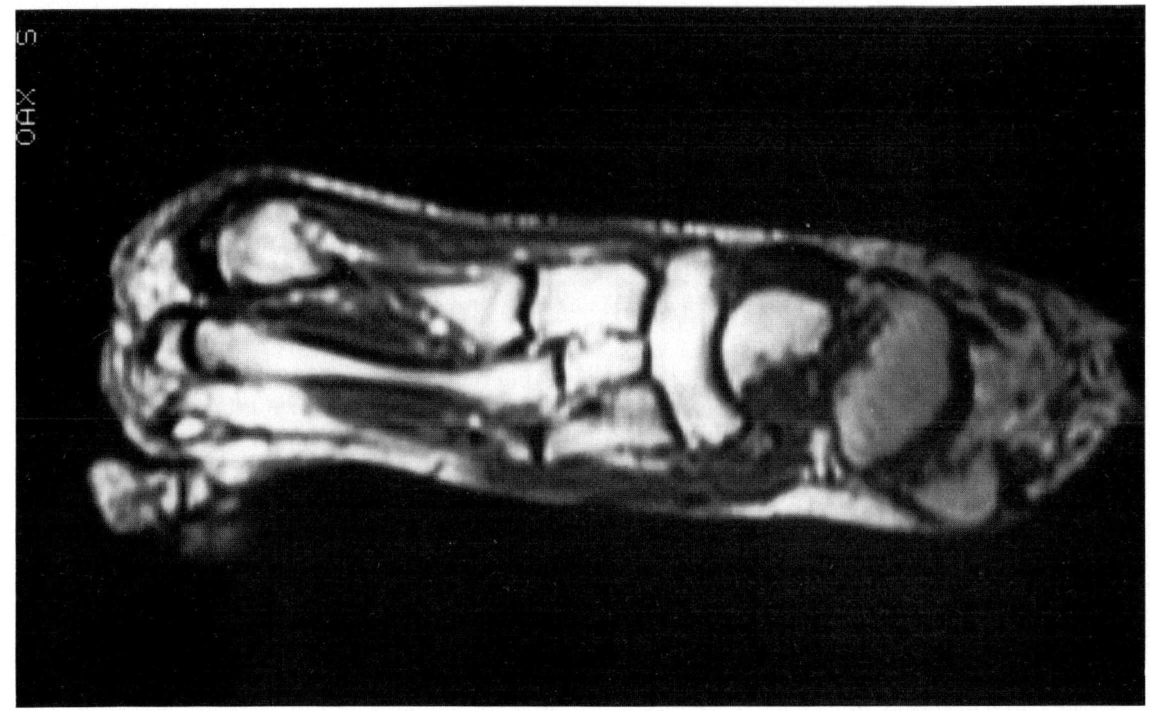

5-59 Foot, axial view (TR 800; TE 20).

Foot, Axial and Coronal

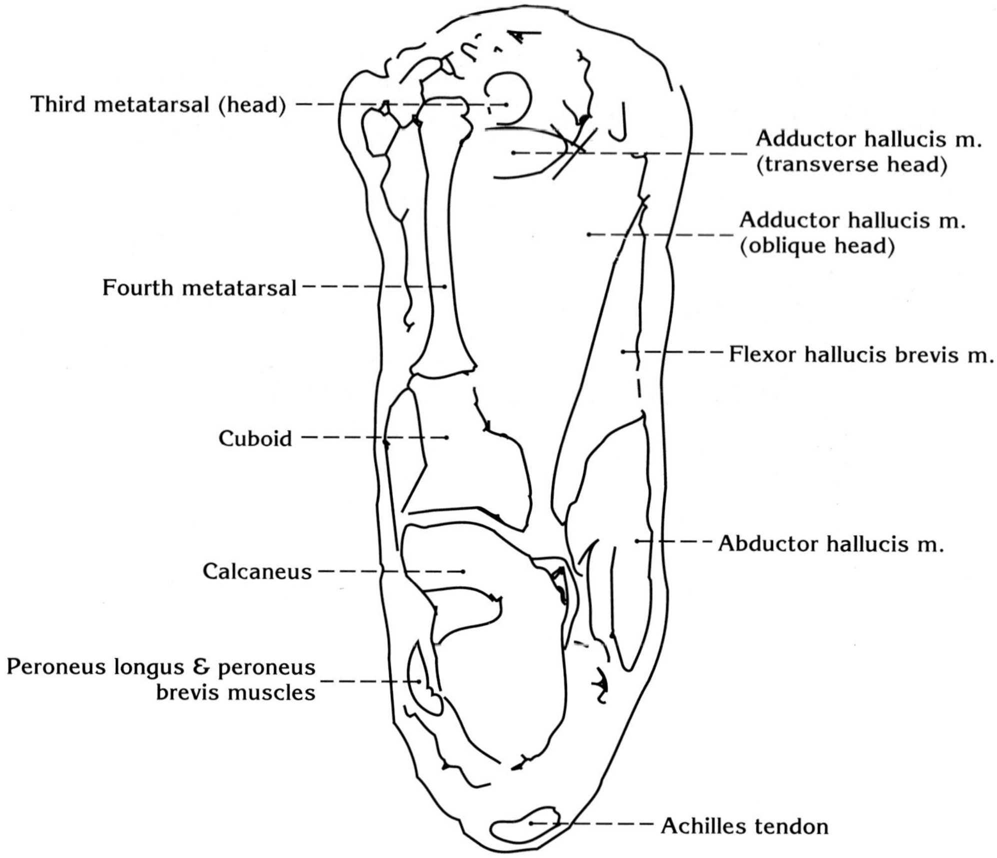

Third metatarsal (head)
Adductor hallucis m. (transverse head)
Adductor hallucis m. (oblique head)
Fourth metatarsal
Flexor hallucis brevis m.
Cuboid
Abductor hallucis m.
Calcaneus
Peroneus longus & peroneus brevis muscles
Achilles tendon

Extensor hallucis longus m.
Flexor digitorum longus muscle
Great saphenous vein
First metatarsal
Second metatarsal
Flexor digitorum brevis m.
Abductor hallucis m.
Third metatarsal
Flexor hallucis brevis m.
Fourth metatarsal
Adductor hallucis longus m. (oblique head)
Fifth metatarsal
Flexor digitorum brevis m.
Opponens digiti minimi m.
Abductor digiti minimi m.
Flexor digiti minimi brevis m.

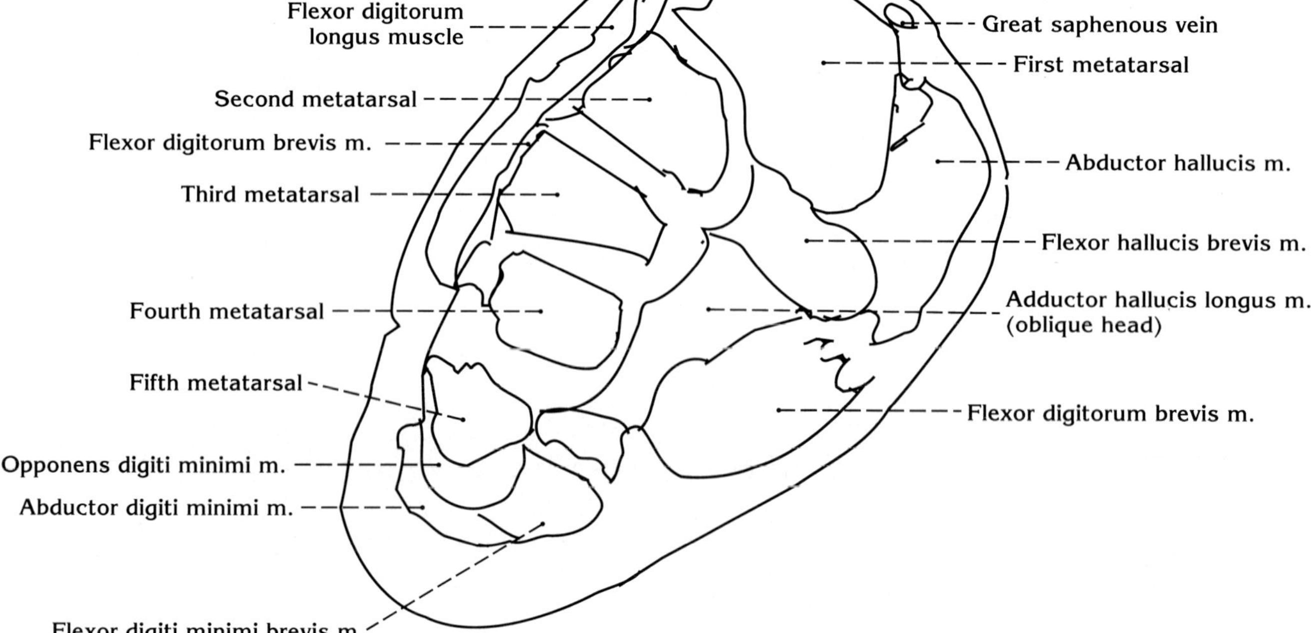

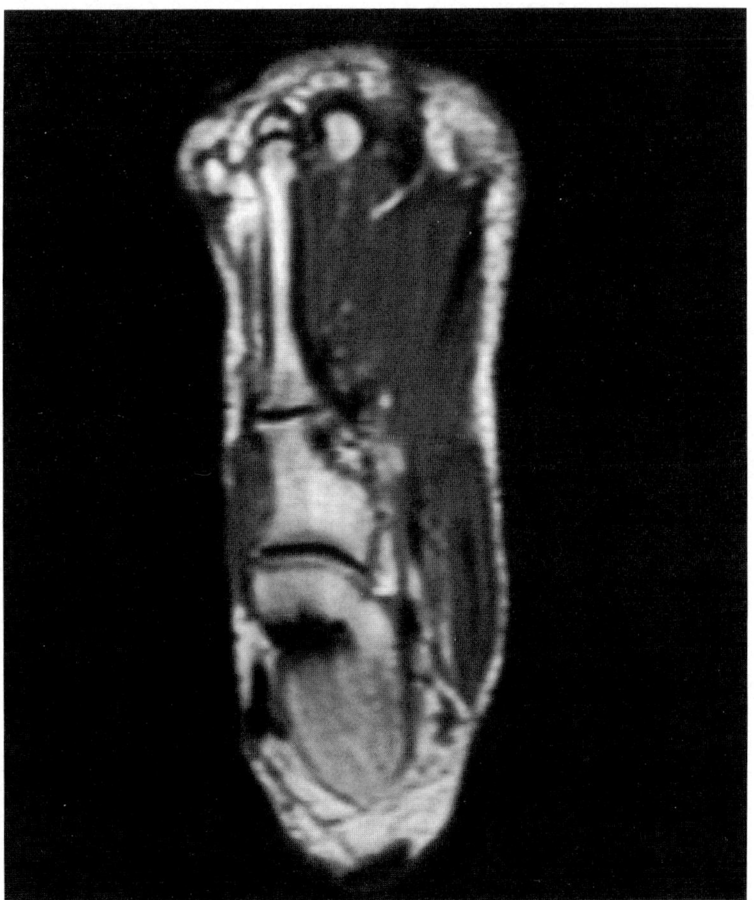

5-60 Foot, axial view (TR 800; TE 20).

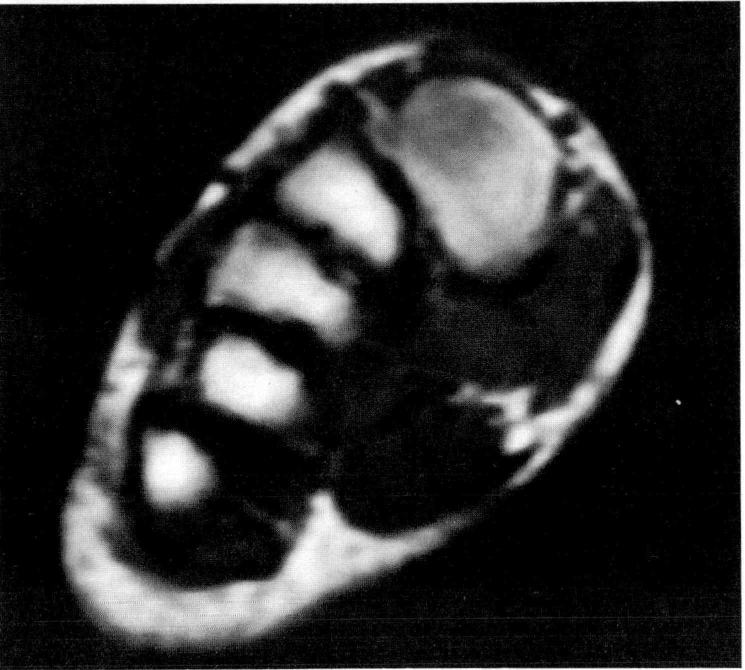

5-61 Foot, coronal view (TR 800; TE 20).

Foot and Ankle, Sagittal

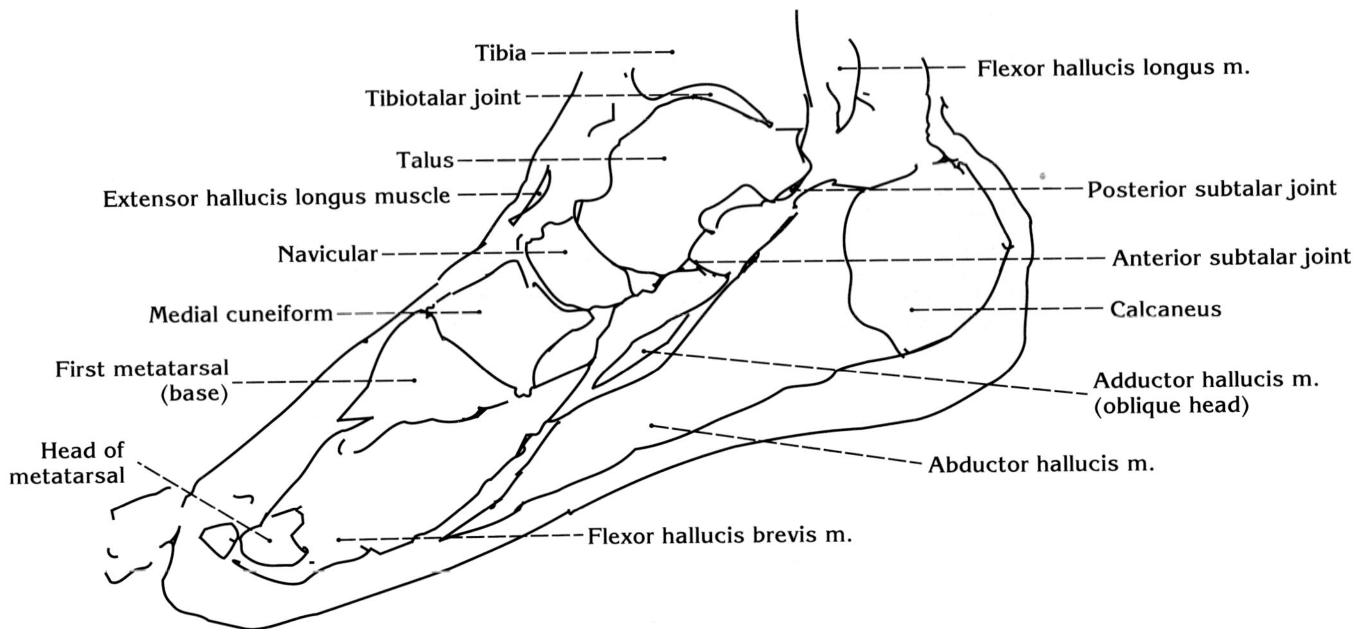

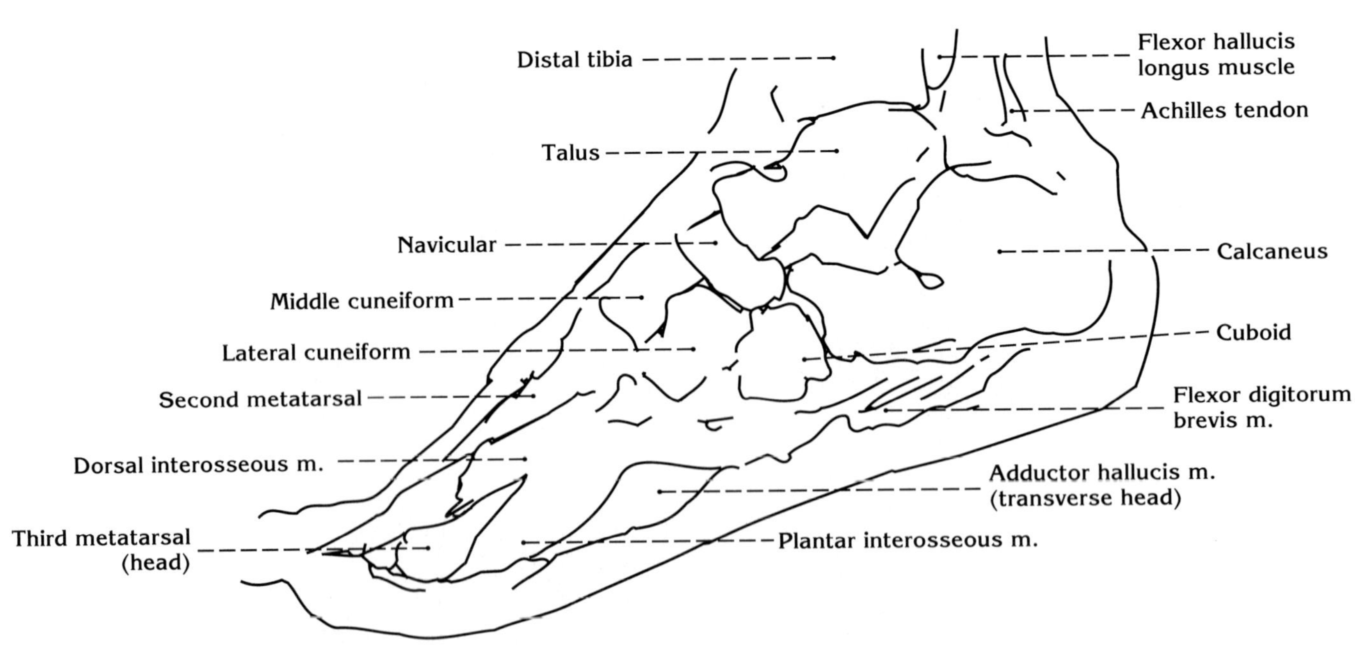

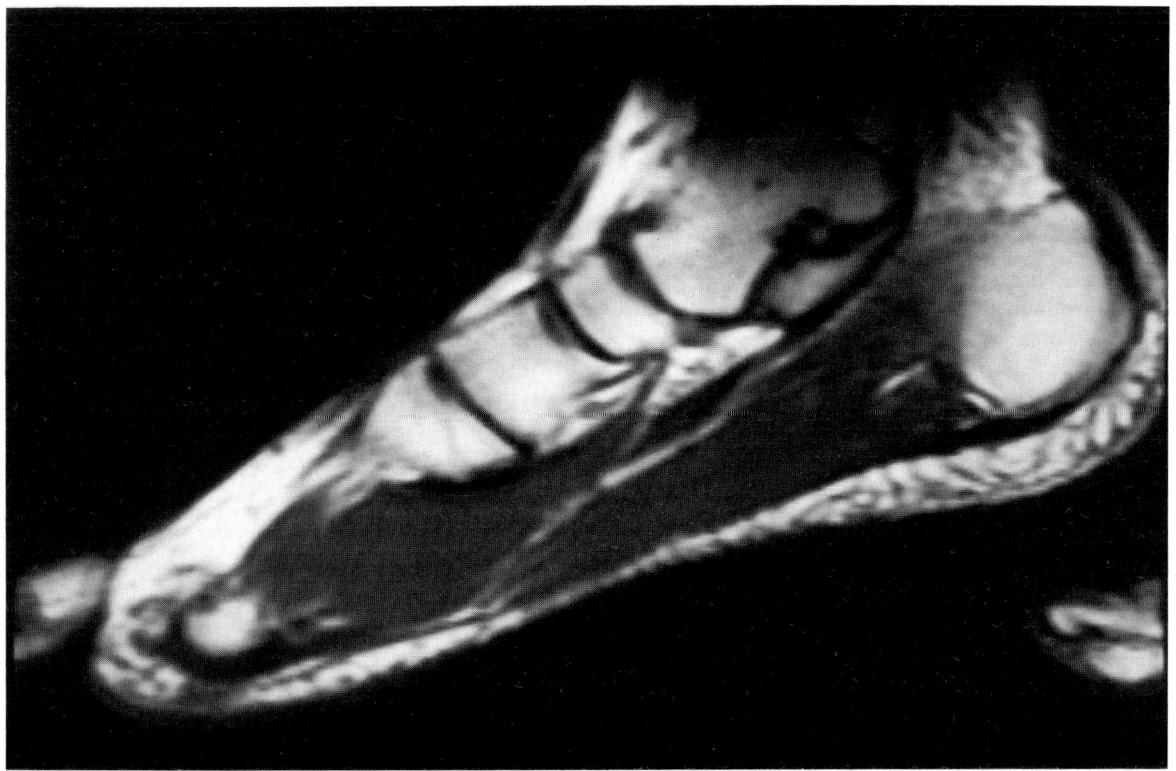

5-62 Foot and ankle, sagittal view (TR 800; TE 20).

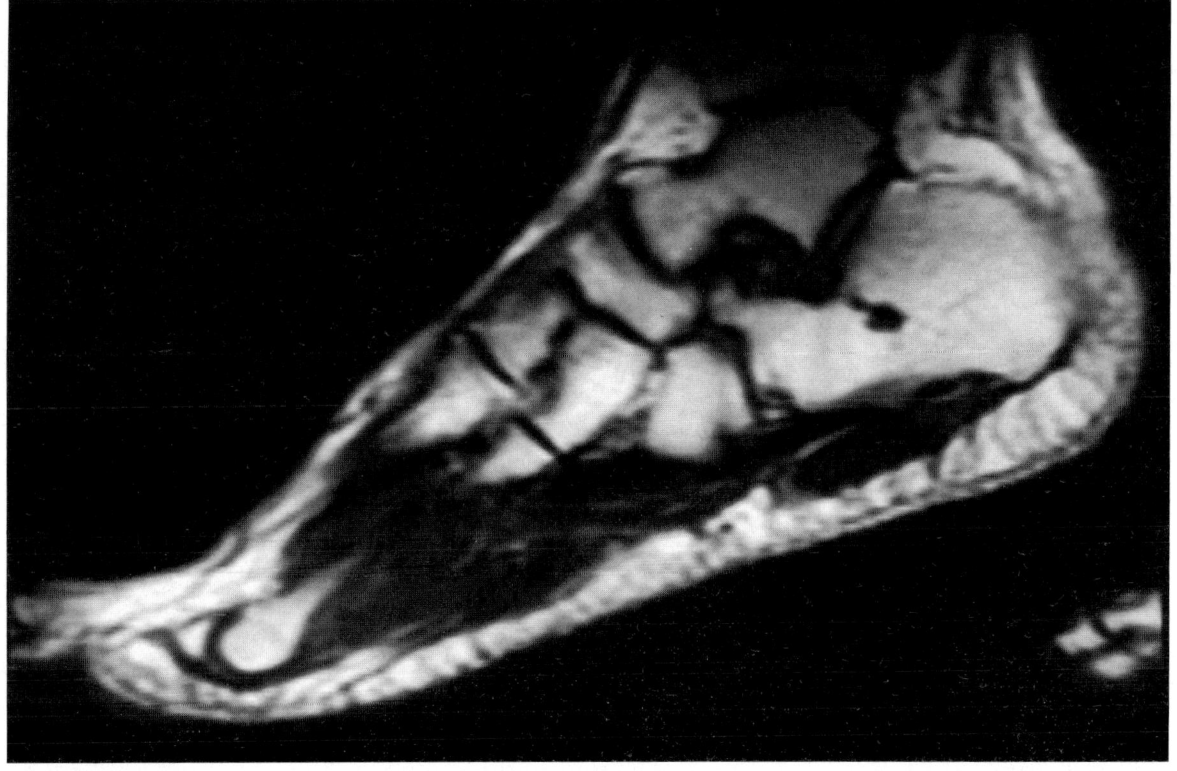

5-63 Foot and ankle, sagittal view (TR 800; TE 20).

Foot and Ankle, Sagittal

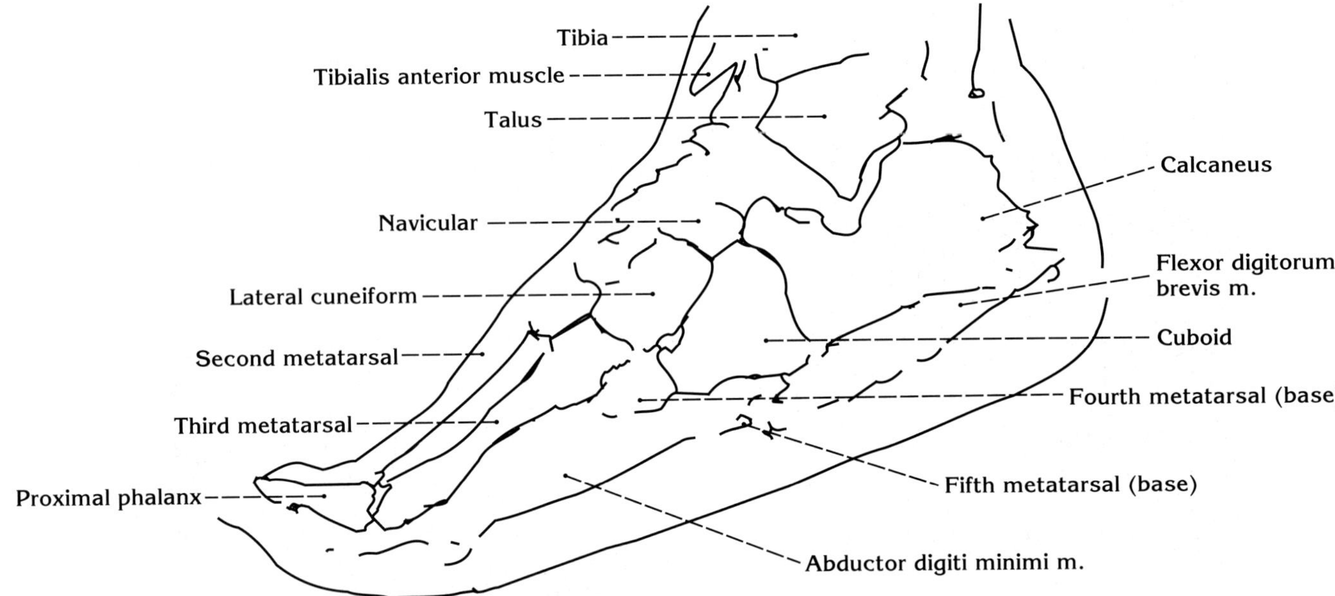

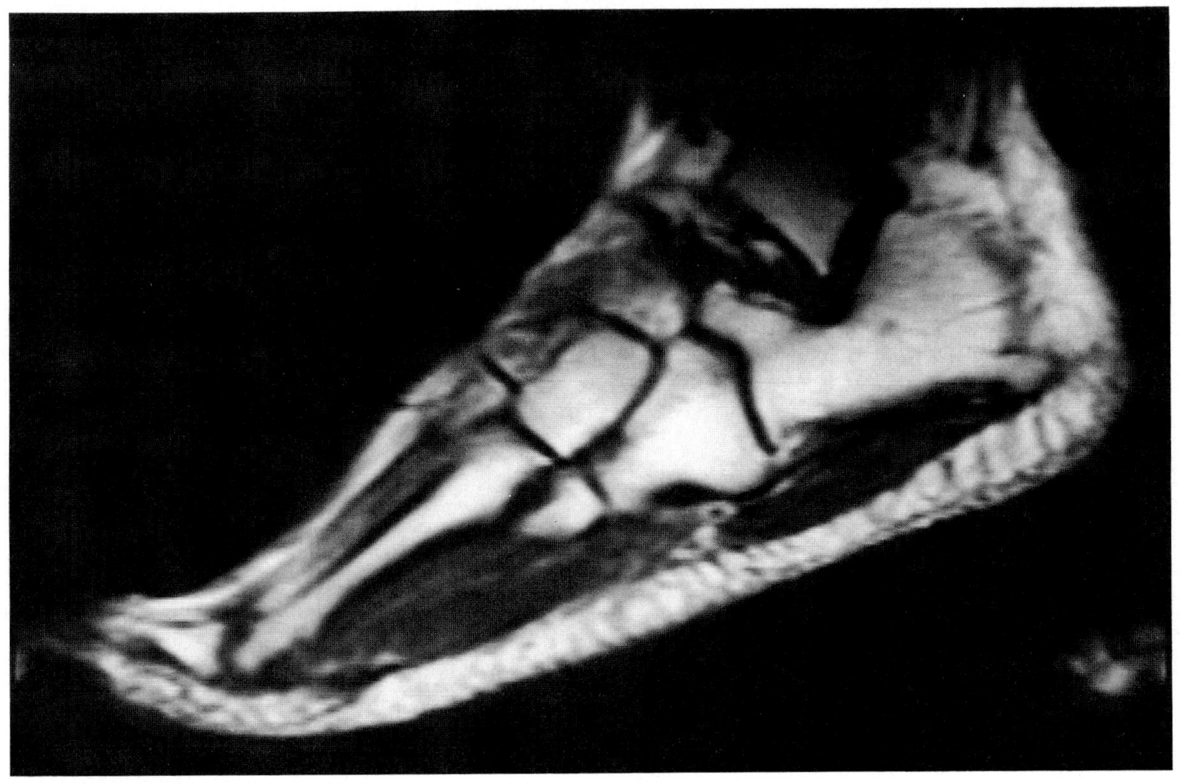

5-64 Foot and ankle, sagittal view (TR 800; TE 20).